EPIDEMIOLOGY

Beyond the Basics
THIRD EDITION

Moyses Szklo, MD, DrPH
Professor of Epidemiology and Medicine
The Johns Hopkins University
Editor-in-Chief, *American Journal of Epidemiology*
Baltimore, MD

F. Javier Nieto, MD, PhD
Helfaer Professor of Public Health
Professor and Chair
Department of Population Health Sciences
University of Wisconsin School of Medicine and Public Health
Madison, WI

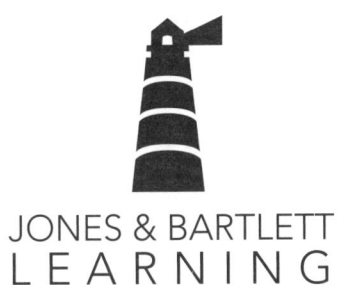

World Headquarters
Jones & Bartlett Learning
5 Wall Street
Burlington, MA 01803
978-443-5000
info@jblearning.com
www.jblearning.com

Jones & Bartlett Learning books and products are available through most bookstores and online booksellers. To contact Jones & Bartlett Learning directly, call 800-832-0034, fax 978-443-8000, or visit our website, www.jblearning.com.

Substantial discounts on bulk quantities of Jones & Bartlett Learning publications are available to corporations, professional associations, and other qualified organizations. For details and specific discount information, contact the special sales department at Jones & Bartlett Learning via the above contact information or send an email to specialsales@jblearning.com.

Copyright © 2014 by Jones & Bartlett Learning, LLC, an Ascend Learning Company

All rights reserved. No part of the material protected by this copyright may be reproduced or utilized in any form, electronic or mechanical, including photocopying, recording, or by any information storage and retrieval system, without written permission from the copyright owner.

Epidemiology: Beyond the Basics, Third Edition is an independent publication and has not been authorized, sponsored, or otherwise approved by the owners of the trademarks or service marks referenced in this product.

Production Credits
Chief Executive Officer: Ty Field
President: James Homer
SVP, Editor-in-Chief: Michael Johnson
SVP, Chief Marketing Officer: Alison M. Pendergast
Publisher: Michael Brown
Associate Editor: Teresa Reilly
Editorial Assistant: Chloe Falivene
Editorial Assistant: Kayla Dos Santos
Director of Production: Amy Rose
Production Manager: Tracey McCrea
Production Assistant: Eileen Worthley
Senior Marketing Manager: Sophie Fleck Teague
Manufacturing and Inventory Control Supervisor: Amy Bacus
Composition: Lapiz, Inc.
Cover Design: Kristin E. Parker
Cover Image: © BioMedical/ShutterStock, Inc.
Printing and Binding: Edwards Brothers Malloy
Cover Printing: Edwards Brothers Malloy

Library of Congress Cataloging-in-Publication Data
Szklo, M. (Moyses)
 Epidemiology : beyond the basics / Moyses Szklo and F. Javier Nieto.—3rd ed.
   p. ; cm.
 Includes bibliographical references and index.
 ISBN 978-1-4496-0469-1 (pbk.) — ISBN 1-4496-0469-2 (pbk.)
 I. Nieto, F. Javier. II. Title.
 [DNLM: 1. Epidemiologic Methods. 2. Epidemiology. WA 950]
 614.4—dc23

2012015799

6048

Printed in the United States of America
16 15 14 13 12   10 9 8 7 6 5 4 3 2 1

To Hilda and Marion

Contents

Preface   ix
Acknowledgments   xii
About the Authors   xiii

PART ONE Introduction   1

CHAPTER 1 Basic Study Designs in Analytical Epidemiology   3

1.1 Introduction: Descriptive and Analytical Epidemiology   3
1.2 Analysis of Age, Birth Cohort, and Period Effects   4
1.3 Ecologic Studies   14
1.4 Studies Based on Individuals as Observation Units   19
References   39
Exercises   42

PART TWO Measures of Disease Occurrence and Association   45

CHAPTER 2 Measuring Disease Occurrence   47

2.1 Introduction   47
2.2 Measures of Incidence   49
2.3 Measures of Prevalence   71
2.4 Odds   73
References   74
Exercises   75

CHAPTER 3 Measuring Associations Between Exposures and Outcomes   79

3.1 Introduction   79
3.2 Measuring Associations in a Cohort Study   79
3.3 Cross-Sectional Studies: Point Prevalence Rate Ratio   90
3.4 Measuring Associations in Case-Control Studies   90
3.5 Assessing the Strength of Associations   101
References   104
Exercises   105

PART THREE — Threats to Validity and Issues of Interpretation — 107

CHAPTER 4 — Understanding Lack of Validity: Bias — 109
- 4.1 Overview — 109
- 4.2 Selection Bias — 111
- 4.3 Information Bias — 116
- 4.4 Combined Selection/Information Biases — 133
- References — 147
- Exercises — 150

CHAPTER 5 — Identifying Noncausal Associations: Confounding — 153
- 5.1 Introduction — 153
- 5.2 The Nature of the Association Between the Confounder, the Exposure, and the Outcome — 156
- 5.3 Theoretical and Graphical Aids to Frame Confounding — 162
- 5.4 Assessing the Presence of Confounding — 164
- 5.5 Additional Issues Related to Confounding — 171
- 5.6 Conclusion — 179
- References — 180
- Exercises — 182

CHAPTER 6 — Defining and Assessing Heterogeneity of Effects: Interaction — 185
- 6.1 Introduction — 185
- 6.2 Defining and Measuring Effect — 186
- 6.3 Strategies to Evaluate Interaction — 186
- 6.4 Assessment of Interaction in Case-Control Studies — 196
- 6.5 More on the Interchangeability of the Definitions of Interaction — 203
- 6.6 Which is the Relevant Model? Additive Versus Multiplicative Interaction — 205
- 6.7 The Nature and Reciprocity of Interaction — 207
- 6.8 Interaction, Confounding Effect, and Adjustment — 211
- 6.9 Statistical Modeling and Statistical Tests for Interaction — 212
- 6.10 Interpreting Interaction — 214
- 6.11 Interaction and Search for New Risk Factors in Low-Risk Groups — 219
- 6.12 Interaction and "Representativeness" of Associations — 221
- References — 222
- Exercises — 224

PART FOUR — Dealing with Threats to Validity — 227

CHAPTER 7 — Stratification and Adjustment: Multivariate Analysis in Epidemiology — 229
- 7.1 Introduction — 229

Contents

    7.2   Stratification and Adjustment Techniques to Disentangle Confounding   230
    7.3   Adjustment Methods Based on Stratification   234
    7.4   Multiple Regression Techniques for Adjustment   248
    7.5   Alternative Approaches for the Control of Confounding   282
    7.6   Incomplete Adjustment: Residual Confounding   293
    7.7   Over-Adjustment   295
    7.8   Conclusion   296
    References   301
    Exercises   305

CHAPTER 8   Quality Assurance and Control   313

    8.1   Introduction   313
    8.2   Quality Assurance   313
    8.3   Quality Control   318
    8.4   Indices of Validity and Reliability   328
    8.5   Regression to the Mean   358
    8.6   Final Considerations   359
    References   360
    Exercises   363

PART FIVE   Issues of Reporting and Application of Epidemiologic Results   367

CHAPTER 9   Communicating Results of Epidemiologic Studies   369

    9.1   Introduction   369
    9.2   What to Report   369
    9.3   How to Report   373
    9.4   Conclusion   385
    References   386
    Exercises   388

CHAPTER 10   Epidemiologic Issues in the Interface with Public Health Policy   391

    10.1   Introduction   391
    10.2   Causality: Application to Public Health and Health Policy   392
    10.3   Decision Tree and Sensitivity Analysis   408
    10.4   Meta-Analysis   413
    10.5   Publication Bias   416
    10.6   Summary   420
    References   421
    Exercises   426

APPENDIX A Standard Errors, Confidence Intervals, and Hypothesis Testing for Selected Measures of Risk and Measures of Association   431

APPENDIX B Test for Trend (Dose Response)   455

APPENDIX C Test of Homogeneity of Stratified Estimates (Test for Interaction)   459

APPENDIX D Quality Assurance and Quality Control Procedures Manual for Blood Pressure Measurement and Blood/Urine Collection in the ARIC Study   461

APPENDIX E Calculation of the Intraclass Correlation Coefficient   469

APPENDIX F Answers to Exercises   473

Index   501

Preface

This book was conceived as an intermediate epidemiology textbook. Similarly to the first and second editions, the third edition explores and discusses key epidemiologic concepts and basic methods in more depth than that found in basic textbooks on epidemiology. For the third edition, new examples and exercises have been added to all chapters. In Chapters 7 and 10, respectively, we included discussions of novel epidemiologic strategies for handling confounding (i.e., instrumental variables and propensity scores) and of decision tree as a decision-making tool.

As an intermediate methods text, this book is expected to have a heterogeneous readership. Epidemiology students may wish to use it as a bridge between basic and more advanced epidemiologic methods. Other readers may desire to advance their knowledge beyond basic epidemiologic principles and methods but are not statistically minded and are thus reluctant to tackle the many excellent textbooks that strongly focus on epidemiology's quantitative aspects. The demonstration of several epidemiologic concepts and methods needs to rely on statistical formulations, and this text extensively supports these formulations with real-life examples, hopefully making their logic intuitively easier to follow. The practicing epidemiologist may find selected portions of this book useful for an understanding of concepts beyond the basics. Thus, the common denominators for the intended readers are familiarity with the basic strategies of analytic epidemiology and a desire to increase their level of understanding of several notions that are insufficiently covered (and naturally so) in many basic textbooks. The way in which this textbook is organized makes this readily apparent.

In Chapter 1, the basic observational epidemiologic research strategies are reviewed, including those based on studies of both groups and individuals. Although descriptive epidemiology is not the focus of this book, birth cohort analysis is discussed in some depth in this chapter because this approach is rarely covered in detail in basic textbooks. Another topic in the interface between descriptive and analytical epidemiology—namely, ecological studies—is also discussed, with a view toward extending its discussion beyond the possibility of inferential (ecological) bias. Next, the chapter reviews observational studies based on individuals as units of observation—that is, cohort and case-control studies. Different types of case-control design are reviewed. The strategy of *matching* as an approach by which to achieve comparability prior to data collection is also briefly discussed.

Chapters 2 and 3 cover issues of measurement of outcome frequency and measures of association. In Chapter 2, absolute measures of outcome frequency and their calculation methods are reviewed, including the person-time approach for the calculation of incidence density, and both the classic life table and the Kaplan-Meier method for the calculation of cumulative incidence. Chapter 3 deals with measures of association, including those based on relative (e.g., relative risk, odds ratio) and absolute (attributable risk) differences. The connections between measures of association obtained in cohort and case-control studies are emphasized. In particular, a description is given of the different measures of association (i.e., odds ratio, relative risk, rate ratio) that can be obtained in case-control studies as a function of the control selection strategies that were introduced in Chapter 1.

Chapters 4 and 5 are devoted to threats to the validity of epidemiologic studies, namely bias and confounding. In Chapter 4, the most common types of bias are discussed, including selection bias and information bias. In the discussion of information bias, simple examples are given to improve the understanding of the phenomenon of misclassification resulting from less-than-perfect sensitivity and specificity of the approaches used for ascertaining exposure, outcome, and/or confounding variables. This chapter also provides a discussion of cross-sectional biases and biases associated with evaluation of screening procedures; for the latter, a simple approach to estimate lead time bias is given, which may be useful for those involved in evaluative studies of this sort. In Chapter 5, the concept of confounding is introduced, and approaches to evaluate confounding are reviewed. Special issues related to confounding are discussed, including the distinction between confounders and intermediate variables, residual confounding, and the role of statistical significance in the evaluation of confounding effects.

Interaction (effect modification) is discussed in Chapter 6. The chapter presents the concept of interaction, emphasizing its pragmatic application as well as the strategies used to evaluate the presence of additive and multiplicative interactions. Practical issues discussed in this chapter include whether to adjust when interaction is suspected and the importance of the additive model in public health.

The next three chapters are devoted to the approaches used to handle threats to the validity of epidemiologic results. In Chapter 7, strategies for the adjustment of confounding factors are presented, including the more parsimonious approaches (e.g., direct adjustment, Mantel-Haenszel) and the more complex (i.e., multiple regression, instrumental variables, Mendelian randomization, and propensity scores). Emphasis is placed on the selection of the method that is most appropriate for the study design used (e.g., Cox proportional hazards for the analysis of survival data or Poisson regression for the analysis of rates per person-time). Chapter 8 reviews the basic quality-control strategies for the prevention and control of measurement error and bias. Both qualitative and quantitative approaches used in quality control are discussed. The most-often used analytic strategies for estimating validity and reliability of data obtained in epidemiologic studies are reviewed (e.g., unweighted and weighted kappa, correlation coefficients) in this chapter. In Chapter 9, the key issue of communication of results of epidemiologic studies is discussed. Examples of common mistakes made when reporting epidemiologic data are given as a way to stress the importance of clarity in such reports.

Chapter 10 discusses—from the epidemiologist's viewpoint—issues relevant to the interface between epidemiology, health policy, and public health, such as Rothman's causality model, proximal and distal causes, and Hill's guidelines. This chapter also includes brief discussions of three topics pertinent to causal inference: sensitivity analysis, meta-analysis, and publication bias; and consideration of the decision tree as a tool to evaluate interventions. As in the previous editions, Appendices A, B, C, and E describe selected statistical procedures (e.g., standard errors and confidence levels, trend test, test of heterogeneity of effects, intraclass correlation) to help the reader to more thoroughly evaluate the measures of risk and association discussed in the text and to expose him or her to procedures that, although relatively simple, are not available in many statistical packages used by epidemiology students and practitioners. Appendix D includes two sections on quality assurance and control procedures taken from the corresponding manual of the Atherosclerosis Risk in Communities (ARIC) Study as examples of real-life applications of some of the procedures discussed in Chapter 8. Finally, Appendix F provides the answers to the exercises.

We encourage readers to advise us of any errors or unclear passages, and to suggest improvements. Please email any such suggestions or comments to: info@jblearning.com.

All significant contributions will be acknowledged in the next edition.

Acknowledgments

This book is an outgrowth of an intermediate epidemiology course taught by the authors at the Johns Hopkins Bloomberg School of Public Health. Over the years, this course has benefited from significant intellectual input of many faculty members, including, among others, George W. Comstock, Helen Abbey, James Tonascia, Leon Gordis, and Mary Meyer. The authors especially acknowledge the late George W. Comstock, a mentor to both of us, who was involved with the course for several decades. His in-depth knowledge of epidemiologic methods and his wisdom over the years has been instrumental to our professional growth. Dr. Comstock also kindly provided many of the materials and examples used in Chapter 9 of this book.

We are indebted to many colleagues, including Leonelo Bautista, Daniel Brotman, Woody Chambless, Steve Cole, Joseph Coresh, Rosa Maria Corona, Ana Diez-Roux, Jingzhong Ding, Manning Feinleib, Leon Gordis, Eliseo Guallar, Jay Kaufman, Kristen Malecki, Alfonso Mele, Paolo Pasquini, Paul Peppard, Patrick Remington, Jonathan Samet, Eyal Shahar, Richey Sharrett, and Michael Silverberg. These colleagues reviewed partial sections of this or previous editions or provided guidance in solving conceptual or statistical riddles. We are especially grateful to our current and former students Gabrielle Detjen, Salwa Massad, Margarete (Grete) Wichmann, and Hannah Yang for their careful review of the exercises. The authors are also grateful to Lauren Wisk for creating the ancillary instructor materials for this text. Finally, we would like to extend our appreciation to Patty Grubb, whose assistance has been instrumental in getting this edition ready, and to Jennifer Seltzer for her administrative help.

To have enjoyed the privilege of teaching intermediate epidemiology for so many years made us realize how much we have learned from our students, to whom we are deeply grateful. Finally, without the support and extraordinary patience of all members of our families, particularly our wives, Hilda and Marion, we could not have devoted so much time and effort to writing the three editions of this text.

About the Authors

Moyses Szklo, MD, DrPH, is a Professor of Epidemiology and Medicine (Cardiology) at the Johns Hopkins University. His current research focuses on risk factors for subclinical and clinical atherosclerosis. He is also Editor-in-Chief of the *American Journal of Epidemiology*.

F. Javier Nieto, MD, PhD, is Helfaer Professor of Public Health, and Professor and Chair at the Department of Population Health Sciences at the University of Wisconsin School of Medicine and Public Health. His current research focuses on epidemiology of cardiovascular and sleep disorders as well as on population-based survey methods.

PART ONE

Introduction

CHAPTER 1 Basic Study Designs in Analytical Epidemiology   3

Basic Study Designs in Analytical Epidemiology

CHAPTER 1

1.1 INTRODUCTION: DESCRIPTIVE AND ANALYTICAL EPIDEMIOLOGY

Epidemiology is traditionally defined as the study of the distribution and determinants of health-related states or events in specified populations and the application of this study to control health problems.[1] Epidemiology can be classified as either "descriptive" or "analytic." In general terms, *descriptive epidemiology* makes use of available data to examine how rates (e.g., mortality) vary according to demographic variables (e.g., those obtained from census data). When the distribution of rates is not uniform according to person, time, and place, the epidemiologist is able to define high-risk groups for prevention purposes—e.g., hypertension is more prevalent in US blacks than in US whites, thus defining blacks as a high-risk group. In addition, disparities in the distribution of rates serve to generate causal hypotheses based on the classic agent–host–environment paradigm—e.g., the hypothesis that environmental factors to which blacks are exposed, such as excessive salt intake or psychosocial stress, are responsible for their higher risk of hypertension.

A thorough review of descriptive epidemiologic approaches can be readily found in numerous sources.[2,3] For this reason and given the overall scope of this book, this chapter focuses on study designs that are relevant to *analytical epidemiology*; that is, designs that allow assessment of hypotheses of associations of suspected risk factor exposures with health outcomes. Moreover, the main focus of this textbook is *observational epidemiology*, even though many of the concepts discussed in subsequent chapters, such as measures of risk, measures of association, interaction/effect modification and quality assurance/control, are also relevant to experimental studies (randomized clinical trials).

In this chapter, the two general strategies used for the assessment of associations in observational studies are discussed: (1) studies using populations or groups of individuals as units of observation—the so-called ecologic studies; and (2) studies using individuals as observation units, which include the prospective (or cohort), the case-control, and the cross-sectional study designs.

Before that, however, the next section briefly discusses the *analysis of birth cohorts*. The reason for including this descriptive technique here is that it often requires the application of an analytical approach with a level of complexity usually not found in descriptive epidemiology; furthermore, this type of analysis is frequently important for understanding the patterns of association between age (a key determinant of health status) and disease in cross-sectional analyses. (An additional, more pragmatic reason for including a discussion of birth cohort analysis here is that it is usually not discussed in detail in basic textbooks.)

CHAPTER 1 | Basic Study Designs in Analytical Epidemiology

1.2 ANALYSIS OF AGE, BIRTH COHORT, AND PERIOD EFFECTS

Health surveys conducted in population samples usually include participants over a broad age range. Age is a strong risk factor for many health outcomes and is also frequently associated with numerous exposures. Thus, even if the effect of age is not among the primary objectives of the study, given its potential confounding effects, it is often important to assess its relationship with exposures and outcomes.

Table 1-1 shows the results of a hypothetical cross-sectional study conducted in 2005 to assess the prevalence rates of a disease Y according to age. (A more strict use of the term "rate" as a measure of the occurrence of incident events is defined in Section 2.2.2. This term is also widely used in a less precise sense to refer to proportions such as prevalence.[1] It is in this more general sense that the term is used here and in other parts of the book.)

In Figure 1-1, these results are plotted at the midpoints of 10-year age groups (e.g., for ages 30–39, at 35 years; for ages 40–49, at 45 years; and so on). These data show that the prevalence of Y in this population decreases with age. Does this mean that the prevalence rates of Y decrease as individuals age? Not necessarily. For many disease processes,

TABLE 1-1 Hypothetical data from a cross-sectional study of prevalence of disease Y in a population, by age, 2005.

Age group (years)	Midpoint (years)	2005 Prevalence (per 1000)
30–39	35	45
40–49	45	40
50–59	55	36
60–69	65	31
70–79	75	27

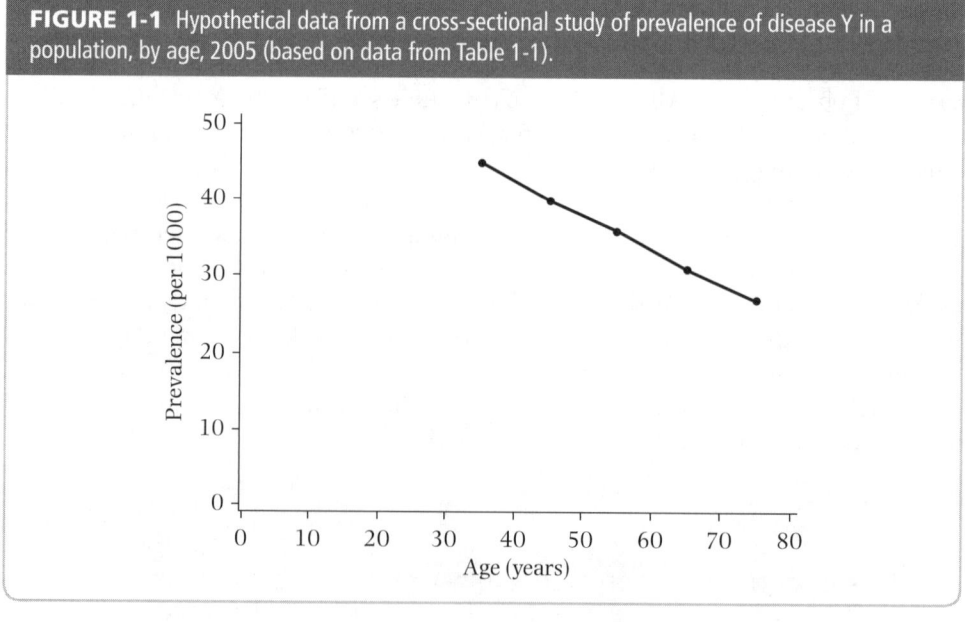

FIGURE 1-1 Hypothetical data from a cross-sectional study of prevalence of disease Y in a population, by age, 2005 (based on data from Table 1-1).

exposures have cumulative effects that are expressed over long periods of time. Long latency periods and cumulative effects characterize, for example, numerous exposure/disease associations, including smoking-lung cancer, radiation-thyroid cancer, and saturated fat intake-atherosclerotic disease. Thus, the health status of a person who is 50 years old at the time of the survey may be partially dependent on this person's past exposures (e.g., smoking during early adulthood). Variability of past exposures across successive generations (birth cohorts*) can distort the apparent associations between age and health outcomes that are observed at any given point in time. This concept can be illustrated as follows.

Suppose that the same investigator who collected the data shown in Table 1-1 is able to recover data from previous surveys conducted in the same population in 1975, 1985, and 1995. The resulting data, presented in Table 1-2 and Figure 1-2, show consistent trends of decreasing prevalence of Y with age in each of these surveys. Consider now plotting these data using a different approach, as shown in Figure 1-3. The dots in Figure 1-3 are at the same places as in Figure 1-2, except that the lines are connected by *birth cohort* (the 2005 survey data are also plotted in Figure 1-3). Each of the dotted lines represents a birth cohort converging to the 2005 survey. For example, the "youngest" age point in the 2005 cross-sectional curve represents the rate of disease Y for individuals aged 30 to 39 years (average of 35 years) who were born between 1965 and 1974—that is, in 1970 on average (the "1970 birth cohort"). Individuals in this 1970 birth cohort were on average 10 years younger—that is, 25 years of age at the time of the 1995 survey and 15 years of age at the time of the 1985 survey. The line for the 1970 birth cohort thus represents how the prevalence of Y changes with increasing age for individuals born, on average, in 1970. Evidently, the cohort pattern shown in Figure 1-3 is very different from that suggested by the cross-sectional data and is consistent for all birth cohorts shown in Figure 1-3 in that it suggests that the prevalence of Y actually

TABLE 1-2 Hypothetical data from a series of cross-sectional studies of prevalence of disease Y in a population, by age and survey date (calendar time), 1975–2005.

Age group (years)	Midpoint (years)	Survey date			
		1975	1985	1995	2005
		Prevalence (per 1000)			
10–19	15	17	28		
20–29	25	14	23	35	
30–39	35	12	19	30	45
40–49	45	10	18	26	40
50–59	55		15	22	36
60–69	65			20	31
70–79	75				27

Birth cohort: From Latin *cohors*, warriors, the 10th part of a legion. The component of the population born during a particular period and identified by period of birth so that its characteristics (e.g., causes of death and numbers still living) can be ascertained as it enters successive time and age periods.[1]

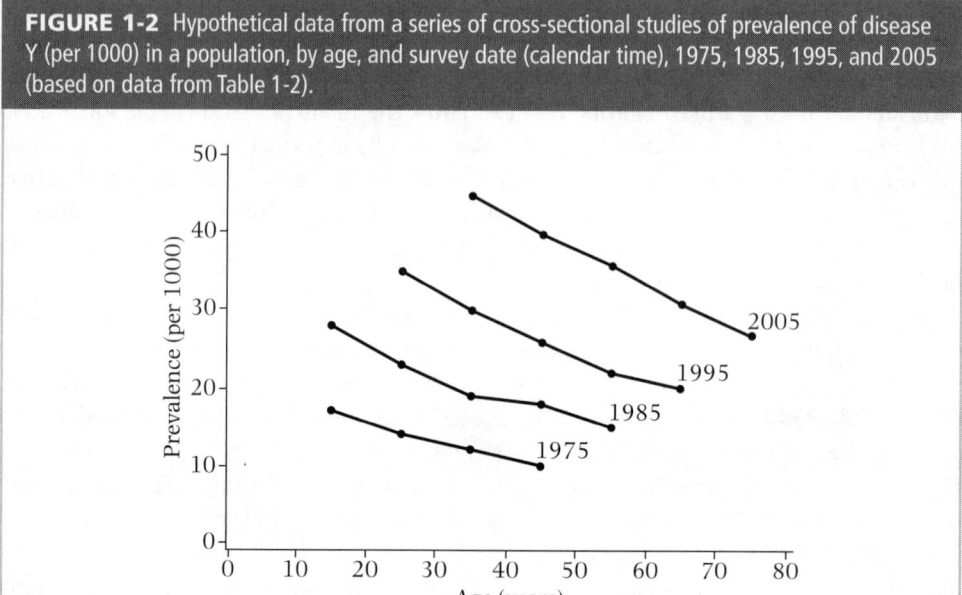

FIGURE 1-2 Hypothetical data from a series of cross-sectional studies of prevalence of disease Y (per 1000) in a population, by age, and survey date (calendar time), 1975, 1985, 1995, and 2005 (based on data from Table 1-2).

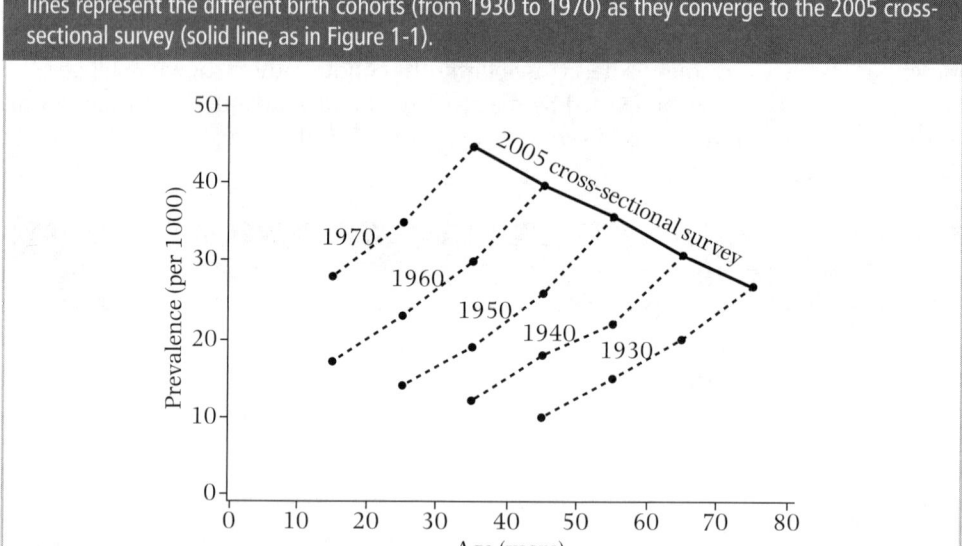

FIGURE 1-3 Plotting of the data in Figure 1-2 by birth cohort (see also Table 1-3). The dotted lines represent the different birth cohorts (from 1930 to 1970) as they converge to the 2005 cross-sectional survey (solid line, as in Figure 1-1).

increases as people age. The fact that the inverse trend is observed in the cross-sectional data is due to a strong "cohort effect" in this example; that is, the prevalence of Y is strongly determined by the year of birth of the person. For any given age, the prevalence rate is higher in younger (more recent) than in older cohorts. Thus, in the 2005 cross-sectional survey (Figure 1-1), the older subjects come from birth cohorts with relatively lower rates, whereas the youngest come from the cohorts with higher rates. This can be seen clearly in Figure 1-3 by selecting one age (e.g., 45 years) and observing that the rate is lowest for the 1930 birth cohort, and increases for each subsequent birth cohort (i.e., the 1940, 1950, and 1960 cohorts, respectively).

1.2 Analysis of Age, Birth Cohort, and Period Effects

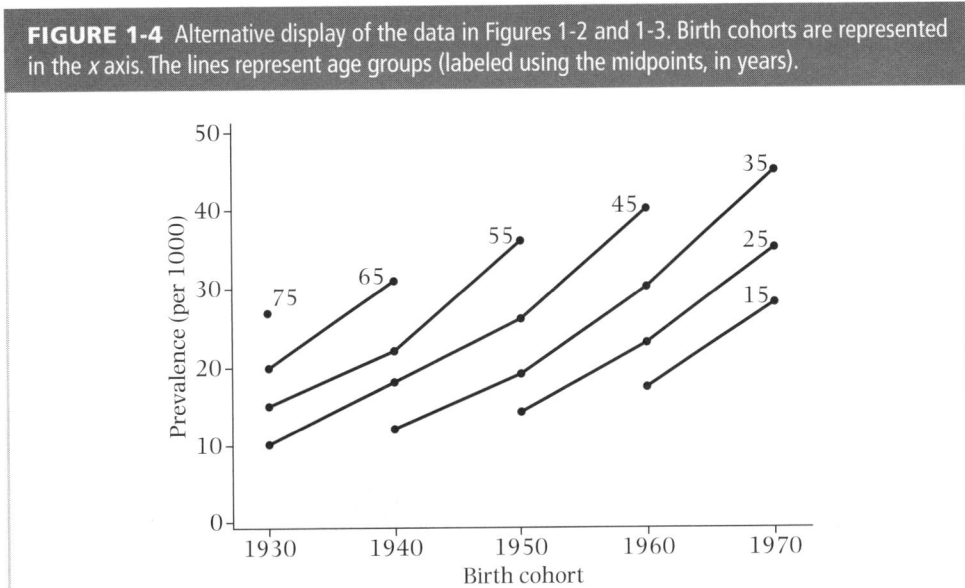

FIGURE 1-4 Alternative display of the data in Figures 1-2 and 1-3. Birth cohorts are represented in the x axis. The lines represent age groups (labeled using the midpoints, in years).

Although the cross-sectional analysis of prevalence rates in this example gives a distorted view of the disease behavior as a birth cohort ages, it is still useful for planning purposes; this is because, regardless of the mix of birth cohorts, cross-sectional data inform the public health authorities about the burden of disease as it exists currently (e.g., the age distribution of disease Y in 2005).

An alternative display of the data from Table 1-2 is shown in Figure 1-4. Instead of age (as in Figures 1-1 to 1-3), the scale in the abscissa (x axis) corresponds to the birth cohort and each line to an age group; thus, the slope of the lines represents the change across birth cohorts for a given age group.

Often the choice among these alternative graphical representations is a matter of personal preference (i.e., which pattern the investigator wishes to emphasize). Whereas Figure 1-4 shows trends according to birth cohorts more explicitly (e.g., for any given age group, there is an increasing prevalence from older to more recent cohorts), Figure 1-3 has an intuitive appeal in that each line represents a birth cohort as it ages. As long as one pays careful attention to the labeling of the graph, any of these displays is appropriate to identify age and birth cohort patterns. The same patterns displayed in Figures 1-3 and 1-4 can be seen in Table 1-2, moving downward to examine cross-sectional trends and diagonally from left to right to examine birth cohort trends. An alternative and somewhat more readable display of the same data for the purpose of detecting trends according to birth cohort is shown in Table 1-3, which allows the examination of trends according to age ("age effect") within each birth cohort (horizontal lines in Table 1-3). Additionally, and in agreement with Figure 1-4, Table 1-3 shows how prevalence rates increase from older to more recent cohorts (cohort effect)—readily visualized by moving one's eyes from the top to the bottom of each age group column in Table 1-3.

Thus, the data in the previous example are simultaneously affected by two strong effects: "cohort effect" and "age effect" (for definitions, see Exhibit 1-1). These two trends are jointly responsible for the seemingly paradoxical trend observed in the cross-sectional analyses in this hypothetical example (Figures 1-1 and 1-2), in which the rates seem

TABLE 1-3 Rearrangement of the data shown in Table 1-2 by birth cohort.

Birth cohort range	Midpoint	Age group (midpoint, in years)						
		15	25	35	45	55	65	75
		Prevalence (per 1000)						
1925–1934	1930				10	15	20	27
1935–1944	1940			12	18	22	31	
1945–1954	1950		14	19	26	36		
1955–1964	1960	17	23	30	40			
1965–1974	1970	28	35	45				

EXHIBIT 1-1 Definitions of age, cohort, and period effects.

Age effect: Change in the rate of a condition according to age, irrespective of birth cohort and calendar time

Cohort effect: Change in the rate of a condition according to year of birth, irrespective of age and calendar time

Period effect: Change in the rate of a condition affecting an entire population at some point in time, irrespective of age and birth cohort

---

to *decrease* with age. The fact that more recent cohorts have substantially higher rates (cohort effect) overwhelms the increase in prevalence associated with age and explains the observed cross-sectional pattern.

In addition to cohort and age effects, patterns of rates can be influenced by the so-called "period effect." The term period effect is frequently used to refer to a global shift or change in trends that affect the rates across birth cohorts and age groups (Exhibit 1-1). Any phenomenon occurring at a specific point in time (or during a specific period) that affects an entire population (or a significant segment of it), such as a war, a new treatment, or massive migration, can produce this change independently of age and birth cohort effects. A hypothetical example is shown in Figure 1-5. This figure shows data similar to those used in the previous example (Figure 1-3), except that in this case the rates level off in 1995 for all cohorts (i.e., when the 1970 cohort is 25 years old on the average, when the 1960 cohort is 35 years old, and so on).

Period effects on prevalence rates can occur, for example, when new medications or preventive interventions are introduced for diseases that previously had poor prognoses, as in the case of the introduction of insulin, antibiotics, and the polio vaccine.

It is important to understand that the so-called birth cohort effects may have little to do with the circumstances surrounding the time of birth of a given cohort of individuals. Rather, cohort effects may result from the lifetime experience (including, but not limited to, those surrounding birth) of the individuals born at a given point in time that influence the disease or outcome of interest. For example, currently observed patterns of association between age and coronary heart disease (CHD) may have resulted from cohort effects related to changes in diet (e.g., fat intake) or smoking habits of adolescent and young adults over time. It is well known that coronary atherosclerotic markers,

1.2 Analysis of Age, Birth Cohort, and Period Effects

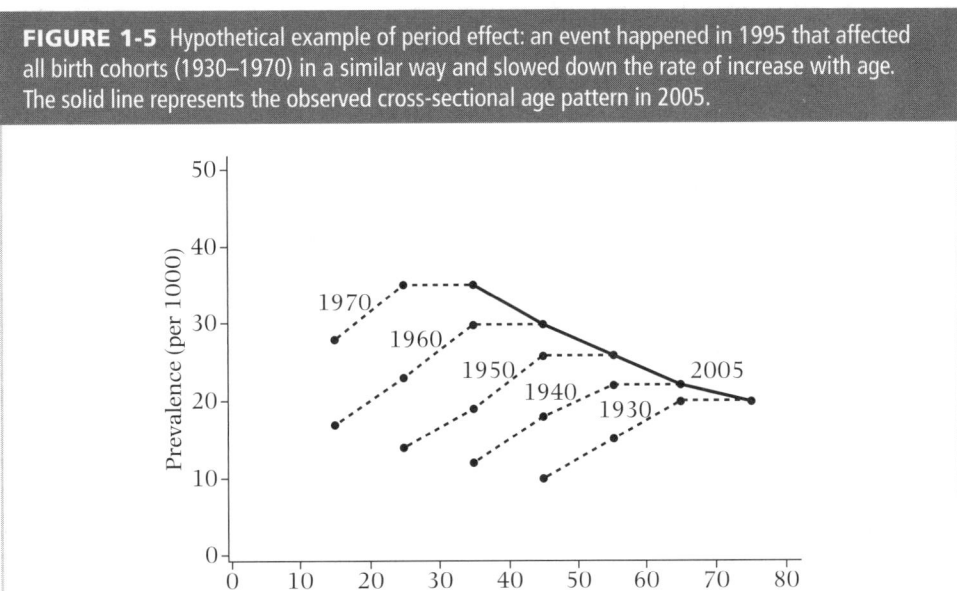

FIGURE 1-5 Hypothetical example of period effect: an event happened in 1995 that affected all birth cohorts (1930–1970) in a similar way and slowed down the rate of increase with age. The solid line represents the observed cross-sectional age pattern in 2005.

such as thickening of the arterial intima, frequently develop early in life.[4] In middle and older ages, some of these early intimal changes may evolve into raised atherosclerotic lesions, eventually leading to thrombosis, lumen occlusion, and the resulting clinically manifest acute ischemic events. Thus, a young adult's dietary and/or smoking habits may influence atherosclerosis development and subsequent coronary risk. If changes in these habits occur in the population over time, successive birth cohorts will be subjected to changing degrees of exposure to early atherogenic factors, which will determine in part future cross-sectional patterns of the association of age with CHD.

Another way to understand the concept of cohort effects is as the result of an *interaction* between age and calendar time. The concept of interaction is discussed in detail in Chapter 6 of this book. In simple terms, it means that a given variable (e.g., calendar time in the case of a cohort effect) *modifies* the strength or the nature of an association between another variable (e.g., age) and an outcome (e.g., coronary atherosclerosis). In the previous example, it means that the way age relates to the development of atherosclerosis changes over time as a result of changes in the population prevalence of key risk factors (e.g., dietary/smoking habits of young adults). In other words, calendar time-related changes in risk factors *modify* the association between age and atherosclerosis.

Cohort–age–period analyses can be applied not only to prevalence data but also to incidence and mortality data. A classic example is Wade Hampton Frost's study of age patterns of tuberculosis mortality.[5] Figure 1-6 presents two graphs from Frost's landmark paper. With regard to Figure 1-6A, Frost[5(p.94)] noted that "looking at the 1930 curve, the impression given is that nowadays an individual encounters his greatest risk of death from tuberculosis between the ages of 50 and 60. But this is not really so; the people making up the 1930 age group 30 to 60 have, in earlier life, passed through *greater* mortality risk" (emphasis in original). This is demonstrated in Figure 1-6B, aptly used by Frost to show how the risk of tuberculosis death after the

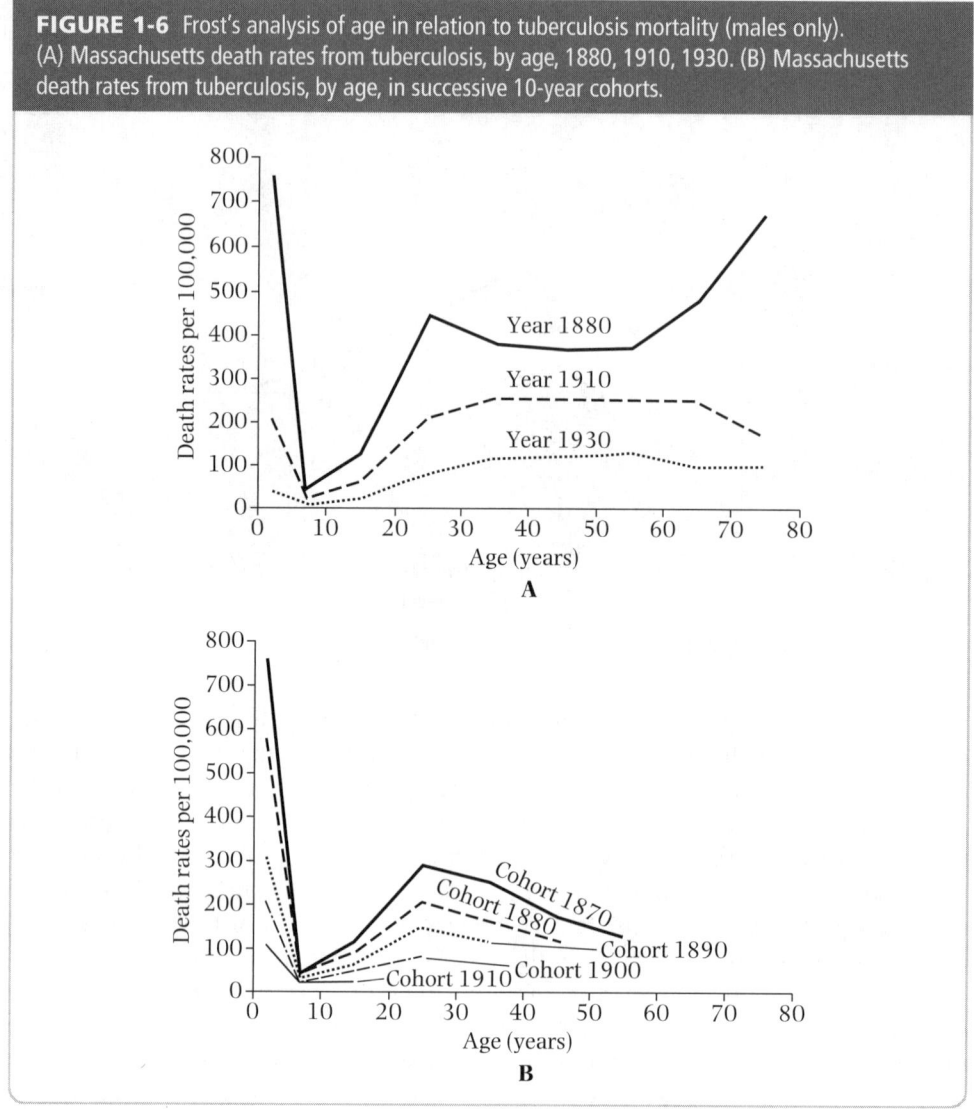

FIGURE 1-6 Frost's analysis of age in relation to tuberculosis mortality (males only). (A) Massachusetts death rates from tuberculosis, by age, 1880, 1910, 1930. (B) Massachusetts death rates from tuberculosis, by age, in successive 10-year cohorts.

Source: Reprinted with permission from WH Frost, The Age-Selection of Tuberculosis Mortality in Successive Decades. *American Journal of Hygiene*, Vol 30, pp. 91–96, © 1939.

first few years of life is actually highest at ages 20 to 30 years for cohorts born in 1870 through 1890.

Another, more recent, example is shown in Figure 1-7, based on an analysis of age, cohort, and period effects on the incidence of colorectal cancer in a region of Spain.[6] In these figures, birth cohorts are placed on the *x* axis (as in Figure 1-4). These figures show strong cohort effects: for each age group, the incidence rates of colorectal cancer tend to increase from older to more recent birth cohorts. An age effect is also evident, as for each birth cohort (for any given year-of-birth value in the horizontal axis) the rates are higher for older than for younger individuals. Note that a logarithmic scale was used in the ordinate in this figure, in part because of the wide range of rates needed to be plotted. (For further discussion of the use of logarithmic vs arithmetic scales, see Chapter 9, Section 9.3.5.)

1.2 Analysis of Age, Birth Cohort, and Period Effects

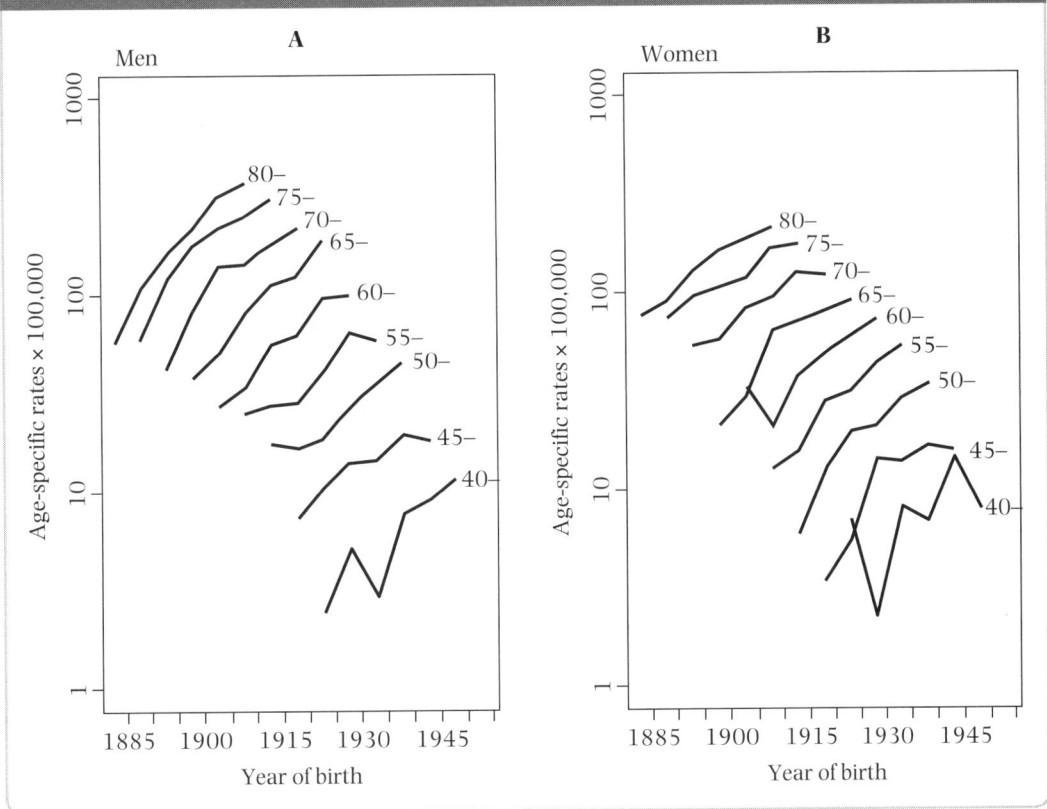

FIGURE 1-7 Trends in age-specific incidence rates of colorectal cancer in Navarra and Zaragoza (Spain). The number next to each line represents the initial year of the corresponding 5-year age group.

Source: Reprinted with permission from G. López-Abente et al., Age-Period-Cohort Modeling of Colorectal Cancer Incidence and Mortality in Spain. *Cancer Epidemiology, Biomarkers, and Prevention,* Vol 6, pp. 999–1005. © 1997.

An additional example of age and birth cohort analysis of incidence data is shown in Figure 1-8. This figure shows the incidence of ovarian cancer in Mumbai, India, by age and year of birth cohort.[7] This is an example in which there is a strong age effect, particularly for the cohorts born from 1940 through 1970—that is, rates increase dramatically with age through age 52 years—but virtually no cohort effect, as indicated by the approximate flat pattern for the successive birth cohorts for each age group (the figure shows the midpoint of each age group). It should be manifest that, with very little cohort effect, the same age patterns for rates are found in cross-sectional and cohort curves (Figure 1-8B).

Period effects associated with incidence rates tend to be more prominent for diseases for which the cumulative effects of previous exposures are relatively unimportant, such as infectious diseases and injuries. Conversely, in chronic diseases such as cancer and cardiovascular disease, cumulative effects are usually important, and thus, cohort effects tend to affect incidence rates to a greater extent than period effects.

These methods can also be used to study variables other than disease rates. An example is the analysis of age-related changes in serum cholesterol levels shown in Figure 1-9, based on data from the Florida Geriatric Research Program, an ongoing program designed to provide free medical screening for older people.[8] This figure reveals a slight cohort effect, in that serum cholesterol levels tend to be lower in older than in more

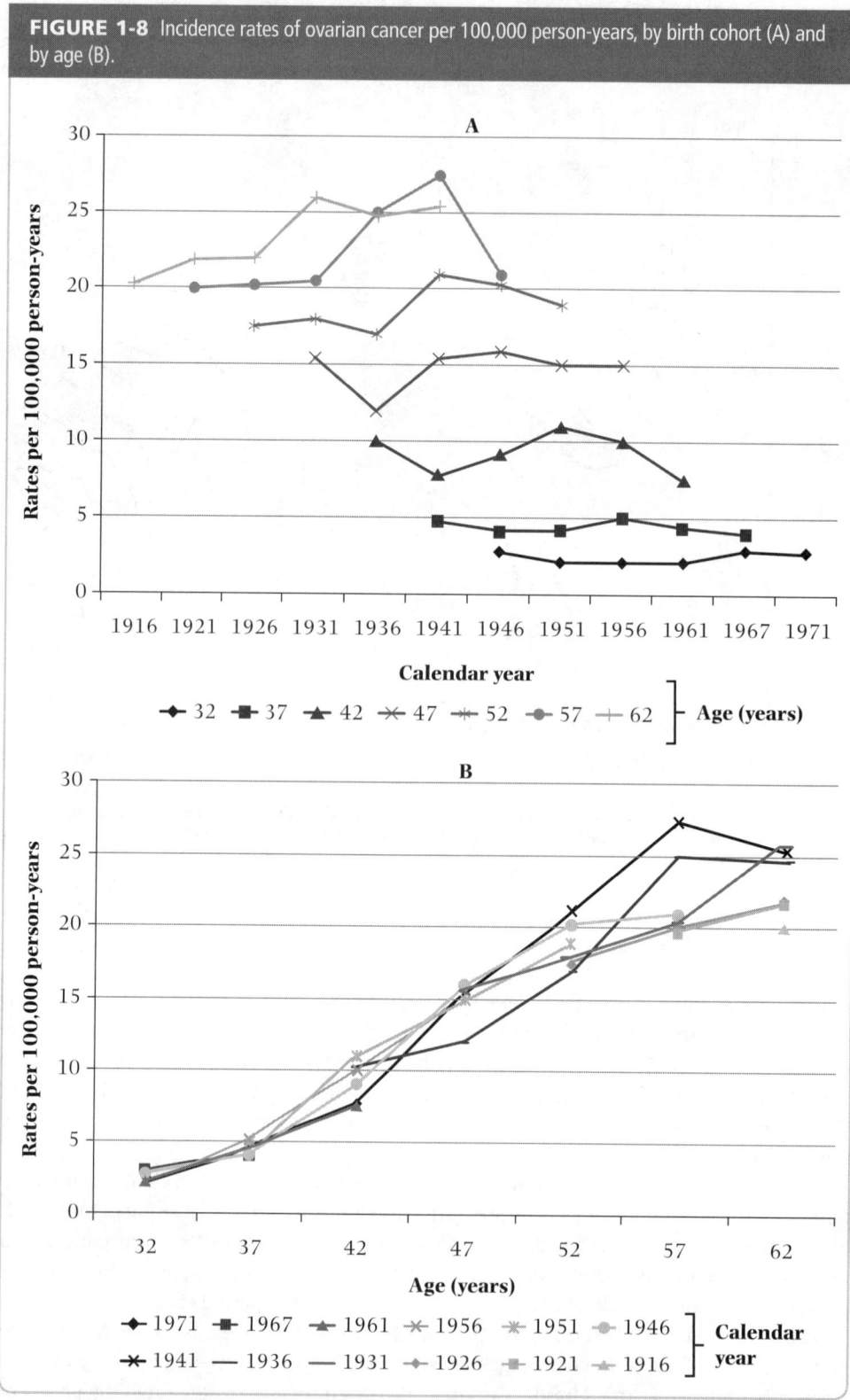

FIGURE 1-8 Incidence rates of ovarian cancer per 100,000 person-years, by birth cohort (A) and by age (B).

Source: Adapted from PK Dhillon et al., Trends in Breast, Ovarian and Cervical Cancer Incidence in Mumbai, India Over a 30-Year Period, 1976–2005: An Age-Period-Cohort Analysis. *British Journal of Cancer,* Vol 105, No 5, pp. 723–730, © 2011.

FIGURE 1-9 Sex-specific mean serum cholesterol levels by age and birth cohort: longitudinal data from the Florida Geriatric Research Program, Dunedin County, Florida, 1976 to 1987.

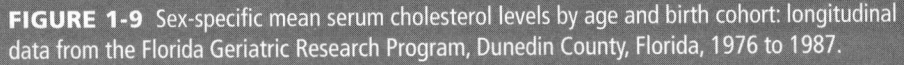

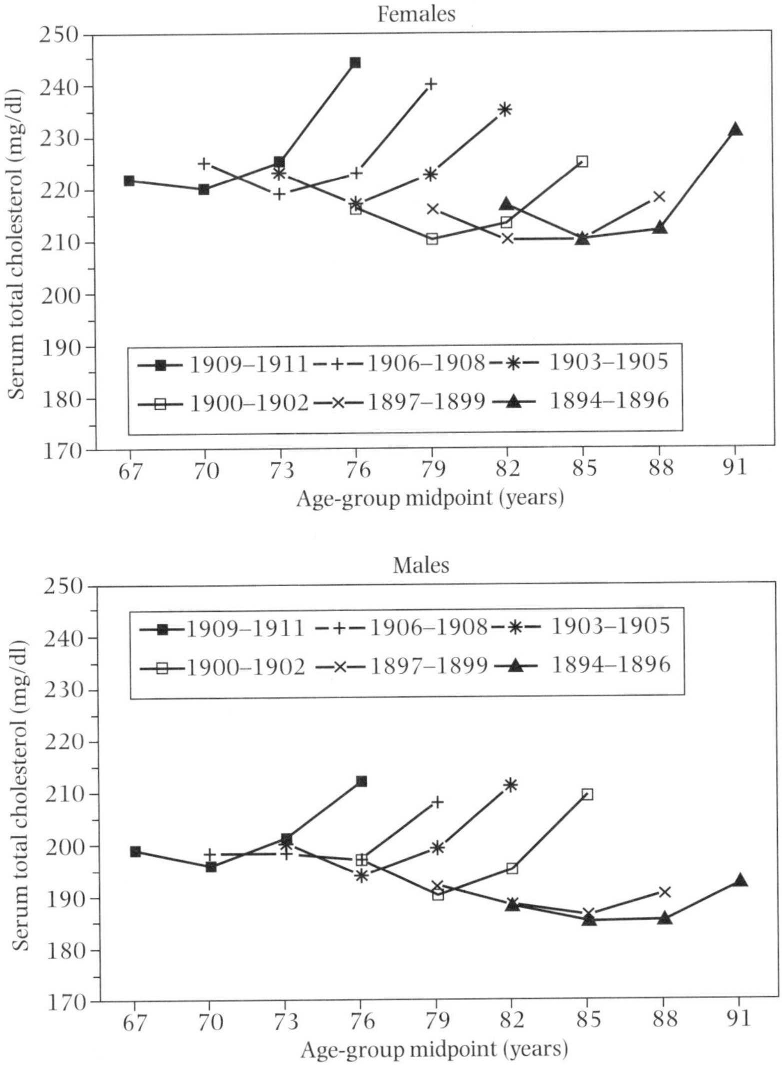

Source: Reprinted with permission from CJ Newschaffer, TL Bush, and WE Hale, Aging and Total Cholesterol Levels: Cohort, Period, and Survivorship Effects. *American Journal of Epidemiology*, Vol 136, pp. 23–34, © 1992.

recent birth cohorts for most age groups. A J- or U-shaped age pattern is also seen; that is, for each birth cohort, serum cholesterol tends to first decrease or remain stable with increasing age and then increase to achieve its maximum value in the oldest members of the cohort. Although at first glance this pattern might be considered an "age effect," for each cohort the maximum cholesterol values in the oldest age group coincide with a single point in calendar time: 1985 through 1987 (i.e., for the 1909–1911 birth cohort at 76 years of age, for the 1906–1908 cohort at 79 years of age, and so on), leading Newschaffer et al. to observe that "a period effect is suggested by a consistent change in curve height at a given time point over all cohorts. . . . Therefore, based on simple visual inspection of the curves, it is not possible to attribute the consistent U-shaped increase in cholesterol to aging, since some of this shape may be accounted for by period effects."[8(p.26)]

In complex situations, it may be difficult to clearly differentiate age, cohort, and period effects. In these situations, such as that illustrated in the preceding discussion, multiple regression techniques can be used to disentangle these effects. Describing these techniques in detail is beyond the scope of this book. (A general discussion of multiple regression methods is presented in Chapter 7, Section 7.4.) The interested reader can find examples and further references in the original papers from the previously cited examples (e.g., López-Abente et al.[6] and Newschaffer et al.[8]).

Finally, it should be emphasized that birth cohort effects may affect associations between disease outcomes and variables other than age. Consider, for example, a case-control study (see Section 1.4.2) in which cases and controls are closely matched by age (see Section 1.4.5). Assume that, in this study, cases are identified over a 10-year span (e.g., from 1960 through 1969) and controls at the end of the accrual of cases. In this study, age *per se* does not act as a confounder, as cases and controls are matched on age (see Section 5.2.2); however, the fact that cases and controls are identified from different birth cohorts may affect the assessment of variables, such as educational level, that may have changed rapidly across birth cohorts. In this case, birth cohort, but not age, would confound the association between education and the disease of interest.

1.3 ECOLOGIC STUDIES

The units of observation in an ecologic study are usually geographically defined populations (such as countries or regions within a country) or the same geographically defined population at different points in time. Mean values* for both a given postulated risk factor and the outcome of interest are obtained for each observation unit for comparison purposes. Typically, the analysis of ecologic data involves plotting the risk factor and outcome values for all observation units to assess whether a relationship is evident. For example, Figure 1-10 displays the death rates for CHD in men from 16 cohorts included in the Seven Countries Study plotted against the corresponding estimates of mean fat intake (percent calories from fat).[9] A positive relationship between these two variables is suggested by these data, as there is a tendency for the death rates to be higher in countries having higher average saturated fat intakes.

Different types of variables can be used in ecologic studies,[10] which are briefly summarized as follows:

- *Aggregate measures* that summarize the characteristics of individuals within a group as the mean value of a certain parameter or the proportion of the population or group of interest with a certain characteristic. Examples include the prevalence of a given disease, average amount of fat intake (Figure 1-10), proportion of smokers, and median income.
- *Environmental measures* that represent physical characteristics of the geographic location for the group of interest. Individuals within the group may have different degrees of exposure to a given characteristic, which could theoretically be measured. Examples include air pollution intensity and hours of sunlight.

---

*A mean value can be calculated for both continuous and discrete (e.g., binary) variables. A proportion is a mean of individual binary values (e.g., 1 for presence of a certain characteristic, 0 if the characteristic is absent).

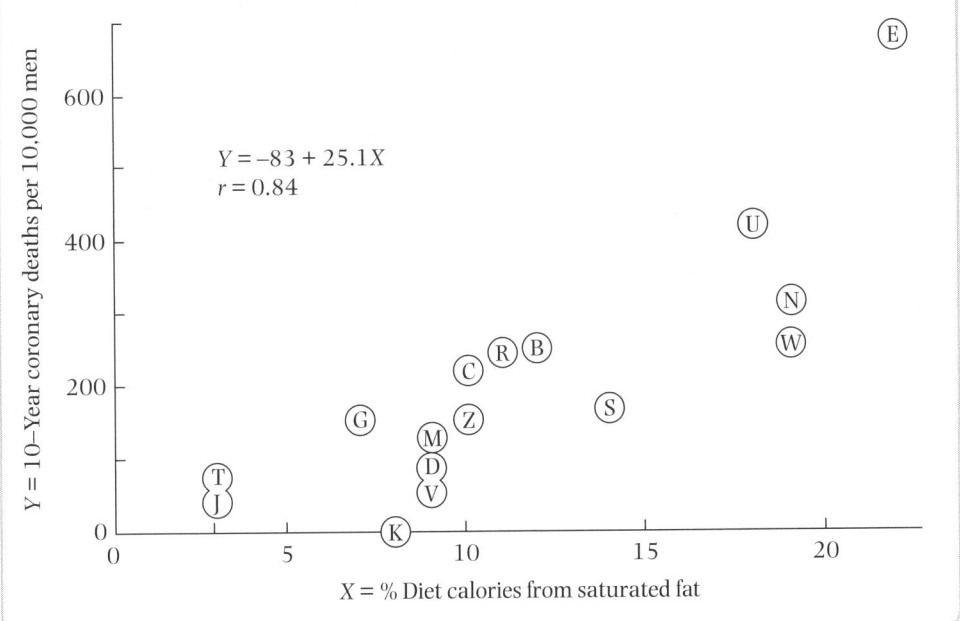

FIGURE 1-10 Example of an ecologic study. Ten-year coronary death rates of the cohorts from the Seven Countries Study plotted against the percentage of dietary calories supplied by saturated fatty acids. Cohorts: B, Belgrade; C, Crevalcore; D, Dalmatia; E, East Finland; G, Corfu; J, Ushibuka; K, Crete; M, Montegiorgio; N, Zuphen; R, Rome railroad; S, Slavonia; T, Tanushimaru; U, American railroad; V, Velika Krsna; W, West Finland; Z, Zrenjanin. Shown in the figure are the correlation coefficient r and the linear regression coefficients (see Chapter 7, Section 7.4.1) corresponding to this plot.

Source: Reprinted with permission from *Seven Countries: A Multivariate Analysis of Death and Coronary Heart Disease*, by A Keys, Cambridge, Mass: Harvard University Press, © 1980.

- *Global measures* that represent characteristics of the group that are not reducible to characteristics of individuals (i.e., that do not have analogues at the individual level). Examples include the type of political or healthcare system in a given region, a certain regulation or law, and the presence and magnitude of health inequalities.

In a traditional ecologic study, two ecologic variables are contrasted to examine their possible association. Typically, an ecologic measure of exposure and an aggregate measure of disease or mortality are compared (Figure 1-10). These ecologic measures can also be used in studies of individuals (see Section 1.4) in which the investigator chooses to define exposure using an ecologic criterion on the basis of its expected superior construct validity.* For example, in a cross-sectional study of the relationship between socioeconomic status and prevalent cardiovascular disease, the investigator may choose to define study participants' socioeconomic status using an aggregate indicator (e.g., median family income in the neighborhood) rather than, for example, his or her own (individual) educational level or income. Furthermore, both individual and aggregate measures can be simultaneously considered in *multilevel analyses*, as when examining

---

*Construct validity is the extent to which an operational variable (e.g., body weight) accurately represents the phenomenon it purports to represent (e.g., nutritional status).

the joint role of individuals' and aggregate levels of income and education in relation to prevalent cardiovascular disease.[11]

An ecologic association may accurately reflect a causal connection between a suspected risk factor and a disease (e.g., the positive association between fat intake and CHD depicted in Figure 1-10). However, the phenomenon of *ecologic fallacy* is often invoked as an important limitation for the use of ecologic correlations as *bona fide* tests of etiologic hypotheses. The ecologic fallacy (or *aggregation bias*) has been defined as "the bias that may occur because an association observed between variables on an aggregate level does not necessarily represent the association that exists at an individual level."[1] The phenomenon of ecologic fallacy is schematically illustrated in Figure 1-11, based on an example proposed by Diez-Roux.[12] In a hypothetical ecologic study examining the relationship between per capita income and the risk of motor vehicle injuries in three populations composed of seven individuals each, a positive correlation between mean income and risk of injuries is observed; however, a close inspection of *individual* values reveals that cases occur exclusively in persons with low income (less than US $20,000). In this extreme example of ecologic fallacy, the association detected when using populations as observation units—for example, higher mean income relates to a higher risk of motor vehicle injuries—has a direction diametrically opposed to the relationship between income and motor vehicle injuries in individuals—in whom higher individual income relates to a lower injury risk. Thus, the conclusion from the ecologic analysis that a higher income is a risk factor for motor vehicle injuries may be fallacious (discussed later in this section).

Another example of a situation in which this type of fallacy may have occurred is given by an ecologic study that showed a direct correlation between the percentage

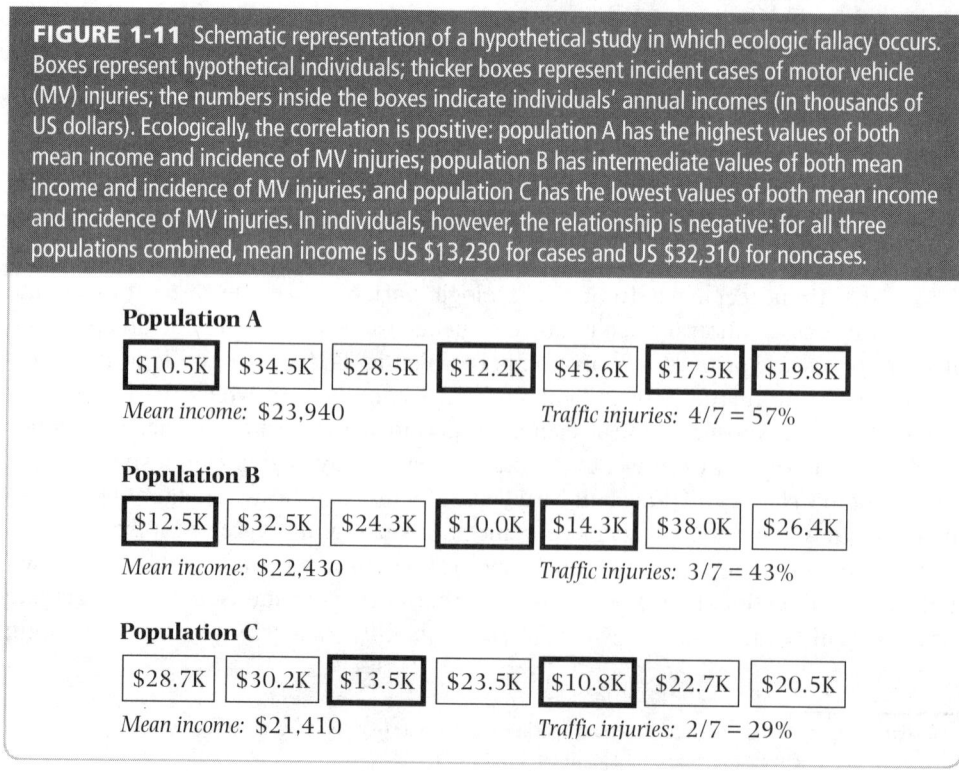

FIGURE 1-11 Schematic representation of a hypothetical study in which ecologic fallacy occurs. Boxes represent hypothetical individuals; thicker boxes represent incident cases of motor vehicle (MV) injuries; the numbers inside the boxes indicate individuals' annual incomes (in thousands of US dollars). Ecologically, the correlation is positive: population A has the highest values of both mean income and incidence of MV injuries; population B has intermediate values of both mean income and incidence of MV injuries; and population C has the lowest values of both mean income and incidence of MV injuries. In individuals, however, the relationship is negative: for all three populations combined, mean income is US $13,230 for cases and US $32,310 for noncases.

Population A

| $10.5K | $34.5K | $28.5K | $12.2K | $45.6K | $17.5K | $19.8K |

Mean income: $23,940   Traffic injuries: 4/7 = 57%

Population B

| $12.5K | $32.5K | $24.3K | $10.0K | $14.3K | $38.0K | $26.4K |

Mean income: $22,430   Traffic injuries: 3/7 = 43%

Population C

| $28.7K | $30.2K | $13.5K | $23.5K | $10.8K | $22.7K | $20.5K |

Mean income: $21,410   Traffic injuries: 2/7 = 29%

of the population that was Protestant and suicide rates in a number of Prussian communities in the late 19th century.[10,13] Concluding from this observation that being Protestant is a risk factor for suicide may well be wrong (i.e., may result from an ecologic fallacy). For example, it is possible that most of the suicides within these communities were committed by Catholic individuals who, when in the minority (i.e., in communities predominantly Protestant), tended to be more socially isolated and therefore at a higher risk of suicide.

As illustrated in these examples, errors associated with ecologic studies are the result of *cross-level inference*, which occurs when aggregate data are used to make inferences at the individual level.[10] The mistake in the example just discussed is to use the correlation between the proportion of Protestants (which is an aggregate measure) and suicide rate to infer that the risk of suicide is higher in Protestant than in Catholic *individuals*. If one were to make an inference at the *population* level, however, the conclusion that predominantly Protestant communities with Catholic minorities have higher rates of suicide would still be valid (provided that other biases and confounding factors were not present). Similarly, in the income/injuries example, the inference from the ecologic analysis is only wrong if intended for the understanding of determinants at the level of the individual. The ecologic information may be valuable if the investigator's purpose is to understand fully the complex web of causality[14] involved in motor vehicle injuries, as it may yield clues regarding the causes of motor vehicle injuries that are not provided by individual-level data. In the previous example (Figure 1-11), higher mean population income may truly be associated with increased traffic volume and, consequently, with higher rates of motor vehicle injuries. At the individual level, however, the inverse association between income and motor vehicle injuries may result from the higher frequency of use of unsafe vehicles among low-income individuals, particularly in the context of high traffic volume.

Because of the prevalent view that inference at the individual level is the "gold standard" when studying disease causation,[15] as well as the possibility of ecologic fallacy, ecologic studies are often considered imperfect surrogates for studies in which individuals are the observation units. Essentially, ecologic studies are seen as preliminary studies that "can suggest avenues of research that may be promising in casting light on etiological relationships."[3(p.206)] That this is often but not always true has been underscored by the examples discussed previously here. Furthermore, the following two situations demonstrate that an ecologic analysis may on occasion lead to *more* accurate conclusions than an analysis using individual-level data—even if the level of inference in the ecologic study is at the individual level.

1. The first situation is when the within-population variability of the exposure of interest is low, but the between-population variability is high. For example, if salt intake of individuals in a given population were above the threshold needed to cause hypertension, a relationship between salt and hypertension might not be apparent in an observational study of individuals in this population, but it could be seen in an ecologic study including populations with diverse dietary habits.[16] (A similar phenomenon has been postulated to explain why ecologic correlations, but not studies of individuals, have detected a relationship between fat intake and risk of breast cancer.[17])

2. The second situation is when, even if the intended level of inference is the individual, the *implications for prevention or intervention are at the population level*. Some examples of the latter situation are as follows:

- In the classic studies on pellagra, Goldberger et al.[18] assessed not only individual indicators of income but also food availability in the area markets. They found that, independently of individual socioeconomic indicators, food availability in local markets in the villages was strongly related to the occurrence of pellagra, leading these authors to conclude the following:

  > The most potent factors influencing pellagra incidence in the villages studied were (a) low family income, and (b) unfavorable conditions regarding the availability of food supplies, suggesting that under conditions obtaining [sic] in some of these villages in the spring of 1916 many families were without sufficient income to enable them to procure an adequate diet, and that improvement in food availability (particularly of milk and fresh meat) is urgently needed in such localities.[18(p.2712)]

  It should be readily apparent in this example that an important (and potentially modifiable) link in the causal chain of pellagra occurrence—namely, food availability—may have been missed if the investigators had focused exclusively on individual income measures.

- Studies of risk factors for smoking initiation and/or smoking cessation may focus on community-level cigarette taxes or regulation of cigarette advertising. Although individual factors may influence the individual's predisposition to smoking (e.g., psychological profile, smoking habits of relatives or friends), regulatory "ecologic" factors may be strong determinants and modifiers of the individual behaviors. Thus, an investigator may choose to focus on these global factors rather than (or in addition to) individual behaviors.

- When studying the determinants of transmission of certain infectious diseases with complex nonlinear infection dynamics (e.g., attenuated exposure-infection relationship at the individual level), ecologic studies may be more appropriate than studies using individuals as observation units.[19]

Because ultimately all risk factors must operate at the individual level, the quintessential reductionistic* approach would focus only on the causal pathways at the biochemical or intracellular level. For example, the study of the carcinogenic effects of tobacco smoking could focus on the effects of tobacco byproducts at the cellular level—that is, alteration of the cell's DNA. However, will that make the study of smoking habits irrelevant? Obviously not. Indeed, from a public health perspective, the use of a comprehensive theoretical model of causality—one that considers all factors influencing the occurrence of disease—often requires taking into account the role of upstream and ecologic factors (including environmental, sociopolitical, and cultural) in the causal chain (see also Chapter 10, Sections 10.2.2 and 10.2.3). As stated at the beginning of this chapter, the ultimate goal of epidemiology is to be effectively used as a tool to improve the health conditions of the public; in this context, the factors that operate at a global level may represent important links in the chain of causation, particularly when they are amenable to intervention (e.g., improving access to fresh foods in villages or establishing laws that limit cigarette advertising). As a result, studies focusing on factors at the individual level may be insufficient in that they fail to address these ecologic links in the causal chain. This important concept

---

*Reductionism is a theory that postulates that all complex systems can be completely understood in terms of their components, basically ignoring interactions between these components.

can be illustrated using the previously discussed example of religion and suicide. A study based on individuals would "correctly" find that the risk of suicide is higher in Catholics than in Protestants.[10] This finding would logically suggest explanations of why the suicide rate differs between these religious groups. For example, is the higher rate in Catholics caused by Catholicism *per se*? Alternatively, is it because of some ethnic difference between Catholics and Protestants? If so, is it due to some genetic component that distinguishes these ethnic groups? The problem is that these questions, which attempt to characterize risk at the individual level, although important, are insufficient to explain fully the "web of causality,"[14] for they fail to consider the ecologic dimension of whether minority status explains and determines the increased risk of suicide. This example underscores the concept that both individual and ecologic studies are often necessary to study the complex causal determination not only of suicide but also of many other health and disease processes.[12] The combination of individual and ecologic levels of analysis poses analytical challenges for which statistical models (hierarchical models) have been developed. Difficult conceptual challenges remain, however, such as the development of causal models that include all relevant risk factors operating from the social to the biological level and that take into consideration their possible multi-level interaction.[12]

1.4 STUDIES BASED ON INDIVIDUALS AS OBSERVATION UNITS

There are three basic types of nonexperimental (observational) study designs in which individuals are the units of observation: the cohort or prospective study, the case-control study, and the cross-sectional study. In this section, key aspects of these study designs are reviewed. The case-crossover study, a special type of case-control study, is also briefly discussed. For a more comprehensive discussion of the operational and analytic issues related to observational epidemiologic studies, the reader is referred to specialized texts.[20–24]

From a conceptual standpoint, the fundamental study design in observational epidemiology—that is, the design from which the others derive and that can be considered as the "gold standard"—is the cohort or prospective study. Cohort data, if unbiased, reflect the "real-life" cause–effect temporal sequence of events, a *sine qua non* criterion to establish causality (see Section 10.2.4). From this point of view, the case-control and the cross-sectional designs are mere variations of the cohort study design and are primarily justified by feasibility, logistical ease, and efficiency.

1.4.1 Cohort Study

In a cohort study, a group of healthy people or a *cohort** is identified and followed up for a certain time period to ascertain the occurrence of health-related events (Figure 1-12). The usual objective of a cohort study is to investigate whether the incidence of an event is related to a suspected exposure.

Study populations in cohort studies can be quite diverse and may include a sample of the general population of a certain geographical area (e.g., the Framingham Study[25]); an occupational cohort, typically defined as a group of workers in a given occupation or industry who are classified according to exposure to agents thought to be occupational

---

*A definition of the term *cohort* broader than that found in the footnote in Section 1.2 is any designated and defined group of individuals who are followed or traced over a given time period.[1]

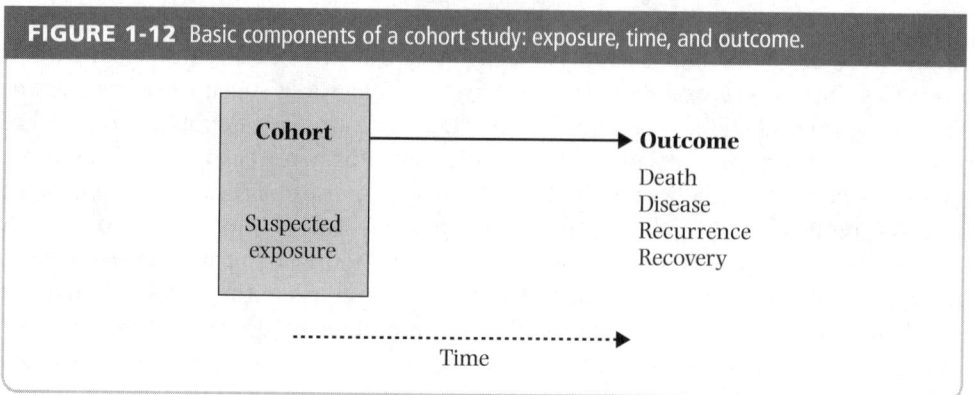

FIGURE 1-12 Basic components of a cohort study: exposure, time, and outcome.

hazards; or a group of people who, because of certain characteristics, are at an unusually high risk for a given disease (e.g., the cohort of homosexual men who are followed in the Multicenter AIDS Cohort Study[26]). Alternatively, cohorts can be formed by "convenience" samples, or groups gathered because of their willingness to participate or because of other logistical advantages, such as ease of follow-up; examples include the Nurses Health Study cohort,[27] the Health Professionals Study cohort,[28] and the American Cancer Society cohort studies of volunteers.[29]

After the cohort is defined and the participants are selected, a critical element in a cohort study is the ascertainment of events during the follow-up time (when the event of interest is a newly developed disease, prevalent cases are excluded from the cohort at baseline). This is the reason why these studies are also known as *prospective studies*.[30] A schematic depiction of a cohort of 1000 individuals is shown in Figure 1-13. In this hypothetical example, cohort members are followed for a given time period during

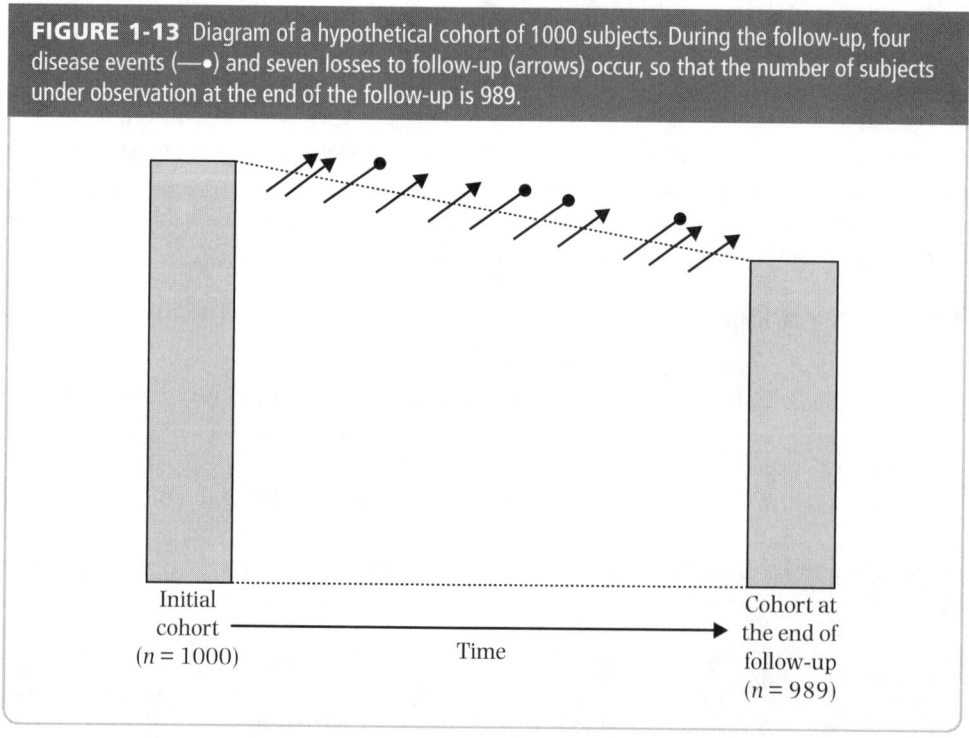

FIGURE 1-13 Diagram of a hypothetical cohort of 1000 subjects. During the follow-up, four disease events (—•) and seven losses to follow-up (arrows) occur, so that the number of subjects under observation at the end of the follow-up is 989.

which four events such as incident disease cases or deaths (which appear in Figure 1-13 as lines ending with a dot) occur. In addition to these four events, seven individuals are lost to follow-up during the study period. These losses (represented in Figure 1-13 as arrows) are usually designated as *censored observations* or *withdrawals*. As described in Chapter 2, these losses to follow-up need to be taken into account for the calculation of incidence. Using the actuarial life-table approach as an example (see Chapter 2, Section 2.2.1), incidence can be estimated as the number of events occurring during the follow-up period divided by the number of subjects in the cohort at baseline minus one-half of the losses. Thus, for the hypothetical cohort in Figure 1-13, the incidence of disease is $4/[1000 - (1/2 \times 7)] = 4.01/1000$.

In the *cohort study*'s most representative format, a defined population is identified. Its subjects are classified according to exposure status, and the incidence of the disease (or any other health outcome of interest) is ascertained and compared across exposure categories (Figure 1-14). For example, based on the hypothetical cohort schematically represented in Figure 1-13 and assuming that the prevalence of the exposure of interest is 50%, Figure 1-15 outlines the follow-up separately for exposed ($n = 500$) and unexposed ($n = 500$) individuals. Data analysis in this simple situation is straightforward, involving a comparison of the incidence of disease between exposed and unexposed persons, using as the denominator the "population at risk." For example, using the actuarial life table approach previously mentioned for the hypothetical cohort study depicted in Figure 1-15, the incidence of disease in exposed individuals is $3/[500 - (1/2 \times 4)] = 6.02/1000$, and in unexposed, $1/[500 - (1/2 \times 3)] = 2.01/1000$. After obtaining incidence in exposed and unexposed, typically the relative risk is estimated (Chapter 3, Section 3.2.1); that is, these results would suggest that exposed individuals in this cohort have a risk approximately three times higher than that of unexposed individuals (relative risk = $6.02/2.01 = 3.0$).

As discussed in Chapter 2, an important assumption for the calculation of incidence in a cohort study is that individuals who are lost to follow-up (the arrows in Figures 1-13 and 1-15) are similar to those who remain under observation with regard to characteristics affecting the outcome of interest. The reason is that even though techniques to "correct" the denominator for the number (and timing) of losses are available (see Section 2.2), if the average risk of those who are lost differs from that of those remaining

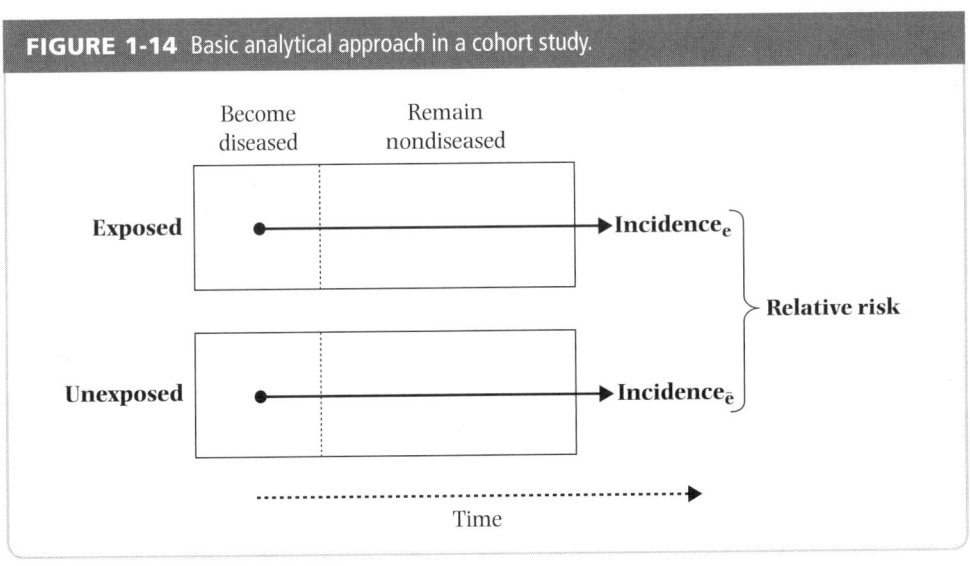

FIGURE 1-14 Basic analytical approach in a cohort study.

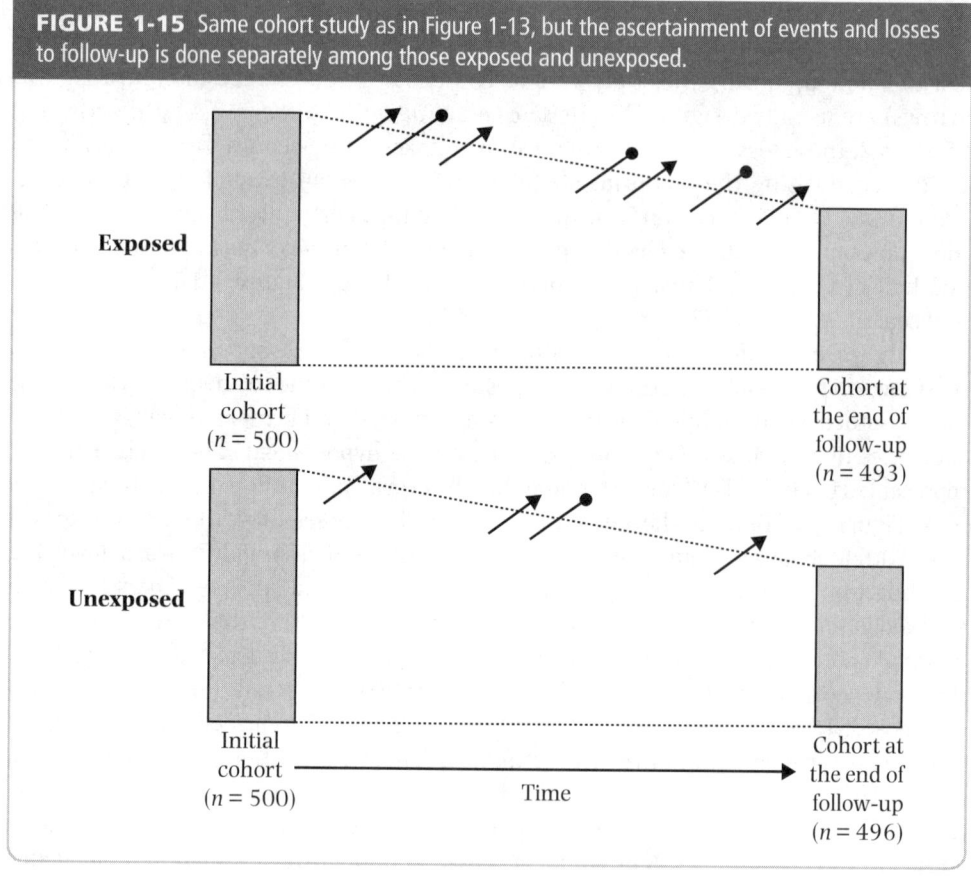

FIGURE 1-15 Same cohort study as in Figure 1-13, but the ascertainment of events and losses to follow-up is done separately among those exposed and unexposed.

in the cohort, the incidence based on the latter will not represent accurately the true incidence in the initial cohort (see Section 2.2.1). If, however, the objective of the study is an *internal comparison* of the incidence between exposed and unexposed subjects, even if those lost to follow-up differ from the remaining cohort members, as long as the biases caused by losses are similar in the exposed and the unexposed, they will cancel out when the relative risk is calculated (see Chapter 4, Section 4.2). Thus, a biased relative risk caused by losses to follow-up is present only when losses are differential in exposed and unexposed subjects with regard to the characteristics influencing the outcome of interest—in other words, when losses are affected by both exposure and disease status.

Cohort studies are defined as *concurrent*[3] (or truly "prospective"[30]) when the cohort is assembled at the present time—that is, the calendar time when the study starts—and is followed up toward the future (Figure 1-16). The main advantage of concurrent cohort studies is that the baseline exam, methods of follow-up, and ascertainment of events are planned and implemented for the purposes of the study, thus best fitting the study objectives; in addition, quality control measures can be implemented as needed (see Chapter 8). The disadvantages of concurrent studies relate to the amount of time needed to conduct them (results are available only after a sufficient number of events is accumulated) and their usually elevated costs. Alternatively, in *nonconcurrent* cohort studies (also known as *historical* or *retrospective* cohort studies), a cohort is identified and assembled in the past on the basis of existing records and is "followed" to the present time (i.e., the time when the study is conducted) (Figure 1-16). An example of this type of design is a 1992 study in which the relationship between childhood body weight and subsequent adult

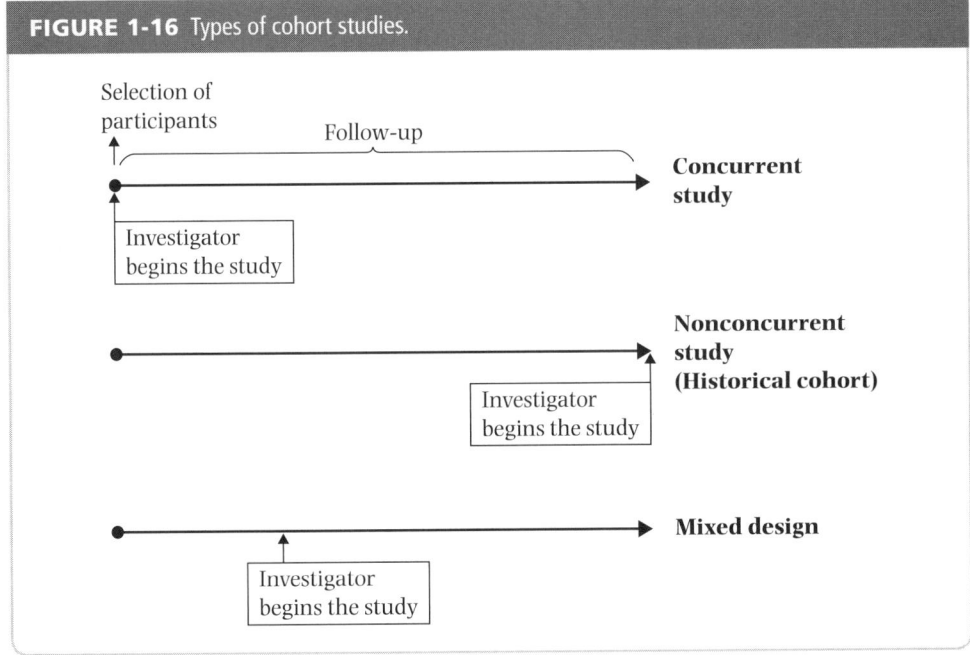

FIGURE 1-16 Types of cohort studies.

mortality was examined nonconcurrently on the basis of existing records of weight and height values obtained from 1933 through 1945 in school-age children that were linked to adult death records.[31] The nonconcurrent design is also useful in occupational epidemiology, as occupational records can be linked to mortality or cancer registries: for example, a cohort of all electricians working in Norway in 1960 was followed nonconcurrently through 1990 to study the relationship of electromagnetic radiation to cancer incidence.[32] *Mixed designs* with both nonconcurrent and concurrent follow-up components are also possible (Figure 1-16). Nonconcurrent cohort studies are obviously less expensive and can be done more expeditiously than concurrent studies. Their main disadvantage is an obligatory reliance on available information; as a result, the type or quality of exposure or outcome data may not be well suited to fulfill the study objectives.

1.4.2 Case-Control Study

As demonstrated by Cornfield[33] and discussed in basic epidemiology textbooks (e.g., Gordis[3]), the case-control design is an alternative to the cohort study for investigating exposure-disease associations. In contrast to a cohort study, in which exposed and unexposed individuals are compared in relationship with the disease incidence (or some other mean value for the outcome) (Figure 1-14), a case-control study compares cases (usually, diseased individuals) and controls (e.g., nondiseased individuals) with respect to their level of exposure to a suspected risk factor. When the risk factor of interest is a binary characteristic (present/absent), the typical analytical approach in case-control studies is to compare the odds of exposure in cases with that in controls by calculating the exposure *odds ratio* (Figure 1-17), which is often an appropriate estimate of the relative risk (see Chapter 3, Section 3.2.1). When the exposure of interest is a continuous trait, its mean levels (e.g., mean blood pressure) can be compared in cases and controls.

The case-control study design has important advantages over the cohort design, particularly over the concurrent cohort study, as the need for a follow-up time is avoided, thus optimizing speed and efficiency.[3]

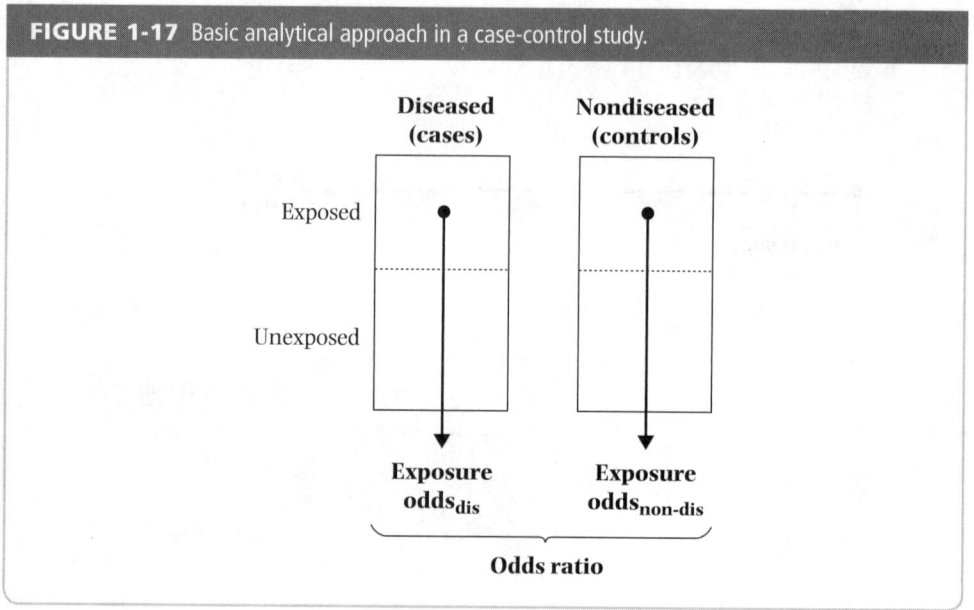

FIGURE 1-17 Basic analytical approach in a case-control study.

Case-Based Case-Control Study

In the simplest strategy for the selection of groups in a case-control study, cases occurring over a specified time period and noncases are identified. An example of this strategy, sometimes called *case-based case-control study*, is a study in which incident cases are identified as the individuals in whom the disease of interest was diagnosed (e.g., breast cancer) in a certain hospital during a given year and controls are selected from among members of the community served by this hospital who did not have a diagnosis of the disease of interest by the end of that same year. If exposure data are obtained through interviews, it is necessary to assume that recall or other biases will not distort the findings (see Chapter 4). If only living cases are included in the study, it must be also assumed that cases that survive through the time when the study is done are representative of all cases with regard to the exposure experience (Figure 1-18). Furthermore, to validly compare cases and controls regarding their exposure status, it is necessary to assume that they originate from the same reference population—that is, from a more or less explicitly identified cohort, as depicted in Figure 1-18. In other words, for a case-control comparison to represent a valid alternative to a cohort study analysis, cases and controls are expected to belong to a common reference population (or to a similar reference population or study base; discussed later in this chapter). It is, however, frequently difficult to define the source cohort in a case-control study, as, for example, in a case-based study in which the cases are ascertained in a single hospital A but controls are selected from a population sample. In this example, it is important to consider the correspondence between the patient population of hospital A and the population of the geographic area from which controls are sampled. Thus, for example, if hospital A is the only institution to which area residents can be admitted and all cases are hospitalized, a sample of the same area population represents a valid control group. If, however, residents use hospitals outside of the area and hospital A admits patients from other areas, alternative strategies have to be considered to select controls who are representative of the theoretical population from which cases originate (e.g., matching controls to cases by neighborhood of residency).

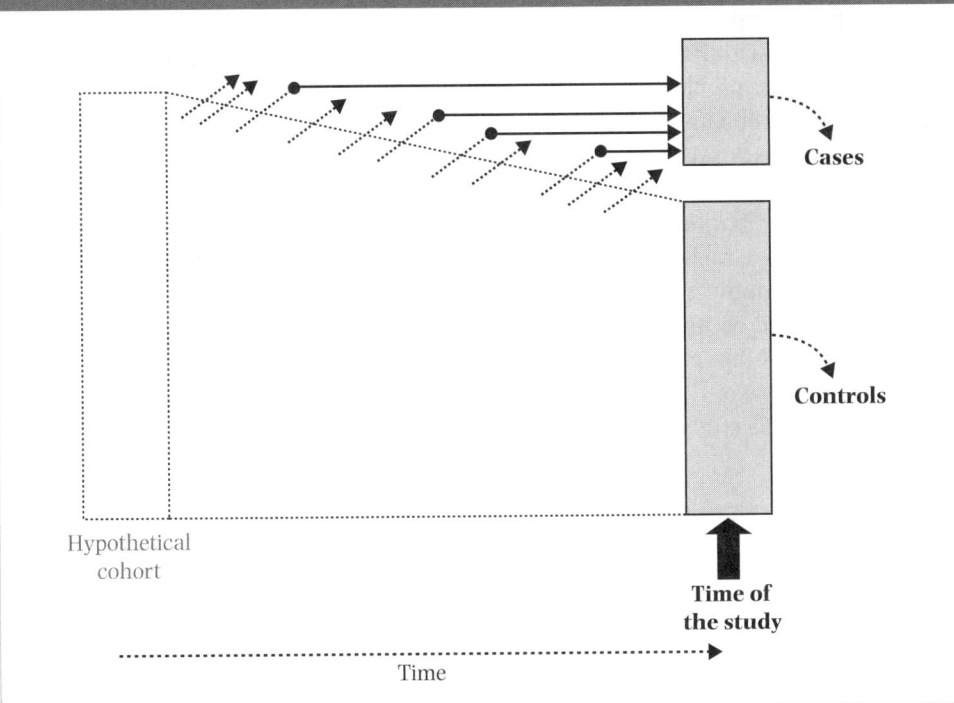

FIGURE 1-18 Hypothetical case-based case-control study, assuming that cases and controls are selected from a hypothetical cohort, as in Figure 1-13. The case group is assumed to include all cases that occurred in that hypothetical cohort up to the time when the study is conducted (dots with horizontal arrows ending at the "case" bar): that is, they are assumed to be all alive and available to participate in the study; controls are selected from among those without the disease of interest (noncases) at the time when the cases are identified and assembled. Broken diagonal lines with arrows represent losses to follow-up.

The assumption that cases and controls originate from the same hypothetical source cohort (even if undefined) is critical when judging the internal validity of case-control data. Ideally, controls should have been eligible to be included in the case group had they developed the disease of interest. Pragmatically, although it is not strictly necessary that cases and controls be chosen from exactly the *same* reference population, both groups must originate from populations having *similar relevant characteristics*. Under these circumstances, the control group can be regarded as a reasonably representative sample of the case reference population.

When cases and controls are not selected from the same (or similar) reference population(s), *selection bias* may ensue, as discussed in detail in Chapter 4. Selection bias may occur even if cases and controls are from the same "hypothetical" cohort; this happens when "losses" occurring *before* the study groups are selected affect their comparability. For example, if losses among potential controls include a higher proportion of individuals with low socioeconomic status than losses among cases, biased associations may be found with exposures related to socioeconomic status. This example underscores the close relationship between selection bias in case-control studies and differential losses to follow-up in cohort studies. In this context, consider the similarity between Figures 1-18 and 1-13, in that the validity of the comparisons made in both cohort (Figure 1-13) and case-control (Figure 1-18) studies depends on whether the losses (represented by diagonal arrows in both figures) affect the representativeness of the baseline cohort (well defined in Figure 1-13, hypothetical in Figure 1-18) with regard to both exposure and outcome variables.

Deaths caused by either other diseases or the disease of interest comprise a particular type of (prior) "loss" that may affect comparability of cases and controls. For the type of design represented in Figure 1-18, characterized by cross-sectional ascertainment of study subjects, those who die before they can be included in the study may have a different exposure experience compared to the rest of the source population. In addition, this design identifies primarily cases that are prevalent at the time of the study (i.e., those with the longest survival) (Figure 1-19). These types of selection bias constitute generic problems affecting cross-sectional ascertainment of study participants; another problem is recall bias, which results from obtaining past exposure data long after disease onset. (For a detailed discussion of these and other biases in case-control studies, see Chapter 4.)

It should be emphasized that although cross-sectional ascertainment of cases and controls is often carried out, it is not a *sine qua non* feature of case-based case-control studies. An alternative strategy, which aims at minimizing selection and recall biases and which should be used whenever possible, is to ascertain cases concurrently (i.e., to identify [and obtain exposure information on] cases as soon as possible after disease onset). An example of this strategy is a study of risk factors for oral clefts conducted in Denmark.[34] In this study, case mothers were women who were hospitalized and gave

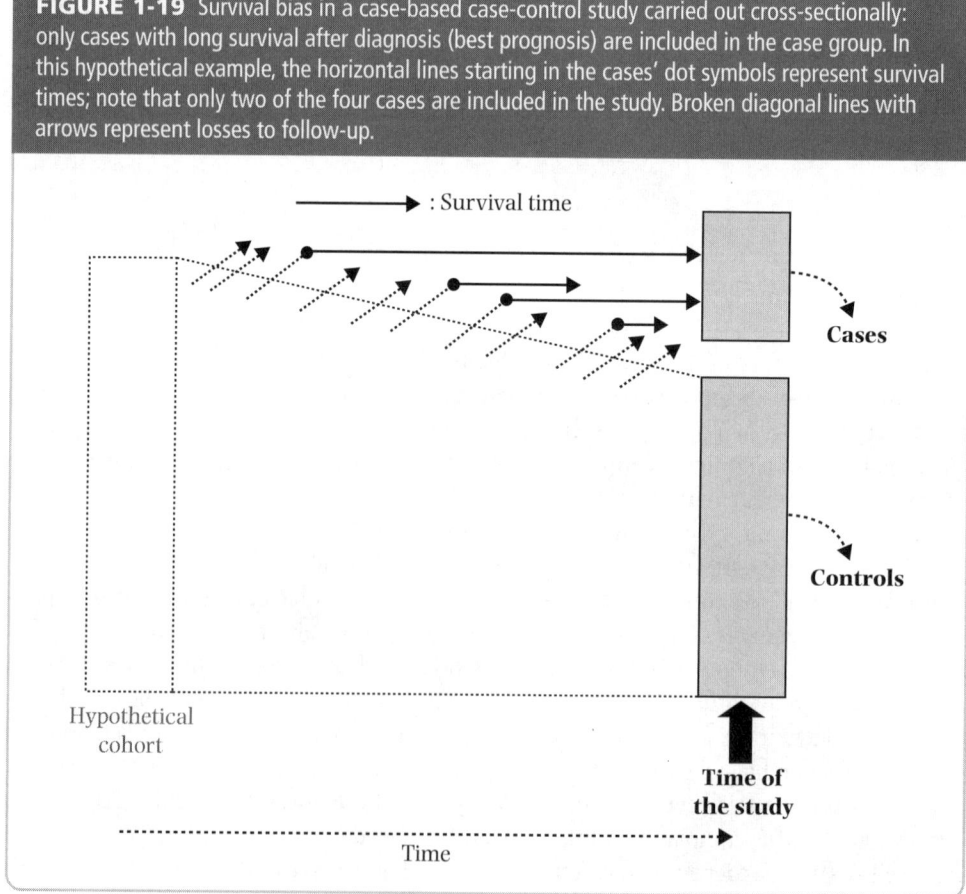

FIGURE 1-19 Survival bias in a case-based case-control study carried out cross-sectionally: only cases with long survival after diagnosis (best prognosis) are included in the case group. In this hypothetical example, the horizontal lines starting in the cases' dot symbols represent survival times; note that only two of the four cases are included in the study. Broken diagonal lines with arrows represent losses to follow-up.

birth to a live child with cleft lip and/or palate (without other malformations) between 1991 and 1994. Controls were the mothers of the two preceding births in the hospital where the case mother had given birth. Both case and control mothers were concurrently interviewed by trained nurses with regard to previous pregnancies, medications, smoking, diet, and other environmental and occupational exposures.

Case-Control Studies Within a Defined Cohort

When cases are identified within a well-defined cohort, it is possible to carry out *nested case-control* or *case-cohort studies*. These designs have received considerable attention in recent years,[35-37] in part because of the increasing number of well-established large cohort studies that have been initiated and continued during the last few decades and in part because of recent methodological and analytical advances.

Case-control studies within a cohort are also known as *hybrid* or *ambidirectional designs*[35] because they combine some of the features and advantages of both cohort and case-control designs. In these studies, although the selection of the participants is carried out using a case-control approach (Figure 1-17), it takes place within a well-defined cohort. The case group consists of all (or a representative sample of) individuals with the outcome of interest occurring in the defined cohort over a specified follow-up period (diagonal lines ending with a dot in Figure 1-13). The control group can be selected either from individuals at risk at the time each case occurs or from the baseline cohort. These two alternatives, respectively known as *nested case-control* and *case-cohort designs*, are described in the next paragraphs.

- Controls are a random sample of the individuals remaining in the cohort at the time each case occurs (Figure 1-20). This *nested case-control design* is based on a sampling

FIGURE 1-20 Nested case-control study in which the controls are selected at each time when a case occurs (incidence density sampling). Cases are represented by a dot connected to a horizontal arrow. Broken diagonal lines with arrows represent losses to follow-up.

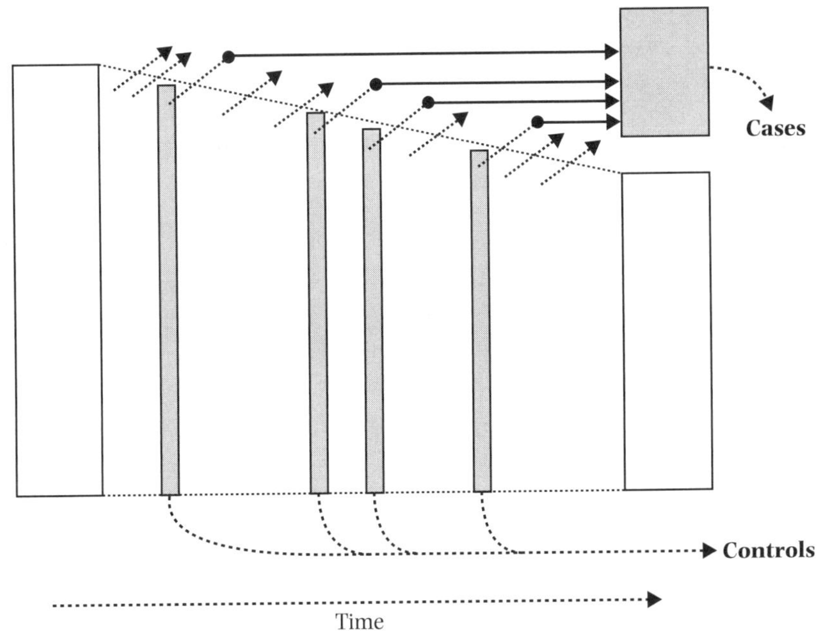

approach known as *incidence density sampling*[35,38] or *risk-set sampling*.[21] Cases are compared with a subset (a sample) of the "risk set," that is, the cohort members who are at risk (i.e., that could become a case) at the time when each case occurs. By using this strategy, cases occurring later in the follow-up are eligible to be controls for earlier cases. Incidence density sampling is the equivalent of matching cases and controls on duration of follow-up (see Section 1.4.5) and permits the use of straight-forward statistical analysis techniques (e.g., standard multiple regression procedures for the analysis of matched and survival data; see Chapter 7, Section 7.4.6).

- Controls are selected as a random sample of the total cohort at baseline (Figure 1-21). In this design, known as *case-cohort*, the control group may include individuals who become cases during the follow-up (diagonal lines ending with a dot in Figure 1-21). Because of the potential overlap between the case and the cohort random sample (control) groups, special techniques are needed for the analysis of this type of study (see Section 7.4.6).[37] An important advantage of the case-cohort design is that a sample of the baseline cohort can serve as a control group for different sets of cases occurring in the same cohort. For example, in a report from the Atherosclerosis Risk in Communities (ARIC) Study, Dekker et al.[39] used a case-cohort approach to analyze the relationship between heart rate variability (a marker of autonomic nervous system function) and several outcomes. ARIC is a cohort study of approximately 15,800 men and women aged 45 to 64 years at the study's outset (1986–1989). During a 6-year follow-up period, 443 deaths from all causes, 140 cardiovascular deaths, 173 cancer deaths, and 395 incident CHD cases were identified. As a comparison group for all of these four case groups, a single sample of 900 baseline cohort participants was identified. Heart rate variability was

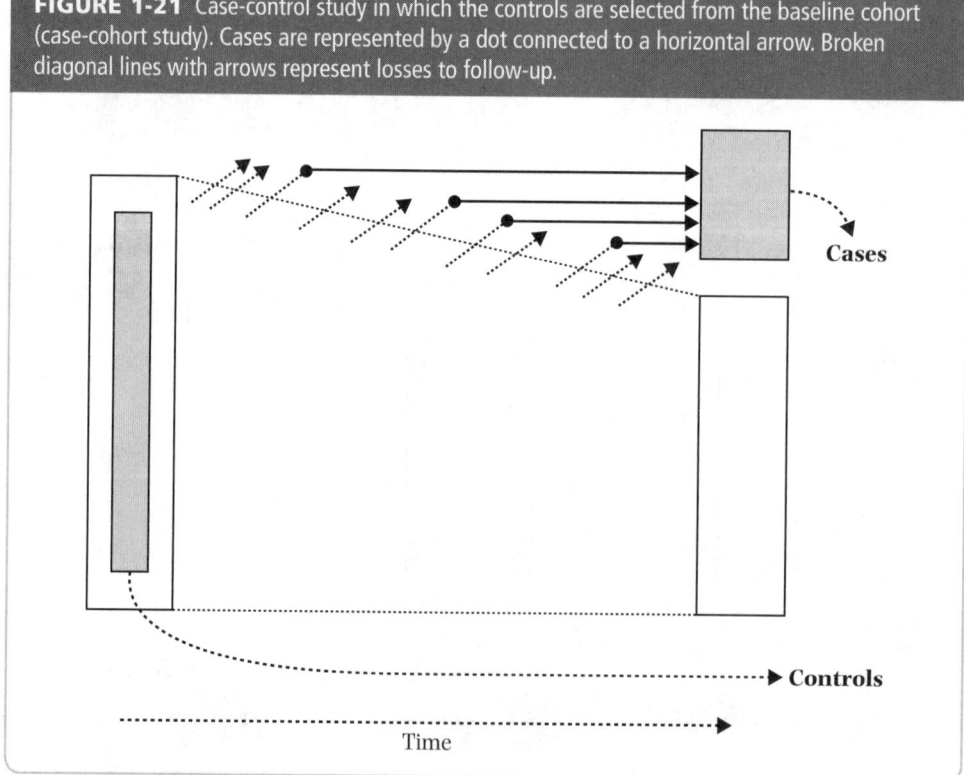

FIGURE 1-21 Case-control study in which the controls are selected from the baseline cohort (case-cohort study). Cases are represented by a dot connected to a horizontal arrow. Broken diagonal lines with arrows represent losses to follow-up.

thus measured in electrocardiography (ECG) records of these 900 controls and on the records of the individuals in each of the four case groups. (An incidence density-type nested case-control design would have required that, for each case group, a separate control group be selected, for a total of four different control groups.)

An additional practical advantage of the case-cohort approach is that if the baseline cohort sample is representative of the source population, risk factor distributions and prevalence rates needed for population attributable risk estimates (Chapter 3, Section 3.2.2) can be obtained.

Another consideration in these types of designs is whether to include or exclude the cases from the pool of eligible controls, that is, the baseline cohort sample or the risk sets in case-cohort and nested case-control designs, respectively. The analytical implications of this choice are discussed in Section 3.4.1.

In general, and regardless of which of the previously mentioned control selection strategies is used (e.g., nested case-control or case-cohort), the likelihood of selection bias tends to be diminished in comparison with the traditional case-based case-control study. This is because cases and controls are selected from the same (defined) source cohort and because (as in any traditional cohort study) exposures are assessed *before* the disease occurs.

When Should a Case-Control Study Within a Cohort Be Used Instead of a Comparison of Exposed and Unexposed in the Full Cohort? If a well-defined cohort with prospectively collected follow-up data is available, why not simply analyze the data from the entire cohort (as in Figure 1-15)? What would be the advantage of limiting the study to a comparison of incident cases and a subset of the cohort (controls)? The answer is that the nested case-control or the case-cohort designs are fundamentally efficient when *additional information that was not obtained* or measured for the whole cohort is needed. A typical situation is a concurrent cohort study in which biological (e.g., serum) samples are collected at baseline and stored in freezers. After a sufficient number of cases are accrued during the follow-up, the frozen serum samples for cases and for a sample of controls can be thawed and analyzed. This strategy not only reduces the cost that would have been incurred if the analyte(s) of interest had been assayed in the entire cohort, but in addition preserves serum samples for future analyses. A similar situation arises when the assessment of key exposures or confounding variables (see Chapter 5) requires labor-intensive data collection activities, such as data abstraction from medical or occupational records. Collecting this additional information in cases and a sample of the total cohort (or of the noncases) is a cost-effective alternative to using the entire cohort. Thus, case-control studies within a cohort combine and take advantage of both the methodological soundness of the cohort design (i.e., limiting selection bias) and the efficiency of the case-control approach. Some examples follow:

- A study was conducted to examine the relationship of military rank and radiation exposure to brain tumor risk within a cohort of male members of the US Air Force who had had at least one year of service between 1970 and 1989.[40] In this study, for each of the 230 cases of brain tumor identified in that 20-year period, four race- and year-of-birth-matched controls (*noncases*) were randomly selected among Air Force employees that were active *at the time the case was diagnosed* (for a total of 920 controls). The reason for choosing a nested case-control design (i.e., a design based on incidence density sampling; see Figure 1-20) instead of using the entire cohort of 880,000 US Air Force members in this study was that labor-intensive abstraction of occupational records was required to obtain accurate data on electromagnetic radiation exposure as well as other relevant information on potentially confounding variables. An alternative strategy would have been not to exclude cases from the eligible control sampling frame (discussed previously). Yet another strategy would have been to use a case-cohort design whereby controls would have been sampled from among Air Force cohort members at the beginning of their employment (i.e., at baseline; see Figure 1-21).

- Dekker et al.'s[39] study on heart rate variability in relation to mortality and CHD incidence in the ARIC study (discussed previously) is an example of the application of a case-cohort design (Figure 1-21). In this study, an elaborate and time-consuming coding of the participant's ECG was required to characterize heart rate variability. Conducting such coding in the entire cohort (approximately 15,800 subjects) would have been prohibitively expensive. By using a case-cohort design, the authors were able to limit the ECG coding to only 900 controls and the individuals in the four case groups.

- Another example of sampling controls from the total baseline cohort (i.e., a case-cohort design) (Figure 1-21) is given by a study conducted by Nieto et al.[41] assessing the relationship of *Chlamydia pneumoniae* antibodies in serum collected at baseline to incident CHD in the ARIC study. Over a 5-year follow-up period, a total of 246 cases of incident CHD (myocardial infarctions or coronary deaths) were identified. The comparison group in this study consisted of a sample of 550 participants of the total baseline cohort, which actually included 10 of the 246 individuals who later developed CHD (incident cases), a fact that needs to be taken into account in the statistical analyses of these data (also see Section 7.4.6). For this study, *C. pneumoniae* IgG antibody levels were determined only in sera of the cases and cohort sample, that is, in only approximately 800 individuals rather than in the approximately 15,800 cohort participants required for a full cohort analysis. In addition to the estimation of risk ratios expressing the relationship between *C. pneumoniae* antibodies and incident CHD, the selection of a random sample of the cohort in Nieto et al.'s study has the advantage over the incidence density nested case-control approach of allowing the estimation of the prevalence of *C. pneumoniae* infection in the cohort (and, by extension, in the reference population) and thus also of population attributable risk (Chapter 3, Section 3.2.2). As in the previous example, the control group could have been used for the assessment of the role of *C. pneumoniae* for a different outcome. For example, after a sufficient number of stroke cases were accrued, a study of the relationship between *C. pneumoniae* infection and stroke incidence could have been conducted; the only additional costs would have been those related to measuring *C. pneumoniae* antibodies in the stroke cases, as the measurements would have been already available in the control group.

1.4.3 Cross-Sectional Studies

In a cross-sectional study design, a sample of (or the total) reference population is examined at a given point in time. Like the case-control study, the cross-sectional study can be conceptualized as a way to analyze cohort data, albeit an often flawed one, in that it consists of taking a "snapshot" of a cohort by recording information on disease outcomes and exposures at a single point in time (Figure 1-22).* Accordingly, the

---

*Cross-sectional studies can also be done periodically for the purpose of monitoring trends in prevalence of diseases, or prevalence or distributions of risk factors, as in the case of the US National Health Surveys.[42,43]

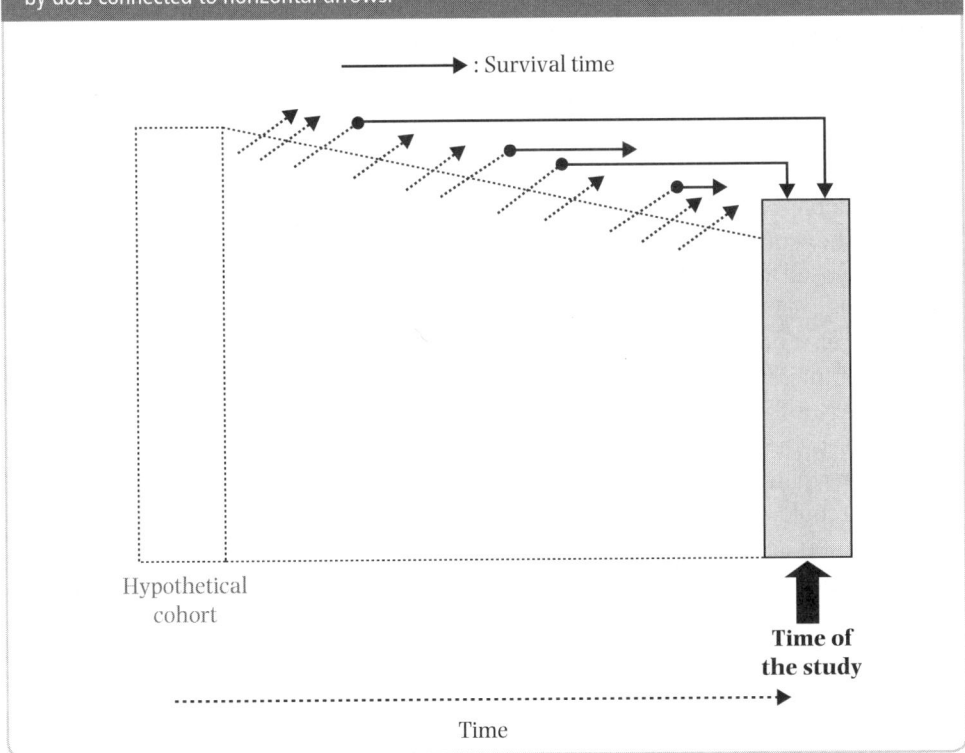

FIGURE 1-22 Schematic representation of a cross-sectional study, conceptually and methodologically analogous to the case-based case-control study represented in Figure 1-19, except that instead of explicitly selecting cases and controls, it selects a sample of the entire population. Broken diagonal lines with arrows represent losses to follow-up. Cases are represented by dots connected to horizontal arrows.

case-based case-control study represented schematically in Figure 1-19 can also be regarded as a cross-sectional study, as it includes cross-sectionally ascertained prevalent cases and noncases (i.e., cohort participants who survived long enough to be alive at the time of the study). It follows that when cross-sectional data are obtained from a defined reference population or cohort, the analytical approach may consist of either comparing point prevalence rates for the outcome of interest between exposed and unexposed individuals or using a "case-control" strategy, in which prevalent cases and noncases are compared with regard to odds of exposure (see Chapters 2 and 3).

Even though any population-based cross-sectional morbidity survey could (at least theoretically) offer the opportunity to examine exposure/outcome associations,[44] cross-sectional analyses of baseline information in cohort studies are especially advantageous. This is particularly the case when examining subclinical outcomes less amenable to survival bias. In the context of baseline data from a cohort study, it may be of interest to verify whether results from cross-sectional analyses are consistent with subsequent analyses of longitudinal data. For example, in the ARIC study, the cross-sectional associations found at baseline of both active and passive smoking with asymptomatic carotid artery atherosclerosis (defined by B-mode ultrasound)[45] were subsequently confirmed by assessing progression of atherosclerosis.[46]

The conditions influencing the validity of associations inferred from cross-sectional data are discussed in detail in Chapter 4 (Section 4.4.2).

1.4.4 Case-Crossover Design

Initially proposed by Maclure,[47] the case-crossover study design consists of comparing the exposure status of a case immediately before its occurrence with that of the same case at some other prior time (e.g., the average level of exposure during the previous year). It is especially appropriate to study acute (brief) exposures that vary over time and that produce a transient change in risk of an acute condition within a short latency (incubation) period. For example, this design has been used to study acute triggers of intracranial aneurysms, such as vigorous physical exercise,[48] and of asthma, such as traffic-related air pollution.[49]

The case-crossover design represents a special type of matching (see Section 1.4.5) in that individuals serve as their own controls. Thus, the analytical unit is time: the time just preceding the acute event ("case" time) is compared with some other time ("control" time). In this design, all fixed individual characteristics that might confound the association (e.g., gender and genetic susceptibility) are controlled for. This design, however, must assume that the disease does not have an undiagnosed stage that could inadvertently affect the exposure of interest. It also assumes that the exposure does not have a cumulative effect, as its strategy is to focus on its acute effect on the suspected outcome. Provided that data are available, other time-related differences that could *confound* the comparison between the case-control times (e.g., differences in the weather or in other varying environmental conditions) could be controlled for in the analyses (see Chapters 5 and 7).

Information on exposures in case-crossover studies are obtained either objectively—as for example in studies of environmental exposures such as particulate matter[50]—or rely on participants' recall, thus being subject to recall bias (see Section 4.3.1).

An example of a case-crossover design is given by a study conducted by Valent et al.,[51] in which the association between sleep (and wakefulness) duration and childhood unintentional injury was examined in 292 children. The "case" and "control" periods were designated as the 24 and the 25–48 hours preceding the injury, respectively. Table 1-4 presents results of the matched-paired analysis, in which the association of the exposure (sleeping less than 10 hours/day) with unintentional injury was found to be present only in boys, thus suggesting the presence of qualitative interaction with gender (see Section 6.7.1). In addition to analyzing data using the ratio of discrepant pairs to estimate the odds ratio (Table 1-4), analysis of case-crossover study data can also be done by means of conditional logistic regression (see Section 7.4.6)—as done by these authors, with additional adjustment for day of the week when injury occurred (weekend vs weekday) and the activity risk level of the child (higher vs lower level of energy).

TABLE 1-4 Odds ratios and 95% confidence intervals (CI) for sleeping less than 10 hours/day in relation to unintentional injuries in children.

Study subjects	n	Ca+, Co+	Ca+, Co−	Ca−, Co+	Ca−, Co−	Odds ratio* (95% CI)
All children	292	62	26	14	190	1.86 (0.97, 3.55)
Boys	181	40	21	9	111	2.33 (1.07, 5.09)
Girls	111	22	5	5	79	1.00 (0.29, 3.45)

*Ratio of number of pairs in which Ca+, Co− to the number of pairs in which Ca−, Co+ (See Section 3.4.1).
Source: Data from F Valent et al., A Case-Crossover Study of Sleep and Childhood Injury. *Pediatrics*, Vol 10, p. E23, © 2001.

1.4.5 Matching

In observational epidemiology, an important concern is that study groups may not be comparable with regard to characteristics that may distort ("confound") the associations of interest. The issue of *confounding* is key in epidemiologic inference and practice and is discussed in detail in Chapter 5. Briefly, this issue arises when spurious factors (*confounding variables*) influence the direction and magnitude of the association of interest. For example, if a case-control study shows an association between hypertension (exposure) and coronary disease (outcome), it can be argued that this association may (at least in part) be due to the fact that coronary disease cases tend to be older than controls: because hypertension is more frequently seen in older people, the difference in age between cases and controls may produce the observed association (or exaggerate its magnitude). Thus, if the question of interest is to assess the net relationship between hypertension and coronary disease (*independently* of age), it makes intuitive sense to select cases and controls with the same or similar ages (i.e., *matched* on age). Similarly, a putative association between serum markers of inflammation (e.g., C-reactive protein) and the risk of CHD may result from confounding by smoking (as smoking increases both the risk of CHD and the levels of inflammatory markers). Recognizing this possibility, researchers matched cases and controls according to smoking status (current, former, or never smoker) in a nested case-control study showing an association between C-reactive protein levels and CHD.[52]

Matching in Case-Control and in Cohort Studies

The practice of matching is particularly common and useful in the context of *case-control studies* when trying to make cases and controls as similar as possible with regard to potential confounding factors. In addition to the two examples just cited, another example is the previously mentioned study of risk factors for oral clefts, in which cases and controls were matched according to place of birth (by selecting controls from the same hospital where the case mother had given birth) and time (by selecting for each case the two preceding births as controls). A special example of matching is given by the nested case-control study design based on incidence density sampling (Section 1.4.2, Figure 1-20). As discussed previously, this strategy results in matching cases and controls on follow-up time. In addition to time in the study, controls may be matched to cases according to other variables that may confound the association of interest. For example, in the US Air Force study of brain tumors mentioned previously,[40] controls sampled from the risk sets at the time of occurrence of each case were additionally matched on birth year and race.

In contrast, in cohort studies, matching on potentially confounding variables is not common. Cohort studies are often large and examine a multitude of exposures and outcomes. Thus, alternative means to control for confounding are usually preferred (e.g., adjustment—see Chapter 7). Among the relatively rare instances in which matching is used in cohort studies are studies of prognostic factors for survival after cancer diagnosis in certain settings. For example, in a study examining age (the "exposure" of interest) as a prognostic factor in multiple myeloma patients following an autologous transplant,[53] older individuals (≥ 65 years old) were matched to younger individuals (< 65 years old) with regard to other factors that affect prognosis and that could thus confound the age-survival association (levels of β_2-microglobulin, albumin, creatinine, C-reactive protein, and the presence/absence of chromosomal abnormalities); the results of this study suggested that after controlling for these variables, age is not a "biologically adverse" prognostic parameter in these patients.

Types of Matching

Previous examples concerned studies in which cases and controls were *individually* matched: that is, for each case, one or more controls with the relevant characteristics matching those of the cases were selected from the pool of eligible individuals. Individual matching according to naturally categorical variables (e.g., gender) is straightforward. When matching is conducted according to continuous variables (e.g., age), a matching range is usually defined (e.g., the matched control's age should be equal to the index case's age plus or minus 5 years). In this situation, as well as when continuous or ordinal variables are arbitrarily categorized (e.g., hypertensive/normotensive or current/former/never smoker), differences between cases and controls may remain, resulting in residual confounding (see Sections 5.5.4 and 7.5).

Individual matching may be logistically difficult in certain situations, particularly when there is a limited number of potentially eligible controls and/or if matching is based on multiple variables. An alternative strategy is to carry out *frequency matching*, which consists of selecting a control group to balance the distributions of the matching variable (or variables) in cases and controls, but without doing a case-by-case individual matching. To carry out frequency matching, advance knowledge of the distribution of the case group according to the matching variable(s) is usually needed so that the necessary sampling fractions within each stratum of the reference population for the selection of the control group can be estimated. For example, if matching is to be done according to gender and age (classified in two age groups, < 45 years and ≥ 45 years), four strata would be defined: females younger than 45 years, females aged 45 years or older, males younger than 45 years, and males aged 45 years or older. After the proportion of cases in each of these four groups is obtained, the number of controls to be selected from each gender-age stratum is chosen so that it is proportional to the distribution in the case group. If the controls are to be selected from a large population frame from which information on the matching variables is available, this can be easily done by stratified random sampling with the desirable stratum-specific sampling fractions. On the other hand, if this information is not available in advance (e.g., when controls are chosen from among persons attending a certain outpatient clinic), control selection can be done by systematic sampling and by successively adding the selected individuals to each stratum until the desired sample size is reached for that stratum. Another strategy, if the distribution of cases according to matching variables is not known in advance but the investigators wish to select and obtain information on cases and controls more or less concurrently, is to obtain (and periodically update) provisional distributions of cases, thus allowing control selection to be carried out before all cases are identified.

When matching for several variables, and particularly when matching for continuous variables is desired, the so-called *minimum Euclidean distance measure method* is a useful alternative.[54] For example, in the study of age as a prognostic factor after transplantation in multiple myeloma patients described previously, older and younger individuals were matched according to five prognostic factors (four of them continuous variables). Matching according to categorical definitions of all of those variables would have been rather cumbersome; furthermore, for some "exposed" individuals, it might have been difficult to find matches among "unexposed" persons. Thus, the authors of this study carried out matching using the minimum Euclidean distance measure method, as schematically illustrated in Figure 1-23. For the purpose of simplification, only two matching factors are considered in the figure. For each exposed case, the closest eligible person (e.g., unexposed patient) in this bidimensional space defined by albumin and creatinine levels is chosen as a control. In Siegel et al.'s study,[53] the authors used this method to match on more than two variables (levels of β_2-microglobulin, albumin, creatinine, and C-reactive protein and the presence/absence of chromosomal abnormalities), which would be hard to represent in a diagram. This method can also be used in the context of either case-based case-control studies and case-control studies within the cohort, as in the original application by Smith et al.,[54] representing a convenient and efficient alternative form of matching on multiple and/or continuous variables.

In situations in which there is a limited pool of cases, it might be desirable to select more than one matched control for each case in order to increase sample size and thus statistical power. For example, in the US Air Force study of brain tumor risk factors cited previously,[40] each case was individually matched to four controls. In general, however, little statistical power is gained beyond four or five controls per case.[55]

Advantages and Disadvantages of Matching

Although there is little doubt that matching is a useful strategy to control for confounding, it is far from being the only one. Chapter 7 is entirely devoted to describing alternative approaches that can be used at the analytical stage to address the problem of confounding—namely, stratification and adjustment. Whether investigators choose to

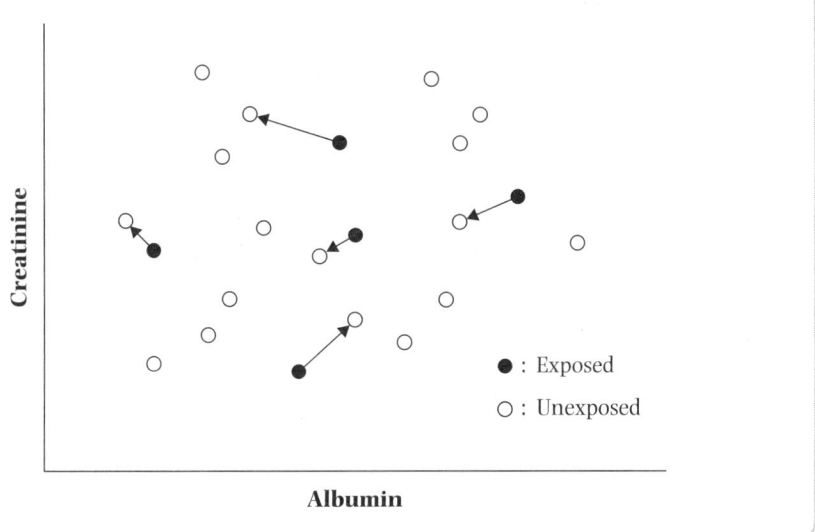

FIGURE 1-23 Matching according to minimal Euclidean distance measure method. Hypothetical example of a cohort study of survival after transplantation in multiple myeloma patients in which exposed individuals (e.g., older individuals) are matched to unexposed (younger) patients according to two prognostic factors: serum albumin and creatinine levels. For each case, the closest unexposed individual in the bidimensional space defined by the two matching variables is chosen as control.

Source: The authors, based on a study by DS Siegel et al. Age Is Not a Prognostic Variable with Autotransplants for Multiple Myeloma. *Blood,* Vol 93, pp. 51–54, © 1999.

deal with confounding before data collection by matching during the recruitment phase of the study rather than by stratification or adjustment at the analysis stage depends on a number of considerations.

The *advantages* of matching include the following:

1. In addition to being easy to understand and describe, matching may be the only way to guarantee some degree of control for confounding in certain situations. This may be particularly important in studies in which a potentially strong confounding variable may produce such an imbalance in the composition of the study groups that adjustment is difficult or outright impossible. For example, in a case-control study of risk factors for prostate cancer, it would make sense to match controls to cases according to age; at the very least, given that most prostate cancer cases are in the older age brackets, the investigator should consider *restricting* the eligibility of the control group to a certain age range. (Restriction is a somewhat "loose" form of matching.) Otherwise, if controls were to be sampled from the general population, the age range could be so broad that there might not be enough overlap with the restricted age range of cases, particularly if the sample size were small (i.e., not enough older subjects in the control sample), to allow for adjustment.

2. If done according to strong confounders (variables that are related to both exposure and outcome; see Chapter 5), matching tends to increase the statistical power (efficiency) of the study.[56,57]

3. Matching (especially individual matching) is a logistically straightforward way to obtain a comparable control group when cases and controls are identified from a reference population for which there is no available sampling frame listing. For example, in a case-control study using cases of diabetes identified in an outpatient clinic, each case can be matched to the next nondiabetic person attending the clinic who has the same characteristics as the index case (e.g., similar age, gender).

Potential *disadvantages* of matching should also be considered. They include the following:

1. In certain situations, particularly when multiple variables are being matched for, it may be difficult or impossible to find a matched control— or controls— for a given case, particularly when sampling from a limited source population, when matching on multiple variables, or when the ratio of controls to cases is greater than 1:1. Furthermore, even if matched controls are available, the process of identifying them may be cumbersome and may add costs to the study's recruitment phase.

2. When matching is done, the association between the matching variable(s) and the outcome cannot be assessed; the reason for this is that, after matching on a certain variable is carried out, the study groups (e.g., cases and controls) are set by design to be equal (or similar) with regard to this variable or set of variables.

3. It follows from number 2 that it is not possible to assess additive interaction in matched case-control studies between the matching variable(s) and the exposure(s) of interest. As discussed in Chapter 6 (Section 6.4.2), the assessment of additive interaction in a case-control study relies on the formula for the joint expected relative risk (RR) of two variables A and Z, $RR_{A+Z+} = RR_{A+Z-} + RR_{A-Z+} - 1.0$ (using the odds ratios as estimates of the relative risks). Assuming that A is the

matching variable, its independent effect (RR_{A+Z-}) cannot be estimated, as it has been set to 1.0 by design (see number 2). Therefore, this formula cannot be applied.

4. Matching implies some kind of tailoring of the selection of the study groups to make them as comparable as possible; this increased "internal validity" (comparability) may, however, result in a reduced "external validity" (representativeness). For example a control group that is made identical to the cases with regard to sociodemographic characteristics and other confounding variables may no longer constitute a representative sample of the reference population. For example, in studies that examine the association between novel risk factors and disease, a secondary, yet important, objective may be to study the distribution or correlates of these factors in the reference population. If controls are matched to cases, it may be a complicated task to use the observed distributions in the control group to make inferences applicable to the population at large (complex weighted analyses taking into account the sampling fractions associated with the matching process would be required). On the other hand, if a random sample of the reference population is chosen (as is done in case-cohort studies), it will be appropriate to generalize the distributions of risk factors in the control group to the reference population. Obtaining these distributions (e.g., the prevalence of exposure in the population) is particularly important for the estimation of the population attributable risk (see Chapter 3, Section 3.4.2). In addition, as mentioned previously in this chapter, a control group that is selected as a random sample of the source population can be used as a comparison group for another case group selected from the same cohort or reference population.

5. Because when matching is done it cannot be "undone," it is important that the matching variables not be strongly correlated with the variable of interest; otherwise, the phenomenon of "overmatching" may ensue. For example, matching cases and controls on ethnic background may to a great extent make them very similar with regard to variables of interest related to socioeconomic status. For further discussion of this topic and additional examples, see Chapter 5 (Section 5.5.3).

6. Finally, no statistical power is gained if the matching variables are weak confounders. If the matching variables are weakly related to exposure, even if these variables are related to the outcome, the gain in efficiency may be very small. Moreover, if the matching variables are weakly or not related to the outcome of interest, matching can result in a loss of power.[56,57]

When matching is conducted according to categorical definitions of continuous or ordinal variables, residual differences between cases and controls may remain (*residual confounding*; see Chapter 5, Section 5.5.4, and Chapter 7, Section 7.6). In these situations, it may be necessary to adjust for the variable in question in the analyses to eliminate variation within the matching categories. For example, in a study on the relationship between cytomegalovirus antibodies in serum samples collected in 1974 (and retrospectively analyzed) and the presence of carotid atherosclerosis measured by B-mode ultrasound of the carotid arteries about 15 years later (1987–1989),[58] 150 controls (selected among individuals with normal carotid arteries) were frequency matched to 150 carotid atherosclerosis cases according to gender and two relatively broad age groups (45–54 years and 55–64 years). Thus, by design, both the case and control groups had an identical number of individuals in all four gender-age groups; however, cases in this study were 58.2 years of age on average, whereas the average age in controls was 56.2 years. Therefore, even though the study groups were matched on two age categories, the residual age difference prompted the authors to adjust for age *as a continuous variable* in the multivariate logistic regression analyses (see Chapter 7, Section 7.4.3).

The same residual differences may remain even in individually matched studies if the matching categories are broadly categorized. The reason for this phenomenon is illustrated in Figure 1-24. Even though the cases and controls are equally represented in both age groups, within each age group cases tend to be older, thus resulting in an overall difference.

In summary, investigators should always consider carefully whether to match. Unlike *post hoc* means to control for confounding (e.g., stratification and adjustment), matching is irreversible after implemented. Although it may be the strategy of choice in studies with limited sample size and a clear-cut set of objectives, it should be avoided in most situations in which a reasonable overlap on potential confounding variables is expected to exist (thus allowing adjustment). If matching is used, the investigators must keep in mind that ignoring the matching during the analysis of the data can lead to bias[59] and that special statistical techniques for analyses of matched data are available (Chapter 7, Section 7.4.6).

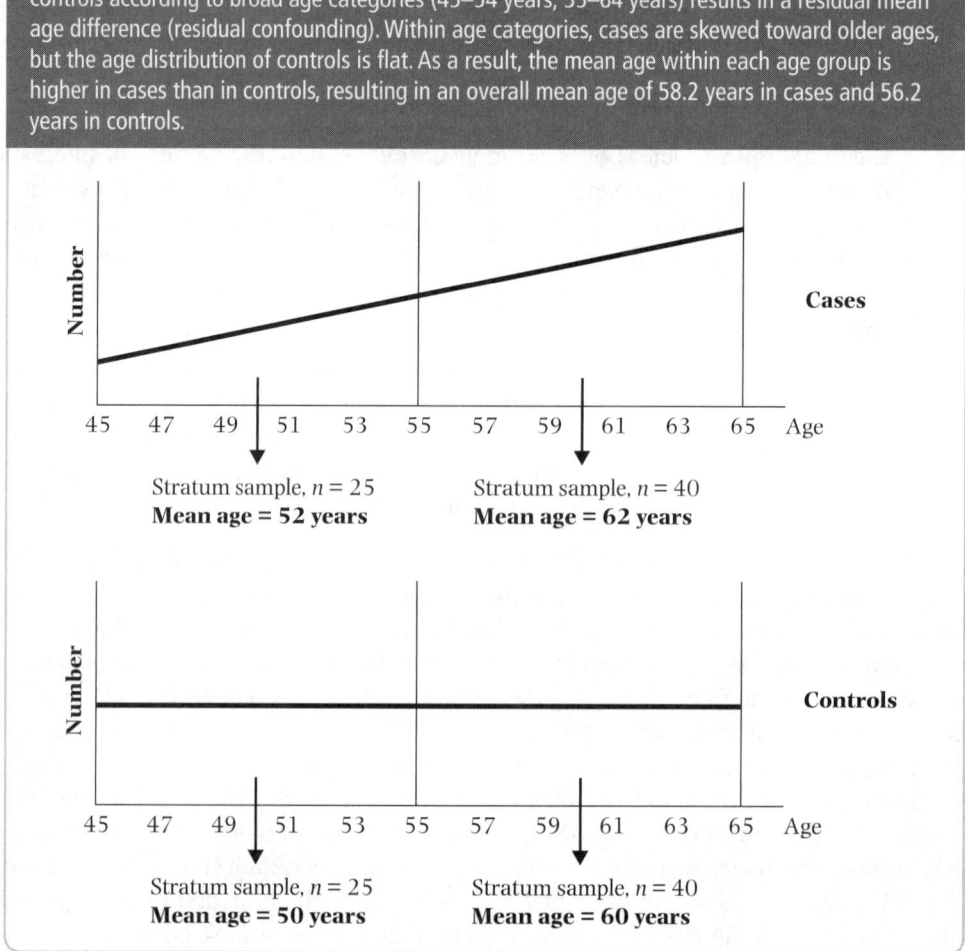

FIGURE 1-24 Schematic representation of a hypothetical situation where matching cases and controls according to broad age categories (45–54 years; 55–64 years) results in a residual mean age difference (residual confounding). Within age categories, cases are skewed toward older ages, but the age distribution of controls is flat. As a result, the mean age within each age group is higher in cases than in controls, resulting in an overall mean age of 58.2 years in cases and 56.2 years in controls.

REFERENCES

1. Porta M. *A Dictionary of Epidemiology*, 5th ed. New York: Oxford University Press; 2008.
2. Koepsell TD, Weiss NS. *Epidemiologic Methods*. New York: Oxford University Press; 2003.
3. Gordis L. *Epidemiology*, 4th ed. Philadelphia: Elsevier Saunders; 2008.
4. Strong JP, McGill HC Jr. The pediatric aspects of atherosclerosis. *J Atheroscler Res*. 1969;9:251–265.
5. Frost WH. The age-selection of tuberculosis mortality in successive decades. *Am J Hyg*. 1939;30:91–96.
6. López-Abente G, Pollan M, Vergara A, et al. Age-period-cohort modeling of colorectal cancer incidence and mortality in Spain. *Cancer Epidemiol Biomar*. 1997;6:999–1005.
7. Dhillon PK, Yeole BB, Dikshit R, et al. Trends in breast, ovarian and cervical cancer incidence in Mumbai, India over a 30-year period, 1976–2005: An age-period-cohort analysis. *Br J Cancer*. 2011;105:723–730.
8. Newschaffer CJ, Bush TL, Hale WE. Aging and total cholesterol levels: Cohort, period, and survivorship effects. *Am J Epidemiol*. 1992;136:23–34.
9. Keys A. *Seven Countries: A Multivariate Analysis of Death and Coronary Heart Disease*. Cambridge, MA: Harvard University Press; 1980.
10. Morgenstern H. Ecologic studies in epidemiology: Concepts, principles, and methods. *Ann Rev Public Health*. 1995;16:61–81.
11. Diez-Roux AV, Nieto FJ, Muntaner C, et al. Neighborhood environments and coronary heart disease: A multilevel analysis. *Am J Epidemiol*. 1997;146:48–63.
12. Diez-Roux AV. Bringing context back into epidemiology: Variables and fallacies in multilevel analysis. *Am J Public Health*. 1998;88:216–222.
13. Durkheim E. *Suicide: A Study in Sociology*. New York: Free Press; 1951.
14. MacMahon B, Pugh TF. *Epidemiology: Principles and Methods*. Boston: Little, Brown and Co.; 1970.
15. Piantadosi S, Byar DP, Green SB. The ecological fallacy. *Am J Epidemiol*. 1988;127:893–904.
16. Elliott P. Design and analysis of multicentre epidemiological studies: The INTERSALT study. In Marmot M, Elliott P, eds. *Coronary Heart Disease Epidemiology: From Aetiology to Public Health*. Oxford: Oxford University Press; 1992:166–178.
17. Wynder EL, Cohen LA, Muscat JE, et al. Breast cancer: Weighing the evidence for a promoting role of dietary fat. *J Natl Cancer Inst*. 1997;89:766–775.
18. Goldberger J, Wheeler GA, Sydenstricker E. A study of the relation of family income and other economic factors to pellagra incidence in seven cotton-mill villages of South Carolina in 1916. *Public Health Rep*. 1920;35:2673–2714.
19. Koopman JS, Longini IM Jr. The ecological effects of individual exposures and nonlinear disease dynamics in populations. *Am J Public Health*. 1994;84:836–842.
20. Breslow NE, Day NE. Statistical methods in cancer research: Volume I: The analysis of case-control studies. *IARC Sci Publ*. 1980.
21. Breslow NE, Day NE. Statistical methods in cancer research: Volume II: The design and analysis of cohort studies. *IARC Sci Publ*. 1987.
22. Samet JM, Munoz A. Perspective: Cohort studies. *Epidemiol Rev*. 1998;20:135–136.
23. Schlesselman J. *Case Control Studies: Design, Conduct, Analysis*. New York: Oxford University Press; 1982.
24. Armenian HK, Lilienfeld DE. Applications of the case-control method: Overview and historical perspective. *Epidemiol Rev*. 1994;16:1–5.

25. Dawber TR. *The Framingham Study: The Epidemiology of Atherosclerotic Disease*. Cambridge, MA: Harvard University Press; 1980.

26. Kaslow RA, Ostrow DG, Detels R, et al. The Multicenter AIDS Cohort Study: Rationale, organization, and selected characteristics of the participants. *Am J Epidemiol*. 1987;126:310–318.

27. Stampfer MJ, Willett WC, Colditz GA, et al. A prospective study of postmenopausal estrogen therapy and coronary heart disease. *N Engl J Med*. 1985;313:1044–1049.

28. Ascherio A, Rimm EB, Stampfer MJ, et al. Dietary intake of marine n-3 fatty acids, fish intake, and the risk of coronary disease among men. *N Engl J Med*. 1995;332:977–982.

29. Garfinkel L. Selection, follow-up, and analysis in the American Cancer Society prospective studies. *Natl Cancer Inst Monogr*. 1985;67:49–52.

30. Vandenbroucke JP. Prospective or retrospective: What's in a name? *Br Med J*. 1991;302:249–250.

31. Nieto FJ, Szklo M, Comstock GW. Childhood weight and growth rate as predictors of adult mortality. *Am J Epidemiol*. 1992;136:201–213.

32. Tynes T, Andersen A, Langmark F. Incidence of cancer in Norwegian workers potentially exposed to electromagnetic fields. *Am J Epidemiol*. 1992;136:81–88.

33. Cornfield J. A method of estimating comparative rates from clinical data: Applications to cancer of the lung, breast, and cervix. *J Natl Cancer Inst*. 1951;11:1269–1275.

34. Christensen K, Olsen J, Norgaard-Pedersen B, et al. Oral clefts, transforming growth factor alpha gene variants, and maternal smoking: A population-based case-control study in Denmark, 1991–1994. *Am J Epidemiol*. 1999;149:248–255.

35. Kleinbaum D, Kupper LL, Morgenstern H. *Epidemiologic Research: Principles and Quantitative Methods*. Belmont, CA: Lifetime Learning Publications; 1982.

36. Langholz B, Thomas DC. Nested case-control and case-cohort methods of sampling from a cohort: A critical comparison. *Am J Epidemiol*. 1990;131:169–176.

37. Thomas D. New techniques for the analysis of cohort studies. *Epidemiol Rev*. 1998;20:122–134.

38. Checkoway H, Pearce, NE, Crawford-Brown, DJ. *Research Methods in Occupational Epidemiology*. New York: Oxford University Press; 1989.

39. Dekker JM, Crow RS, Folsom AR, et al. Low heart rate variability in a 2-minute rhythm strip predicts risk of coronary heart disease and mortality from several causes: The ARIC Study: Atherosclerosis risk in communities. *Circulation*. 2000;102:1239–1244.

40. Grayson JK. Radiation exposure, socioeconomic status, and brain tumor risk in the US Air Force: A nested case-control study. *Am J Epidemiol*. 1996;143:480–486.

41. Nieto FJ, Folsom AR, Sorlie PD, et al. Chlamydia pneumoniae infection and incident coronary heart disease: The Atherosclerosis Risk in Communities Study. *Am J Epidemiol*. 1999;150:149–156.

42. Flegal KM, Carroll MD, Kuczmarski RJ, Johnson CL. Overweight and obesity in the United States: Prevalence and trends, 1960–1994. *Int J Obes Relat Metab Disord*. 1998;22:39–47.

43. Hickman TB, Briefel RR, Carroll MD, et al. Distributions and trends of serum lipid levels among United States children and adolescents ages 4–19 years: Data from the Third National Health and Nutrition Examination Survey. *Prev Med*. 1998;27:879–890.

44. Lister SM, Jorm LR. Parental smoking and respiratory illnesses in Australian children aged 0–4 years: ABS 1989–90 National Health Survey results. *Aust N Z J Public Health*. 1998;22:781–786.

45. Howard G, Burke GL, Szklo M, et al. Active and passive smoking are associated with increased carotid wall thickness: The Atherosclerosis Risk in Communities Study. *Arch Intern Med*. 1994;154:1277–1282.

46. Howard G, Wagenknecht LE, Burke GL, et al. Cigarette smoking and progression of atherosclerosis: The Atherosclerosis Risk in Communities (ARIC) Study. *J Am Med Assoc.* 1998;279:119–124.
47. Maclure M. The case-crossover design: A method for studying transient effects on the risk of acute events. *Am J Epidemiol.* 1991;133:144–153.
48. Vlak MH, Rinkel GJE, Greebe P, et al. Trigger factors and their attributable risk for rupture of intracranial aneurysms. A case-crossover study. *Stroke* 2011;42:1878-1882.
49. Pereira G, Cook A, De Vos AJ, Holman CD. A case-crossover analysis of traffic-related air pollution and emergency department presentations for asthma in Perth, Western Australia. *Med J Aust* 2010;193:511–514.
50. Rich KE, Petkau J, Vedal S, Brauer M. A case-crossover analysis of particulate air pollution and cardiac arrhythmia in patients with implantable cardioverter defibrillators. *Inhal Toxicol.* 2004;16:363–372.
51. Valent F, Brusaferro S, Barbone F. A case-crossover study of sleep and childhood injury. *Pediatrics.* 2001;107:E23.
52. Ridker PM, Cushman M, Stampfer MJ, et al. Inflammation, aspirin, and the risk of cardiovascular disease in apparently healthy men. *N Engl J Med.* 1997;336:973–979.
53. Siegel DS, Desikan KR, Mehta J, et al. Age is not a prognostic variable with autotransplants for multiple myeloma. *Blood.* 1999;93:51–54.
54. Smith AH, Kark JD, Cassel JC, Spears GF. Analysis of prospective epidemiologic studies by minimum distance case-control matching. *Am J Epidemiol.* 1977;105:567–574.
55. Breslow N. Case-control studies. In: Ahrens W, Pigeot I, eds. *Handbook of Epidemiology.* Heidelberg, Germany: Springer-Verlag Berlin; 2005:287–319.
56. Samuels M. Matching and design efficiency in epidemiological studies. *Biometrika.* 1981;68:577–588.
57. Thompson WD, Kelsey JL, Walter SD. Cost and efficiency in the choice of matched and unmatched case-control study designs. *Am J Epidemiol.* 1982;116:840–851.
58. Nieto FJ, Adam E, Sorlie P, et al. Cohort study of cytomegalovirus infection as a risk factor for carotid intimal-medial thickening, a measure of subclinical atherosclerosis. *Circulation.* 1996;94:922–927.
59. Breslow N. Design and analysis of case-control studies. *Annu Rev Public Health.* 1982;3:29–54.

EXERCISES

1. The table shows a series of cross-sectional incidence rates of cancer Y per 100,000 by age and calendar year.

	Calendar year							
Age	1950	1955	1960	1965	1970	1975	1980	1985
20–24	10	15	22	30	33	37	41	44
25–29	8	17	20	24	29	38	40	43
30–34	5	12	22	25	28	35	42	45
35–39	3	12	15	26	30	32	39	42
40–44	2	10	17	19	28	32	39	42
45–49	2	12	15	18	21	33	40	42
50–54	2	10	16	20	25	32	42	44
55–59	2	15	17	19	22	27	43	44

a. After observing the incidence rates by age at any given year, it is concluded that "aging is not related to an increase in the incidence of Y and may even be related to a decrease in the incidence." Do you agree with this observation? Justify your answer.
b. What are the purposes of examining birth cohort vis-à-vis cross-sectional rates?

2. Chang et al. carried out a birth cohort analysis of epilepsy mortality in Taiwan from 1971 through 2005.* The figure shows the epilepsy mortality rates per

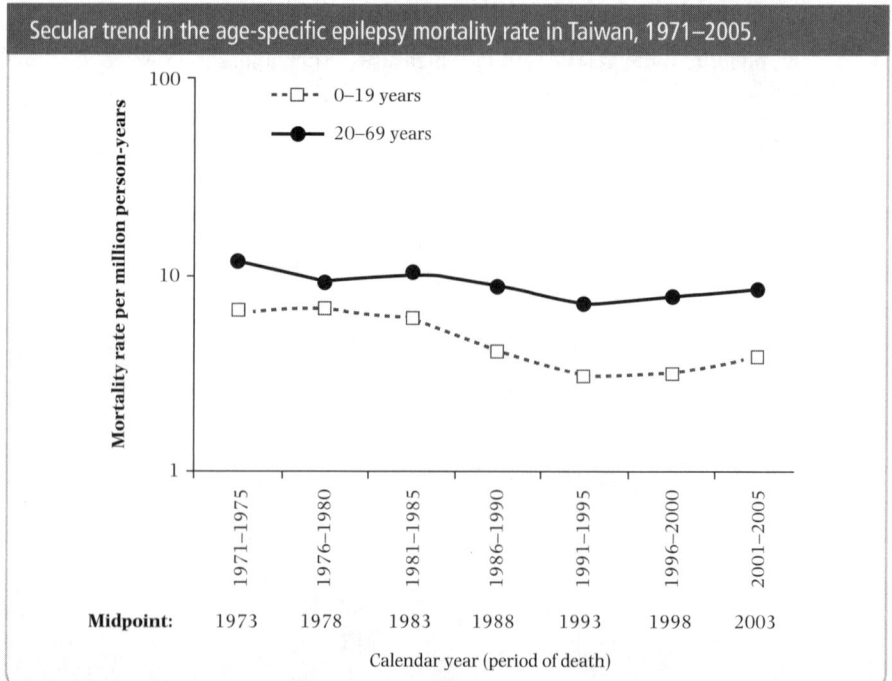

Secular trend in the age-specific epilepsy mortality rate in Taiwan, 1971–2005.

*Chang Y, Li C, Tung T, et al. Age-period-cohort analysis of mortality from epilepsy in Taiwan, 1971–2005. *Seizure*. 2011;20:240–243.

million person-years by calendar year for two of the three age groups examined by the authors.

Assume that year of death for people dying in each calendar year category is the midpoint for that period, e.g., for the calendar year category of 1971–1975, the assumed year of death is 1973; for the category 1976–1980, it is 1978, and so on. The same should be assumed for the age groupings, e.g., for ages 0–19, assume that the age of death is 10 years, for the age group 20–69 years it is 45 years, and so on.

   a. Is the use of the midpoint value a reasonable approach to analyzing birth cohorts?
   b. To which cohort do individuals dying in 1973 at ages 0–19 years belong?
   c. Is there a birth cohort effect?
   d. Is there an age effect?

3. The figure shows the incidence of dementia and Alzheimer's disease per 100,000 person-years by age and birth cohort, both sexes combined, in residents of Rochester, Minnesota, from 1975 through 1984.[†]

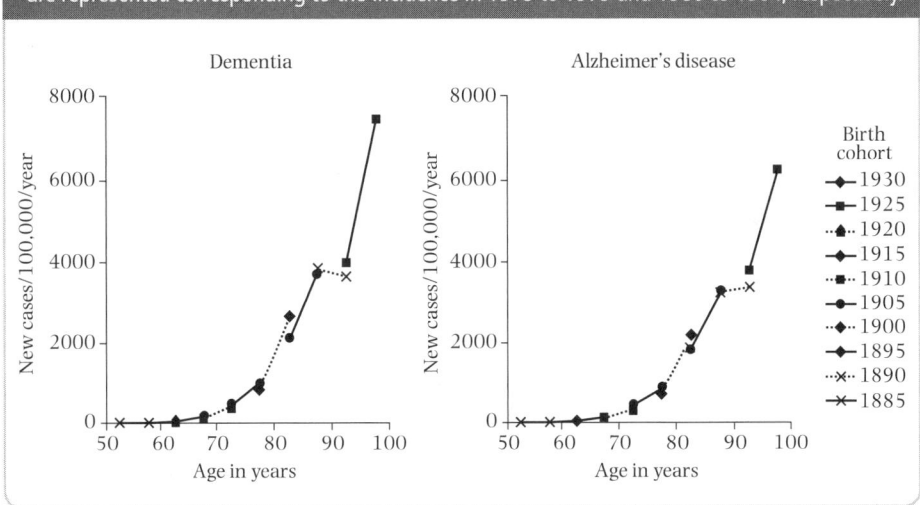

Five-year average incidence rates of dementia (new cases per 100,000 person-years) by age and birth cohort, both sexes combined, Rochester, Minnesota. For each birth cohort, two points are represented corresponding to the incidence in 1975 to 1979 and 1980 to 1984, respectively.

Source: Reprinted with permission from WA Rocca et al., Incidence of Dementia and Alzheimer's Disease: A Reanalysis of the Rochester, Minnesota 1975–1984 Data. *American Journal of Epidemiology*, Vol 148, No 1, pp. 51–62. © 1998.

   a. Are age effects apparent in the figure? Justify your answer.
      ☐ Yes   ☐ No
   b. Are cohort effects apparent in the figure? Justify your answer.
      ☐ Yes   ☐ No
   c. From your answer to question (b), would you expect age patterns to be similar in cross-sectional and cohort analyses? Justify your answer.
      ☐ Yes   ☐ No

[†]Rocca WA, Cha RH, Waring SC, et al. Incidence of dementia and Alzheimer's disease: A reanalysis of data from Rochester, Minnesota, 1975–1984. *Am J Epidemiol*. 1998;148:51–62.

4. A case-control study is conducted within a well-defined cohort. The reason for this is that expensive additional data collection is needed, and the budget is not sufficient to obtain these data from all cohort participants.

   a. What type of case-control study within this cohort would be ideal to study multiple outcomes, and why is the alternative case-control design not recommended?
   b. In this cohort study, prevalent cases were not excluded at baseline and, thus, the investigators chose to use baseline data to examine associations between suspected risk factors and prevalent disease. What type of approach is this, and what are its main advantages and disadvantages?

5. In planning an individually matched case-based case-control study to test the hypothesis that air pollution (measured by individually placed monitors) is related to a certain type of respiratory cancer, the investigators decide to match cases and controls on age, gender, ethnic background, and smoking (yes or no).

   a. In addition to general logistical difficulties usually associated with matching, what is the main undesirable consequence that may result from matching cases and controls in this study?
   b. Because the disease of interest is rare, the investigators decide to individually match 10 controls for each case. Is this a reasonable strategy, considering the additional costs involved and the tight budget to conduct this study?

PART TWO

Measures of Disease Occurrence and Association

CHAPTER 2 Measuring Disease Occurrence 47

CHAPTER 3 Measuring Associations Between Exposures and Outcomes 79

CHAPTER 2

Measuring Disease Occurrence

2.1 INTRODUCTION

The outcomes of epidemiologic research have been traditionally defined in terms of disease, although the growing application of epidemiology to public health and preventive medicine increasingly requires the use of outcomes measuring health in general (e.g., outcome measures of functional status in epidemiologic studies related to aging). Outcomes can be expressed as either discrete (e.g., disease occurrence or severity) or continuous variables.

Continuous variables, such as blood pressure and glucose levels, are commonly used as outcomes in epidemiology. The main statistical tools used to analyze correlates or predictors of these types of outcomes are the correlation coefficients, analysis of variance, and linear regression analysis, which are discussed in numerous statistical textbooks. Linear regression is briefly reviewed in Chapter 7 (Section 7.4.1) as a background for the introduction to multivariate regression analysis techniques in epidemiology. Other methodological issues regarding the analysis of continuous variables in epidemiology, specifically as they relate to quality control and reliability measures, are covered in Chapter 8.

Most of the present chapter deals with *categorical* dichotomous outcome variables, which are the most often used in epidemiologic studies. The frequency of this type of outcome can be generically defined as the number of individuals with the outcome (the numerator) divided by the number of individuals at risk for that outcome (the denominator). There are two types of absolute measures of outcome frequency: incidence and prevalence (Table 2-1).

Although the term *incidence* has been traditionally used to indicate a proportion of newly developed (incident) cases of a disease, in fact, it encompasses the frequency of any new health- or disease-related event, including death, recurrent disease among

TABLE 2-1 Absolute measures of disease frequency.

Measure	Expresses	Types of events
Incidence	Frequency of a new event	Newly developed disease Death in the total population at risk (mortality) Death in patients (case fatality) Recurrence of a disease Development of a side effect of a drug
Prevalence	Frequency of an existing event	Point prevalence: cases at a given point in time Period prevalence: cases during a given period (e.g., 1 year) Cumulative (lifetime) prevalence: cases at any time in the past (up to present time)

patients, disease remission, menopause, and so forth. Incidence is a particularly important measure for analytical epidemiologic research, as it allows the estimation of risk necessary to assess causal associations (Chapter 10, Section 10.2.4).

Prevalence, on the other hand, measures the frequency of an existing outcome either at one point in time—point prevalence, or during a given period—period prevalence. A special type of period prevalence is the lifetime prevalence, which measures the cumulative lifetime frequency of an outcome up to the present time (i.e., the proportion of people who have had the event at any time in the past).

For both prevalence and incidence, it is necessary to have a clear definition of the outcome as an *event* (a "noteworthy happening," as defined in an English dictionary[1]). In epidemiology, an event is typically defined as the occurrence of any phenomenon of disease or health that can be discretely characterized. For incidence (see Section 2.2), this characterization needs to include a precise definition of the time of occurrence of the event in question. Some events are easily defined and time of occurrence easily located in time, such as "birth," "death," "surgery," and "trauma." Others are not easily defined and require some more or less arbitrary operational definition for study, such as "menopause," "recovery," "dementia," or cytomegalovirus (CMV) disease (Table 2-2). An example of the complexity of defining certain clinical events is given by the widely adopted definition of a case of AIDS, which uses a number of clinical and laboratory criteria.[2]

The next two sections of this chapter describe the different alternatives for the calculation of incidence and prevalence. The last section describes the *odds*, another measure of disease frequency that is the basis for a measure of association often used in epidemiology,

TABLE 2-2 Examples of operational definitions of events in epidemiologic studies.

Event	Definition	Reference
Natural menopause	Date of last menstrual period after a woman has stopped menstruating for 12 months	Bromberger et al. 1997*
Remission of diarrhea	At least two days free of diarrhea (diarrhea = passage of ≥ 3 liquid or semisolid stools in a day)	Mirza et al. 1997†
Dementia	A hospital discharge, institutionalization or admission to a day care center in a nursing home or psychiatric hospital with a diagnosis of dementia (ICD-9-CM codes 290.0–290.4, 294.0, 294.1, 331.0–331.2)	Breteler et al. 1995‡
CMV disease	Evidence of CMV infection (CMV antigen on white blood cells, CMV culture, or seroconversion) accompanied by otherwise unexplained spiking fever over 48 hours and either malaise or a fall in neutrophil count over 3 consecutive days.	Gane et al. 1997§

*JT Bromberger, KA Matthews, KA Kuller, et al. Prospective Study of the Determinants of Age at Menopause. *American Journal of Epidemiology*, Vol 145, pp. 124–133, © 1997.

†NM Mirza, LE Caulfield, RE Black, et al. Risk Factors for Diarrheal Duration. *American Journal of Epidemiology*, Vol 146, pp. 776–785, © 1997.

‡MMB Breteler, RRM de Groot, LKJ van Romunde, and A Hofman. Risk of Dementia in Patients with Parkinson's Disease, Epilepsy, and Severe Head Trauma: A Register-Based Follow-up Study. *American Journal of Epidemiology*, Vol 142, pp. 1300–1305, © 1995.

§E Gane, F Salilba, JC Valdecasas, et al. Randomised Trial of Efficacy and Safety or Oral Ganciclovir in the Prevention of Cytomegalovirus Disease in Liver-Transplant Recipients. *Lancet*, Vol 350, pp. 1729–1333, © 1997.

particularly in case-based case-control studies (Chapter 1, Section 1.4.2)—namely, the odds ratio (Chapter 3, Section 3.4.1).

2.2 MEASURES OF INCIDENCE

Incidence is best understood in the context of prospective (cohort) studies (Chapter 1, Section 1.4.1). The basic structure of any incidence indicator is represented by the number of events occurring in a defined population over a specified period of time (numerator), divided by the population at risk for that event over that time (denominator). There are two types of measures of incidence defined by the type of denominator: (1) incidence based on persons at risk and (2) incidence based on person-time units at risk.

2.2.1 Incidence Based on Individuals at Risk

This is an index defined in terms of the probability of the event, also known as *cumulative incidence* (or *incidence proportion*[3]), which is the basis for the statistical techniques collectively known as *survival analysis*.

If follow-up is complete on every individual in the cohort, the estimation of the cumulative incidence is simply the number of events occurring during the follow-up time divided by the initial population. Often in epidemiologic studies, however, the follow-up is incomplete for many or all individuals in the study. In a typical cohort study, there are individuals lost to follow-up, those dying from causes other than the outcome of interest, and those whose follow-up is shorter because they are recruited later in the accrual period for the study; the latter are all called *censored observations*, and they require special analytical approaches. The traditional techniques for the estimation of cumulative incidence (or its complement, *cumulative survival* or *survival function*) in the presence of censored observations are the life table of the actuarial type (interchangeably referred to in this chapter as the *classic*, *actuarial*, or *interval-based life table*) and the Kaplan-Meier method.[4]

As an example, Figure 2-1 provides a schematic representation of a study for which the outcome of interest is death, in which 10 individuals are followed for up to 2 years (2010–2011). Each horizontal line in the figure represents the follow-up time of a unique individual. Follow-up can be terminated either by the event (D) or by a loss (withdrawal) from the study, also referred to as *censored observation* (denoted in the figure as an arrow ending at the time when follow-up ended). Individuals are recruited at different points in time and also leave the study (because of either death or censoring) at different times. For example, individual 1 is recruited in November 2010 and dies in December 2010, after only 1 month of follow-up, and individual 5 lives throughout the entire follow-up period (2 years). Figure 2-2 shows a reorganization of the data in Figure 2-1, where the time scale has been changed to reflect follow-up time rather than calendar time. Thus, time 0 now represents the beginning of the follow-up for each individual (regardless of the actual date of the start of follow-up). Much of the discussion of incidence indexes that follows is based on Figure 2-2.

Cumulative Incidence Based on the Life Table Interval Approach (Classic Life Table)

The cumulative probability of the event during a given interval (lasting m units of time and beginning at time x) is the proportion of new events during that period of time (with events noted as $_m d_x$), in which the denominator is the initial population (l_x) corrected for losses ($_m c_x$). In the classic life table, this measure corresponds to the interval-based

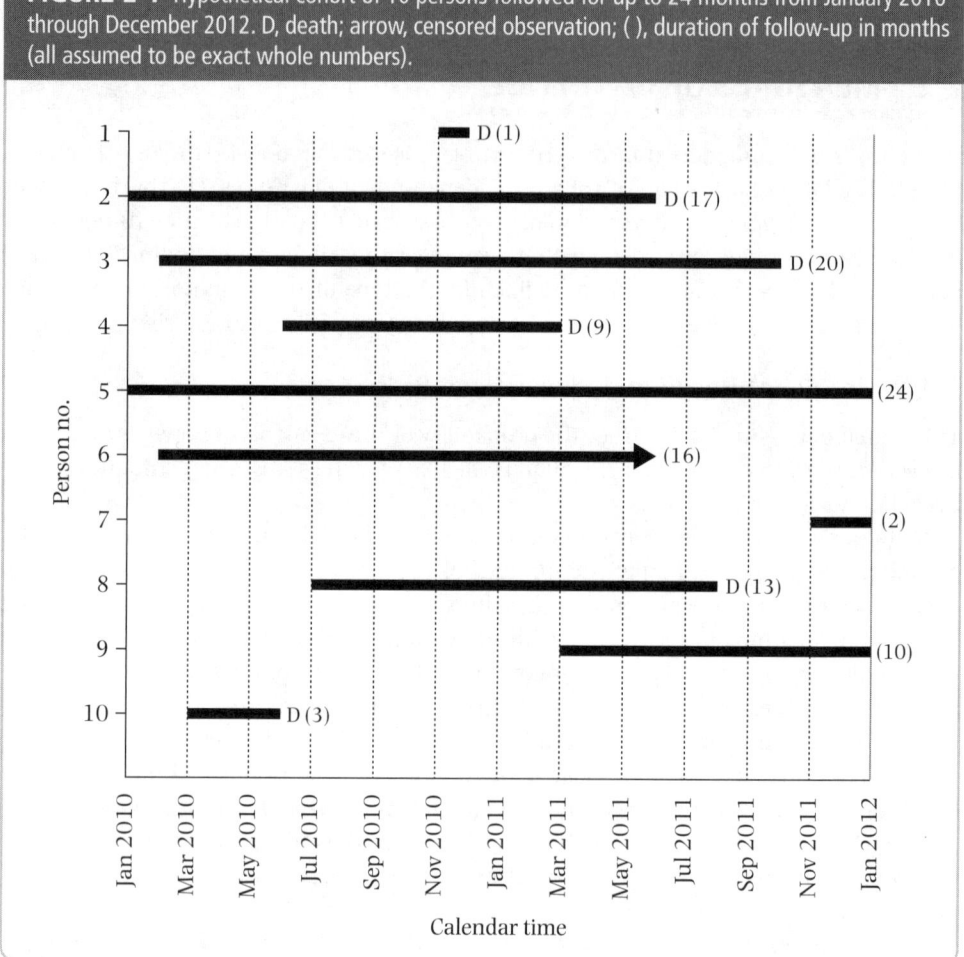

FIGURE 2-1 Hypothetical cohort of 10 persons followed for up to 24 months from January 2010 through December 2012. D, death; arrow, censored observation; ( ), duration of follow-up in months (all assumed to be exact whole numbers).

probability of the event $_mq_x$.[5] Its calculation is straightforward. As seen in Figure 2-2, six deaths occurred among the 10 individuals who were alive at the beginning of the follow-up. If no individual had been lost to observation, $_2q_0$ (with times specified in years) would be simply the number of deaths over this 2-year interval ($_2d_0$) divided by the number of individuals at the beginning of the interval (l_0): that is, 6 ÷ 10 = 0.60, or 60%. Because the three individuals lost to observation (censored, $_2c_0$) were not at risk during the entire duration of the follow-up, however, their limited participation must be accounted for in the denominator of the cumulative probability. By convention, half of these individuals are subtracted from the denominator, and the probability estimate is then calculated as follows:

$$_2q_0 = \frac{_2d_0}{l_0 - 0.5 \times {_2c_0}} = \frac{6}{10 - 0.5 \times 3} = 0.71 \qquad \text{(Eq. 2.1)}$$

The conventional approach of subtracting one-half of the total number of censored observations from the denominator is based on the assumption that censoring occurred uniformly throughout that period and thus, on average, these individuals were at risk for only one-half of the follow-up period.

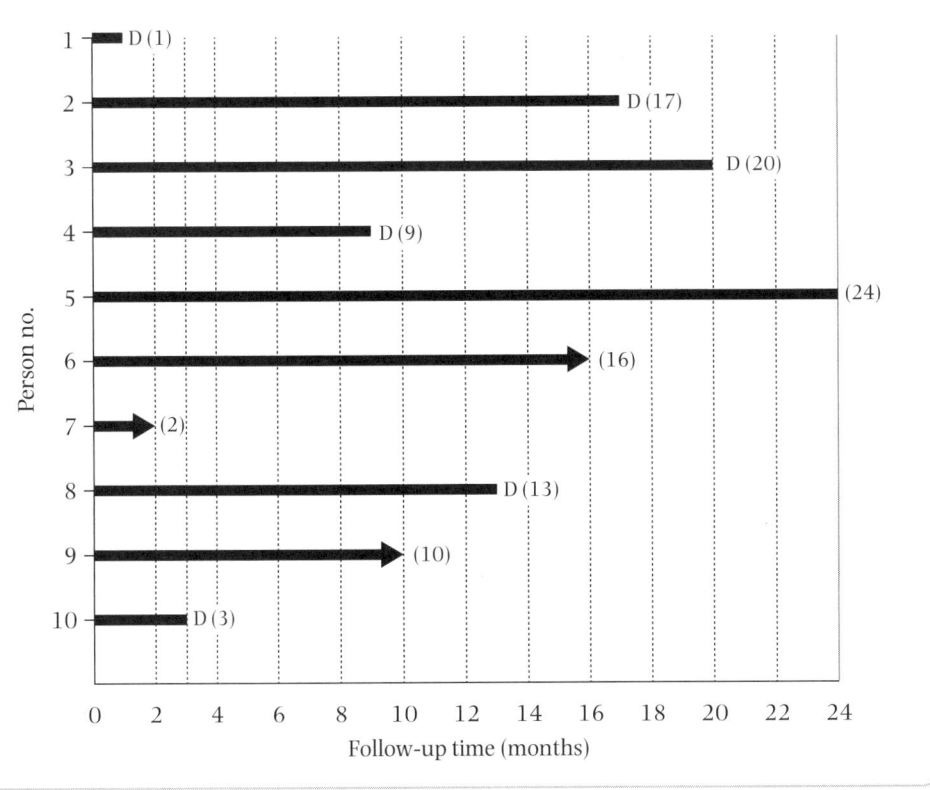

FIGURE 2-2 Same cohort as in Figure 2-1, with person-time represented according to time since the beginning of the study. D, death; arrow, censored observation; ( ), duration of follow-up in months (all assumed to be exact whole numbers).

The complement of this cumulative probability of the event (q) is the cumulative probability of survival (p), that is,

$$_2p_0 = 1 - {_2q_0} = 0.29$$

It is important to note that the cumulative probability of an event (or the cumulative survival) has no time period intrinsically attached to it: time must be specified. Thus, in this example, one has to describe q as the "*2-year* cumulative probability of death."

Usually, the classic life table uses multiple intervals—for example, five intervals of 2 years for a total follow-up of 10 years. Within each interval, the probability of survival is calculated using as denominator the number of individuals under observation *at the beginning* of the interval corrected for losses during the interval as described previously. In order to be part of the denominator for the calculation of the survival probability in the second interval ($_2p_2$), for example, one has to survive through the first interval; likewise, the survival probability for the third interval (starting at year 4, or $_2p_4$) is calculated only among those who survived both the first and second time interval. This is the reason why these interval-specific probabilities are technically called "conditional probabilities." A cumulative probability of survival over more than one interval—for example, the full 10-year follow-up with five 2-year intervals—is obtained by multiplying the conditional survival probabilities over all the intervals:

$$_{10}p_0 = {_2p_0} \times {_2p_2} \times {_2p_4} \times {_2p_6} \times {_2p_8}$$

The cumulative probability of having the event is the complement of this joint probability of survival:

$$_{10}q_0 = 1 - {_{10}p_0} = 1 - (_2p_0 \times {_2p_2} \times {_2p_4} \times {_2p_6} \times {_2p_8}) \quad \text{(Eq. 2.2)}$$

This is analogous to the calculation of the cumulative survival function using the Kaplan-Meier method illustrated in the section that follows.

It is not necessary that the intervals in a classic (interval-based) life table be of the same duration. The length of the interval should be determined by the pace at which incidence changes over time so that, within any given interval, events and withdrawals occur at an approximately uniform rate (discussed later). For example, to study survival after an acute myocardial infarction, the intervals should be very short soon after onset of symptoms, when the probability of death is high and rapidly changing. Subsequent intervals could be longer, however, as the probability of a recurrent event and death tends to stabilize.

Examples of the use of the actuarial life table method can be found in reports from classic epidemiologic studies (e.g., Pooling Project Research Group[6]). More details and additional examples can be found in other epidemiology textbooks (e.g., Gordis[7] and Kahn and Sempos[8]).

Cumulative Incidence Based on the Kaplan-Meier (Exact Event Times) Approach

The Kaplan-Meier approach involves the calculation of the probability of each event at the time it occurs. The denominator for this calculation is the population at risk at the time of each event's occurrence.[4] As for the actuarial life table, these are "conditional probabilities"; in other words, they are conditioned on being at risk (alive and not censored) at each event time. If each event (first, second, etc.) is designated by its time of occurrence i, then the formula for the conditional probability is simply

$$q_i = \frac{d_i}{n_i}$$

where d_i is the number of deaths (or other type of event) occurring at time i, and n_i is the number of individuals still under observation (i.e., at risk of the event) at time i. (Usually $d_i = 1$, unless more than one event is occurring simultaneously—something that will only occur when nonexact discrete measures of time are used.)

In order to facilitate the calculations, Figure 2-3 shows the same data as in Figures 2-1 and 2-2 but with the individuals' follow-up times arranged from shortest to longest. When the first death occurs exactly at the end of the first month (person 1), there are 10 individuals at risk; the conditional probability is then

$$q_1 = \frac{1}{10}$$

When the second death occurs after 3 months of follow-up (person 10), there are only eight persons at risk; this is because in addition to the one previous death (D), one individual had been lost to observation after 2 months (person 7) and therefore was not at risk when the second death occurred. Thus, the conditional probability at the time of the second death is estimated as follows:

$$q_3 = \frac{1}{8} = 0.125$$

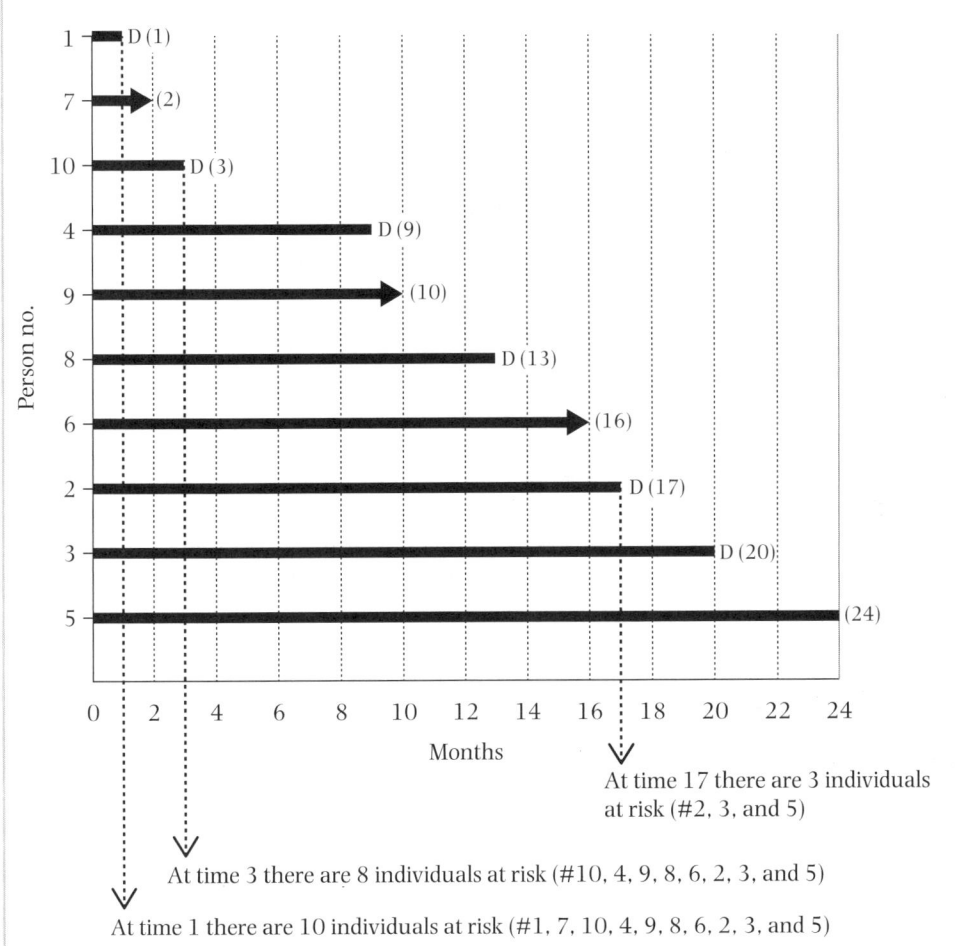

FIGURE 2-3 Same cohort as in Figures 2-1 and 2-2, with individuals sorted according to follow-up time from shortest to longest. D, death; arrow, censored observation; ( ), duration of follow-up in months (all assumed to be exact whole numbers). As examples, the vertical arrows mark the individuals who were at risk for the calculations of the conditional probabilities of death at three of the event times: 1 month, 3 months, and 17 months (see text).

These calculations are repeated for all the event times. For example, for the fifth event, when person 2 dies at 17 months of follow-up, there were three individuals still under observation (Figure 2-3) and thus the conditional probability of the death at month 17 can be estimated as:

$$q_{17} = \frac{1}{3} = 0.333$$

Table 2-3 (column 4) shows the calculation of these conditional probabilities for each and every six event times in this example. The censored observations are skipped in these calculations, as they do not represent an identified event. Censored observations, however, are counted in the denominator for the calculation of conditional probabilities corresponding to events occurring up to the time when the censoring occurs. This represents the most efficient use of the available information.[4]

TABLE 2-3 Calculation of Kaplan-Meier survival estimates for the example in Figure 2-3.

Time (months) (1) i	Number of individuals at risk (2) n_i	Number of events (3) d_i	Conditional probability of the event (4) $q_i = d_i/n_i$	Conditional probability of survival (5) $p_i = 1 - q_i$	Cumulative probability of survival* (6) S_i
1	10†	1	1/10 = 0.100	9/10 = 0.900	0.900
3	8†	1	1/8 = 0.125	7/8 = 0.875	0.788
9	7	1	1/7 = 0.143	6/7 = 0.857	0.675
13	5	1	1/5 = 0.200	4/5 = 0.800	0.540
17	3†	1	1/3 = 0.333	2/3 = 0.667	0.360
20	2	1	1/2 = 0.500	1/2 = 0.500	0.180

*Obtained by multiplying the conditional probabilities in column (5)—see text.
†Examples of how to determine how many individuals were at risk at three of the event times (1, 3, and 17) are shown with vertical arrows in Figure 2-3.

Column 5 in Table 2-3 shows the complements of the conditional probabilities of the event at each time—that is, the conditional probabilities of survival (p_i) which, as in the classic life table method, represent the probability of surviving beyond time i among those who were still under observation at that time (i.e., conditioned on having survived up to time i). Column 6, also shown graphically in Figure 2-4, presents the cumulative probabilities of survival—that is, the so-called Kaplan-Meier *survival function* (usually notated as S_i). This represents the probability of surviving beyond time i for all

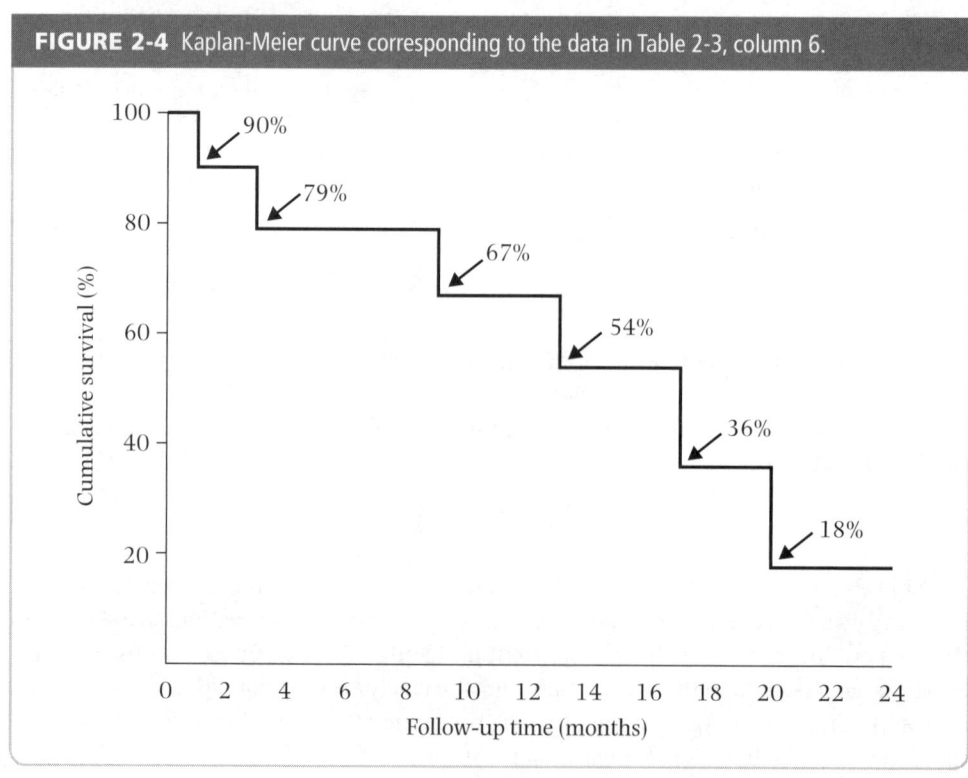

FIGURE 2-4 Kaplan-Meier curve corresponding to the data in Table 2-3, column 6.

of those present at the beginning of follow-up, calculated as the product of all conditional survival probabilities up to time *i*. In the example, the cumulative probability of surviving beyond the end of the follow-up period of 2 years (S_i, where $i = 24$ months) is

$$S_{24} = \frac{9}{10} \times \frac{7}{8} \times \frac{6}{7} \times \frac{4}{5} \times \frac{2}{3} \times \frac{1}{2} = 0.180$$

Thus, the estimate of the cumulative probability of the event $(1 - S_i)$ is

$$1 - S_{24} = 1 - 0.18 = 0.82$$

As for the cumulative probability based on the actuarial life table approach (Equation 2.2), the time interval for the cumulative probability using the Kaplan-Meier approach also needs to be specified (in this example, 24 months or 2 years). For a method to calculate confidence limits for a cumulative survival probability estimate, see Appendix A, Section A.1.

Regardless of the method used in the calculation (actuarial or Kaplan-Meier), the cumulative incidence is a proportion in the strict sense of the term. It is unitless, and its values can range from 0 to 1 (or 100%).

Assumptions in the Estimation of Cumulative Incidence Based on Survival Analysis

The following assumptions must be met when conducting survival analysis:

Uniformity of Events and Losses Within Each Interval (Classic Life Table). Implicit in the classic life table calculation (discussed previously) is the generic assumption that events and losses are approximately uniform during each defined interval. If risk changes rapidly within a given interval, then calculating an average risk over the interval is not very informative. The rationale underlying the method to correct for losses—that is, subtracting one-half of the losses from the denominator (Equation 2.1)—also depends on the assumption that losses occur uniformly. The assumption of uniformity of events and losses within a given interval is entirely related to the way the life table is defined and can be met by adjusting the interval definitions to appropriately uniform risk intervals (i.e., by shortening them). Furthermore, this assumption does not apply to the Kaplan-Meier calculation, where intervals are not defined *a priori*.

Whereas this interval-based assumption applies only to classic life table estimates, the two following assumptions apply to both classic life table and Kaplan-Meier estimates, and are key to survival analysis techniques and analyses of cohort data in general: (1) independence between censoring and survival; and (2) lack of secular trends during the study's accrual period.

Independence Between Censoring and Survival. For the calculations of the conditional and cumulative incidences using the previously described methods, censored individuals are included in the denominator during the entire time when they are under observation; after censored, they are ignored in subsequent calculations. Thus, if one wants to infer that the estimated overall cumulative survival (e.g., $S_{24} = 18\%$, as in Figure 2-4) is generalizable to the entire population present at the study's outset (at time 0), one needs to assume that *the censored observations have the same probability of the event after censoring as those remaining under observation*. In other words, censoring needs to be independent of survival; otherwise, bias will ensue. For example, if the risk were higher for censored than for noncensored observations (e.g., study subjects withdrew because they were sicker) over time, the study population would include a

TABLE 2-4 Relationship between reason for censoring and the assumption of independence between censoring and survival in survival analysis.

Type of censoring	May violate assumption of independence of censoring/survival	If assumption is violated, likely direction of bias on the cumulative incidence estimate
Deaths from other causes when there are common risk factors*	Yes	Underestimation
Participants' refusal to follow up contacts	Yes	Underestimation
Migration	Yes	Variable
Administrative censoring	Unlikely†	Variable

*In cause-specific incidence or mortality studies.
†More likely in studies with a prolonged accrual period in the presence of secular trends.

progressively greater proportion of lower risk subjects; as a result, the (true) overall cumulative incidence would be underestimated (i.e., survival would be overestimated). The opposite bias would occur if censored observations tended to include healthier individuals. The likely direction of the bias according to the reason why censoring occurred is summarized in Table 2-4. With regard to censored observations caused by *death from other causes* in cause-specific outcome studies, if the disease of interest shares strong risk factors with other diseases that are associated with mortality, censoring may not be independent of survival. An example is a study in which the outcome of interest is coronary heart disease death, and participants dying from other causes, including respiratory diseases (such as lung cancer and emphysema), are censored at the time of their death (as they are no longer at risk of dying from coronary heart disease). Because coronary heart disease and respiratory diseases share an important risk factor (smoking) and because, in addition, respiratory disease deaths are common in smokers, individuals dying from respiratory diseases may have had a higher risk of coronary heart disease if they had not died from respiratory diseases, resulting in a violation of the assumption of independence between censoring and survival.

Other frequent reasons for censoring include *refusal* of study participants to allow subsequent follow-up contacts (in a study where assessment of the outcome events depends on such contacts), and inability to contact participants due to migration out of the study area. Individuals who refuse follow-up contacts may have a less healthy lifestyle than individuals who agree to continuing participation in a prospective study; if that were the case, censoring for this reason may lead to an underestimation of the cumulative incidence. The direction of the bias resulting from the loss to follow-up of individuals because of *migration* is a function of the sociodemographic context in which the migration occurs—for example, whether the individuals who migrate are of higher or lower socioeconomic status (SES). If losses occurred mainly among those in the upper SES, who tend to be healthier, those remaining in the study would tend to have poorer survival. On the other hand, if the losses occurred primarily among individuals with a lower SES, and thus poorer health, the survival of those remaining in the study would be overestimated. For the so-called *administrative* losses, defined as those that occur because the follow-up ends (e.g., persons 7 and 9 in Figure 2-1), the assumption of independence between censoring and survival is regarded as more justified, as these losses are usually thought to be independent of the characteristics of the individuals *per se*. (Administrative losses are, however, amenable to temporal changes occurring during the accrual period; see the following section "Lack of Secular Trends.")

In summary, whether the key *assumption* of independence between censoring and survival for the calculation of cumulative incidence/survival estimates is met depends on the reasons why censoring occurred (Table 2-4). This assumption is particularly relevant when the magnitude of the absolute incidence estimate is the focus of the study; it may be less important if the investigator is primarily interested in a relative estimate (e.g., when comparing incidence/survival in two groups defined by exposure levels in a cohort study), provided that biases resulting from losses are reasonably similar in the groups being compared. (For a discussion of a related bias, the so-called compensating bias, see "Selection Bias" in Chapter 4, Section 4.2.) Finally, this assumption can often be verified. For example, it is usually possible to compare baseline characteristics related to the outcome of interest between individuals lost and those not lost to observation. In addition, if relevant study participant identifying information is available, linkage to the National Death Index can be used to compare the mortality experience of those lost and those not lost to follow-up.

Lack of Secular Trends. In studies in which the accrual of study participants occurs over an extended time period, the decision to pool all individuals at time 0 (as in Figure 2-2) assumes a lack of secular trends with regard to the characteristics of these individuals that affect the outcome of interest. This, however, may not be the case in the presence of *birth cohort* and *period* (calendar time) effects (see Chapter 1, Section 1.2). Changes over time in the characteristics of recruited participants as well as significant secular changes in relevant exposures and/or treatments may introduce bias in the cumulative incidence/survival estimates, the direction and magnitude of which depend on the characteristics of these cohort or period effects. Thus, for example, it would not have been appropriate to estimate survival from diagnosis of all patients identified with insulin-dependent diabetes from 1915 through 1935 as a single group, as this extended accrual period would inappropriately combine two very heterogeneous patient cohorts: those diagnosed before and those diagnosed after the introduction of insulin. Similarly, it would not be appropriate to carry out a survival analysis pooling at time 0 all HIV-seropositive individuals recruited into a cohort accrued between 1995 and 1999—that is, both before and after a new effective treatment (protease inhibitors) became available.

2.2.2 Incidence Rate Based on Person-Time

Rather than individuals, the denominator for the incidence *rate* is formed by time units (t) contributed to the follow-up period by the individuals at risk (n). For example, consider a hypothetical cohort in which 12 events occur and the total amount of follow-up time for all individuals is 500 days. The incidence rate in this example is $12 \div 500 = 0.024$ per person-day or 2.4 per 100 person-days. The number of individuals who were followed up with is not provided; thus, the "person-time" estimate in the example could have originated from 50 individuals seen during 10 days each (50×10), 5 individuals observed for 100 days (5×100), and so on.

Incidence rates are *not* proportions. They are obtained by dividing the number of events by the amount of time at risk (pooling all study participants) and are measured in units of time^{-1}. As a result, a rate can range from 0 to infinity, depending on the unit of time being used. For example, the previously mentioned incidence rate could be expressed in a number of ways: 12 ÷ 500 person-days = 12 ÷ 1.37 person-years = 8.76 per person-year (or 876 per 100 person-years). The latter value exceeds 1 (or 100%) only because of the arbitrary choice of the time unit used in the denominator. If a person has the event of interest after a follow-up of 6 months and the investigator chooses to express the rate per person-years, the rate will be 1 ÷ 0.5 or 200 per 100 person-years.

The time unit used is at the discretion of the investigator and is usually selected on the basis of the frequency of the event under study. The main reason that many epidemiologic studies use person-*years* as the unit of analysis is because it is a convenient way to express rare events. On the other hand, when one is studying relatively frequent health or disease events, it may be more convenient to use some other unit of time (Table 2-5). The choice is entirely arbitrary and will not affect the inferences derived from the study.

Rather than a unitless proportion of individuals who develop the event among those at risk (see cumulative incidence described previously in this chapter), incidence based on person-time expresses the "rate" at which the events occur in the population at risk at any given point in time. This type of rate is also called *incidence density*, a concept analogous to that of velocity: the instantaneous rate of change or the "speed" at which individuals develop the event (disease, death, etc.) in the population. This concept is the basis for some of the mathematic modeling techniques used for the analysis of incidence rates (e.g., Poisson regression models; see Chapter 7, Section 7.4.5). Because the instantaneous rate for each individual cannot be directly calculated, however, the average incidence over a period of time for a population is usually used as a proxy. The average incidence can be calculated based on individual or aggregate follow-up data, as is discussed later in this chapter. Epidemiologists often use the terms *rate* and *density* interchangeably; however, in the discussion that follows, the term *rate* will be primarily used in the context of grouped data, whereas *density* will denote a rate based on data obtained from each individual in the study.

Incidence Rate Based on Aggregate Data

This type of incidence is typically obtained for a geographic location by using as the denominator the average population estimated for a certain time period. Provided that this period is not excessively long and that the population and its demographic composition in the area of interest are relatively stable, the average population can be estimated

TABLE 2-5 Examples of person-time units according to the frequency of events under investigation.

Population	Event studied	Person-time unit typically used
General	Incident breast cancer	Person-years
General	Incident myocardial infarction	Person-years
Malnourished children	Incident diarrhea	Person-months
Lung cancer cases	Death	Person-months
Influenza epidemic	Incident influenza	Person-weeks
Children with acute diarrhea	Recovery	Person-days

as the population at the middle of the period (e.g., July 1 for a 1-year period). In a cohort study, the average of the population at the beginning and at the end of the period can be obtained for a given follow-up interval. Thus, for a given time interval,

$$\text{Incidence rate} = \frac{\text{Number of events}}{\text{Average population}}$$

In Figure 2-2 for example, 10 individuals are alive and present in the study at the beginning of the follow-up period ("point zero"). Only one person is alive and present in the study when the 2-year follow-up ends (person 5). Thus, the average population (n) for the total 2-year follow-up period is

$$n = \frac{10 + 1}{2} = 5.5$$

The average population n can be also calculated by subtracting one-half of the events (d) and losses (c) from the initial population:

$$n = 10 - \frac{1}{2}(6 + 3) = 5.5$$

As for all mean values, the underlying assumption when using this approach is that, on the average, there were 5.5 persons for the duration of the study (2 years). For this assumption to be met, events and withdrawals must occur uniformly throughout the follow-up period. The rate of new events in relationship to the average population is then calculated as follows:

$$\text{Incidence rate} = \frac{6}{5.5} = 1.09 \text{ per person} - 2 \text{ years}$$

In this example, the rate is based on a time unit of 2 years and not on the number of individuals. The assumption underlying the use of the average population is that the same rate would have been obtained if 5.5 individuals had been followed for the entire 2-year period, during which six events were observed. This example again highlights the fact that this type of incidence is not a proportion and, thus, is not bound to be 1 (100%) or less. In this particular instance, the seemingly counterintuitive rate of 109 per 100 person-time obviously resulted from the fact that "2 years" is being used as the time unit; if a "person-year" unit had been used instead, the rate would have been 1.09 ÷ 2 years = 0.545 per person-year (or 54.5 per 100 person-years).

This example illustrates the estimation of the incidence rate using the average population of a defined cohort (i.e., the hypothetical cohort represented in Figure 2-2); however, this is not its usual application. Instead, the calculation of incidence based on grouped data is typically used to estimate mortality based on vital statistics information or incidence of newly diagnosed disease based on population-based registries (e.g., cancer registries); in other words, when incidence needs to be estimated for a *population* or an *aggregate* defined by residence in a given geographic area over some time period. These aggregates are called *open* or *dynamic cohorts* because they include individuals who are added or withdrawn from the pool of the population at risk as they migrate in or out of the area (i.e., a situation more clearly represented by the diagram in Figure 2-1 than that in Figure 2-2).

Incidence Density Based on Individual Data

When relatively precise data on the timing of events or losses are available for each individual from a defined cohort, it is possible to estimate *incidence density*. The total person-time for the study period is simply the sum of the person-time contributed by each individual. The average incidence density is then calculated as follows:

$$\text{Incidence density} = \frac{\text{Number of events}}{\text{Total person-time}}$$

For each individual in the example shown in Figures 2-1, 2-2, and 2-3, the length of the horizontal line represents the length of time between the beginning of the follow-up and the point when the individual either had the event, which in this hypothetical example is death (D) or was lost to observation. For example, for individual 1, death occurred after exactly 1 month. Thus, this individual's contribution to the total number of person-years in the first follow-up year (see Figure 2-3) would be $1 \div 12 = 0.083$; obviously, this person made no contribution to the follow-up during the second year. On the other hand, individual 2 died after remaining in the study for 17 months, or 1 year and 5 months. Thus, his or her contribution to the first follow-up year was $12 \div 12$ and to the second year was $5 \div 12$, for a total of 1.417 person-years.

The contribution of censored individuals is calculated in an identical fashion. For example, the contribution of individual 6 to the total number of person-years was equivalent to 16 months, or 1 full person-year in the first year and $4 \div 12$ person-years in the second year, for a total of 1.333 person-years. The calculation of person-years for all 10 study participants is shown in Table 2-6. In this example, the incidence density applicable to the total follow-up period is, therefore, $6 \div 9.583 = 0.63$ per person-year (or 63 per 100 person-years). Alternatively, the incidence density could be expressed as $6 \div (9.583 \times 12 \text{ months}) = 0.052$ per person-month (or 5.2 per 100 person-months). For a method to estimate confidence limits of incidence rates, see Appendix A, Section A.2.

Assumptions in the Estimation of Incidence Based on Person-Time

The assumptions of independence between censoring and survival and of lack of secular trends discussed in Section 2.2.1 are also relevant in the context of person-time analysis. The former assumption relates to absence of selection bias resulting from losses to follow-up. Both assumptions actually apply to any type of cohort study analysis. Furthermore, as for incidence based on the actuarial life table (Equation 2.1), an important assumption when using the person-time approach is that the risk of the event remains approximately constant over time during the interval of interest or, in other words, that the estimated rate should apply equally to *any point in time within the interval*. This means that n persons followed during t units of time are equivalent to t persons observed during n units of time; for example, the risk of an individual living five units of time within the interval is equivalent to that of five individuals living one unit each (Figure 2-5). When individuals are exposed to a given risk factor, another interpretation of this assumption is that the effect resulting from the exposure is not cumulative within the follow-up interval of interest. Often this assumption is difficult to accept, as, for example, when doing studies of chronic respiratory disease in smokers: the risk of chronic bronchitis for 1 smoker followed for 30 years is certainly not the same as that of 30 smokers followed for 1 year, in view of the strong cumulative effect of smoking and the latency period needed for disease initiation. To decrease the dependency of the person-time approach on this assumption, the follow-up period can be divided

2.2 Measures of Incidence

TABLE 2-6 Calculation of the number of person-years based on Figure 2-2.

Person no.	Total follow-up (in months)	Contribution to the total number of person-years by participants in:		Total follow-up period
		1st Year of follow-up	2nd Year of follow-up	
1	1	1/12 = 0.083	0	0.083
2	17	12/12 = 1.000	5/12 = 0.417	1.417
3	20	12/12 = 1.000	8/12 = 0.667	1.667
4	9	9/12 = 0.750	0	0.750
5	24	12/12 = 1.000	12/12 = 1.000	2.000
6	16	12/12 = 1.000	4/12 = 0.333	1.333
7	2	2/12 = 0.167	0	0.167
8	13	12/12 = 1.000	1/12 = 0.083	1.083
9	10	10/12 = 0.833	0	0.833
10	3	3/12 = 0.250	0	0.250
Total	115 months	7.083 years	2.500 years	9.583 years

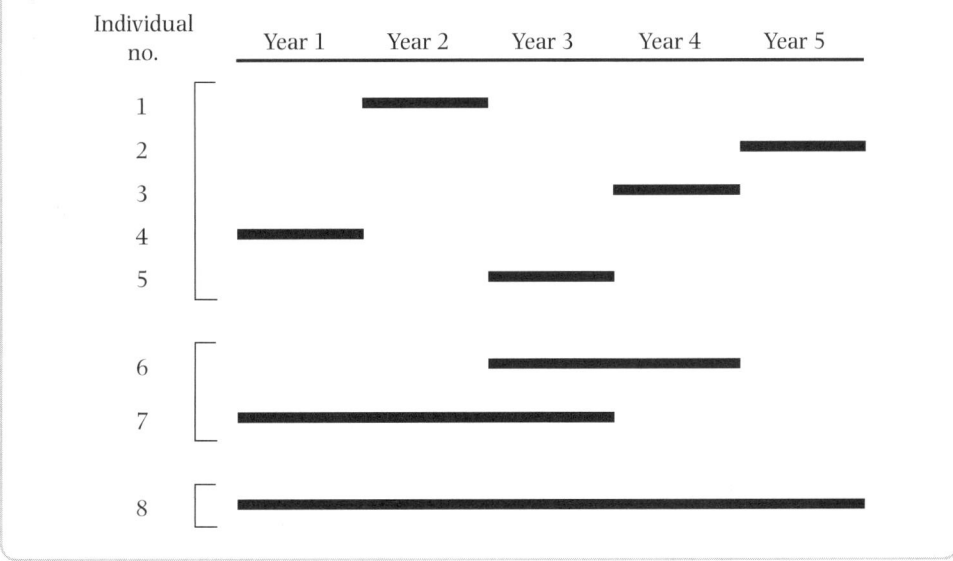

FIGURE 2-5 Follow-up time for eight individuals in a hypothetical study. It is assumed that the sum of the person-time units for individuals no. 1 to 5 (with a short follow-up time of 1 year each) is equivalent to the sum for individuals no. 6 and 7 (with follow-up times of 2 and 3 years, respectively) and to the total time for individual no. 8 (who has the longest follow-up time, 5 years). For each group of individuals (no. 1–5, 6 and 7, and 8) the total number of person-years of observation is 5.

into smaller intervals and incidence densities calculated for each interval. For example, using data from Table 2-6 and Figure 2-3, it is possible to calculate densities separately for the first and the second years of follow-up, as follows:

First follow-up year: $3 \div 7.083 = 42.4$ per 100 person-years
(or $3 \div 85 = 3.5$ per 100 person-months)

Second follow-up year: $3 \div 2.500 = 120$ per 100 person-years
(or $3 \div 30 = 10$ per 100 person-months)

The fact that the densities differ markedly between the first and second follow-up years in this example strongly implies that it would not be reasonable to estimate an incidence density for the overall 2-year period.

Relationship Between Density (Based on Individual Data) and Rate (Based on Grouped Data)

It is of practical interest that when withdrawals (and additions in an open population or dynamic cohort) and events occur uniformly, rate (based on grouped data) and density (based on individual data) are virtually the same. The following equation demonstrates the equivalence between the rate per average population and the density (per person-time), when the former is averaged with regard to the corresponding time unit (e.g., yearly average).

$$\text{Rate} = \frac{\dfrac{\text{No. events } (x)}{\text{average population } (n)}}{\text{time } (t)} = \frac{x}{n \times t} = \text{Density}$$

This idea can be understood intuitively. For a given time unit, such as 1 year, the denominator of the rate (the average population) is analogous to the total number of time units lived by all of the individuals in the population in that given time period. An example is given in Table 2-7, based on data for four persons followed for a maximum of 2 years. One individual is lost to follow-up (censored) after 1 year; two individuals die, one after 0.5 years and the other after 1.5 years, and the fourth individual survives through the end of the study. There is, therefore, perfect symmetry in the distribution of withdrawals or events, which occurred after 0.5, 1, 1.5, and 2 years after the onset of the study. Summing the contribution to the follow-up time made by each participant yields a total of 5 person-years. Density is thus two deaths per 5 person-years, or 0.40.

The average population (n) in this example can be estimated as [(initial population + final population) $\div$ 2], or [(4 + 1) $\div$ 2 = 2.5]. The rate for the total time (t = 2 years) is then $2 \div 2.5$. The average *yearly* rate is thus equivalent to the density using person-time as the denominator:

$$\text{Yearly rate} = \frac{\dfrac{x}{n}}{t} = \frac{x}{n \times t} = \frac{x}{\text{person-years}}$$

$$= \text{Density} = \frac{2}{2.5 \times 2} = \frac{2}{5} = 0.40$$

On the other hand, when losses and events do not occur in an approximate uniform fashion, the incidence rate based on the average study population and the incidence density for a given population and time period may be discrepant. For example, based on the hypothetical data in Figure 2-3, the estimate of the mean yearly incidence based on the average population was 54.5/100 person-years, whereas that based on the incidence

TABLE 2-7 Hypothetical data for four individuals followed for a maximum of 2 years.

Individual no.	Outcome	Timing of event/loss	No. of person-years
1	Death	At 6 months	0.5
2	Loss to observation	At 1 year	1.0
3	Death	At 18 months	1.5
4	Administrative censoring	At 2 years	2.0
	Total no. of person years:		5.0

density was 63/100 person-years. In real life, when the sample size is large and provided that the time interval is reasonably short, the assumption of uniformity of events/losses is likely to be met.

The notion that the average population is equivalent to the total number of person-time when events and withdrawals are uniform is analogous to the assumption regarding uniformity of events and withdrawals in the actuarial life table (see Section 2.2.1, Equation 2.1). When it is not known exactly when the events occurred in a given time period, each person in whom the event occurs or who enters or withdraws from the study is assumed to contribute one-half the follow-up time of the interval. (It is expected that this will be the average across a large number of individuals entering/exiting at different times throughout each time period for which person-time is estimated.)

The correspondence between rate (based on grouped data) and density (based on individual person-time) is conceptually appealing as it allows the comparison of an average yearly rate based on an average population—which, in vital statistics, is usually the midpoint, or July 1, population estimate—with a density based on person-years. It is, for example, a common practice in occupational epidemiology studies to obtain an expected number of events needed for the calculation of the standardized mortality ratio by applying population vital statistics age-specific rates to the age-specific number of person-years accumulated by an exposed cohort (see Chapter 7, Section 7.3.2).

Stratifying Person-Time and Rates According to Follow-up Time and Covariates

The calculation of person-time contributed by a given population or group is simply the sum of the person-time contributed by each individual in the group during the follow-up period. In most analytical prospective studies relevant to epidemiology, the risk of the event changes with time. For example, the incidence of fatal or nonfatal events may increase with time, as when healthy individuals are followed up with as they age. In other situations, risk diminishes as follow-up progresses, as in a study of complications after surgery or of case fatality after an acute myocardial infarction. Because calculating an overall average rate over a long time period when the incidence is not uniform violates the assumptions discussed previously in this chapter (and ultimately does not make a lot of sense), it is necessary to estimate the event rate for time intervals within which homogeneity of risk can be assumed. Thus, it is often important to stratify the follow-up time and calculate the incidence rate for each time stratum (as seen in the example based on the data in Table 2-6). Furthermore, in a cohort study, one may additionally wish to control for potentially confounding variables (see Chapter 5). Time and confounders can be taken into account by stratifying the follow-up time for each individual according to other time variables (e.g., age) and categories of the confounder(s), and then summing up the person-time within each stratum.

The following examples illustrate the calculation of person-time and the corresponding incidence rates based on the data shown in Table 2-8, from a hypothetical study of four postmenopausal women followed for mortality after breast cancer surgery (2000 to 2010). Table 2-8 provides the dates of surgery ("entry"), the date of the event (death or censoring), ages at surgery and at menopause, and smoking status.

One Time Scale. Based on the data from Table 2-8, the follow-up of these four women is displayed in Figure 2-6. The top panel of Figure 2-6 displays the follow-up according to calendar time for each of the four women; the bottom panel displays the follow-up time after surgery. In Figure 2-6 (top), because the precise dates of surgery and events are not known, it is assumed that these occur in the middle of the corresponding year (discussed previously in this chapter).

If it could be assumed that the risk of the event was approximately uniform within 5-year intervals, it would be justified to calculate person-time separately for the first and the second 5-year calendar period (Figure 2-6, top); the calculation of the rates is shown in Table 2-9. Individuals whose follow-up starts or ends sometime during a given year are assigned one-half of a person-year: for example, a contribution of 0.5 person-year is made by woman 1 in 2003, as her surgery was carried out at some time in 2003. Thus, the total person-time for the period 2000 to 2004 is 1.5 years (woman 1) + 4.5 years (woman 3) + 2 years (woman 4) = 8 person-years.

Alternatively, one might be interested in examining the rates in this study according to follow-up time, as shown in Table 2-10. For example, because woman 1 was followed from 2003.5 to 2009.5, she can be assumed to have a full 6-year follow-up (Figure 2-6, bottom).

Two or More Time Scales. Epidemiologic cohorts are often constituted by free-living individuals who interact and are the subject of multiple and varying biological and environmental circumstances. Thus, it is frequently important to take into consideration more than one time scale; the choice of time scales used for the stratification of follow-up time varies according to the characteristics and goals of the study (Table 2-11).

TABLE 2-8 Hypothetical data for four postmenopausal women followed for mortality after breast cancer surgery.

	Woman no. 1	Woman no. 2	Woman no. 3	Woman no. 4
Date of surgery	2003	2005	2000	2002
Age at surgery	58	50	48	54
Age at menopause	54	46	47	48
Smoking at time of surgery	Yes	No	Yes	No
Change in smoking status (year)	Quits (2006)	No	No	Starts (2003)
Type of event	Death	Loss	Withdrawal alive	Death
Date of event	2009	2008	2010	2004

FIGURE 2-6 Schematic representation of person-time for the hypothetical data in Table 2-8, according to one time scale: calendar time (top) and follow-up time (bottom) (censored observations are shown with arrows; D = death).

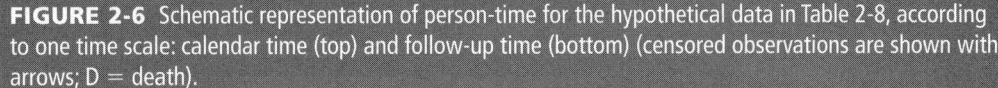

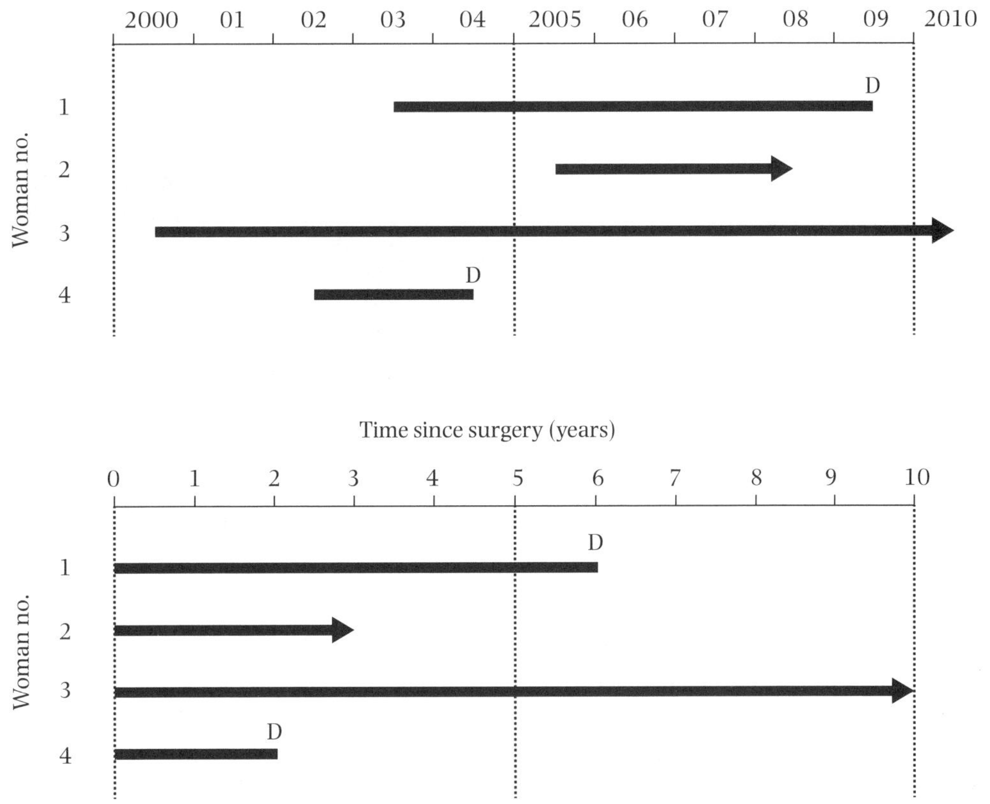

TABLE 2-9 Stratification of person-time and rates according to calendar time, based on Table 2-8 and Figure 2-6, top.

Calendar time	Person-years	Events	Incidence rate
2000–2004	8	1	0.125
2005–2009	12.5	1	0.080
(2010–2014)	(0.5)	(0)	(0)

In Figure 2-7, the person-time and outcomes of the four women from Table 2-8 are represented according to two time scales, age and calendar time. In this type of graphic representation (known as a *Lexis diagram*), each individual's trajectory is represented by diagonals across the two time scales. As in the previous example and given that the time data are approximate (in whole years), it is assumed that entry, censoring, and event of interest occur at the midpoint of the 1-year interval.

Table 2-12 shows the corresponding estimates of total person-time in each two-dimensional stratum. These are obtained by adding up the total time lived by the individuals in the study in each age/calendar time stratum represented by eight squares

TABLE 2-10 Stratification of person-time and rates according to follow-up time (time since surgery), based on Table 2-8 and Figure 2-6, bottom.

Time since surgery	Person-years	Events	Rate
0–4 years	15	1	0.0667
5–9 years	6	1	0.1667

TABLE 2-11 Examples of time scales frequently relevant in the context of cohort studies.

Time scale	Type of study
Follow-up time (time since recruitment)	All studies
Age	All studies
Calendar time	All studies (especially if recruitment is done over an extended period)
Time since employment	Occupational studies
Time since menarche	Studies of reproductive outcomes
Time since seroconversion	Follow-up of patients with HIV infection

in Figure 2-7; for example, for those 55 to 59 years old between 2000 and 2004, it is the sum of the 1.5 years lived by woman 4 (between age 55 and age 56.5 years, the assumed age of her death) and the 1.5 years lived by woman 1 in that stratum. The relevant events (deaths) are also assigned to each corresponding stratum, thus allowing the calculation of calendar- and age-specific incidence rates, also shown in Table 2-12.

Other time scales may be of interest. In occupational epidemiology, for example, it may be of interest to obtain incidence rates of certain outcomes taking into account three time scales simultaneously; for example, age (if the incidence depends on age), calendar time (if there have been secular changes in exposure doses), and time since employment (so as to consider a possible cumulative effect). For this situation, one could conceive a tridimensional analogue to Figure 2-7: cubes defined by strata of the three time scales and each individual's person-time displayed across the tridimensional diagonals.

The layout for the calculation of person-time and associated incidence rates described in this section can be used for the internal or external comparison of stratified rates by means of standardized mortality or incidence ratios (see Chapter 7, Section 7.3.2).

Time and Fixed or Time-Dependent Covariates. Stratification according to other variables, in addition to time, may be necessary in certain situations. For example, the data in Table 2-8 could be further stratified according to an additional time scale (e.g., time since menopause) and additional covariates (e.g., smoking status at the time of surgery). Thus, instead of eight strata, as in Figure 2-7 and Table 2-12, one would need to stratify the person-time into 32 strata defined by the combination of all four variables (calendar time, age, time since menopause, and smoking). Individuals under observation would shift from stratum to stratum as their status changes. For example, woman 1 (Table 2-8) is a smoker who enters the study in 2003 at the age of 58 years (that is assumed to be 2003.5 and 58.5 years, respectively; discussed previously), 4 years after menopause. Thus, as she enters the study in stratum "2000–2004/55–59 years of

FIGURE 2-7 Schematic representation of person-time for the four women in Table 2-8 according to two time scales, age and calendar time, categorized in 5-year intervals. Because time data are given in whole years, entry, events, and withdrawals are assumed to occur exactly at the middle of the year. Censored observations are represented by an arrow. The total time within each time stratum for all four women is shown in parentheses. The entry and exit times for woman no. 1 are given in italics; D = death.

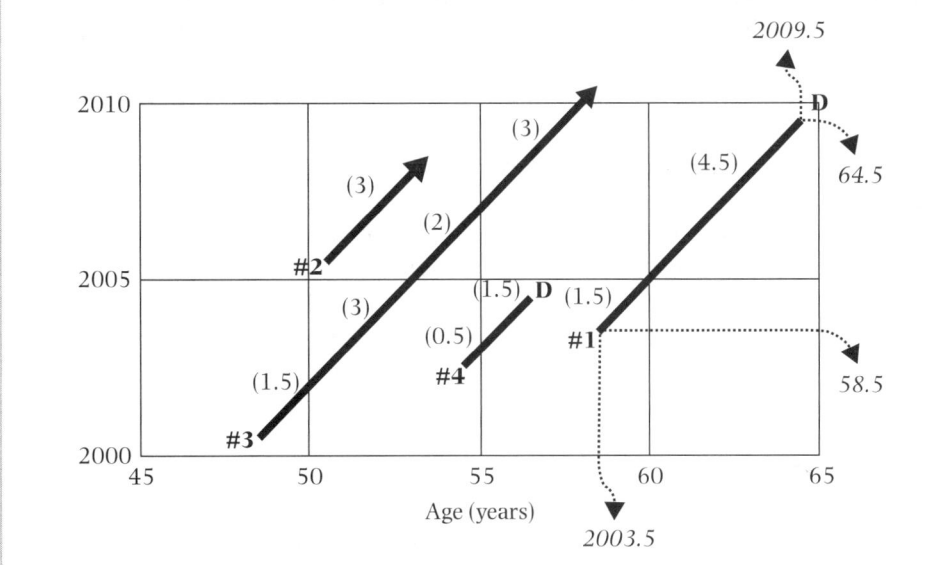

TABLE 2-12 Stratification of person-time and rates according to calendar time and age (see Figure 2-7).

Calendar time	Age (years)	Person-years	Events	Rate
2000–2004	45–49	1.5	0	0
	50–54	3.5	0	0
	55–59	3	1	0.3333
	60–64	0	-	-
2005–2009	45–49	0	-	-
	50–54	5	0	0
	55–59	3	0	0
	60–64	4.5	1	0.2222

age/smoker-at-baseline/menopause < 5 years," after contributing 1 person-year to this stratum (i.e., in 2004.5 at age 59.5 years), she becomes " ≥ 5 years after menopause" and thus shifts to a new stratum: "2000–2004/55–59 years of age/smoker-at-baseline/menopause ≥ 5 years." Half a year later, she turns 60 and enters a new stratum ("2005–2009/60–64 years of age/smoker-at-baseline/menopause ≥ 5 years") to contribute her last 4.5 person-years of observation before her death in 2009.5.

In the preceding example, smoking is treated as a fixed covariate, as only baseline status is considered; however, information on smoking status change is available in the hypothetical study data shown in Table 2-8. Changes in exposure status for certain covariates can easily be taken into account when using the person-time strategy. For example, using the information at baseline and change in smoking status shown in Table 2-8, assignment of person-time according to smoking as a time-dependent covariate can be represented as illustrated in Figure 2-8. Using this approach, each relevant event is assigned to the exposure status at the time of the event. Thus, woman 1's death is assigned to the "nonsmoking" group, whereas that of woman 4 is assigned to the "smoking" group. (The latter assignments are opposite to those based on smoking status at baseline described in the preceding paragraph.)

To use the person-time approach to take into account changing exposures involves an assumption akin to that used in crossover clinical trials: that after the exposure status changes, so does the associated risk. This is merely another way to state that there is no *accumulation* of risk and thus that the effect of a given exposure is "instantaneous." Whether this assumption is valid depends on the specific exposure or outcome being considered. For example, for smoking, the assumption may be reasonable when studying thromboembolic events likely to result from the acute effects of smoking (e.g., those leading to sudden cardiac death). On the other hand, given the well-known latency and cumulative effects leading to smoking-related lung cancer, the assumption of an "instantaneous" effect would be unwarranted if lung cancer were the outcome of interest. (The cumulative effect of smoking on lung cancer risk can be easily inferred from the fact that the risk in smokers who quit decreases yet never becomes the same as that in people who have never smoked.) If there is cumulative effect, the approach illustrated in Figure 2-8 (e.g., assigning the event in woman 1 to the nonsmoking category) will result in misclassification of exposure status (see Chapter 4, Section 4.3).

The cumulative effects of exposure can be taken into account with more complex exposure definitions; for example, total pack-years of smoking could be considered even among former smokers. Moreover, lag or latency times could also be introduced in the definition of person-time in relation to events, a frequent practice in occupational or environmental epidemiology studies.[9(pp.150–155)] Obviously, when the study requires stratification according to more than one time scale and several covariates, person-time and rates will need to be calculated for dozens or hundreds of multidimensional strata, which will require the use of computer programs.[10–12]

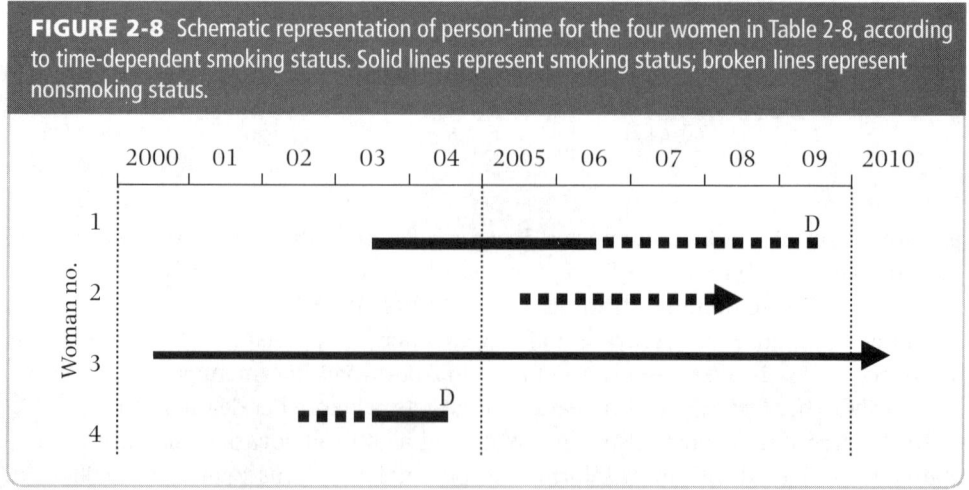

FIGURE 2-8 Schematic representation of person-time for the four women in Table 2-8, according to time-dependent smoking status. Solid lines represent smoking status; broken lines represent nonsmoking status.

2.2.3 Comparison Between Measures of Incidence

For the estimation of the different incidence measures, the numerator (number of deaths) is constant; the differentiation between the measures is given by the way the denominator is calculated. The main features that distinguish cumulative probability on the one hand and density or rate on the other are shown in Exhibit 2-1. As discussed previously, the upper limit of values for a rate or a density may exceed 100%, whereas values for probabilities cannot be greater than 100%.

Rates are often calculated as *yearly average rates* or, for example, as *rates per 1000 person-years*, the latter implying a rate per 1000 persons per year, which underscores the correspondence between a vital statistics-derived rate and a rate per person-time, as discussed previously. On the other hand, no time unit whatsoever is attached to a cumulative incidence (a probability), thus requiring that the relevant time period always be specified (e.g., "the cumulative probability *for the initial 3 years of follow-up*").

Another practical difference between the two types of incidence measures is that, although it is possible to calculate a cumulative incidence over time (using any of the survival analysis techniques described in Section 2.2.1), it is obviously not possible to obtain an overall *cumulative* rate over several time intervals (using either an average population or a person-time approach); this is, of course, a consequence of the "instantaneous" character of rate estimates.

With regard to their numerical value, a cumulative incidence and a rate can only be compared if they are based on the same time unit (e.g., cumulative incidence over a 1-year period and rate per person-year). Under this circumstance, the general rule is that, in absolute value, *the rate will always be larger than the cumulative incidence*. The rationale for this rule is best explained when comparing a rate with a cumulative incidence based on the classic life table, as illustrated in Exhibit 2-2. Although losses because of censoring are similarly taken into account in the denominator of both cumulative incidence and rate, the observation time "lost" by the cases is subtracted from the denominator of the rate but not from the probability-based cumulative incidence (which uses number of observations at the start of the interval corrected for losses, regardless of how many cases occur subsequently). As a result, the denominator for the rate will always tend to be smaller than

EXHIBIT 2-1 Comparing measures of incidence: cumulative incidence vs incidence rate.

	Cumulative incidence		Incidence rate	
	If follow-up is complete	*If follow-up is incomplete*	*Individual data (cohort)*	*Grouped data (area)*
Numerator	Number of cases	Classic life table Kaplan-Meier	Number of cases	Number of cases
Denominator	Initial population		Person-time	Average population*
Units	Unitless		Time^{-1}	
Range	0 to 1		0 to infinity	
Synonyms	Proportion Probability		Incidence density[†]	

*Equivalent to person-time when events and losses (or additions) are homogeneously distributed over the time interval of interest.
[†]In the text, the term *density* is used to refer to the situation in which the exact follow-up time for each individual is available; in real life, however, the terms *rate* and *density* are often used interchangeably.

that of the cumulative incidence and thus the larger absolute value of the former when compared with the latter. When events are relatively rare, the discrepancy is very small (e.g., example in Exhibit 2-2); as the frequency of the event increases, so will the numerical discrepancy between cumulative incidence and rate pertaining to the same time unit.

Finally, regarding assumptions, all methods for the calculation of incidence share the fundamental assumptions in the analysis of cohort data that were discussed in previous sections and are summarized in Exhibit 2-3: independence between censoring and survival, and lack of secular trends. Additional assumptions are needed depending on the specific requirements of the method (e.g., uniformity of risk across defined interval in classic life table and/or person-time-based analyses).

Experienced epidemiologists have learned that whereas each approach has advantages and disadvantages, the ultimate choice on how to present incidence data is dictated by pragmatism (and/or personal preference). Thus, in a cohort study without an "internal" unexposed group—as may be the case in occupational epidemiology research—estimation of densities, rather than probabilities, allows using available population rates as control rates. On the other hand, probabilities are typically estimated in studies with a focus on the temporal behavior (or "natural history") of a disease, as in studies of survival after diagnosis of disease.

2.2.4 The Hazard Rate

An alternative definition of an instantaneous incidence rate (density) is the so-called *hazard rate* or instantaneous conditional incidence or *force of morbidity* (or *mortality*). In the context of a cohort study, the hazard rate is defined as each individual's instantaneous probability of the event at precisely time t (or at a small interval

---

EXHIBIT 2-2 Comparing absolute numerical values of cumulative incidence based on the actuarial life table and rate (assuming that follow-up interval equals person-time unit). Notice that (as long as $x > 0$) the denominator of the rate will always be smaller than that of the cumulative incidence (960 vs 985 in the example), thus explaining the larger absolute value of the rate.

	In the absence of censoring	In the presence of censoring (C)	Example: N=1000 individuals followed for 1 year, x=50 events, C=30 censored observations
Cumulative incidence (q) is calculated based on number of individuals at risk *at the beginning* of the interval (N)	$q = \dfrac{x}{N}$	$q = \dfrac{x}{N - 1/2 C}$	$= \dfrac{50}{1000 - 1/2 \cdot 30}$ $= \dfrac{50}{985} = .0508$
Rate is calculated based on person-time of observation over the follow-up, subtracting person-time lost by the cases (x)	Rate $= \dfrac{x}{N - 1/2 x}$	Rate $= \dfrac{x}{N - 1/2 C - 1/2 x}$	$= \dfrac{50}{1000 - 1/2 \cdot 50 - 1/2 \cdot 30}$ $= \dfrac{50}{960} = .0521$

EXHIBIT 2-3 Assumptions necessary for survival and person-time analyses.

	Survival analysis	Person-time
If there are losses to follow-up:	Censored observations have an outcome probability that is similar to that of individuals remaining under observation.	
If intervals are used, and there are losses during a given interval:	Losses are uniform over the interval.	
If risk is calculated over intervals:	Risk is uniform during the interval.	N individuals followed for T units of time have the same risks as T individuals followed for N units of time.
If accrual of study subjects is done over a relatively long time period:	There are no secular trends over the calendar period covered by the accrual.	

$[t, t+\Delta t])$, given (or "conditioned" on) the fact that the individual was at risk at time t. The hazard rate is defined for each particular point in time during the follow-up. In mathematical terms, this is defined for a small time interval (Δt close to zero) as follows:

$$h(t) = \frac{P(\text{event in interval between } t \text{ and } [t+\Delta t] \mid \text{alive at } t)}{\Delta t}$$

The hazard is analogous to the conditional probability of the event that is calculated at each event time using Kaplan-Meier's approach (Table 2-3, column 4); however, because its denominator is "time-at-risk," it is a rate measured in units of time^{-1}. Another important difference is that, in contrast with the Kaplan-Meier's conditional probability, the hazard rate *cannot* be directly calculated, as it is defined for an infinitely small time interval; however, the hazard *function* over time can be estimated using available parametric survival analysis techniques.[13]

The hazard rate is a useful concept when trying to understand some of the statistical techniques used in survival analysis, particularly those pertaining to proportional hazards regression (see Chapter 7, Section 7.4.4). It is outside of the scope of this textbook, however, to discuss the complex mathematical properties of the hazard rate; the interested reader should consult more advanced statistical textbooks such as Collett's.[13]

2.3 MEASURES OF PREVALENCE

Prevalence is defined as the frequency of *existing* cases of a disease or other condition in a given population at a certain time or period. Depending on how "time" is defined, there are two kinds of prevalence, point prevalence and period prevalence (Table 2-1). *Point prevalence* is the frequency of a disease or condition at a point in time; it is the measure estimated in the so-called prevalence or cross-sectional surveys, such as the National Health and Nutrition Examination Surveys conducted by the US National Center for Health Statistics. For the calculation of point prevalence, it is important to emphasize that all existing cases at a given point in time are considered prevalent, regardless of whether they are old or more recent. *Period prevalence* is less commonly used and is defined as the frequency of an existing disease or condition during a defined time period. For example, the period prevalence of condition Y in year 2010 includes all existing cases on January 1, 2010, plus the new (incident) cases occurring during the year. A special type of period prevalence is the *cumulative lifetime prevalence*, which provides an estimate of the occurrence of a condition at any time during an individual's past (up to the present time). For example, the US-based 2003 National Youth Risk Behavior Survey estimated the lifetime prevalence of asthma among high school students to be 18.9%, whereas the estimated point prevalence at the time of the survey was estimated to be 16.1%.[14]

In the case of period prevalence, the denominator is defined as the average reference population over the period. In general, when the term *prevalence* is not specified, it can be taken to mean *point prevalence*. As a descriptive measure, point prevalence is a useful index of the magnitude of current health problems and is particularly relevant to public health and health policy (Chapter 10). In addition, prevalence is often used as the basis for the calculation of the *point prevalence rate ratio*, a measure of association in cross-sectional studies or in cohort studies using baseline data. Because the point prevalence rate ratio is often used as a "surrogate" of the incidence ratio in the absence of prospective cohort data (see Chapter 3, Section 3.3), it is important to understand prevalence's dependence on *both* incidence and duration of the disease after onset—duration is, in turn, determined by either survival for fatal diseases or recovery for nonfatal diseases. In a population in a steady-state situation (i.e., no major migrations or changes over time in incidence/prevalence of the condition of interest), the relationship between prevalence and disease incidence and duration can be expressed by the following formula:*

$$\frac{\text{Point prevalence}}{(1 - \text{Prevalence})} = \text{Incidence} \times \text{Duration} \qquad (\text{Eq. 2.3})$$

The term [Point prevalence ÷ (1 − Point prevalence)] is the odds of point prevalence (see Section 2.4). Also, in this equation and those derived from it, the time unit for incidence and duration should be the same: that is, if incidence is given as a yearly average, duration should be given using year(s) or a fraction thereof. Equation 2.3 can be rewritten as follows:

$$\text{Point prevalence} = \text{Incidence} \times \text{Duration} \times (1 - \text{Point prevalence}) \qquad (\text{Eq. 2.4})$$

As discussed in Chapters 3 and 4, Equation 2.4 underscores the two elements of a disease that are responsible for the difference between incidence and point prevalence:

---

*The derivation of this formula is fairly straightforward. Under the assumption that the disease is in steady state, the incidence and the number of existing cases at any given point (e.g., X) are approximately constant. For an incurable disease, this implies that the number of *new cases* during any given time period is approximately equal to the *number of deaths* among the cases. If N is the population size, I is the incidence, and F is the case fatality rate, the number of new cases can be estimated by multiplying the incidence times the number of potentially "susceptible" ($N − X$); in turn, the number of deaths can be estimated by multiplying the case fatality rate (F) times the number of prevalent cases. Thus, the above assumption can be formulated as follows: $I \times (N − X) \approx F \times X$. If there is no immigration, the case fatality rate is the inverse of the duration (D).[3] Thus, after a little arithmetical manipulation and dividing numerator and denominator of the right-hand side term by N:

$$I \times D \approx \frac{X}{(N - X)} = \frac{\text{Prevalence}}{(1 - \text{Prevalence})}$$

An analogous reasoning can be applied to nonfatal diseases, for which F is the proportion cured.

its duration and the magnitude of its point prevalence. When the point prevalence is relatively low (e.g., 0.05 or less), the term (1 − Point prevalence) is almost equal to 1.0, and the following well-known simplified formula defining the relationship between prevalence and incidence is obtained:

$$\text{Point prevalence} \approx \text{Incidence} \times \text{Duration}$$

For example, if the incidence of a disease that has remained stable over the years (e.g., diabetes) is 1% per year, and its approximate duration (survival after diagnosis) is 15 years, its point prevalence will be approximately 15%.

2.4 ODDS

Odds are the ratio of the probability of the event of interest to that of the nonevent. This can be defined both for incidence and for prevalence. For example, when dealing with incidence probabilities, the odds are

$$\text{Incidence odds} = \frac{q}{1-q}$$

(Alternatively, knowing the odds allows the calculation of probability: $q = \text{Odds} \div [1 + \text{Odds}]$.)

The point prevalence odds are as follows (see also Equation 2.3):

$$\text{Point prevalence odds} = \frac{\text{Point prevalence}}{1 - \text{Point prevalence}}$$

Both odds and proportions can be used to express "frequency" of the disease. An odds approximates a proportion when the latter is small (e.g., less than 0.1). For example,

$$\text{Proportion} = 0.05$$
$$\text{Odds} = 0.05/(1 - 0.05) = 0.05/0.95 = 0.0526$$

It is easier to grasp the intuitive meaning of the proportion than that of the odds, perhaps because in a description of odds, the nature of the latter as a ratio is often not clearly conveyed. For example, if the proportion of smokers in a population is 0.20, the odds are

$$\text{Odds} = \frac{\text{Proportion of smokers}}{1 - \text{Proportion of smokers}} = \frac{\text{Proportion of smokers}}{\text{Proportion of nonsmokers}}$$

or $0.20 \div (1 - 0.20) = 0.20 \div 0.80 = 1:4 = 0.25$.

Thus, there are two alternative ways to describe an odds estimate: either as an isolated number, 0.25, implying that the reader understands that it intrinsically expresses a ratio, 0.25:1.0, or clearly as a ratio—in the example, 1:4—conveying more explicitly the message that, in the study population, for every smoker there are four nonsmokers.

As an isolated absolute measure of disease occurrence, the odds are rarely if ever used by epidemiologists; however, the ratio of two odds (the odds ratio) is a very popular measure of association both because the logistic regression adjustment method is widely used and because the odds ratio allows the estimation of the easier-to-grasp relative risk in case-based case-control studies (see Chapter 1, Section 1.4.2; Chapter 3, Sections 3.2.1 and 3.4.1; and Chapter 7, Section 7.4.3).

REFERENCES

1. *Webster's Ninth New Collegiate Dictionary*. Springfield, MA: Merriam-Webster Inc.; 1988.
2. Centers for Disease Control. Revision of the CDC surveillance case definition for acquired immunodeficiency syndrome. *J Am Med Assoc*. 1987;258:1143–1145.
3. Rothman K, Greenland S. *Modern Epidemiology*, 3rd ed. Philadelphia: Wolters Kluwer Health/Lippincott Williams & Wilkins; 2008.
4. Kaplan EL, Meier P. Nonparametric estimation from incomplete observations. *J Am Stat Assoc*. 1958;53:457–481.
5. Reed LJ, Merrell M. A short method for constructing an abridged life table: 1939. *Am J Epidemiol*. 1995;141:993–1022; discussion 1991–1022.
6. Pooling Project Research Group. Relationship of blood pressure, serum cholesterol, smoking habit, relative weight and ECG abnormalities to incidence of major coronary events: Final report of the Pooling Project. *J Chron Dis*. 1978;31:201–306.
7. Gordis L. *Epidemiology*, 4th ed. Philadelphia: Elsevier Saunders; 2008.
8. Kahn HA, Sempos CT. *Statistical Methods in Epidemiology*. New York: Oxford University Press; 1989.
9. Checkoway H, Pearce, NE, Crawford-Brown, DJ. *Research Methods in Occupational Epidemiology*. New York: Oxford University Press; 1989.
10. Monson RR. Analysis of relative survival and proportional mortality. *Comput Biomed Res*. 1974;7:325–332.
11. Macaluso M. Exact stratification of person-years. *Epidemiology*. 1992;3:441–448.
12. Pearce N, Checkoway H. A simple computer program for generating person-time data in cohort studies involving time-related factors. *Am J Epidemiol*. 1987;125:1085–1091.
13. Collett D. *Modelling Survival Data in Medical Research*, 2nd ed. Boca Raton, FL: Chapman & Hall; 2003.
14. Centers for Disease Control and Prevention. Self-reported asthma among high school students: United States, 2003. *MMWR* 2005;54:765–767.

EXERCISES

1. A prospective study with a 2-year (24-month) follow-up was conducted. Results are shown in the table for individuals who either died or were censored before the end of the follow-up period.

Survival data for 20 participants of a hypothetical prospective study.	
Follow-up time (months)	**Event**
2	Death
4	Censored
7	Censored
8	Death
12	Censored
15	Death
17	Death
19	Death
20	Censored
23	Death

   a. Using the data from the table, calculate for all deaths: (a) the probability of death at the exact time when each death occurred, (b) the probability of survival beyond the time when each death occurred, and (c) the cumulative probabilities of survival.
   b. What is the cumulative survival probability at the end of the follow-up period?
   c. Using an arithmetic graph paper, plot the cumulative probabilities of survival.
   d. What is the simple proportion of individuals apparently surviving (i.e., not observed to die) through the end of the study's observation period?
   e. Why are the simple proportion surviving and the cumulative probability of survival different?
   f. Using the same data, calculate the overall death rate per 100 person-years. (To facilitate your calculations, you may wish to calculate the number of person-months and then convert it to the number of person-years.)
   g. Calculate the rates separately for the first and the second years of follow-up. (For this calculation, assume that the individual who withdrew at month 12 did it just after midnight on the last day of the month.)
   h. Assuming that there was no random variability, was it appropriate to calculate the rate per person-year for the total 2-year duration of follow-up?
   i. What is the most important assumption underlying the use of both survival analysis and the person-time approach?
   j. Now assume that the length of follow-up was the same for all individuals (except those who died). Calculate the proportion dying and the odds of death in this cohort.
   k. Why are these figures so different in this study?

2. In a cohort study of individuals aged 65 years and older and free of dementia at baseline,* the associations of age and APOE ε4 with the risk of incidence Alzheimer's disease (AD) were investigated. The table shows the number of individuals, person-years, and probable cases of AD, overall and according to age (< 80 and ≥ 80 years old) and, separately, to presence of APOE ε4.

Probable Alzheimer's disease (AD) by age and APOE ε4.				
	Number of individuals	Number with probable AD/person-years	Density of AD per 100 person-years	Average duration of follow-up
All subjects	3,099	263/18,933		
<80 years	2,343	157/15,529		
≥80 years	756	106/3,404		
APOE ε4(+)	702	94/4,200		
APOE ε4(−)	2,053	137/12,894		

   a. Calculate the densities of AD per 100 person-years, and the average durations of follow-up for all subjects and for each subgroup.
   b. Why is it important that the follow-up durations be similar for the "exposed" and "unexposed" categories, particularly in this study?
   c. When calculating a density for a given long follow-up period, the assumption is that the risk remains the same throughout the duration of follow-up. Is this a good assumption in the case of Alzheimer's Disease? Why or why not?

3. In a case-based case-control study of risk factors for uterine leiomyoma, the authors assessed a history of hypertension in cases and controls, as shown in the table here.

	Cases		Controls	
History of hypertension	Number	Percentage	Number	Percentage
Absent	248	78.0	363	92.4
Present	70	22.0	30	7.6
Total	318	100.0	393	100.0

   a. Using the absolute numbers of cases and controls with and without a history of hypertension, calculate the absolute odds of history of hypertension separately in cases and in controls.
   b. Now calculate the odds of hypertension using the percentages of cases and controls with a history of hypertension.

---

*Li G, Shofer JB, Rhew IC, et al. Age-varying association between statin use and incident Alzheimer's disease. J Am Geriatr Soc 2010; 58:1311–1317.

c. What can you conclude from comparing the response to question 2a to the response to question 2b?

d. Why are the odds of a history of hypertension more similar to the proportion of individuals with a history of hypertension in controls than in cases?

4. The baseline point prevalence of hypertension in African-American women aged 45–64 years included in the Atherosclerosis Risk in Communities (ARIC) cohort study was found to be 56%.[†] In this study, over a follow-up period of 6 years, the average yearly incidence of hypertension in African-American women was estimated to be about 5% and stable over the years.[‡] Using these data, estimate the average duration of hypertension in African American women in the ARIC study.

[†]Harris MM, Stevens J, Thomas N, et al. Associations of fat distribution and obesity with hypertension in a biethnic population: The ARIC study. *Obesity Res.* 2000;8:516–524.
[‡]Fuchs FD, Chambless LE, Whelton PK, et al. Alcohol consumption and the incidence of hypertension: The Atherosclerosis Risk in Communities Study. *Hypertension* 2001;37:1242–1250.

Measuring Associations Between Exposures and Outcomes

CHAPTER 3

3.1 INTRODUCTION

Epidemiologists are often interested in assessing the presence of associations expressed by differences in disease frequency. Measures of association can be based on either *absolute differences* between measures of disease frequency in groups being compared (e.g., exposed vs unexposed) or *relative differences* or ratios (Table 3-1). Measures based on absolute differences are often preferred when public health or preventive activities are contemplated, as their main goal is often an absolute reduction in the risk of an undesirable outcome. In contrast, etiologic studies that are searching disease determinants (causes) usually rely on relative differences in the occurrence of discrete outcomes, with the possible exception of instances in which the outcome of interest is continuous; in this situation, the assessment of mean absolute differences between exposed and unexposed individuals is also a frequently used method for evaluating an association (Table 3-1).

3.2 MEASURING ASSOCIATIONS IN A COHORT STUDY

In traditional prospective or cohort studies, study participants are selected in one of two ways: (1) a defined population or population sample is included in the study and classified according to level of exposure; or (2) exposed and unexposed individuals are specifically identified and included in the study. These individuals are then followed concurrently or nonconcurrently[1,2] for ascertainment of the outcome(s), allowing for the estimation of an incidence measure in each group (see also Chapters 1 and 2).

To simplify the concepts described in this chapter, only two levels of exposure are considered in most of the examples that follow—exposed and unexposed. Furthermore,

TABLE 3-1 Types of measures of association used in analytical epidemiologic studies.

Type	Examples	Usual application
Absolute difference	Attributable risk in exposed	Primary prevention impact; search for causes
	Population attributable risk	Primary prevention impact
	Effectiveness, efficacy	Impact of intervention on recurrences, case fatality, etc.
	Mean differences (continuous outcomes)	Search for causes
Relative difference	Relative risk/rate	Search for causes
	Relative odds	Search for causes

the length of follow-up is assumed to be complete in all individuals in the cohort (i.e., no censoring occurs). (The discussion that follows, however, also generally applies to risk and rate estimates that take into account incomplete follow-up and censoring, described in the previous chapter; Section 2.2.) For simplification purposes, this chapter focuses almost exclusively on the ratio of two simple incidence probabilities (proportions/risks) or odds (which are generically referred to in this chapter as relative risk and odds ratio, respectively) or on the absolute difference between two incidence probabilities (i.e., the attributable risk); however, concepts described in relationship to these measures also apply to a great extent to the other related association measures, such as the rate ratio and the hazard ratio. Finally, for the purposes of simplifying the description of measures of association, it is generally assumed that the estimates are not affected by either confounding or bias.

3.2.1 Relative Risk (Risk Ratio) and Odds Ratio

A classic two-by-two cross-tabulation of exposure and disease in a cohort study is shown in Table 3-2. Of a total of $(a + b)$ exposed and $(c + d)$ unexposed individuals, a exposed and c unexposed develop the disease of interest during the follow-up time. The corresponding risk and odds estimates are shown in the last two columns of Table 3-2. The probability odds of the disease (the ratio of the probability of disease to the probability of no disease) arithmetically reduces to the ratio of the number of cases divided by the number of individuals who do not develop the disease for each exposure category.

The *relative risk* of developing the disease is expressed as the ratio of the risk (incidence) in exposed individuals (q_+) to that in unexposed (q_-):

$$\text{Relative risk (RR)} = \frac{q_+}{q_-} = \frac{\dfrac{a}{a+b}}{\dfrac{c}{c+d}} \qquad \text{(Eq. 3.1)}$$

For methods on estimating confidence limits and p values for a relative risk, see Appendix A, Section A.3.

The *odds ratio* (or *relative odds*) of disease development is the ratio of the odds of developing the disease in exposed individuals divided by that in unexposed individuals. In Table 3-2, the odds of disease are based on incidence proportions or probabilities; thus, it is occasionally designated *probability odds ratio*. The ratio of the probability odds of disease is equivalent to the *cross-product ratio*, $(a \times d)/(b \times c)$. Using the notation in Table 3-2:

TABLE 3-2 Cross-tabulation of exposure and disease in a cohort study.

Exposure	Diseased	Nondiseased	Disease incidence (risk)	Probability odds of disease	
Present	a	b	$q_+ = \dfrac{a}{a+b}$	$\dfrac{q_+}{1-q_+} = \dfrac{\dfrac{a}{a+b}}{1-\left(\dfrac{a}{a+b}\right)}$	$= \dfrac{a}{b}$
Absent	c	d	$q_- = \dfrac{c}{c+d}$	$\dfrac{q_-}{1-q_-} = \dfrac{\dfrac{c}{c+d}}{1-\left(\dfrac{c}{c+d}\right)}$	$= \dfrac{c}{d}$

$$\text{Probability odds ratio (OR)} = \frac{\frac{q_+}{1-q_+}}{\frac{q_-}{1-q_-}} = \frac{\frac{a}{a+b}}{1-\left(\frac{a}{a+b}\right)} \div \frac{\frac{c}{c+d}}{1-\left(\frac{c}{c+d}\right)} = \frac{\frac{a}{a+b}}{\frac{b}{a+b}} \div \frac{\frac{c}{c+d}}{\frac{d}{c+d}} = \frac{a}{b} \div \frac{c}{d}$$

Thus,

$$\text{OR} = \frac{a \times d}{b \times c} \quad \text{(Eq. 3.2)}$$

For methods on obtaining confidence limits and p values for an odds ratio, see Appendix A, Section A.4.

In the hypothetical example shown in Table 3-3, severe hypertension and acute myocardial infarction are the exposure and the outcome of interest, respectively. The sample size for each level of exposure was arbitrarily set at 10,000 to facilitate the calculations. For these data, because the probability (risk, incidence) of myocardial infarction is low for both the exposed and the unexposed groups, the probability odds of developing the disease approximate the probabilities; as a result, the probability odds ratio of disease (exposed vs unexposed) approximates the relative risk:

$$\text{RR} = \frac{\frac{180}{10{,}000}}{\frac{30}{10{,}000}} = \frac{0.018}{0.003} = 6.00$$

$$\text{Probability OR} = \frac{\frac{180}{9820}}{\frac{30}{9970}} = \frac{0.01833}{0.00301} = 6.09$$

A different situation emerges when the probabilities of developing the outcome are high in exposed and unexposed individuals. For example, Seltser et al.[3] examined the incidence of local reactions in individuals assigned randomly to either an injectable

TABLE 3-3 Hypothetical cohort study of the 1-year incidence of acute myocardial infarction in individuals with severe systolic hypertension ($\geq$ 180 mm Hg) and normal systolic blood pressure (< 120 mm Hg).

Blood pressure status	Number	Myocardial infarction			Probability odds$_{dis}$
		Present	Absent	Probability	
Severe hypertension	10,000	180	9820	180/10,000 = 0.018	180/(10,000 − 180) = 180/9820 = 0.01833
Normal	10,000	30	9970	30/10,000 = 0.003	30/(10,000 − 30) = 30/9970 = 0.00301

influenza vaccine or a placebo group. Table 3-4, based on this study, shows that as the probability (incidence) of local reactions is high, the probability odds estimates of local reactions do not approximate the probabilities (particularly in the group assigned to the vaccine). Thus, the probability odds ratio of local reactions (vaccine vs placebo) is fairly different from the relative risk:

$$\text{RR} = \frac{\frac{650}{2570}}{\frac{170}{2410}} = \frac{0.2529}{0.0705} = 3.59 \qquad \text{OR} = \frac{\frac{650}{1920}}{\frac{170}{2240}} = \frac{0.3385}{0.0759} = 4.46$$

When the condition of interest has a high incidence and when prospective data are available, as was the case in this vaccination trial, the common practice is to report the relative risk because it is a more easily understood measure of association between the risk factor and the outcome.

Although, as discussed later, the odds ratio is a valid measure of association in its own right, it is often used as an approximation of the relative risk in situations when the latter cannot be calculated (i.e., case-control studies, see Section 3.4.1).

In any case, when used as an *estimate of the relative risk*, the odds ratio is biased in a direction opposite to the null hypothesis. In other words, when compared to the relative risk, the numerical value of the odds ratio tends to exaggerate the magnitude of the association. When the disease is relatively rare, this "built-in" bias is negligible, as in the previous example from Table 3-3. When the incidence is high, however, as in the vaccine trial example (Table 3-4), the bias can be substantial.

An expression of the mathematical relationship between the odds ratio on the one hand and the relative risk on the other can be derived as follows. Assume that q_+ is the incidence (probability) in exposed (e.g., vaccinated) and q_- the incidence in unexposed individuals. The odds ratio is then

$$\text{OR} = \frac{\left(\frac{q_+}{1-q_+}\right)}{\left(\frac{q_-}{1-q_-}\right)} = \frac{q_+}{1-q_+} \times \frac{1-q_-}{q_-} = \frac{q_+}{q_-} \times \left(\frac{1-q_-}{1-q_+}\right) \qquad \text{(Eq. 3.3)}$$

TABLE 3-4 Incidence of local reactions in the vaccinated and placebo groups, influenza vaccination trial.

		Local reaction			
Group	Number	Present	Absent	Probability	Probability odds$_{dis}$
Vaccine	2570	650	1920	650/2570 = 0.2529	650/(2570 − 650) = 650/1920 = 0.3385
Placebo	2410	170	2240	170/2410 = 0.0705	170/(2410 − 170) = 170/2240 = 0.0759

Note: Based on data for individuals 40 years old or older in Seltser et al.[3] To avoid rounding ambiguities in subsequent examples based on these data (Figure 3-4, Tables 3-7 and 3-9), the original sample sizes in Seltser et al.'s study (257 vaccinees and 241 placebo recipients) were multiplied by 10.
Source: Data from R Seltser, PE Sartwell, and JA Bell, A Controlled Test of Asian Influenza Vaccine in Population of Families. *American Journal of Hygiene*, Vol 75, pp. 112–135, © 1962.

The term q_+/q_- in Equation 3.3 is the relative risk. Thus, the term

$$\left(\frac{1-q_-}{1-q_+}\right)$$

defines the *bias* responsible for the discrepancy between the relative risk and the odds ratio estimates (*built-in bias*). If the association between the exposure and the outcome is positive, $q_- < q_+$, thus $(1-q_-) > (1-q_+)$. The bias term will therefore be greater than 1.0, leading to an overestimation of the relative risk by the odds ratio. By analogy, if the factor is related to a decrease in risk, the opposite occurs (i.e., $[1-q_-] < [1-q_+]$), and the odds ratio will again overestimate the strength of the association (in this case, by being smaller than the relative risk in absolute value). In general, the odds ratio tends to yield an estimate further away from 1.0 than the relative risk on both sides of the scale (above or below 1.0).

In the hypertension/myocardial infarction example (Table 3-3), the bias factor is of a small magnitude, and the odds ratio estimate, albeit a bit more distant from 1.0, still approximates the relative risk; using Equation 3.3:

$$\text{OR} = \text{RR} \times \text{"built-in bias"} = 6.0 \times \frac{1-0.003}{1-0.018} = 6.0 \times 1.015 = 6.09$$

In the example of local reactions to the influenza vaccine (Table 3-4), however, there is a considerable bias when using the odds ratio to estimate the relative risk:

$$\text{OR} = 3.59 \times \frac{1-0.0705}{1-0.2529} = 3.59 \times 1.244 = 4.46$$

Regardless of whether the odds ratio can properly estimate the relative risk, it is, as mentioned previously, a *bona fide* measure of association. Thus, a *built-in bias* can only be said to exist when the odds ratio is used as an estimate of the relative risk. The odds ratio is especially valuable because it can be measured in case-control (case–noncase) studies and because it is directly derived from logistic regression models (see Chapter 7, Section 7.4.3). In addition, unlike the relative risk, the odds ratio of an event is the exact reciprocal of the odds ratio of the nonevent. For example, in the study of local reactions to the influenza vaccine discussed previously,[3] the odds ratio of a local reaction

$$\text{OR}_{\text{local reaction }(+)} = \frac{\frac{650}{1920}}{\frac{170}{2240}} = 4.46$$

is the exact reciprocal of the odds ratio of not having a local reaction

$$\text{OR}_{\text{local reaction }(-)} = \frac{\frac{1920}{650}}{\frac{2240}{170}} = 0.224 = \frac{1}{4.46}$$

This feature is not shared by the relative risk: using the same example

$$\text{RR}_{\text{local reaction }(+)} = \frac{\frac{650}{2570}}{\frac{170}{2410}} = 3.59$$

and

$$\text{RR}_{\text{local reaction }(-)} = \frac{\frac{1920}{2570}}{\frac{2240}{2410}} = 0.8 \neq \frac{1}{3.59}$$

This seemingly paradoxical finding results from the sensitivity of the relative risk to the absolute frequency of the condition of interest, with relative risks associated with *very* common endpoints approaching 1.0. This is easily appreciated when studying the complement of rare outcomes. For example, if the case fatality rates of patients undergoing surgery using a standard surgical technique and a new technique were 0.02 and 0.01, respectively, the relative risk for the relatively rare outcome "death" would be $0.02/0.01 = 2.0$. The relative risk for survival (a common outcome), however, would be 0.98/0.99, which is virtually equal to 1.0, suggesting that the new surgical technique did not affect survival. On the other hand, the odds ratio of death would be

$$\text{OR}_{\text{death}} = \frac{\frac{0.02}{1.0 - 0.02}}{\frac{0.01}{1.0 - 0.01}} = 2.02$$

and that of survival would be

$$\text{OR}_{\text{survival}} = \frac{\frac{0.98}{1.0 - 0.98}}{\frac{0.99}{1.0 - 0.99}} = 0.495 = \frac{1}{2.02}$$

3.2.2 Attributable Risk

The *attributable risk* is a measure of association based on the absolute difference between two risk estimates. Thus, the attributable risk estimates the absolute excess risk associated with a given exposure. Because the attributable risk is often used to imply a cause–effect relationship, it should be interpreted as a true *etiologic fraction* only when there is reasonable certainty of a causal connection between exposure and outcome.[4,5] The term *excess fraction* has been suggested as an alternative term when causality has not been firmly established.[4] Also, although the formulas and examples in this section generally refer to attributable "risks," they are also applicable to attributable rates or densities; that is, if incidence data based on person-time are used, an attributable rate among the exposed can be calculated in units of rate per person-time.

As extensively discussed by Gordis,[2] the attributable risk assumes the following different formats.

Attributable Risk in Exposed Individuals

The attributable risk in the exposed is merely the difference between the risk estimates of different exposure levels and a reference exposure level; the latter is usually formed by the unexposed (or the lowest exposure level) category. Assuming a binary exposure

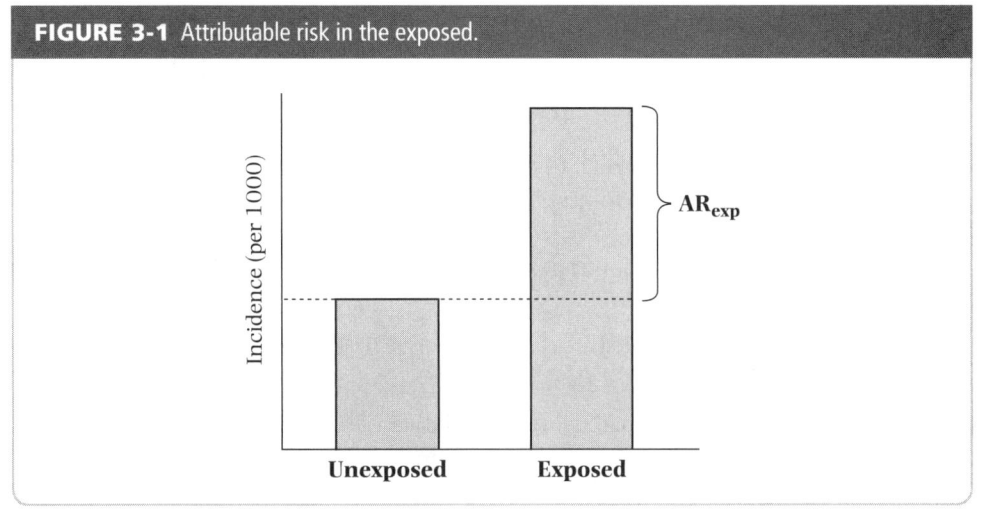

FIGURE 3-1 Attributable risk in the exposed.

variable and letting risk in exposed equal q_+ and risk in unexposed equal q_-, the attributable risk in the exposed (AR_{exp}) is simply

$$AR_{exp} = q_+ - q_- \qquad (Eq.\ 3.4)$$

The attributable risk in the exposed measures the excess risk associated with a given exposure category. For example, based on the example in Table 3-3, the cumulative incidence of myocardial infarction among the severely hypertensive individuals (q_+) is 0.018 (or 1.8%), and that for normotensives (reference or unexposed category) (q_-) is 0.003 (or 0.3%); thus, the excess risk associated with exposure to severe hypertension is 0.018 − 0.003 = 0.015 (or 1.5%). That is, assuming a causal association (and thus, no confounding or bias—see Chapters 4 and 5) and if the excess incidence were completely reversible, the cessation of the exposure (severe systolic hypertension) would lower the risk in the exposed group from 0.018 to 0.003. In Figure 3-1, the two bars represent the cumulative incidence in exposed and unexposed individuals; thus, the attributable risk in the exposed (Equation 3.4) is the difference in height between these bars. Because it is the difference between two incidence measures, the attributable risk in the exposed is also an absolute incidence magnitude and therefore is measured using the same units. The estimated attributable risk in the exposed of 1.5% in the previous example represents the absolute excess incidence that would be prevented by eliminating severe hypertension.

Because most exposure effects are cumulative, cessation of exposure (even if causally related to the disease) usually does not reduce the risk in exposed individuals to the level found in those who were never exposed. Thus, the maximum risk reduction is usually achieved only through prevention of exposure rather than its cessation.

Percent Attributable Risk in Exposed Individuals

A percent attributable risk in the exposed (%AR_{exp}) is merely the AR_{exp} expressed as a percentage of the q_+ (i.e., the percentage of the total q_+ that can be attributed to the exposure). For a binary exposure variable, it is calculated as follows:

$$\%AR_{exp} = \left(\frac{q_+ - q_-}{q_+}\right) \times 100 \qquad (Eq.\ 3.5)$$

In the example shown in Table 3-3, the percent attributable risk in the exposed is

$$\%AR_{exp} = \frac{0.018 - 0.003}{0.018} \times 100 = 83.3\%$$

If causality had been established, this measure can be interpreted as the percentage of the total risk of myocardial infarction among hypertensives that is attributable to hypertension.

It may be useful to express Equation 3.5 in terms of the relative risk:

$$\%AR_{exp} = \left(\frac{q_+ - q_-}{q_+}\right) \times 100 = \left(1 - \frac{1}{RR}\right) \times 100 = \left(\frac{RR - 1.0}{RR}\right) \times 100$$

Thus, in the previous example, using the relative risk (0.018/0.003 = 6.0) in this formula produces the same result as when applying Equation 3.5:

$$\%AR_{exp} = \left(\frac{6.0 - 1.0}{6.0}\right) \times 100 = 83.3\%$$

The obvious advantage of the formula

$$\%AR_{exp} = \left(\frac{RR - 1.0}{RR}\right) \times 100 \qquad \text{(Eq. 3.6)}$$

is that it can be used in case-control studies, in which incidence data (i.e., q_+ or q_-) are unavailable, but the odds ratio can be used as an estimate of the relative risk if the disease is relatively rare (see Section 3.2.1).

The percent attributable risk in the exposed is analogous to percentage *efficacy* when assessing an intervention such as a vaccine. The usual formula for efficacy is equivalent to the formula for percent attributable risk in the exposed (Equation 3.5) when q_+ is replaced by q_{cont} (risk in the control group, e.g., the group receiving a placebo) and q_- is replaced by q_{interv} (risk in those undergoing intervention):

$$\text{Efficacy} = \left(\frac{q_{cont} - q_{interv}}{q_{cont}}\right) \times 100 \qquad \text{(Eq. 3.7)}$$

For example, in a randomized trial to evaluate the efficacy of a vaccine, the risks in persons receiving the vaccine and the placebo are 5% and 15%, respectively. Using Equation 3.7, efficacy is found to be 66.7%:

$$\text{Efficacy} = \left(\frac{15\% - 5\%}{15\%}\right) \times 100 = 66.7\%$$

Alternatively, Equation 3.6 can be used to estimate efficacy. In the previous example, the relative risk (placebo/vaccine) is 15% ÷ 5% = 3.0. Thus,

$$\text{Efficacy} = \left(\frac{3.0 - 1.0}{3.0}\right) \times 100 = 66.7\%$$

The use of Equation 3.6 for the calculation of efficacy requires that, when calculating the relative risk, the group not receiving the intervention (e.g., placebo) be regarded as "exposed" and the group receiving the active intervention (e.g., vaccine) be regarded as "unexposed." A mathematically equivalent approach would consist of first obtaining the relative risk, but this time with the risk of those receiving the active intervention (e.g., vaccine) in the numerator and those not receiving it in the denominator (e.g., placebo). In this case, efficacy is calculated as the complement of the relative risk, that is, $(1.0 - RR) \times 100$. In the previous example, using this approach, the vaccine efficacy would be

$$\text{Efficacy} = \left[1.0 - \left(\frac{5\%}{15\%}\right)\right] \times 100 = 66.7\%$$

As for percent attributable risk, the correspondence between the relative risk and the odds ratio in most practical situations allows the estimation of efficacy in case-control studies using Equation 3.6.

Levin's Population Attributable Risk

Levin's population attributable risk estimates the proportion of the disease risk in the total population associated with the exposure.[6] For example, let the exposure prevalence in the target population (p_e) be 0.40 (and, thus, prevalence of *nonexposure*, $[1 - p_e]$, be 0.60), and the risks in exposed and unexposed be $q_+ = 0.20$ and $q_- = 0.15$, respectively. Thus, the risk in the total population (q_{pop}) is as follows:

$$q_{pop} = [q_+ \times p_e] + [q_- \times (1 - p_e)] \quad \text{(Eq. 3.8)}$$

representing the weighted sum of the risks in the exposed and unexposed individuals in the population. In the example

$$q_{pop} = (0.20 \times 0.40) + (0.15 \times 0.60) = 0.17$$

The population attributable risk (Pop AR) is the difference between the risk in the total population and that in unexposed subjects:

$$\text{Pop AR} = q_{pop} - q_-$$

Thus, in the example, the population attributable risk is $0.17 - 0.15 = 0.02$. That is, if the relationship were causal and if the effect of the exposure were completely reversible, exposure cessation would be expected to result in a decrease in total population risk (q_{pop}) from 0.17 to 0.15 (i.e., to the level of risk of the unexposed group).

The Pop AR is usually expressed as the percent population attributable risk (%Pop AR):

$$\%\text{Pop AR} = \frac{(q_{pop} - q_-)}{q_{pop}} \times 100 \quad \text{(Eq. 3.9)}$$

In the previous example, the percent population attributable risk is $(0.02/0.17) \times 100$, or approximately 12%.

As seen in Equation 3.8, the incidence in the total population is the sum of the incidence in the exposed and that in the unexposed, weighted for the proportions of exposed and unexposed individuals in the population. Thus, when the exposure prevalence is low, the population incidence will be closer to the incidence among the unexposed (Figure 3-2A). On the other hand, if the exposure is highly prevalent (Figure 3-2B), the population incidence will be closer to the incidence among the exposed. As a result, the population attributable risk approximates the attributable risk in exposed individuals when exposure prevalence is high.

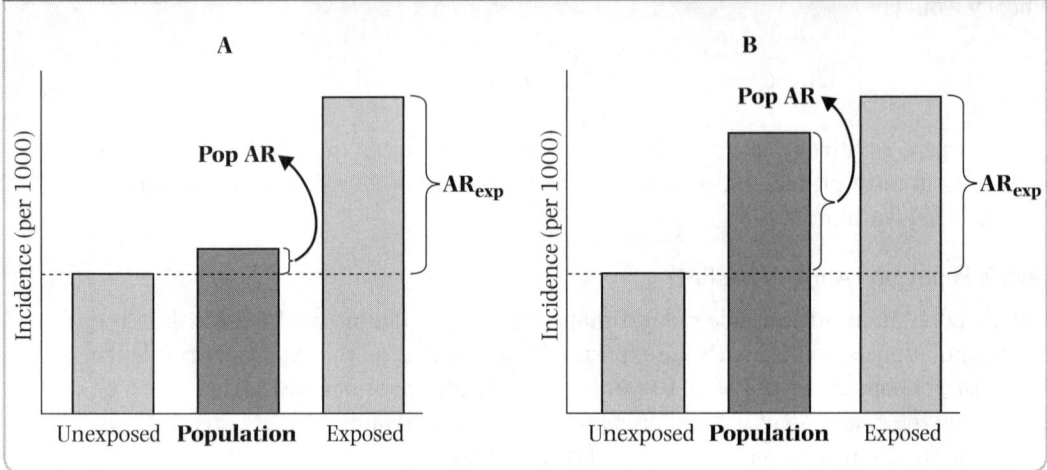

FIGURE 3-2 Population attributable risk and its dependence on the population prevalence of the exposure. As the population is composed of exposed and unexposed individuals, the incidence in the population is similar to the incidence in the unexposed when the exposure is rare (A) and is closer to that in the exposed when the exposure is common (B). Thus, for a fixed relative risk (eg, RR ≈ 2 in the figure) the population attributable risk is heavily dependent on the prevalence of exposure.

After simple arithmetical manipulation,* Equation 3.9 can be expressed as a function of the exposure prevalence in the population and the relative risk, as first described by Levin:[6]

$$\%\text{Pop AR} = \frac{p_e \times (\text{RR} - 1)}{p_e \times (\text{RR} - 1) + 1} \times 100 \qquad \text{(Eq. 3.10)}$$

Using the same example of a population with an exposure prevalence of 0.40 and a relative risk = 0.20/0.15 = 1.33, Equation 3.10 yields the same percent population attributable risk estimated previously:

$$\%\text{Pop AR} = \frac{0.40 \times (1.33 - 1.0)}{0.40 \times (1.33 - 1.0) + 1.0} \times 100 = \frac{0.40 \times 0.33}{0.40 \times 0.33 + 1.0} = 12\%$$

---

*Using Equation 3.8, Equation 3.9 can be rewritten as a function of the prevalence of exposure (p_e) and the incidence in exposed (q_+) individuals as follows

$$\%\text{Pop AR} = \frac{[q_+ \times p_e] + [q_- \times (1 - p_e)] - q_-}{[q_+ \times p_e] + [q_- \times (1 - p_e)]} \times 100$$

$$= \frac{[q_+ \times p_e] - [q_- \times p_e]}{[q_+ \times p_e] - [q_- \times p_e] + q_-} \times 100$$

This expression can be further simplified by dividing all the terms in numerator and denominator by q_-

$$\%\text{Pop AR} = \frac{\frac{q_+}{q_-} \times p_e - p_e}{\frac{q_+}{q_-} \times p_e - p_e + 1} \times 100 = \frac{p_e \times \left(\frac{q_+}{q_-} - 1\right)}{p_e \times \left(\frac{q_+}{q_-} - 1\right) + 1} \times 100$$

$$= \frac{p_e \times (\text{RR} - 1)}{p_e \times (\text{RR} - 1) + 1} \times 100$$

For a method of calculating the confidence limits of the population attributable risk, see Appendix A, Section A.5.

Levin's formula underscores the importance of the two critical elements contributing to the magnitude of the population attributable risk: the relative risk and the prevalence of exposure. The dependence of the population attributable risk on the exposure prevalence is further illustrated in Figure 3-3, which shows that for all values of the relative risk, the population attributable risk increases markedly as the exposure prevalence increases.

The application of Levin's formula in case-control studies requires using the odds ratio as an estimate of the relative risk and obtaining an estimate of exposure prevalence in the reference population, as discussed in more detail in Section 3.4.2.

All of the preceding discussion relates to a binary exposure variable (i.e., exposed vs unexposed). When the exposure has more than two categories, an extension of Levin's formula has been derived by Walter.[7]

$$\%\text{Pop AR} = \frac{p_i \times (RR_i - 1)}{1 + \sum_{i=0}^{k} p_i \times (RR_i - 1)} \times 100$$

The subscript i denotes each exposure level; p_i is the proportion of the study population in the exposure level i, and "RR_i" is the relative risk for the exposure level i compared with the unexposed (reference) level.

It is important to emphasize that both Levin's formula and Walter's extension for multilevel exposures assume that there is no confounding (see Chapter 5). If confounding

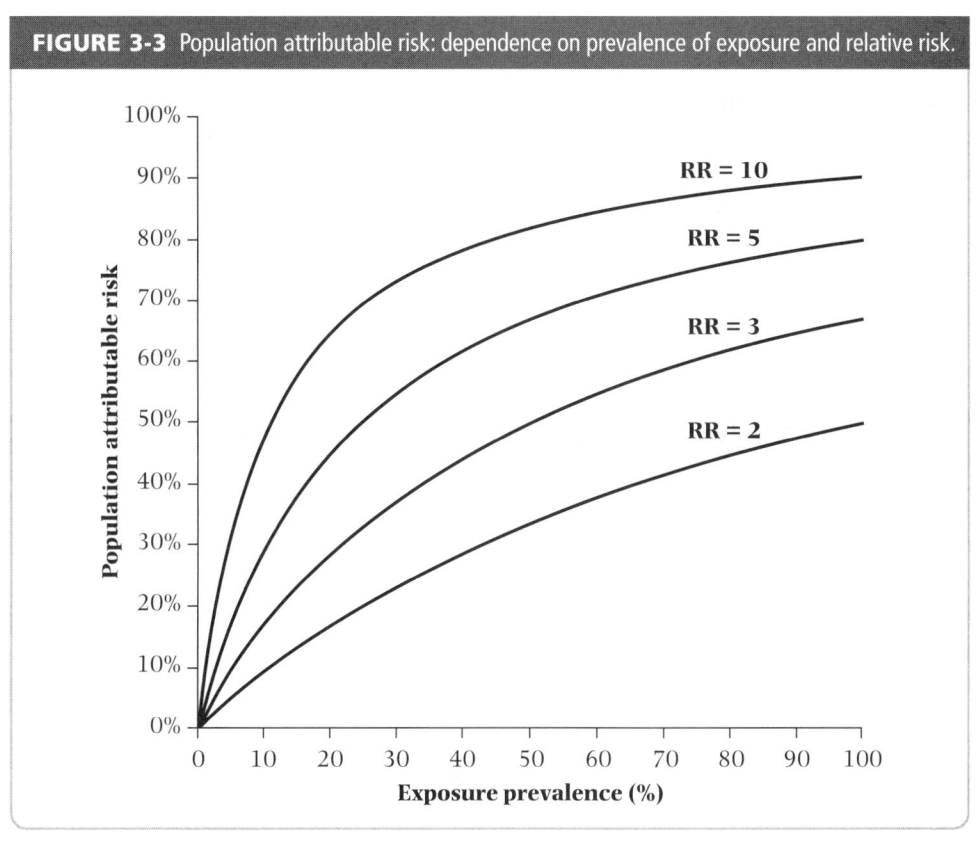

FIGURE 3-3 Population attributable risk: dependence on prevalence of exposure and relative risk.

is present, it is not appropriate to calculate the adjusted relative risk (using any of the approaches described in Chapter 7) and plug it into Levin's or Walter's formulas in order to obtain an "adjusted" population attributable risk.[8] Detailed discussions on the estimation of the population attributable risk in the presence of confounding can be found elsewhere.[7,9]

3.3 CROSS-SECTIONAL STUDIES: POINT PREVALENCE RATE RATIO

When cross-sectional data are available, often associations are assessed using the *point prevalence rate ratio*. The ability of the point prevalence ratio to estimate the relative risk is a function of the relationship between incidence and point prevalence, as discussed previously in Chapter 2 (Section 2.3, Equation 2.4):

$$\text{Point prevalence} = \text{Incidence} \times \text{Duration} \times (1 - \text{Point prevalence})$$

Using the notations "Prev" for point prevalence, "q" for incidence, and "Dur" for duration and denoting presence or absence of a given exposure by "+" or "−," the point prevalence rate ratio (PRR) can be formulated as follows:

$$\text{PRR} = \frac{\text{Prev}_+}{\text{Prev}_-} = \frac{q_+ \times \text{Dur}_+ \times [1.0 - \text{Prev}_+]}{q_- \times \text{Dur}_- \times [1.0 - \text{Prev}_-]}$$

Because one of the components of this formula (q_+/q_-) is the relative risk, this equation can be written as

$$\text{PRR} = \text{RR} \times \left(\frac{\text{Dur}_+}{\text{Dur}_-}\right) \times \left(\frac{1 - \text{Prev}_+}{1 - \text{Prev}_-}\right) \quad \text{(Eq. 3.11)}$$

Thus, if the point prevalence rate ratio is used to estimate the relative risk (e.g., in a cross-sectional study), two types of potential bias will differentiate these two measures: the ratio of the disease durations ($\text{Dur}_+/\text{Dur}_-$), and the ratio of the complements of the point prevalence estimates in the exposed and unexposed groups:

$$\frac{(1 - \text{Prev}_+)}{(1 - \text{Prev}_-)}$$

Chapter 4 (Section 4.4.2) provides a discussion and examples of these biases.

3.4 MEASURING ASSOCIATIONS IN CASE-CONTROL STUDIES

3.4.1 Odds Ratio

One of the major advances in risk estimation in epidemiology occurred in 1951 when Cornfield pointed out that the *odds ratio of disease and the odds ratio of exposure are mathematically equivalent*.[10] This is a simple concept, yet with important implications for the epidemiologist, as it is the basis for estimating the odds ratio of disease in case-control studies.

As seen previously in Equation 3.2, the ratio of the odds of disease development in exposed and unexposed individuals results in the cross-product ratio, $(a \times d)/(b \times c)$. Using the hypothetical *prospective* data shown in Table 3-3, now reorganized as shown in Table 3-5, and assuming that the cells in the table represent the distribution of cohort

TABLE 3-5 Hypothetical case-control study of myocardial infarction in relation to systolic hypertension, based on a 1-year complete follow-up of the study population from Table 3-3.

Systolic blood pressure status*	Myocardial infarction			
	Present		Absent	
Severe hypertension	180	(a)	9820	(b)
Normal	30	(c)	9970	(d)
Total	210	(a + c)	19,790	(b + d)

*Severe systolic hypertension ≥ 180 mm Hg, and normal systolic blood pressure < 120 mm Hg.

participants during a 1-year follow-up, it is possible to carry out a case-control analysis comparing the 210 individuals who developed a myocardial infarction (cases) with the 19,790 individuals who remained free of clinical coronary heart disease during the follow-up (controls). The *absolute* odds of exposure ($Odds_{exp}$) among cases and the analogous odds of exposure among controls are estimated as the ratio of the proportion of individuals exposed to the proportion of individuals unexposed:

$$Odds_{exp\ cases} = \frac{\frac{a}{a+c}}{1 - \left(\frac{a}{a+c}\right)} = \frac{a}{c}$$

$$Odds_{exp\ controls} = \frac{\frac{b}{b+d}}{1 - \left(\frac{b}{b+d}\right)} = \frac{b}{d}$$

The following derivation demonstrates that the odds ratio of exposure (OR_{exp}) is identical to the odds ratio of disease (OR_{dis}), i.e., the ratio of odds of disease in exposed (a/b) to that in unexposed (c/d):

$$OR_{exp} = \frac{\frac{a}{c}}{\frac{b}{d}} = \frac{a \times d}{b \times c} = \frac{\frac{a}{b}}{\frac{c}{d}} = OR_{dis} \quad (Eq.\ 3.12)$$

For the example shown in Table 3-5, the odds ratio of exposure is

$$OR_{exp} = \frac{\frac{180}{30}}{\frac{9820}{9970}} = \frac{180 \times 9970}{9820 \times 30} = 6.09 = OR_{dis}$$

In this example based on prospective data, all cases and noncases (controls) have been used for the estimation of the odds ratio; however, case-control studies are typically based on samples. If the total number of cases is small, as in the example shown in Table 3-5, the investigator may attempt to include all cases and a sample of controls. For example, if 100% of cases and a sample of approximately 10% of the noncases were

TABLE 3-6 Case-control study of the relationship of myocardial infarction to presence of severe systolic hypertension including all cases and a 10% sample of noncases from Table 3-5.

	Myocardial infarction			
Systolic blood pressure status*	Present		Absent	
Severe hypertension	180	(a)	982	(b)
Normal	30	(c)	997	(d)
Total	210	(a + c)	1979	(b + d)

*Severe systolic hypertension ≥ 180 mm Hg, and normal systolic blood pressure < 120 mm Hg.

studied (Table 3-6), assuming no random variability, results would be identical to those obtained when including all noncases, as in Table 3-5:

$$OR_{exp} = \frac{\frac{180}{30}}{\frac{982}{997}} = \frac{180 \times 997}{982 \times 30} = 6.09 = OR_{dis}$$

This example underscores the notion that the sampling fractions do not have to be the same in cases and controls. To obtain unbiased estimates of the absolute odds of exposure for cases and controls, however, sampling fractions must be independent of exposure: that is, they should apply equally to cells (*a*) and (*c*) for cases and cells (*b*) and (*d*) for controls. (Chapter 4, Section 4.2, presents a more detailed discussion of the validity implications for the OR estimate resulting from differential sampling fractions according to case and exposure status.)

In the example of local reactions to vaccination (Table 3-4), a case-control study could have been carried out including, for example, 80% of the cases that had local reactions and 50% of the controls. Assuming no random variability, data would be obtained as outlined in Figure 3-4 and shown in Table 3-7. If the sampling fractions apply equally to exposed (vaccinated) and unexposed (unvaccinated) cases and controls, the results are again identical to those seen in the total population, in which the (true) odds ratio is 4.46:

$$OR_{exp} = \frac{\frac{520}{136}}{\frac{960}{1120}} = 4.46 = OR_{dis}$$

The fact that the odds ratio of exposure is identical to the odds ratio of disease permits a "prospective" interpretation of the odds ratio in case-control studies (i.e., as a *disease odds ratio*—which, in turn, is an approximation of the relative risk, as discussed later in this chapter). Thus, in the previous example based on a case-control strategy (and assuming that the study is unbiased and free of confounding), the interpretation of results is that for individuals who received the vaccine, the odds of developing local reactions is 4.46 times greater than the odds for those who received the placebo.

The use of the ratio of the odds of exposure for cases to that for controls,

$$OR_{exp} = \frac{Odds_{exp\,cases}}{Odds_{exp\,controls}}$$

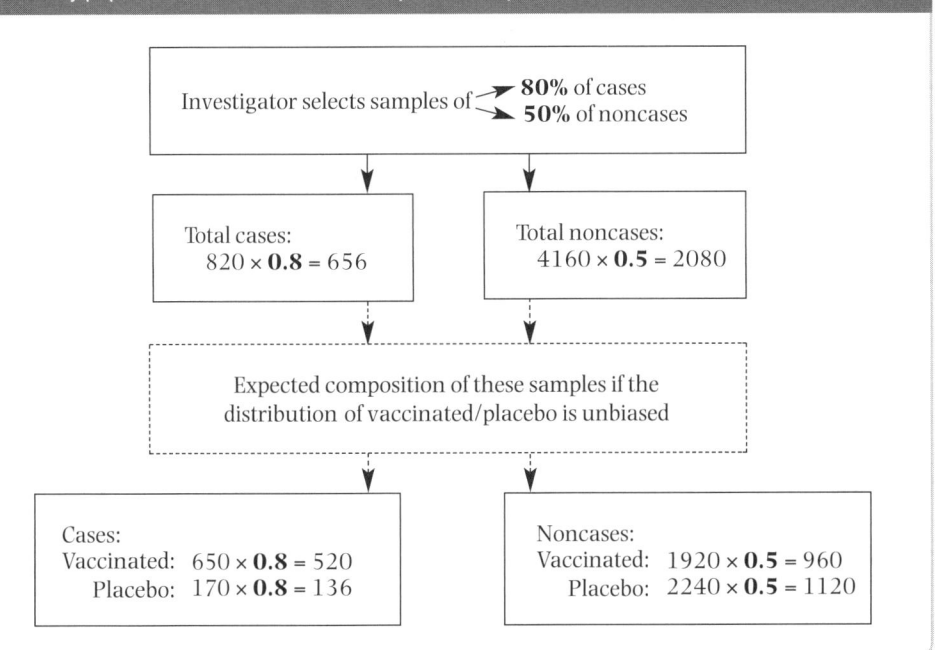

FIGURE 3-4 Selection of 80% of total cases and 50% of noncases in a case-control study from the study population shown in Table 3-4. Expected composition assumes no random variability.

Source: Data from R Seltser, PE Sartwell, and JA Bell, A Controlled Test of Asian Influenza Vaccine in a Population of Families, *American Journal of Hygiene*, Vol 75, pp. 112–135, © 1962.

TABLE 3-7 Case-control study of the relationship between occurrence of local reaction and previous influenza immunization.

Vaccination	Cases of local reaction	Controls without local reaction
Yes	520	960
No	136	1120
Total	820 × 0.8 = 656	4160 × 0.5 = 2080

Note: Based on a perfectly representative sample of 80% of the cases and 50% of the controls from the study population shown in Table 3-4 (see Figure 3-4).
Source: Data from R Seltser, PE Sartwell, and JA Bell, A Controlled Test of Asian Influenza Vaccine in a Population of Families. *American Journal of Hygiene*, Vol 75, pp. 112–135, © 1962.

is strongly recommended for the calculation of the odds ratio of exposure, rather than the cross-products ratio, so as to avoid confusion over different arrangements of the table, as, for example, when placing control data on the left and case data on the right:

Exposure	*Controls*	*Cases*
Yes	"a"	"b"
No	"c"	"d"

In this example, the mechanical application of the cross-product ratio, $(a \times d)/c \times d$, would result in an incorrect estimate of the odds ratio—actually, the exact inverse of the true relative odds. On the other hand, making sure that one divides the exposure odds in cases (b/d) by that in controls (a/c) results in the correct odds ratio.

Odds Ratio in Matched Case-Control Studies

In a matched paired case-control study in which the ratio of controls to cases is 1:1, an unbiased estimate of the odds ratio is obtained by dividing the number of pairs in which the case, but not the matched control, is exposed (case [+], control [−]), by the number of pairs in which the control, but not the case, is exposed (case [−], control [+]). The underlying logic for this calculation and an example of this approach are discussed in Chapter 7, Section 7.3.3.

Odds Ratio as an Estimate of the Relative Risk in Case-Control Studies: The Rarity Assumption

In a case-control study, the use of the odds ratio to estimate the relative risk is based on the assumption that the disease under study has a low incidence, thus resulting in a small built-in bias (Equation 3.3). As a corollary to the discussion in Section 3.2.1, it follows that when the disease that defines case status in a case-control study is sufficiently rare, the estimated odds ratio will likely be a good approximation to the relative risk. On the other hand, when studying relatively common conditions, the built-in bias might be large, and case-control studies may yield odds ratios that substantially overestimate the strength of the association vis-à-vis the relative risk. Based on Equation 3.3, the following expression of the relative risk value as a function of the odds ratio can be derived:

$$\text{RR} = \frac{\text{OR}}{1 - [q_- - (\text{OR} \times q_-)]} \quad \text{(Eq. 3.13)}$$

It is evident from this equation that the relationship between the relative risk and odds ratio depends on the incidence of the outcome of interest (specifically q_-, i.e., the incidence in the unexposed, in this particular formulation). As a corollary of this, Equation 3.13 also implies that, in order to estimate the actual value of the relative risk from an odds ratio obtained in a case-control study, an estimate of incidence obtained from prospective data will be necessary. This could be available from outside sources (e.g., published data from another cohort study judged to be comparable to the source population for the study in question); if the study is nested within a cohort, incidence data may be available from the parent cohort from which the case and comparison groups were drawn (see examples later in this chapter). Table 3-8 illustrates examples of this relationship for a range of incidence and odds ratio values. For outcomes with incidence in the range of less than 1% or 1 per 1000 (e.g., the majority of chronic or infectious diseases), the value of the relative risk is very close to that of the odds ratio. Even for fairly common outcomes with frequency ranging between 1% and 5%, the values of the relative risk and odds ratio are reasonably similar.

Table 3-8, however, shows that when the condition of interest (that defining case status) is more common (e.g., incidence > 10% to 20%), the numerical value of the odds ratio obtained in a case-control study will be substantially different than that of the relative risk. This is not a limitation of the case-control design *per se*, but rather, it is a result of the mathematical relation between the odds ratio and the relative risk, irrespective of study design. Nevertheless, this should be kept in mind when interpreting odds ratio values in studies of highly frequent conditions such as, for example, 5-year mortality among lung cancer cases or smoking relapse in a smoking cessation study.

TABLE 3-8 Relative risk equivalency to a given odds ratio as a function of the incidence of the condition that defined case status in a case-control study.

Incidence in the unexposed population	Odds ratio = 0.5	Odds ratio = 1.5	Odds ratio = 2.0	Odds ratio = 3.0
		Relative risk equivalent		
0.001	0.50	1.50	2.00	2.99
0.01	0.50	1.49	1.98	2.94
0.05	0.51	1.46	1.90	2.73
0.1	0.53	1.43	1.82	2.50
0.2	0.56	1.36	1.67	2.14
0.3	0.59	1.30	1.54	1.88
0.4	0.63	1.25	1.43	1.67*

*Example of calculation: if OR = 3 and q_- = 0.4, and using Equation 3.13, the relative risk is:

$$RR = \frac{3}{1 - (0.4 - 3 \times 0.4)} = 1.67$$

Additional examples of case-control studies assessing relatively common events in situations in which incidence data were also available are as follows:

- In a nested case-control study of predictors of surgical site infections after breast cancer surgery, 76 cases of infection were compared with 154 controls (no infection) with regard to obesity and other variables.[11] Data were available on the incidence of infection in the nonobese group (q_-), which was estimated to be approximately 30%. The study reported that the odds ratio of infection associated with obesity was 2.5. Thus, using Equation 3.13, the corresponding relative risk of infection comparing obese and nonobese can be estimated as 1.72.
- A case-control study investigated the relationship between genetic changes and prostate cancer progression.[12] Cases were individuals with a biochemical marker of cancer progression (prostate-specific agent, PSA > 0.4 ng/mL, n = 26) and were compared with 26 controls without biochemical progression. Loss of heterozygosity (LOH) was associated with an odds ratio of 5.54. Based on data from the study report, the approximate incidence of progression among the non-LOH group was 60%; as a result, it is estimated that the 5.54 odds ratio obtained in the study corresponds to a relative risk of approximately 1.5.
- In a case-control study conducted among nondiabetic and otherwise healthy obese adults,[13] the odds ratio of hypertension comparing male subjects whose waist circumference was ≥ 102 cm to those with waist circumference < 94 cm was 3.04. Assuming that the overall prevalence of hypertension among obese adults in the US is around 40%,[14] that odds ratio translates into a relative risk of approximately 1.7.

As in prospective studies (see Section 3.2.1), the rare-disease assumption *applies only to situations in which the odds ratio is used to estimate the relative risk*. When the odds ratio is used as a measure of association in itself, this assumption is obviously not needed. In the previous examples, there is nothing intrinsically incorrect about the odds ratio estimates; assuming no bias or random error, LOH is indeed associated with an odds ratio of biochemical prostate cancer progression of 5.54. Although it would be a mistake to interpret this estimate as a relative risk, it is perfectly correct to conclude that, compared with non-LOH, LOH multiplies the *odds* of biochemical progression by 5.54; this is as accurate as concluding the LOH multiplies the *risk (incidence)* of biochemical progression by 1.5.

When the Rarity Assumption Is Not Necessary: Selecting Population Controls

The rare-disease assumption is irrelevant in situations in which the control group is a sample of the total population,[15] which is the usual strategy in case-control studies within a defined cohort (Chapter 1, Section 1.4.2). In this situation, the odds ratio is a *direct estimate of the relative risk*, irrespective of the frequency of the outcome of interest.

The irrelevance of the rare-disease assumption when the control group is a sample of the total reference population can be demonstrated by comparing the calculation of the odds ratio using different types of control groups. Referring to the cross-tabulation, including all cases and all noncases in a defined population shown in Table 3-9, when noncases are used as the control group, as seen previously (Equation 3.12), the odds ratio of exposure is used to estimate the odds ratio of disease by dividing the odds of exposure in cases by that in controls:

$$OR_{exp} = \frac{Odds_{exp\ cases}}{Odds_{exp\ noncases}} = \frac{\frac{a}{c}}{\frac{b}{d}} = OR_{dis}$$

Another option is to use as a control group the total study population at baseline (last column in Table 3-9), rather than only the noncases. If this is done in the context of a cohort study, the case-control study is usually called a *case-cohort study* (Chapter 1, Section 1.4.2), and the division of the odds of exposure in cases by that in controls (i.e., the total population) yields the relative risk:

$$OR_{exp} = \frac{Odds_{exp\ cases}}{Odds_{exp\ total\ population}} = \frac{\left(\frac{a}{c}\right)}{\left(\frac{a+b}{c+d}\right)} = \frac{\left(\frac{a}{a+b}\right)}{\left(\frac{c}{c+d}\right)} = RR \quad (Eq.\ 3.14)$$

Using again the local reaction/influenza vaccination investigation as an example (Table 3-4), a case-cohort study could be conducted using all cases and the total study population as the control group. The ratio of the exposure odds in cases ($Odds_{exp\ cases}$) to the exposure odds in the total study population ($Odds_{exp\ pop}$) yields the relative risk:

TABLE 3-9 Cross-tabulation of a defined population by exposure and disease development.

Exposure	Cases	Noncases	Total population (cases + noncases)
Present	a	b	$a + b$
Absent	c	d	$c + d$

$$\text{OR}_{\text{exp}} = \frac{\text{Odds}_{\text{exp cases}}}{\text{Odds}_{\text{exp pop}}} = \frac{\left(\dfrac{650}{170}\right)}{\left(\dfrac{2570}{2410}\right)} = \frac{\left(\dfrac{650}{2570}\right)}{\left(\dfrac{170}{2410}\right)} = \frac{q_+}{q_-} = 3.59 = \text{RR}$$

where q_+ is the incidence in exposed and q_- the incidence in unexposed individuals.

In the estimation of the relative risk in the previous example, all cases and the total study population were included. Because unbiased sample estimates of $\text{Odds}_{\text{exp cases}}$ and $\text{Odds}_{\text{exp pop}}$ provide an unbiased estimate of the relative risk, a sample of cases and a sample of the total study population can be compared in a case-cohort study. For example, assuming no random variability, unbiased samples of 40% of the cases and 20% of the total population would produce the results shown in Table 3-10; the product of the division of the odds of exposure in the sample of cases by that in the study population sample can be shown to be identical to the relative risk obtained prospectively for the total cohort, as follows:

$$\text{OR}_{\text{exp}} = \frac{\dfrac{260}{68}}{\dfrac{514}{482}} = 3.59 = \text{RR}$$

Again, more commonly, because the number of cases is usually small relative to the study population size, case-cohort studies try to include all cases and a sample of the reference population.

One of the advantages of the case-cohort approach is that it allows direct estimation of the relative risk and thus does not have to rely on the rarity assumption. Another advantage is that because the control group is a sample of the total reference population, an unbiased estimate of the exposure prevalence (or distribution) needed for the estimation of Levin's population attributable risk (Equation 3.10) can be obtained. A control group formed by an unbiased sample of the cohort also allows the assessment of relationships between different exposures or even between exposures and outcomes other than the outcome of interest in the cohort sample. To these analytical advantages can be added the practical advantage of the case-cohort design discussed in Chapter 1, Section 1.4.2, namely, the efficiency of selecting a single control group that can be compared with different types of cases identified on follow-up (e.g., myocardial infarction, stroke, and low-extremity arterial disease).

TABLE 3-10 Case-cohort study of the relationship of previous vaccination to local reaction.

Previous vaccination	Cases of local reaction	Cohort sample
Yes	260	514
No	68	482
Total	328	996

Note: Based on a random sample of the study population in Table 3-4, with sampling fractions of 40% for the cases and 20% for the cohort.
Source: Data from R Seltser, PE Sartwell, and JA Bell, A Controlled Test of Asian Influenza Vaccine in a Population of Families. *American Journal of Hygiene*, Vol 75, pp. 112–135, © 1962.

In addition to these advantages connected with the choice of a sample of the cohort as the control group, there are other reasons why the traditional approach of selecting noncases as controls may not always be the best option. There are occasions when excluding cases from the control group is logistically difficult and can add costs and burden participants. For example, in diseases with a high proportion of a subclinical phase (e.g., chronic cholecystitis, prostate cancer), excluding cases from the pool of eligible controls (e.g., apparently healthy individuals) would require conducting more or less invasive and expensive examinations (e.g., contrasted X-rays, biopsy). Thus, in these instances, a case-cohort approach will be more convenient: i.e., selecting "controls" from the reference population irrespective of (i.e., ignoring) the possible presence of the disease (clinical or subclinical).

It is appropriate to conduct a case-cohort study only when a defined population (study base) from which the study cases originated can be identified, as when dealing with a defined cohort in the context of a prospective study. On the other hand, conducting case-cohort studies when dealing with "open" cohorts or populations at large requires assuming that these represented the source populations from which the cases originated (see Chapter 1, Section 1.4.2).

It should also be emphasized that when the disease is rare, the strategy of ignoring disease status when selecting controls would most likely result in few, if any, cases being actually included in the control group; thus, in practice, Equation 3.14 will be almost identical to Equation 3.12 because $(a + b) \approx b$ and $(c + d) \approx d$. For example, in the myocardial infarction/hypertension example shown in Table 3-3, the "case-cohort" strategy selecting, for example, a 50% sample of cases and a 10% sample of total cohort as controls, would result in the following estimate of the odds ratio:

$$OR_{exp} = \frac{Odds_{exp\,cases}}{Odds_{exp\,pop}} = \frac{\frac{90}{15}}{\frac{1000}{1000}} = 6.00 = RR$$

In this same example, a case–noncase strategy would result in the following estimate:

$$OR_{exp} = \frac{Odds_{exp\,cases}}{Odds_{exp\,noncases}} = \frac{\frac{90}{15}}{\frac{982}{997}} = 6.09 = OR_{dis}$$

That is, a situation analogous to that discussed in Section 3.2.1 with regard to the similarity of the odds ratio and the relative risk when the disease is rare.

Influence of the Sampling Frame for Control Selection on the Parameter Estimated by the Odds Ratio of Exposure: Cumulative Incidence Vs Density Sampling

In addition to considering whether controls are selected from either noncases or the total study population, it is important to specify further the sampling frame for control selection. As discussed in Chapter 1 (Section 1.4.2), when controls are selected from a defined total cohort, sampling frames may consist of either (1) individuals at risk when cases occur during the follow-up period (density or risk-set sampling) or (2) the baseline cohort. The first alternative has been designated *nested case-control design* and the latter (exemplified by the "local reaction/influenza vaccination" analysis discussed previously) *case-cohort design*.[16] As demonstrated next, the nested case-control study and case-cohort designs allow the estimation of the rate ratio and the relative risk, respectively. An intuitive way to conceptualize which of these two parameters is being estimated by the odds ratio of exposure (i.e., rate ratio or relative risk) is to think of cases as the "numerator" and controls as the "denominator" of the absolute measure of disease frequency to which the parameter relates (see Chapter 2).

Density Sampling: The Nested Case-Control Design. As described previously (Section 1.4.2), the nested case-control design is based on incidence density sampling (also known as risk-set sampling). It consists of selecting a control group that represents the sum of the subsamples of the cohort selected during the follow-up at the approximate times when cases occur (*risk sets*) (Figure 1-20). These controls can also be regarded as a population sample "averaged" over all points in time when the events happen (see Chapter 2, Section 2.2.2) and could potentially include the case that defined the risk set, or cases that develop in a given risk set after its selection. Therefore, the odds ratio of exposure thus obtained represents an estimate of the *rate* or *density ratio* (or relative rate or relative density). This strategy explicitly recognizes that there are losses (censored observations) during the follow-up of the cohort, in that cases and controls are chosen from the same reference populations excluding previous losses, thus matching cases and controls on duration of follow-up. When cases are excluded from the sampling frame of controls for each corresponding risk set, the odds ratio of exposure estimates the *density odds ratio*.

Selecting Controls From the Cohort at Baseline: The Case-Cohort Design. In the case-cohort design (also described in Chapter 1, Section 1.4.2), the case group is composed of cases identified during the follow-up period, and the control group is a sample of the total cohort at baseline (Figure 1-21). The cases and the sampling frame for controls can be regarded, respectively, as the type of numerator and denominator that would have been selected to calculate a probability of the event based on the initial population, q. Thus, when these controls are selected, the odds ratio of exposure yields a ratio of the probability of the outcome in exposed (q_+) to that in unexposed (q_-) individuals (i.e., the *cumulative incidence ratio* or *relative risk*) (Equation 3.14). Because the distribution of follow-up times in the sample of the initial cohort—which by definition includes those not lost as well as those subsequently lost to observation during follow-up—will be different from that of cases (whose "risk sets" by definition exclude previous losses), it is necessary to use survival analysis techniques to correct for losses that occur during the follow-up in a case-cohort study (see Section 2.2.1).

It is also possible to exclude cases from the control group when sampling the cohort at baseline: that is, the sampling frame for controls would be formed by individuals who have remained disease-free through the duration of the follow-up. These are the persons who would have been selected as the denominator of the *odds based on the initial population*:

$$\left(\frac{q}{1-q}\right)$$

Thus, the calculation of the odds ratio of exposure when carrying out this strategy yields an estimate of the *odds ratio of disease* (i.e., the ratio of the odds of developing the disease during the follow-up in individuals exposed and unexposed at baseline).

A summary of the effect of the specific sampling frame for control selection on the parameter estimated by the odds ratio of exposure is shown in Table 3-11.

Calculation of the Odds Ratio When There Are More Than Two Exposure Categories

Although the examples given so far in this chapter have referred to only two exposure categories, often more than two levels of exposure are assessed. Among the advantages

TABLE 3-11 Summary of the influence of control selection on the parameter estimated by the odds ratio of exposure in case-control studies within a defined cohort.

Design	Population frame for control selection	Exposure odds ratio estimates
Nested case-control	Population at approximate times when cases occur during follow-up	Rate (density) ratio
	(Population during follow-up minus cases)	(Density odds ratio)
Case-cohort	Total cohort at baseline	Cumulative incidence ratio (relative risk)
	(Total cohort at baseline minus cases that develop during follow-up)	(Probability odds ratio)

of studying multiple exposure categories is the assessment of different exposure dimensions (e.g., "past" vs "current") and of graded ("dose-response") patterns.

In the example shown in Table 3-12, children with craniosynostosis undergoing craniectomy were compared with normal children in regard to maternal age.[17] To calculate the odds ratio for the different maternal age categories, the youngest maternal age was chosen as the reference category. Next, for cases and controls separately, the odds for each maternal age category (vis-à-vis the reference category) were calculated (columns 4 and 5). The odds ratio is calculated as the ratio of the odds of each maternal age category in cases to the odds in controls (column 6). In this study, a graded and positive (direct) relationship was observed between maternal age and the odds of craniosynostosis. Note that the odds ratio for each category can also be calculated as the odds of "caseness" for a given category divided by the odds of "caseness" for the reference category. For example in Table 3-12, the odds ratio for the age category 25–29 would be $(56/255)/(12/89) = 1.63$, i.e., the same as in Table 3-12.

When the multilevel exposure variable is ordinal (e.g., age categories in Table 3-12), it may be of interest to perform a trend test (see Appendix B).

TABLE 3-12 Distribution of cases of craniosynostosis and normal controls according to maternal age.

Maternal age (years) (1)	Cases (2)	Controls (3)	Odds of specified maternal age vs reference in cases (4)	Odds of specified maternal age vs reference in controls (5)	Odds ratio (6) = (4)/(5)
< 20*	12	89	12/12	89/89	1.00*
20–24	47	242	47/12	242/89	1.44
25–29	56	255	56/12	255/89	1.63
> 29	58	173	58/12	173/89	2.49

*Reference category.

Source: Data from BW Alderman et al., An Epidemiologic Study of Craniosynostosis: Risk Indicators for the Occurrence of Craniosynostosis in Colorado. *American Journal of Epidemiology*, Vol 128, pp. 431–438. © 1988.

3.4.2 Attributable Risk in Case-Control Studies

As noted previously (Section 3.2.2), percent attributable risk in the exposed can be obtained in traditional case-control (case–noncase) studies when the odds ratio is a reasonable estimate of the relative risk by replacing its corresponding value in Equation 3.6:

$$\%AR_{exp} = \left(\frac{OR - 1.0}{OR}\right) \times 100 \quad \text{(Eq. 3.15)}$$

In studies dealing with preventive interventions, the analogous measure is efficacy (see Section 3.2.2, Equation 3.7). The fact that the odds ratio is usually a good estimate of the relative risk makes it possible to use Equation 3.15 in case-control studies of the efficacy of an intervention such as screening.[18]

The same reasoning applies to the use of case-control studies to estimate the population attributable risk using a variation of Levin's formula:

$$\%Pop\ AR = \frac{p_e^* \times (OR - 1)}{p_e^* \times (OR - 1) + 1} \times 100 \quad \text{(Eq. 3.16)}$$

In Equation 3.16, the proportion of exposed subjects in the reference population (p_e in Equation 3.10) is represented as p_e^* because in the context of a case-control study this is often estimated by the exposure prevalence among controls. Such an assumption is appropriate as long as the disease is rare and the control group is reasonably representative of all noncases in the reference population. Obviously, if a case-cohort study is conducted, the rarity assumption is not needed (Section 3.4.1), as both the relative risk and the exposure prevalence can be directly estimated.

As shown by Levin and Bertell,[19] if the odds ratio is used as the relative risk estimate, Equation 3.16 reduces to a simpler equation:

$$\%Pop\ AR = \frac{p_{e\ case} - p_{e\ control}}{1.0 - p_{e\ control}} \times 100$$

where $p_{e\ case}$ represents the prevalence of exposure among cases—that is, $a/(a + c)$ in Table 3-9—and $p_{e\ control}$ represents the prevalence of exposure among controls—that is, $b/(b + d)$ in Table 3-9.

3.5 ASSESSING THE STRENGTH OF ASSOCIATIONS

The values of the measures of association discussed in this chapter are often used to rank the relative importance of risk factors. However, because risk factors vary in terms of their physiological modus operandi as well as their exposure levels and units, such comparisons are often unwarranted. Consider, for example, the absurdity of saying that systolic blood pressure is a more important risk factor for myocardial infarction than total cholesterol, based on comparing the odds ratio associated with a 50-mm/Hg increase in systolic blood pressure with that associated with a 1-mg/dL increase in total serum cholesterol. In addition, regardless of the size of the units used, it is hard to compare association strengths, given the unique nature of each risk factor.

An alternative way to assess the strength of the association of a given risk factor with an outcome is to estimate the *exposure intensity* necessary for that factor to produce an association of the same magnitude as that of well-established risk factors or vice-versa. For example, Tverdal et al.[20] evaluated the level of exposure of four well-known risk factors for coronary heart disease mortality necessary to replicate the relative risk of 2.2 associated with a coffee intake of nine or more cups per day. As seen in Exhibit 3-1, a relative risk of 2.2 corresponds to smoking about 4.3 cigarettes per day or having an increase in systolic blood pressure of about 6.9 mm Hg, and so on.

Another example comes from a study by Howard et al.,[21] who evaluated the cross-sectional association between passive smoking and subclinical atherosclerosis measured by B-mode ultrasound-determined intimal-medial thickness of the carotid artery walls. Because passive smoking had not been studied previously in connection with directly visualized atherosclerosis, its importance as a risk factor was contrasted with that of a known atherosclerosis determinant, age (Exhibit 3-2). As seen in the exhibit, the cross-sectional association between passive smoking and atherosclerosis is equivalent to an age difference of 1 year. That is, assuming that the cross-sectional association adequately represents the prospective relationship between age and atherosclerosis and that the data are valid, precise, and free of confounding, the average thickness of the carotid arteries of passive smokers looks like that of never smokers who are 1 year older. This inference was extended by Kawachi and Colditz,[22] who, on the basis of data from Howard et al.'s study, estimated that the change in intimal-medial thickness related to passive smoking would result in an increase in the risk of clinical cardiovascular events equivalent to an increment of 7 mm/Hg of systolic blood pressure, or 0.7 mmol/L of total cholesterol—thus, not negligible.

EXHIBIT 3-1 A possible way to describe the strength of an association between a risk factor and an outcome.

A relative risk of 2.2 for coronary heart disease mortality comparing men drinking 9+ or more cups of coffee per day vs < one cup per day corresponds to:

Smoking:	4.3 cigarettes/day
Systolic blood pressure:	6.9 mm/Hg
Total serum cholesterol:	0.47 mmol/L
Serum high-density lipoprotein:	−0.24 mmol/L

Source: Data from A Tverdal et al., Coffee Consumption and Death From Coronary Heart Disease in Middle-Aged Norwegian Men and Women. *British Medical Journal*, Vol 300, pp. 566–569, © 1990.

EXHIBIT 3-2 Cross-sectionally determined mean intimal-medial thickness (IMT) of the carotid arteries (mm) by passive smoking status in never active smokers, the Atherosclerosis Risk in Communities Study, 1987–1989.

	Passive smoking status in never-active smokers		Estimated increase by year of age
	Absent ($n = 1,774$)	Present ($n = 3,358$)	
Mean IMT (mm) →	0.700	0.711	0.011

Age-equivalent excess attributable to passive smoking:
$(0.711 − 0.700)/0.011 = 1$ year

Source: Data from G Howard et al., Active and Passive Smoking are Associated with Increased Carotid Wall Thickness. The Atherosclerosis Risk in Communities Study. *Archives of Internal Medicine*, Vol. 154, pp. 1277–1282, © 1994.

Using a somewhat similar approach, Sharrett et al. examined low-density cholesterol (LDL) equivalents when comparing the roles of diabetes and smoking in atherosclerosis progression in participants of the Multi-Ethnic Study of Atherosclerosis.[23] Because lipids are a necessary component of atherosclerosis, these authors defined LDL equivalent as the concentration of LDL necessary to replicate the magnitudes of the associations of smoking and diabetes with each phase of the natural history of atherosclerosis. They defined as *minimal atherosclerosis* a carotid intimal-medial thickness below the 75th percentile of the total cohort distribution with no clinical manifestations; *moderate atherosclerosis* as intimal-medial thickness equal to or greater than the 75th percentile without clinical manifestations; and *severe atherosclerosis* as the presence of peripheral arterial disease (ankle-brachial index < 0.90). These authors observed that the level of serum LDL concentration that replicated the strength of the associations of both diabetes and smoking with atherosclerosis increased as the natural history progressed from minimal to moderate to severe phases. For minimal and moderate atherosclerosis (as defined), the LDL equivalent seems to be greater for diabetes than for smoking (115 and 117 mg/dL vs 40 and 85 mg/dL, respectively (Figure 3-5). However, for severe atherosclerosis, the LDL concentration that replicated the association with smoking was greater than that with diabetes (238 vs 178 mg/dL, respectively). It can be concluded that, while diabetes seems to be more important in minimal and moderate atherosclerosis, peripheral vascular disease (defined as severe atherosclerosis) appeared to be more strongly related to smoking than to diabetes.

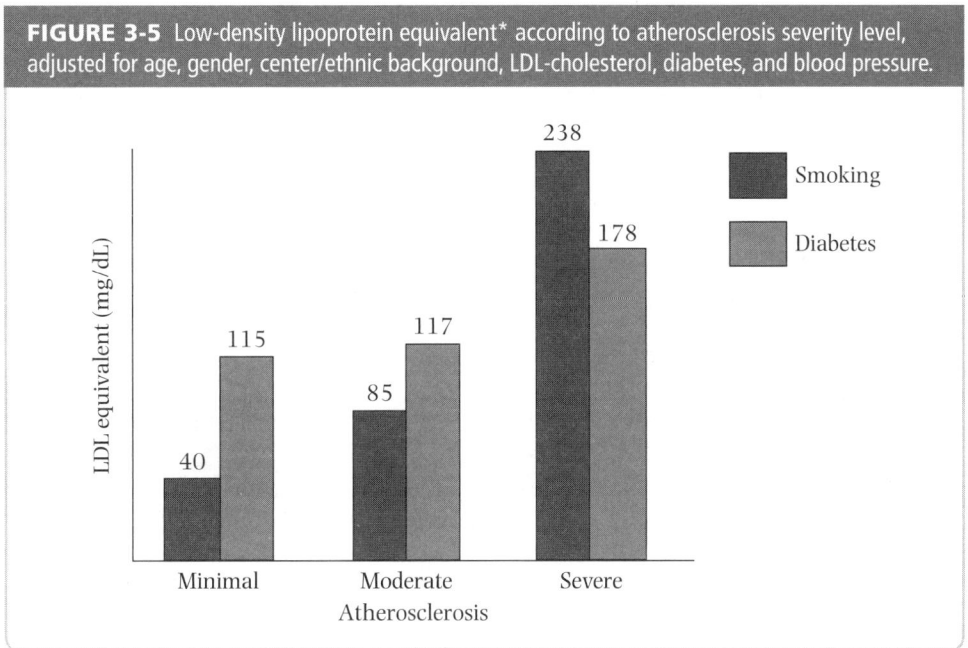

FIGURE 3-5 Low-density lipoprotein equivalent* according to atherosclerosis severity level, adjusted for age, gender, center/ethnic background, LDL-cholesterol, diabetes, and blood pressure.

*LDL equivalent: serum LDL concentration that replicates the strength of the association of diabetes or smoking with atherosclerosis.
Source: Data from Sharrett AR, et al., Smoking, Diabetes and Blood Cholesterol Differ in Their Associations with Subclinical Atherosclerosis: The Multiethnic Study of Atherosclerosis (MESA). *Atherosclerosis*, Vol 186, p. 443 © 2006.

REFERENCES

1. Lilienfeld DE, Stolley, PD. *Foundations of Epidemiology*, 3rd ed. New York: Oxford University Press; 1994.
2. Gordis L. *Epidemiology*, 4th ed. Philadelphia: Elsevier Saunders; 2008.
3. Seltser R, Sartwell PE, Bell JA. A controlled test of Asian influenza vaccine in a population of families. *Am J Hygiene*. 1962;75:112–135.
4. Greenland S, Robins JM. Conceptual problems in the definition and interpretation of attributable fractions. *Am J Epidemiol*. 1988;128:1185–1197.
5. Rothman K, Greenland S. *Modern Epidemiology*, 3rd ed. Philadelphia: Wolters Kluwer Health/Lippincott; 2008.
6. Levin ML. The occurrence of lung cancer in man. *Acta Unio Int Contra Cancrum*. 1953;9:531–541.
7. Walter SD. The estimation and interpretation of attributable risk in health research. *Biometrics*. 1976;32:829–849.
8. Rockhill B, Newman B, Weinberg C. Use and misuse of population attributable fractions. *Am J Public Health*. 1998;88:15–19.
9. Walter SD. Effects of interaction, confounding and observational error on attributable risk estimation. *Am J Epidemiol*. 1983;117:598–604.
10. Cornfield J. A method of estimating comparative rates from clinical data: Applications to cancer of the lung, breast, and cervix. *J Natl Cancer Inst*. 1951;11:1269–1275.
11. Vilar-Compte D, Jacquemin B, Robles-Vidal C, Volkow P. Surgical site infections in breast surgery: Case-control study. *World J Surg*. 2004;28:242–246.
12. Valeri A, Fromont G, Sakr W, et al. High frequency of allelic losses in high-grade prostate cancer is associated with biochemical progression after radical prostatectomy. *Urol Oncol*. 2005;23:87–92.
13. Guagnano MT, Ballone E, Colagrande V, et al. Large waist circumference and risk of hypertension. *Int J Obes* 2001;25:1360–1364.
14. Keenan NL, Rosendorf KA. Prevalence of hypertension and controlled hypertension—United States, 2005–2008. *MMWR* 2011;60:94–97.
15. Prentice RL. A case-cohort design for epidemiologic cohort studies and disease prevention trials. *Biometrika*. 1986;73:1–11.
16. Langholz B, Thomas DC. Nested case-control and case-cohort methods of sampling from a cohort: A critical comparison. *Am J Epidemiol*. 1990;131:169–176.
17. Alderman BW, Lammer EJ, Joshua SC, et al. An epidemiologic study of craniosynostosis: Risk indicators for the occurrence of craniosynostosis in Colorado. *Am J Epidemiol*. 1988;128:431–438.
18. Coughlin SS, Benichou J, Weed DL. Attributable risk estimation in case-control studies. *Epidemiol Rev*. 1994;16:51–64.
19. Levin ML, Bertell R. RE: "simple estimation of population attributable risk from case-control studies." *Am J Epidemiol*. 1978;108:78–79.
20. Tverdal A, Stensvold I, Solvoll K, et al. Coffee consumption and death from coronary heart disease in middle aged Norwegian men and women. *Br Med J*. 1990;300:566–569.
21. Howard G, Burke GL, Szklo M, et al. Active and passive smoking are associated with increased carotid wall thickness: The Atherosclerosis Risk in Communities Study. *Arch Intern Med*. 1994;154:1277–1282.
22. Kawachi I, Colditz GA. Invited commentary: Confounding, measurement error, and publication bias in studies of passive smoking. *Am J Epidemiol*. 1996;144:909–915.
23. Sharrett AR, Ding J, Criqui MH, et al. Smoking, diabetes, and blood cholesterol differ in their associations with subclinical atherosclerosis: The Multi-Ethnic Study of Atherosclerosis (MESA). *Atherosclerosis* 2006;186:441–447.

EXERCISES

1. The following results were obtained in an occupational cohort study of the risk of cancer associated with exposure to radiation.

Radiation dose (rem)	Total population (baseline)	Cancer cases	Cumulative* incidence	Relative risk	Odds ratio (comparing cases to noncases)	Odds ratio (comparing cases to total population)
0–0.99	3642	390				
1–4.99	1504	181				
5+	1320	222				

   *Assume no losses to follow-up.

   a. Fill in the empty cells in this table. For the calculation of relative risks and odds ratios, use the lowest radiation category as the reference category.
   b. How do you explain the difference (or the similarity) between each of the two types of odds ratios calculated here and the corresponding relative risks?
   c. Assuming that an association between exposure and disease is actually present, which of the following statements is true? Why?
      (1) The odds ratio is always smaller in absolute value than the relative risk.
      (2) The odds ratio is always bigger in absolute value than the relative risk.
      (3) The odds ratio is always closer to 1 than the relative risk.
      (4) The odds ratio is always farther away from 1 than the relative risk.
   d. Progressively higher relative risks (or odds ratios) with increasing radiation dose are observed. Which traditional causality criterion is met when progressively higher relative risks (or odds ratios) are observed?

2. A cohort study to examine the relationships of inflammatory markers (such as interleukin-6 and C-reactive protein) to incident dementia was conducted within the Rotterdam Study cohort ($n = 6713$).* A random sample of the total cohort at baseline ($n = 727$) and the 188 individuals who developed dementia on follow-up were compared. Serum inflammatory markers were measured in cases and in the random sample.

   a. Which type of study have the authors conducted?
   b. If the authors wished to study the relationship of inflammatory markers to stroke, could they use the same control group? Why or why not?
   c. The relative risk of dementia associated with an interleukin-6 value in the highest quintile compared with that in the lowest quintile was found to be about 1.9. Assume that there is no random variability; that the relationship is causal; and that the relative risks of the second, third, and fourth quintiles compared with the lowest quintile are all 1.0. Calculate the percentage of dementia incidence in the population that might be explained by the values in the highest quintile.

---

*Engelhart MJ, Geerlings MJ, Meijer J, et al. Inflammatory proteins in plasma and risk of dementia: The Rotterdam Study. *Arch Neurol.* 2004;61:668–672.

3. A recent case-control study assessed the relationship of hepatitis C virus (HCV) infection to B-cell non-Hodgkin lymphomas (B-NHL).[†] Cases of B-NHL were identified in the hematology department wards of 10 hospitals located in different cities throughout Italy. The control group consisted of non-B-NHL patients admitted to other departments of the same hospitals (e.g., ophthalmology, general surgery, internal medicine). For both cases and controls, only patients with newly diagnosed diseases were included in the study. Testing for HCV was done after cases and controls were hospitalized.

   a. What type of case-control study have the authors conducted?

   The numbers of cases and controls as well as the numbers who tested positive for HCV by age (55 or less, and more than 55 years old) are seen in this table:

	Cases		Controls	
Age (years)	Number	HCV positive	Number	HCV positive
≤ 55	163	18	231	6
> 55	237	52	165	16

   b. Calculate the exposure odds ratio reflecting the HCV/B-NHL association for each age group.
   c. Describe in words the meaning of the odds ratio for age group >55 years.
   d. What is an important shortcoming of this study?

4. Melkonian et al. conducted a cohort study of the synergistic association of arsenic exposure with selected environmental factors, including sun exposure and fertilizer use.[‡] As part of their preliminary analyses, they examined the unadjusted relationship of body mass index to skin lesions, as shown in the table:

Body mass index (kg/m^2)	Developed skin lesions (n = 613)	Did not develop skin lesions (n = 3378)	Incidence proportion*	Odds	Odds ratio	Relative risk
< 18.5	285	1451				
18.5 – 24.9	304	1684				
≥ 25	21	231			1.0	1.0

   *Assume no losses to follow-up.

   a. For each category of BMI, calculate the incidence proportions and odds of developing skin lesions as well as odds ratios and relative risks. For the calculation of odds ratios and relative risk, use ≥ 25 as the reference category.
   b. Considering the magnitude of the incidence of skin lesions, what can be inferred with regard to the assumption that the odds ratio is a good estimate of the relative risk when the disease is rare?

[†]Mele A, Pulsoni A, Bianco E, et al. Hepatitis C virus and B-cell non-Hodgkin lymphomas: An Italian multicenter case-control study. *Blood.* 2003;102:996–999.
[‡]Melkonian S, Argos M, Pierce BL, et al. A prospective study of the synergistic effects of arsenic exposure and smoking, sun exposure, fertilizer use, and pesticide use on risk of premalignant skin lesions in Bangladeshi men. *Am J Epidemiol.* 2011;173:183–191.

PART THREE

Threats to Validity and Issues of Interpretation

CHAPTER 4 Understanding Lack of Validity: Bias 109

CHAPTER 5 Identifying Noncausal Associations: Confounding 153

CHAPTER 6 Defining and Assessing Heterogeneity of Effects: Interaction 185

Understanding Lack of Validity: Bias

CHAPTER 4

4.1 OVERVIEW

Bias can be defined as the result of a *systematic* error in the design or conduct of a study. This systematic error results from flaws either in the method of selection of study participants or in the procedures for gathering relevant exposure and/or disease information; as a consequence, the observed study results will *tend* to be different from the true results. This *tendency* toward erroneous results is called bias. As discussed in this chapter, many types of bias can affect the study results. The possibility of bias, in addition to that of confounding (see Chapter 5), is an important consideration and is often a major limitation in the interpretation of results from observational epidemiologic studies. Systematic error (bias) needs to be distinguished from error due to random variability (sampling error), which results from the use of a population sample to estimate the study parameters in the reference population. The sample estimates may differ substantially from the true parameters because of random error, especially when the study sample is small.

The definition of bias relates to the process—that is, the design and procedures—and not the results of any particular study. If the design and procedures of a study are unbiased, the study is considered to be *valid* because, on average, its results will tend to be correct. A faulty study design is considered to be biased (or *invalid*) because it will produce an erroneous result *on average*. Because of sampling variability, however, a given study using "biased" methods can produce a result close to the truth (Figure 4-1). Conversely, an unbiased study can produce results that are substantially different from the truth because of random sampling variability.

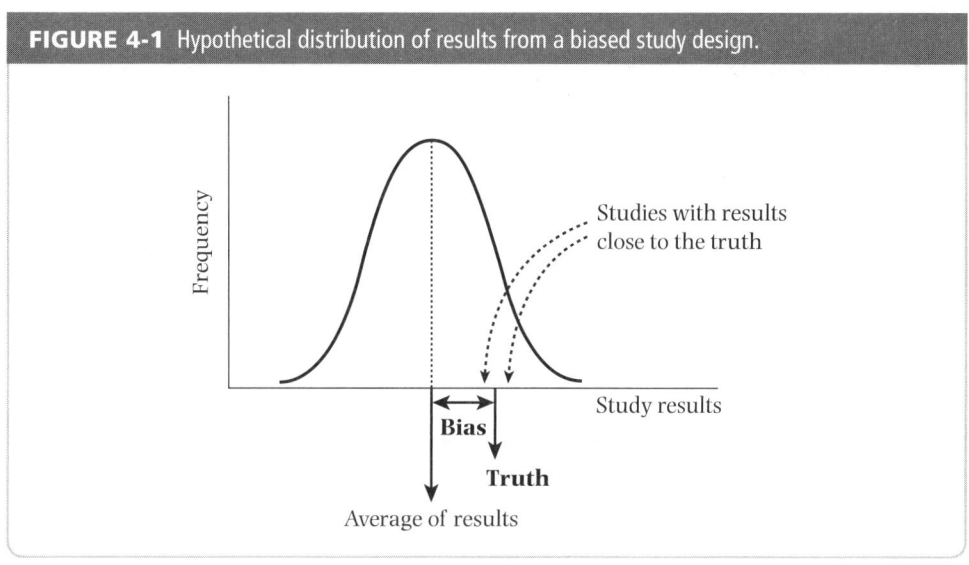

FIGURE 4-1 Hypothetical distribution of results from a biased study design.

109

Bias is said to exist when, *on average*, the results of a hypothetically infinite number of studies (related to a specific association and reference population) differ from the true result—for example, when the average relative odds of a large (theoretically infinite) number of case-control studies on a certain association in a given population is 2.0 but in fact there is no association (Figure 4-1). This definition of bias, however, is of little use to the epidemiologist who must infer from the results of his or her only study. Even when the epidemiologist carries out an overview or meta-analysis, the available published studies are but a fraction of what, by any definition, can be regarded as "an infinite number of studies." (A related problem is publication bias—e.g., the tendency to publish studies in which results are "positive"; see Chapter 10, Section 10.5.) Bias, therefore, has to be assessed in the context of a careful evaluation of the specific study design, methods, and procedures.

Prevention and control of bias are accomplished on three levels: (1) ensuring that the study design—including the procedures for selection of the study sample—is appropriate for addressing the study hypotheses; (2) establishing and carefully monitoring procedures of data collection that are valid and reliable; and (3) using appropriate analytic procedures.

Many types of bias have been described in the epidemiologic literature (see, e.g., Sackett[1]). However, most biases related to the study design and procedures can be classified in two basic categories: *selection* and *information*.

Selection bias is present when individuals have different probabilities of being included in the study sample according to relevant study characteristics—namely, the exposure and the outcome of interest. Figure 4-2 illustrates a general situation where exposed cases have a higher probability of being selected for the study than other categories of individuals. An instance of this type of bias is *medical surveillance bias*, which one might encounter, for example, when conducting a case-control study to examine the relationship of the use of oral contraceptives to any disease with an important subclinical component, such as diabetes. Because oral contraceptive use is likely to be related to a higher average frequency of medical encounters, any subclinical disease is

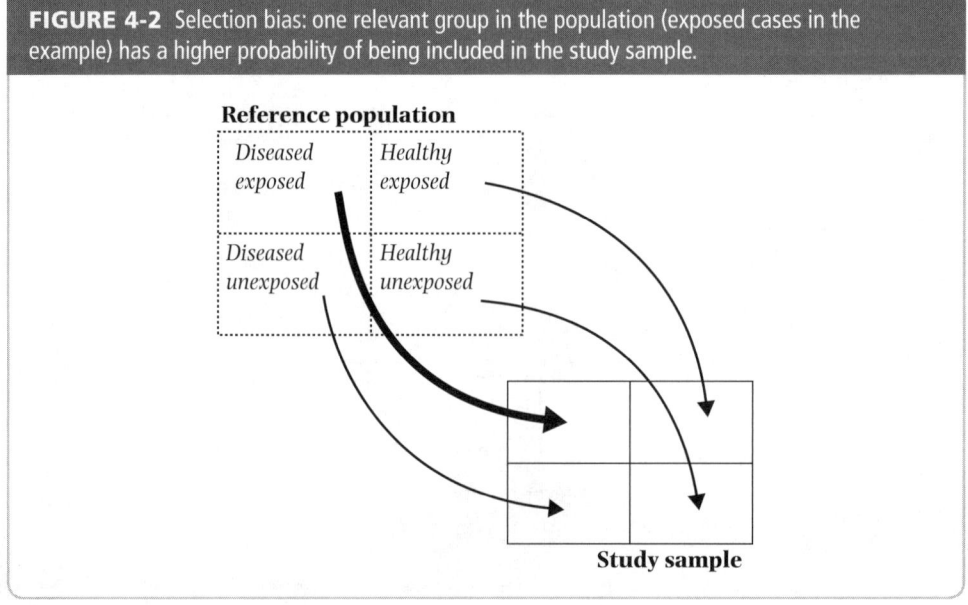

FIGURE 4-2 Selection bias: one relevant group in the population (exposed cases in the example) has a higher probability of being included in the study sample.

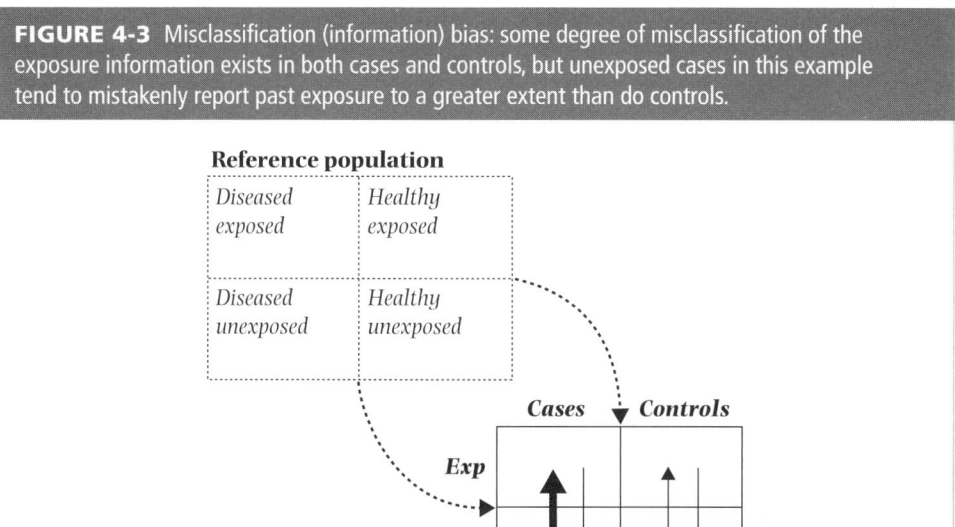

FIGURE 4-3 Misclassification (information) bias: some degree of misclassification of the exposure information exists in both cases and controls, but unexposed cases in this example tend to mistakenly report past exposure to a greater extent than do controls.

more likely to be diagnosed in oral contraceptive users than in nonusers. As a result, in a study comparing cases of diabetes and controls without diabetes, a spurious association with oral contraceptive use may ensue. The effect of selection bias on the direction of the measure of association is, of course, a function of which cell(s) in an $n \times k$ table (e.g., a 2×2 table such as that shown in Figure 4-2) is subject to a spuriously higher or lower probability of selection.

Information bias results from a systematic tendency for individuals selected for inclusion in the study to be erroneously placed in different exposure/outcome categories, thus leading to *misclassification*. The classic example of information bias leading to misclassification is *recall bias*, in which the ability to recall past exposures may be dependent on case-control status. In the hypothetical example sketched in Figure 4-3, cases are more likely than controls to overstate past exposure.

What follows is a discussion of the most common selection and information biases affecting exposure—outcome associations in observational epidemiologic studies. Inevitably, because different types of bias overlap, any attempt to classify bias entails some duplication; as will be readily noted, some types of bias may be categorized as either selection or information bias(or as both). The classification of the different types of biases discussed in the following sections is thus mainly set up for didactic purposes and is by no means intended to be a rigid and mutually exclusive taxonomy.

4.2 SELECTION BIAS

Selection bias occurs when a systematic error in the recruitment or retention of study subjects—cases or controls in case-control studies, or exposed or unexposed subjects in cohort studies—results in a tendency toward distorting the measure expressing the association between exposure and outcome. When this bias occurs in case-control studies of hospitalized patients, it is often referred to as *Berksonian bias*.[2,3]

A hypothetical depiction of selection bias in the context of a case-control study is seen in Tables 4-1 through 4-4. In these tables, for ease of understanding, it is assumed that confounding is absent and that there is neither random variability nor information bias (i.e., that there is no misclassification of either exposure or case-control status; see Section 4.3).

In Table 4-1, all true cases and true noncases in a reference population of 10,000 subjects are included in a case-control study assessing the relationship of risk factor A with disease Y. Table 4-1 thus shows the "true" results that can be used as the "gold standard" for assessing the results shown in Tables 4-2 through 4-4.

TABLE 4-1 Hypothetical case-control study including all cases and all noncases of a defined population; assume no confounding effects and no information bias.

Risk factor A	Total population	
	Cases	Noncases (controls)
Present	500	1800
Absent	500	7200
Total	1000	9000
Exposure odds	500:500 = 1.0:1.0	1800:7200 = 1.0:4.0
Odds ratio		$\dfrac{\left(\dfrac{500}{500}\right)}{\left(\dfrac{1800}{7200}\right)} = 4.0$

Note: The results in this table represent the "gold standard" against which results in Tables 4-2, 4-3, and 4-4 are compared.

TABLE 4-2 Hypothetical case-control study including a 50% unbiased sample of cases and a 10% unbiased sample of noncases of the reference population shown in Table 4-1.

Risk factor A	Sample of the total population	
	50% of Cases	10% of Noncases (controls)
Present	250	180
Absent	250	720
Total	1000 × 0.50 = 500	9000 × 0.10 = 900
Exposure odds	250:250 = 1.0:1.0	180:720 = 1.0:4.0
Odds ratio		$\dfrac{\left(\dfrac{250}{250}\right)}{\left(\dfrac{180}{720}\right)} = 4.0$
Consequences	Unbiased exposure odds in cases and controls Unbiased odds ratio	

In Table 4-2, a 50% unbiased sample of cases and a 10% unbiased sample of controls are chosen from the total population shown in Table 4-1. The use of a larger sampling fraction for cases than for controls in Table 4-2 is typical of many case-control studies for which a limited pool of cases is available (see Chapter 3, Section 3.4.1); however, as long as the sampling fraction *within* the group of cases and that *within* the group of controls are unaffected by exposure, selection bias does not occur, and this sampling strategy yields unbiased exposure odds in cases and controls and, thus, an unbiased odds ratio.

In contrast to the unbiased approach shown in Table 4-2, Table 4-3 provides an example of selection bias, whereby, *unintended and unbeknownst to the investigator*, selection of cases, but not that of controls, is biased in that it varies according to exposure status. In the hypothetical example shown in Table 4-3, the investigator decides to select 50% of cases and 10% of controls, as done in Table 4-2; however, the selection of cases is not independent of exposure status. As a consequence, even though the overall sampling fraction for cases is the intended 50%, a greater sampling fraction is applied to exposed than to unexposed cases, biasing the exposure odds in cases but not in controls, and thus yielding a biased odds ratio. It is important to emphasize that the erroneous dependence of the selection of cases on their exposure status is unintended by the investigator, who is under the impression that both exposed and unexposed cases are subjected to the same preestablished sampling fraction of 50% applied to the total case pool. The examples shown in Tables 4-1 through 4-3 apply to a hypothetical situation in which there is a defined reference population list from which to sample cases and noncases. Often, population listings are unavailable, and thus epidemiologists use convenience samples of cases and controls, making the occurrence of selection bias more likely.

TABLE 4-3 Example of selection bias in choosing cases in a hypothetical case-control study including a 50% sample of cases and a 10% sample of noncases of the reference population shown in Table 4-1.

	Total population	
Risk factor A	Cases	Noncases (controls)
Present	500 × 0.60* = 300	180
Absent	500 × 0.40* = 200	720
Total	1000 × 0.50 = 500	9000 × 0.10 = 900
Exposure odds	300:200 × 1.5:1.0	180:720 = 1.0:4.0
Odds ratio	$\dfrac{\left(\dfrac{300}{200}\right)}{\left(\dfrac{180}{720}\right)} = 6.0$	
Consequences	Biased exposure odds in cases Unbiased exposure in controls Biased odds ratio	

*Differential sampling fractions unintended by, and unknown to, the investigator.

A hypothetical example of selection bias is a study of aplastic anemia in which cases are identified in a major referral hospital and controls are patients with nonmalignant, nonhematologic disorders identified in the same hospital. Because aplastic anemia patients may often be referred to this hospital for a bone marrow transplant, some of their characteristics will differ from those of other patients—for example, these patients may be more likely both to come from large families (as they often have a genetically matched sibling donor) and to have health insurance or a higher income in order to defray the considerable costs involved in this procedure. As a result, exposures related to having a large family and/or a higher socioeconomic status might be differentially distributed between cases and controls, leading to a distortion of the exposure-disease association.

Because differential bias of the type exemplified in Table 4-3 distorts the nature or magnitude of an association, investigators often attempt to "equalize" bias between the groups under comparison. In retrospective studies, for example, attempts are often made to obtain samples of cases and controls undergoing the same selection processes. Thus, for cases identified only in hospitals H1 and H2 out of several hospitals serving a given population A, an appropriate control group would be a sample of the population subset that, if diseased, would have chosen or been referred to hospitals H1 and H2. (This strategy is occasionally called *case-based, clinic-based,* or *hospital-based control selection.*[4,5]) Choice of controls ignoring the selection process that made study cases seek hospitals H1 and H2 (e.g., selecting controls from total population A) may produce selection bias if, for example, the two hospitals where cases are identified cater to patients having characteristics related to the exposure being evaluated.

Possibly the best example of successful equalization of selection processes is given by case-control studies in which both cases and controls are identified from among women attending a screening program.[6] Women participating in a screening program of breast cancer are more likely to have higher prevalence rates of known breast cancer risk factors, such as family history. Thus, if cases diagnosed by screening were compared with a sample of noncases drawn from the general population, overestimation of the magnitude of the association with certain risk factors might occur. Selecting both case and control groups from among screened women, however, makes both groups equally prone to the higher likelihood of exposure to known risk factors. This process is schematically illustrated in the hypothetical example shown in Table 4-4. In this table, bias of the same magnitude resulted in the inclusion of higher proportions of exposed subjects in both the case and the control groups. As a consequence, although exposure odds are biased in both cases and controls vis-à-vis the true exposure odds shown in Tables 4-1 and 4-2, the odds ratio is unbiased.

The magnitude of bias in the selection of cases is the same as for controls in Table 4-4, leading to what Schlesselman[4(p128)] has defined as "*compensating bias*":

$$\text{Bias} = \frac{\text{Observed odds}_{cases}}{\text{True odds}_{cases}} = \frac{\frac{1.5}{1.0}}{\frac{1.0}{1.0}} = \frac{\text{Observed odds}_{controls}}{\text{True odds}_{controls}} = \frac{\frac{1.0}{2.67}}{\frac{1.0}{4.0}} = 1.5$$

For compensating bias to occur, the same bias factor (in this example, "× 1.5") needs to be present in both the numerator (exposure odds of cases, $\text{Odds}_{exp/cases}$) and the denominator (exposure odds of controls, $\text{Odds}_{exp/controls}$) of the odds ratio so as to be canceled out:

$$\frac{\text{Odds}_{exp/cases} \times [\text{bias}]}{\text{Odds}_{exp/controls} \times [\text{bias}]} = \frac{\text{Odds}_{exp/cases}}{\text{Odds}_{exp/controls}} = \text{True odds ratio (OR)}$$

TABLE 4-4 Example of the same level of selection bias in choosing cases and controls in a hypothetical case-control study including a 50% sample of cases and a 10% sample of noncases of the defined population shown in Table 4-1.

Risk factor A	Total population	
	Cases	Noncases (controls)
Present	500 × 0.60* = 300	1800 × 0.136* = 245
Absent	500 × 0.40* = 200	7200 × 0.091* = 655
Total	1000 × 0.50 = 500	9000 × 0.10 = 900
Exposure odds	300:200 = 1.5:1.0	245:655 = 1.0:2.67
Odds ratio	$\dfrac{\left(\dfrac{300}{200}\right)}{\left(\dfrac{245}{655}\right)} = 4.0$	
Consequences	Exposure odds biased to the same extent in cases and controls Unbiased odds ratio	

*Differential sampling fractions unknown to the investigator.

In the example,

$$OR = \frac{\left(\dfrac{1.0}{1.0}\right) \times 1.5}{\left(\dfrac{1.0}{4.0}\right) \times 1.5} = \frac{\left(\dfrac{1.5}{1.0}\right)}{\left(\dfrac{1.0}{2.67}\right)} = 4.0$$

In practice, it is usually difficult to know for sure that the same bias applies to the exposure odds of both cases and controls, and attempts to introduce a compensating bias may even backfire, such as in the study examining the association of coffee intake and pancreatic cancer by MacMahon et al.,[7] in which controls were selected from a group of patients seen by the same physicians who had diagnosed the cases' disease. In addition to ease of logistics, the likely reason why the investigators chose this design was to make the selection process (including attending biases) of cases and controls similar. As the exposure of interest was coffee intake and as patients seen by physicians who diagnose pancreatic cancer often have gastrointestinal disorders and are thus advised not to drink coffee, however, the investigators' attempt to introduce a compensating bias led to the selection of controls with an unusually low odds of exposure. This resulted in a (spurious) positive association between coffee intake and cancer of the pancreas that could not be subsequently confirmed.[8]

Whenever possible, study subjects should be chosen from defined reference populations. In case-control studies, a sample of the defined population from which cases originated (as when doing a case-cohort study) constitutes the best type of control group. Efforts to introduce a compensating bias when the control group selection is driven by the case characteristics may or may not be successful, although they underscore the possibility of obtaining valid measures of association even in situations when it is not possible to obtain valid absolute measures of exposure frequency (odds).

All of the preceding examples are from case-control studies because these studies (along with cross-sectional studies) provide the most likely setting in which the sampling probabilities of the different disease-exposure groups may turn out to be differential (Figure 4-2). In a cohort study, because study participants (exposed or unexposed) are selected *before* the disease actually occurs, differential selection according to disease status is less likely to occur. Nevertheless, selection bias may occur at the outset of a cohort study when, for example, a group of persons exposed to an occupational hazard is compared with a sample of the general population (*healthy worker effect*).[9]

The more significant analogue of selection bias in the context of most cohort studies, however, relates to *differential losses to follow-up*, that is, whether individuals who are lost to follow-up over the course of the study are different from those who remain under observation up to the event occurrence or termination of the study. This analogy was discussed in Section 1.4.2, and Figures 1-13 and 1-18 underscore the theoretical equivalence between issues of selection of cases and controls (from a defined or a hypothetical cohort) and those related to differential losses in a cohort study. The biases on the estimates of incidence that can occur as a consequence of losses were discussed in Section 2.2. Individuals who are lost to follow-up (particularly when losses are due to mortality from causes other than the outcome of interest, refusal, or migration—see Table 2-4) tend to have different probabilities of the outcome than those who remain in the cohort over the entire span of the study. Thus, incidence estimates tend to be biased. However, as in the case-control study situation (Table 4-4), relative measures of association (relative risk, rate ratio) will be unbiased if the bias on the incidence estimates is of similar magnitude in exposed and unexposed individuals (compensating bias). In other words, a biased relative risk or rate ratio estimate will only ensue if losses to follow-up are biased according to *both* outcome and exposure.

4.3 INFORMATION BIAS

Information bias in epidemiologic studies results from either imperfect definitions of study variables or flawed data collection procedures. These errors may result in misclassification of exposure and/or outcome status for a significant proportion of study participants. Throughout this section, the terms *validity, sensitivity, specificity,* and *reliability* are frequently used. These concepts are defined in basic epidemiology texts (Exhibit 4-1) and are also frequently used in Chapter 8, which is closely related to this chapter.

EXHIBIT 4-1 Definitions of terms related to the classification of individuals in epidemiologic studies.

- **Validity:** the ability of a test to distinguish between who has a disease (or other characteristic) and who does not.
  - *Sensitivity:* the ability of a test to identify correctly those who have the disease (or characteristic) of interest.
  - *Specificity:* the ability of a test to identify correctly those who do not have the disease (or characteristic) of interest.
- **Reliability (repeatability):** the extent to which the results obtained by a test are replicated if the test is repeated.

Source: Adapted from L. Gordis, *Epidemiology*, © 2008, Philadelphia: Elsevier Saunders.

A *valid study* is equivalent to an "unbiased" study—a study that, based on its design, methods, and procedures, will produce (on average) overall results that are close to the truth. *Sensitivity* and *specificity* are defined as the two main components of validity. In basic textbooks or chapters discussing issues related to *diagnosis* and *screening* (e.g., Gordis[10]), these terms typically refer to the correct classification of *disease* status (i.e., diagnosis). In this chapter (as well as in Chapter 8), however, *sensitivity* and *specificity* also refer to the classification of *exposure* status. In addition to the main exposure variable (e.g., the main risk factor of interest in the study), misclassification of other variables, such as confounders, may also occur (see Chapter 7, Section 7.6).

4.3.1 Exposure Identification Bias

Problems in the collection of exposure data or an imperfect definition of the level of exposure may lead to bias. Exposure identification bias can affect cohort studies (e.g., when there are technical or other sorts of errors in the baseline measurements of exposure). However, because exposure in a cohort study is usually ascertained before the outcome (disease) of interest occurs, such errors tend to be similar with regard to disease status and thus result in the so-called nondifferential misclassification with somewhat predictable consequences (see Section 4.3.3). Potentially more serious exposure identification biases may occur in case-control studies, where exposure is assessed *after* case (disease) status is ascertained and thus may vary according to case-control status. Depending on the circumstances of each particular study, this can result in *nondifferential* or in *differential* misclassification, leading to less predictable results (see Section 4.3.3). Thus, most examples dealing with this type of information bias come from case-control studies. Two of the main subcategories of exposure identification bias are recall bias and interviewer bias.

Recall Bias

Recall bias resulting from inaccurate recall of past exposure is perhaps the most often cited type of exposure identification bias. It is a concern especially in the context of case-control studies, when cases and controls are asked about exposures in the past. Errors in recall of these past exposures result in misclassification of exposure status, thus biasing the results of the study. An empirical example of recall bias was documented by Weinstock et al.,[11] who collected information on hair color and tanning ability both at baseline and after the occurrence of melanoma in cohort participants of the Nurses' Health Study. In this study, cases of melanoma tended to over report "low tanning ability" in the postmelanoma diagnosis interview, as compared with the interview carried out before the occurrence of the disease, a difference that was not seen among controls (results from this study are discussed in detail in Section 4.3.3).

Methods used to prevent recall bias include verification of responses from study subjects, use of diseased controls in case-control studies, use of objective markers of exposure, and the conduct of case-control studies within the cohort (Chapter 1, Section 1.4.2).

Verification of exposure information obtained from participants by review of pharmacy or hospital charts (or other sources), is occasionally done in case-control studies. Examples include the studies examining the relationship of past use of estrogens to breast cancer,[12] in which responses from samples of cases and controls were verified by contacting physicians. In cohort studies, a similar strategy can be used to confirm participant information pertaining to event outcomes (e.g., myocardial infarction) or to identify and exclude prevalent cases from the baseline cohort in order to estimate incidence on follow-up. As an example, in the Atherosclerosis Risk in Communities Study and in the Multi-ethnic Study of Atherosclerosis, information provided by cohort members during the periodic telephone interviews on admissions for the main outcomes (e.g., myocardial infarction) has been systematically verified by review of relevant medical charts.[13,14]

Because, on occasion in case-control studies, recall bias may be caused by "rumination" by cases regarding the causes of their disease, *a control group formed by diseased subjects* is sometimes selected as an attempt to introduce a similar bias in the exposure odds of controls. An example is a study by Mele et al.[15] in which cases of leukemia were compared with a control group formed by symptomatic patients who, after evaluation in the same hematology clinics as the cases, were not found to have hematological disorders. The problem with using a diseased control group, however, is that it is often unclear whether the "rumination" process related to the controls' diseases is equivalent to that of cases with regard to the magnitude of recall bias.

Compared with *subjective markers, objective markers* of exposure or susceptibility are less prone to recall bias from study subjects, which, however, may still occur. In one of the earliest studies addressing the issue of information bias, Lilienfeld and Graham compared information on circumcision obtained by physical examination with that provided by the participants (Table 4-5).[16] In this study, of 84 truly circumcised participants, only 37 said that they had been circumcised; of the 108 noncircumcised participants, 89 mentioned that they had not been circumcised. Thus, in this study, the sensitivity and specificity of participants' statements on whether they had been circumcised were 44% and 82.4%, respectively. On the other hand, an example in which a reasonably objective exposure (hair color) resulted in the virtual absence of information bias can be found in the study of melanoma risk factors cited previously.[11] In contrast to the bias in reporting "tanning ability" after the disease diagnosis, the responses of cases and controls regarding hair color did not show any significant change when the responses to the questionnaires applied before and after the disease diagnosis were compared (see Section 4.3.3). A likely reason for this is that hair color is more objectively assessed than tanning ability.

Certain genetic markers constitute "exposures" that are not time-dependent and can be measured even after the disease has occurred, thus possibly being less prone to bias (assuming that the genetic marker is not related to survival; see Section 4.3.3). An example is the assessment of DNA repair capabilities as a genetic marker for susceptibility

TABLE 4-5 Patients' statements and examination findings regarding circumcision status, Roswell Park Memorial Institute, Buffalo, New York.

Participants' statements on circumcision	Physical examination finding			
	Circumcised		Noncircumcised	
	Number	%	Number	%
Yes	37	44.0	19	17.6
No	47	56.0	89	82.4
Total	84	100.0	108	100.0

Adapted from: AM Lilienfeld and S Graham. Validity of Determining Circumcision Status by Questionnaire as Related to Epidemiological Studies of Cancer of the Cervix. *Journal of the National Cancer Institute.* Vol 21, pp. 713–720, © 1958.

to ultraviolet light-induced nonmelanoma skin cancer in young cases and controls.[17] Regrettably, however, most environmental exposures that can be assessed by means of objective biologic markers represent current or very recent, rather than past, exposures, such as the levels of serum cotinine to indicate exposure to cigarette smoking, and are thus of limited usefulness.[18]

When a well-defined cohort is available, nested case-control or case-cohort studies (see Section 1.4.2) allow the evaluation of certain hypotheses free of recall bias (or temporal bias; see Section 4.3.3). Typically, in these case-control studies, information on exposure and confounders is collected at baseline (i.e., before the incident cases occur), thus reducing the likelihood of systematic recall differences between cases and controls. The study discussed previously examining the relationship of tanning ability to melanoma[11] (see previously here and Section 4.3.3) is an example of a case-control study within a cohort (the Nurses Health Study cohort); the application of the premelanoma diagnosis questionnaire avoids the recall bias that was observed when the analysis was based on information obtained from the postmelanoma questionnaire.[11]

Although exposure recall bias is typically a problem of case-control studies, it may also occur in cohort studies. In the latter type of study, it may be present at the outset of the study when categorization of individuals by level of exposure relies on recalled information from the distant or recent past, as when attempts are made to classify cohort participants at baseline by duration of exposure.

Interviewer Bias

When data collection in a case-control study is not masked with regard to the disease status of study participants, *observer bias* in ascertaining exposure, such as *interviewer bias*, may occur. Interviewer bias may be a consequence of trying to "clarify" questions when such clarifications are not part of the study protocol, failing to follow either the protocol-determined probing or skipping rules of questionnaires. Although it is often difficult to recognize interviewer bias, it is important to be aware of it and to implement procedures to minimize the likelihood of its occurrence. Attempts to prevent interviewer bias involve the careful design and conduct of quality assurance and control activities (see Chapter 8), including development of a detailed manual of operations, training of staff, standardization of data collection procedures, and monitoring of data collection activities. Even when these methods are in place, however, subtle deviations from the protocol (e.g., emphasizing certain words when carrying out the case, but not the control, interviews—or vice versa) might be difficult to identify. Additional measures to recognize and prevent this bias are the performance of reliability/validity sub-studies and the masking of interviewers with regard to case-control status.

Reliability and validity sub-studies in samples are described in more detail in Chapter 8, Section 8.3. They constitute an important strategy that needs to be carried out systematically, with quick feedback to interviewers who do not follow the protocol or who have encountered problems. Reliability sub-studies of interviews are not as straightforward as those aimed at assessing the reproducibility of laboratory measurements, such as those described in many of the examples in Chapter 8. Assessing the reliability of interview data is difficult because of intraparticipant variability and because when interviews are done at separate points in time, interviewees or interviewers may recall previous responses, with the resultant tendency to provide/record the same, albeit mistaken, responses.

As for recall bias, validity studies using independent sources (e.g., medical charts) can be conducted to assess accuracy of data collection by interviewers.

Masking of interviewers with regard to case-control status of study participants is difficult, but when feasible, it may remove an important source of bias, particularly when the interviewer is familiar with the study hypothesis. On occasion, by including a health question for which a frequent affirmative response is expected from both cases and controls, it is possible to mask the interviewers with regard to the main study hypothesis and have them believe that the hypothesis pertains to the "misleading" question. Such a strategy was employed in a case-control study of psychosocial factors and myocardial infarction in women, in which questions about hysterectomy, which were often answered positively in view of the high frequency of this intervention in the United States, led the interviewers to believe that the study was testing a hormonal hypothesis.[19]

A mistake made in an early study of lung cancer and smoking conducted by Doll and Hill,[20] in which some controls were erroneously classified as cases, suggests an additional strategy for assessing occurrence of interviewer bias. In this study, the odds of exposure to smoking in the misclassified controls was very similar to that of the nonmisclassified controls and much lower than that of cases, thus confirming the absence of interviewer bias. This example suggests the possibility of using "phantom" cases and controls and/or purposely misleading interviewers to believe that some cases are controls and vice versa in order to assess interviewer bias.

4.3.2 Outcome Identification Bias

Outcome (e.g., disease) *identification bias* may occur in both case-control and cohort studies. This bias may result from either differential or nondifferential misclassification of disease status, which in turn may be due to an imperfect definition of the outcome or to errors at the data collection stage.

Observer Bias

In a cohort study, the decision as to whether the outcome is present may be affected by knowledge of the exposure status of the study participant. This may happen particularly when the outcome is "soft," such as, for example, when reporting migraine episodes or psychiatric symptoms. There may be *observer bias* at different stages of the ascertainment of the outcome, including at the stage of applying pathologic or clinical criteria. A fairly crude example of observer bias is the assignment of a histologic specimen to a diagnosis of "alcoholic cirrhosis" when the pathologist knows that the patient is an alcoholic. A documented example of observer bias is the effect of the patient's race on the diagnosis of hypertensive end-stage renal disease (ESRD). In a study conducted by Perneger et al.,[21] a sample of nephrologists were sent case histories of seven patients with ESRD. For each case history, the simulated race of each patient was randomly assigned to be "black" or "white." Case histories that identified the patient's race as "black" were twice as likely to result in a diagnosis of hypertensive ESRD as case histories in which the patient's race was said to be "white."

This type of observer bias occurs when the ascertainment of outcome is not independent from the knowledge of the exposure status and results in *differential* misclassification of the outcome. Thus, measures aimed at *masking observers in charge of deciding whether the outcome is present by exposure status* would theoretically prevent observer bias. When masking of observers by exposure status is not practical, observer bias can be assessed by stratifying on certainty of diagnosis. For example, exposure levels can be assessed in relationship to incidence of "possible," "probable," or "definite" disease.

Observer bias should be suspected if an association is seen only for the "softer" categories (e.g., "possible" disease).

Another strategy to prevent observer bias is to perform diagnostic classification with *multiple observers*. For example, two observers could independently classify an event, and if disagreement occurred, a third observer would adjudicate; that is, decision on the presence or absence of the outcome would have to be agreed on by at least two of three observers.

Respondent Bias

Recall and other informant biases are usually associated with identification of exposure in case-control studies; however, outcome ascertainment bias may occur during follow-up of a cohort when information on the outcome is obtained by participant response; for example, when collecting information on events for which it is difficult to obtain objective confirmation, such as episodes of migraine headaches.

Whenever possible, information given by a participant on the possible occurrence of the outcome of interest should be confirmed by more objective means, such as hospital chart review. Objective confirmation may, however, not be possible—for example, for nonhospitalized events or for events in which laboratory verification is impossible, such as pain or acute panic attacks. For these types of outcomes, detailed information not only on presence versus absence of a given event, but also on related symptoms that may be part of a diagnostic constellation, may be of help in preventing *respondent bias*. For example, the questionnaire on the occurrence of an episode of migraine headaches in a study by Stewart et al.[22] included questions not only on whether a severe headache had occurred but also on the presence of aura, nausea, and fatigue accompanying the headache. This strategy allowed more objectivity in classifying migraines than the simple determination of the presence or absence of pain. For several outcomes, such as angina pectoris and chronic bronchitis, standardized questionnaires are available (see Chapter 8). The validity and limitations of some of these instruments, such as, for example, the Rose questionnaire for the diagnosis of angina pectoris,[23] have been assessed.[24–26]

4.3.3 The Result of Information Bias: Misclassification

Information bias leads to *misclassification* of exposure and/or outcome status. For example, when there is recall bias in a case-control study, some exposed subjects are classified as unexposed and vice versa. In a cohort study, a positive outcome may be missed. Alternatively, a pseudo-event may be mistakenly classified as an outcome (a "false positive"). The examples of both differential and nondifferential misclassification in this section refer to exposure levels in case-control studies. Misclassification of case-control status in case-control studies and of exposure and outcome in cohort studies can be readily inferred, although they are not specifically discussed so as to avoid repetition.

There are two types of misclassification bias: nondifferential and differential.

Nondifferential Misclassification

In a case-control study, *nondifferential misclassification* occurs when the degree of misclassification of exposure is independent of case-control status (or vice versa).

Nondifferential Misclassification When There Are Two Categories. A simplistic hypothetical example of nondifferential misclassification of (dichotomous) exposure

> **EXHIBIT 4-2** Hypothetical example of the effect of nondifferential misclassification of two categories of exposure, with 30% of both exposed cases and exposed controls misclassified as unexposed.
>
> **No misclassification**
>
> | Exposure | Cases | Controls |
> |---|---|---|
> | Yes | 50 | 20 |
> | No | 50 | 80 |
>
> $$OR = \frac{\left(\frac{50}{50}\right)}{\left(\frac{20}{80}\right)} = 4.0$$
>
> **30% Exposure misclassification in each group**
>
> | Exposure | Cases | Controls |
> |---|---|---|
> | Yes | 50 − **15** = 35 | 20 − **6** = 14 |
> | No | 50 + **15** = 65 | 80 + **6** = 86 |
>
> $$OR = \frac{\left(\frac{35}{65}\right)}{\left(\frac{14}{86}\right)} = 3.3$$
>
> Effect of nondifferential misclassification with two exposure categories: to bias the OR toward the null value of 1.0. (It "dilutes" the association.)

Note: Bold numbers represent misclassified individuals.

in a case-control study is shown in Exhibit 4-2. In this example, misclassification of exposed subjects as unexposed occurs in 30% of cases and 30% of controls. In this simpler situation when there are only two exposure categories (for instance, "yes" or "no"), nondifferential misclassification tends to bias the association toward the null hypothesis.

In the hypothetical example shown in Exhibit 4-2, misclassification occurs in only one direction: exposed individuals are misclassified as unexposed. Often, however, misclassification occurs in both directions: that is, exposed individuals are classified as unexposed or "false negatives" (i.e., the correct classification of the truly exposed, or sensitivity, is less than 100%), and unexposed individuals are classified as exposed or "false positives" (i.e., the correct classification of the unexposed, or specificity, is less than 100%). In a case-control study, nondifferential misclassification occurs when the *both* sensitivity *and* specificity of the classification of exposure are the same for cases and controls but either (or both) is less than 100%. Estimation of the total numbers of individuals classified as "exposed" or "unexposed" by using a study's data collection procedures and exposure level definitions is akin to the estimation of "test-positive" and "test-negative" individuals when applying a screening test. Thus, the notions of sensitivity and specificity, schematically represented in Figure 4-4, can be used to explore the issue of misclassification in more depth.

A hypothetical example showing nondifferential misclassification of exposure in a case-control study in both directions—that is, when exposed subjects are misclassified as unexposed and unexposed subjects are misclassified as exposed—is presented

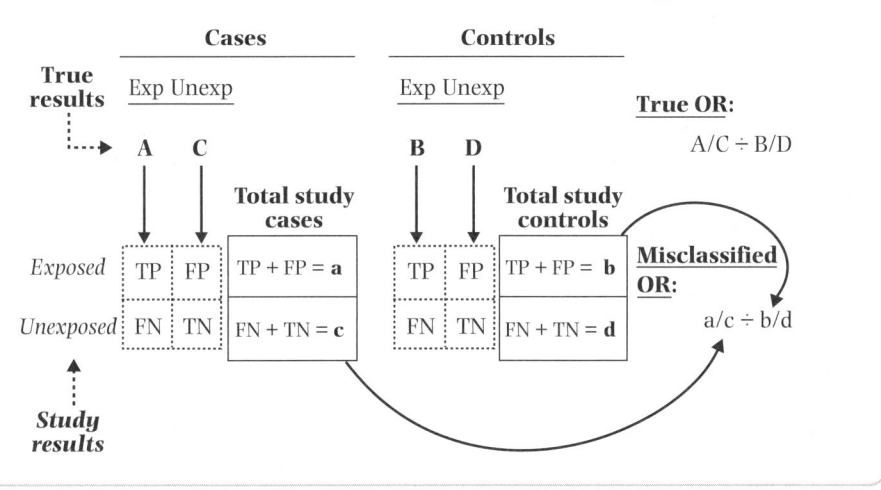

FIGURE 4-4 Application of sensitivity/specificity concepts in misclassification of exposure: schematic representation of true and misclassified relative odds. Sensitivity of exposure ascertainment = TP ÷ (TP + FN); specificity of exposure ascertainment = TN ÷ (TN + FP).

Note: Exp: Exposure; TP: True positive; FP: False positive; FN: False negative; TN: True negative

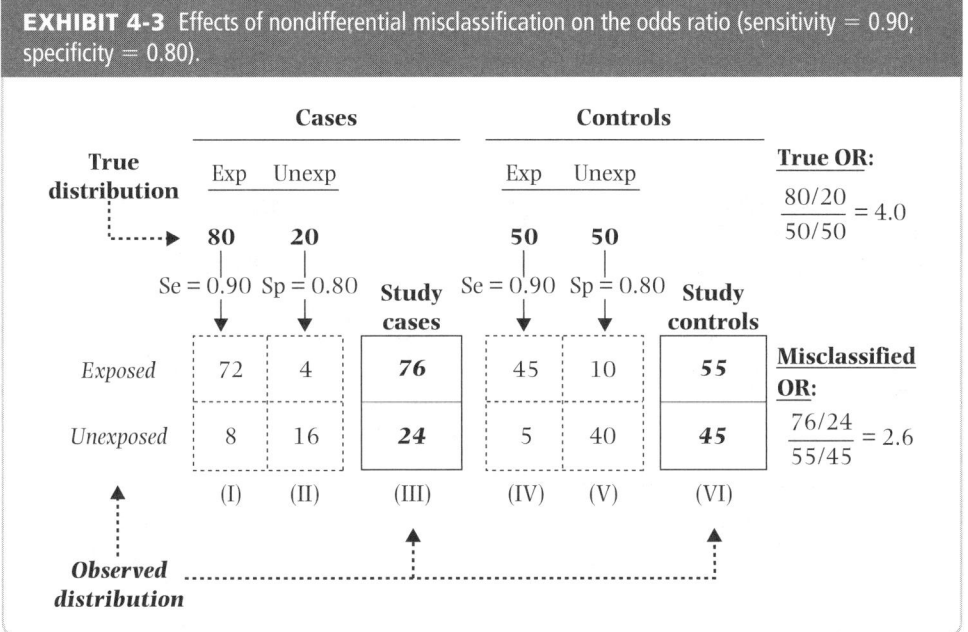

EXHIBIT 4-3 Effects of nondifferential misclassification on the odds ratio (sensitivity = 0.90; specificity = 0.80).

Note: Exp: Exposed; Unexp: Unexposed; Se: Sensitivity; Sp: Specificity; OR: Odds ratio

in Exhibit 4-3. The exhibit shows the effects of nondifferential misclassification resulting from an exposure ascertainment with a sensitivity of 90% and a specificity of 80%. The fact that these sensitivity and specificity values are the same for cases and controls identifies this type of misclassification as nondifferential.

The net effect of misclassifying cases at a sensitivity of 90% and a specificity of 80% is shown in column (III) of Exhibit 4-3. The totals in column (III) indicate the numbers of cases classified as "exposed" or "unexposed" in the study and reflect the misclassification due to the less-than-perfect sensitivity and specificity values. Thus, cases classified as "exposed" include both the 72 persons truly exposed ("true positives") and the 4 cases which, although unexposed, are misclassified as exposed ("false positives") due to a specificity less than 100% (see also Figure 4-4). Similarly, cases classified in the study as "unexposed" include both the 16 truly unexposed cases ("true negatives") and the 8 exposed cases misclassified as unexposed ("false negatives") because the sensitivity is less than 100%. Exhibit 4-3 also shows similar data for *controls*. The net effect of the classification of controls by exposure at the same sensitivity (90%) and specificity (80%) levels as those of cases is shown in column (VI). The observed (biased) odds ratio of 2.6 in the study underestimates the true odds ratio of 4.0, as expected when misclassification of a dichotomous exposure is nondifferential between cases and controls.

In the example shown in Exhibit 4-3, nondifferential misclassification of a dichotomous exposure is shown to be affected by sensitivity and specificity levels, such that the net effect is to bias the odds ratio toward 1.0. In addition to reflecting sensitivity and specificity of the procedures for exposure definition and ascertainment, the magnitude of the bias also depends on the exposure prevalence, particularly in the presence of a large control group. For example, Exhibit 4-4 shows a hypothetical situation where the true strength of the association between exposure and disease is identical to that in Exhibit 4-3 (odds ratio = 4.0) as are the sensitivity and specificity of exposure measurement (90% and 80%, respectively). However, because of the lower prevalence of exposure (i.e., 20/820 or 2.4% among controls, compared to 50% in Exhibit 4-3), the bias is substantially more pronounced (biased odds ratio = 1.3 versus

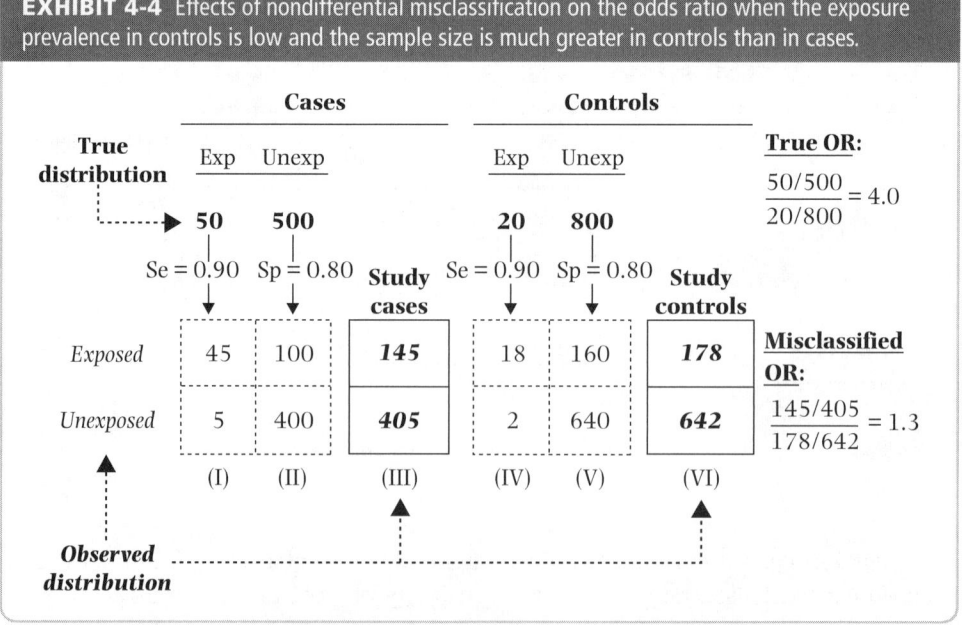

EXHIBIT 4-4 Effects of nondifferential misclassification on the odds ratio when the exposure prevalence in controls is low and the sample size is much greater in controls than in cases.

Notes: Exp: Exposed; Unexp: Unexposed; Se: Sensitivity; Sp: Specificity; OR: Odds ratio

TABLE 4-6 Nondifferential misclassification: hypothetical examples of the effects of sensitivity and specificity of exposure identification and of exposure prevalence in controls on a study's odds ratio when the true odds ratio is 4.0.

Sensitivity*	Specificity†	Prevalence of exposure in controls	Observed odds ratio
0.90	0.85	0.200	2.6
0.60	0.85	0.200	1.9
0.90	**0.95**	0.200	3.2
0.90	**0.60**	0.200	1.9
0.90	0.90	**0.368**	3.0
0.90	0.90	**0.200**	2.8
0.90	0.90	**0.077**	2.2

Note: Bold figures represent the factor (sensitivity, specificity, or exposure prevalence) that is allowed to vary, for fixed values of the other two factors.
*Sensitivity of the exposure identification is defined as the proportion of all truly exposed correctly classified by the study.
†Specificity of the exposure identification is defined as the proportion of all truly unexposed correctly classified by the study.

2.6 in Exhibit 4-3). In general, low exposure prevalence tends to be associated with a higher degree of bias when the specificity is low. If specificity is high but sensitivity is low, however, a higher degree of bias will result from a situation in which exposure is common. The complex relationships between bias, sensitivity/specificity of exposure definition, and its prevalence is illustrated in Table 4-6, showing examples of the effects of sensitivity, specificity, and exposure prevalence in controls on the observed odds ratio in several hypothetical situations where the true odds ratio is 4.0.

Nondifferential Misclassification When There Are More Than Two Exposure Categories. The rule that the direction of a nondifferential misclassification bias dilutes the strength of the association may not hold in certain nondifferential misclassification situations involving more than two exposure categories. A hypothetical example involving three exposure levels in a case-control study ("none," "low," and "high") is discussed by Dosemeci et al.[27] (Table 4-7). In this example, 40% of both cases and controls in the "high" exposure category were misclassified as belonging to the adjacent category, "low"; the net effect was an increase in the odds ratio for the "low" category without a change for the "high." Misclassification for nonadjacent categories of exposure in the example—that is, between "high" and "none"—resulted in the disappearance of the truly graded relationship and, assuming no random error, the emergence of a J-shaped pattern. Additionally, as shown by Dosemeci et al.,[27] misclassification of nonadjacent exposure categories may invert the direction of the graded relationship.

Differential Misclassification

Differential misclassification occurs when the degree of misclassification differs between the groups being compared; for example, in a case-control study, the sensitivity and/or the specificity of the classification of exposure status are different between cases and controls. (Note that differential misclassification may occur even when only one of these validity indices differ.) Whereas the general tendency of nondifferential misclassification of a dichotomous exposure factor is to weaken a true association, differential misclassification may bias the association either toward or away from the

TABLE 4-7 Examples of the effects of nondifferential misclassification involving three exposure categories; misclassification of 40% between "high" and "low" (A) and between "high" and "none" (B).

Case-control status	True exposure status		
	None	Low	High
Cases	100	200	600
Controls	100	100	100
Odds ratio	1.00	2.00	6.00

Misclassified exposure status (in situations A and B)

A. Adjacent categories: 40% of cases and controls in "high" misclassified as "low"

Cases	100	200 CC + 240 MC = 440	600 CC − 240 MC = 360
Controls	100	100 CC + 40 MC = 140	100 CC − 40 MC = 60
Odds ratio	1.00	3.14	6.00

B. Nonadjacent categories: 40% of cases and controls in "high" misclassified as "none"

Cases	100 CC + 240 MC = 340	200	600 CC − 240 MC = 360
Controls	100 CC + 40 MC = 140	100	100 CC − 40 MC = 60
Odds ratio	1.00	0.82	2.47

Note: CC: correctly classified; MC: misclassified.
Source: Data from M Dosemeci, S Wacholder, and JH Lubin, Does Nondifferential Misclassification of Exposure Always Bias a True Effect Toward the Null Value? *American Journal of Epidemiology*, Vol 132, pp. 746–748, © 1990.

null hypothesis. Thus, it is difficult to predict the direction of the bias when differential misclassification occurs, as it is the result of a complex interplay involving differences between cases and controls in sensitivity, specificity, and prevalence of exposure.

A hypothetical example of differential misclassification is given in Exhibit 4-5, in which the sensitivity of capturing the exposure in cases is 96% and that in controls is only 70%. Specificity in the example is 100% for both cases and controls. The better sensitivity among cases leads to a higher proportion of truly exposed subjects being identified in cases than in controls, yielding a biased odds ratio further away from 1.0 than the true odds ratio (true odds ratio = 4.0, biased odds ratio = 5.7). To underscore the difficulties in predicting results when there is differential misclassification, if the same calculations are done using a higher specificity in cases (100%) than in controls (80%), the odds ratio is biased toward the null hypothesis (Exhibit 4-6), as a poorer specificity in controls offsets the higher sensitivity in cases.

Exhibit 4-7 shows a hypothetical example that illustrates a shortcut to the calculation of misclassified odds ratios. The table shows the complements to sensitivity and specificity values, and their application to the relevant cells in cases and controls. In this example, misclassification is differential and yet the misclassified odds ratio is biased toward the null hypothesis.

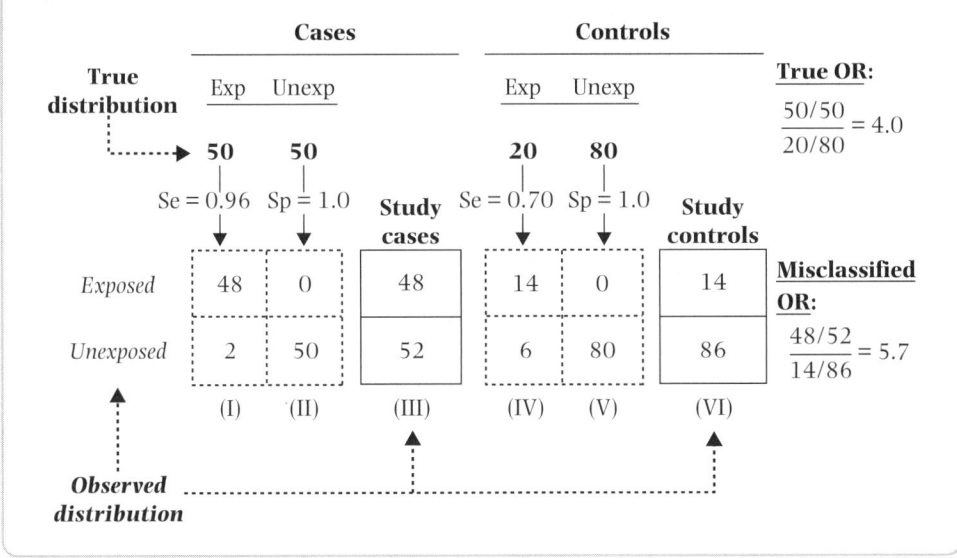

EXHIBIT 4-5 Hypothetical example of the effects of differential misclassification on the odds ratio, in which, for sensitivity, cases > controls, and for specificity, cases = controls.

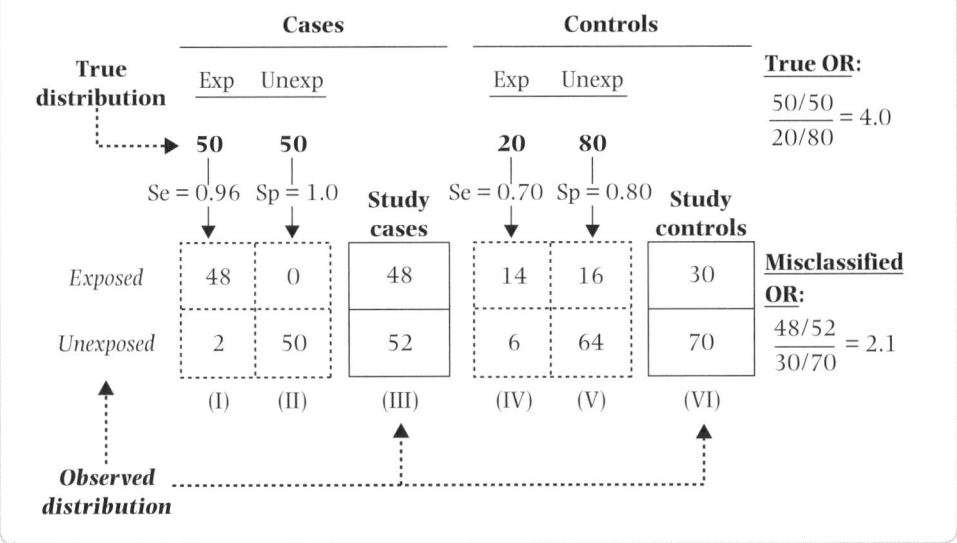

EXHIBIT 4-6 Hypothetical example of the effects of differential misclassification on the odds ratio, in which for both sensitivity and specificity, cases > controls.

Note: Exp: Exposed; Unexp: Unexposed; Se: Sensitivity; Sp: Specificity; OR: Odds ratio

EXHIBIT 4-7 Shortcut calculation of misclassified odds ratios in a case-control study. Exposure information sensitivity: cases = 0.96; controls = 0.85; specificity: cases = 0.80; controls = 0.70. Application of complements of sensitivity and specificity values estimates the number of false negatives and false positives in each exposure category. For example, 1 − sensitivity (0.04) for cases results in 2 exposed cases being misclassified as unexposed (false negatives); 1 − specificity for cases (0.20) results in 10 unexposed cases being misclassified as exposed (false positives). Similar calculations are done for controls.

	Cases (n = 100)				Controls (n = 100)			
		1 - Se	1 - Sp			1 - Se	1 - Sp	
	True distribution	0.04	0.20	Total misclassified	True distribution	0.15	0.30	Total misclassified
Exposed	50	−2	+10 (FP)	58	20	−3	+24 (FP)	41
Unexposed	50	+2 (FN)	−10	42	80	+3 (FN)	−24	59

This differential misclassification biases the odds ratios toward the null hypothesis.

$$\text{True odds ratio}: \frac{50/50}{20/80} = 4.0$$

$$\text{Misclassified odds ratio}: \frac{58/42}{41/59} = 1.98$$

Note: Se: Sensitivity; Sp: Specificity; FN: False negative; FP: False positive

Examples of the isolated effects of sensitivity (for a specificity of 100%) or specificity (for a sensitivity of 100%) on the odds ratio in a hypothetical case-control study with differential misclassification of exposure and a control exposure prevalence of 10% are shown in Table 4-8.

An example of differential misclassification of exposure was documented by Weinstock et al.[11] This example was used previously here to illustrate the concept of recall bias (see Section 4.3.1). In this study, melanoma cases and controls selected from participants of the Nurses Health Study cohort and matched for duration of follow-up were compared with regard to their report of "hair color" and "tanning ability" both at baseline and after the case was diagnosed. In this example, the differential misclassification in the postdiagnosis interview probably occurred because the disease status was known to the case and had the potential to affect recall of exposure. Therefore, the premelanoma diagnosis interview is assumed to accurately reflect the true association. The main results of the study are summarized in Table 4-9. For the discussion that follows, the categories associated with an increase in odds using the case-control data obtained after the occurrence of melanoma were regarded as "exposed" ("red or blond" and "no tan or light tan" for hair color and tanning ability, respectively).

Compared with the predisease development data, the odds for hair color among cases did not change when the postmelanoma interview data were used (11:23 in both interviews) and increased only slightly among controls (from 37:197 to 41:193); as a result, the odds ratio changed relatively little (prediagnosis odds ratio = 2.5; postdiagnosis odds ratio = 2.3). The effect of differential misclassification of tanning

TABLE 4-8 Examples of the effects of differential sensitivity and specificity of exposure ascertainment on the odds ratio (OR) for a true OR of 3.86 and a control exposure prevalence of 0.10.

Exposure ascertainment				
Sensitivity*		Specificity†		
Cases	Controls	Cases	Controls	Odds ratio
0.90	0.60	1.00	1.00	5.79
0.60	0.90	1.00	1.00	2.22
1.00	1.00	0.90	0.70	1.00
1.00	1.00	0.70	0.90	4.43

*Sensitivity of the exposure identification is defined as the proportion of all truly exposed correctly classified by the study.
†Specificity of the exposure identification is defined as the proportion of all truly unexposed correctly classified by the study.

TABLE 4-9 Reported hair color and tanning ability among incident cases and controls in a case-control study of melanoma within the Nurses Health Study cohort.

	Premelanoma diagnosis information ("gold standard")		Postmelanoma diagnosis information	
	Cases	Controls	Cases	Controls
Hair color				
Red or blond (exposed)	11	37	11	41
Brown or black (unexposed)	23	197	23	193
Odds ratio	2.5		2.3	
Tanning ability				
No tan, practically no tan, or light tan (exposed)	9	79	15	77
Medium, average, deep, or dark tan (unexposed)	25	155	19	157
Odds ratio	0.7		1.6	

Source: Data from MA Weinstock et al., Recall (Report) Bias and Reliability in the Retrospective Assessment of Melanoma Risk. *American Journal of Epidemiology*, Vol 133, pp. 240–245, © 1991.

ability, however, was severe, leading to a reversal of the direction of the association. Assuming no random variability, the true association (i.e., that detected using the premelanoma diagnosis information) suggests a protective effect (odds ratio = 0.7), whereas the observed postdiagnosis association (odds ratio = 1.6) indicates a greater melanoma odds associated with a low tanning ability. It is of interest that the misclassification of exposure as measured by tanning ability seems to have resulted in only a slight change in odds of exposure in controls (from 79:155 to 77:157).

In cases, however, the misclassification effect was substantial, with the number of individuals classified as "exposed" increasing from 9 to 15 between the first and the second interviews.

The cross-tabulation of the premelanoma and postmelanoma diagnosis data enables a more detailed analysis of this situation by the calculation of sensitivity and specificity of tanning ability ascertainment in cases.* As shown in Table 4-10, the sensitivity of 89% of the postmelanoma diagnosis interviews resulted in the correct classification of eight of the nine truly exposed cases. However, a specificity of only 72% led to a relatively large number of unexposed persons in the "false-positive" cell and thus to a marked increase in the postdiagnosis exposure odds (true exposure odds in cases, 9:25 or 0.36:1.0; biased exposure odds, 15:19 or 0.79:1.0). Such change resulted in an odds ratio in the postdiagnosis study in a direction opposite to that of the true value. As mentioned previously (Section 4.3.1), differential misclassification in the study by Weinstock et al.[11] probably occurred because of recall bias. Additional misclassification may have occurred because the questions on hair color and tanning ability were not exactly the same in the interviews conducted before and after diagnosis. The latter, however, would be expected to result in nondifferential misclassification (equally affecting cases and controls). (In addition, if the misclassification had been nondifferential, that is, if the sensitivity and specificity values observed among the cases had been the same in controls, the odds ratio would have changed from the true [premelanoma diagnosis] value of 0.7 to a misclassified value of 0.83—that is, an estimate of the association biased toward the null value.)

TABLE 4-10 Distribution of incident cases in the Nurses Health Study cohort, 1976 to 1984, according to responses given with regard to tanning ability prior to the development of melanoma and after diagnosis was made.

	Premelanoma diagnosis information ("gold standard")		
Postmelanoma diagnosis information	No tan, practically no tan, or light tan ("exposed")	Medium, average, deep, or dark tan ("unexposed")	Total (case-control classification)
No tan, practically no tan, or light tan ("exposed")	8 (TP)	7 (FP)	15
Medium, average, deep, or dark tan ("unexposed")	1 (FN)	18 (TN)	19
Total ("true classification")	9 Sensitivity: 8/9 = 89%	25 Specificity: 18/25 = 72%	34

Note: TP: True positives; FP: False positives; FN: False negatives; TN: True negatives.
Source: Data from MA Weinstock et al., Recall (Report) Bias and Reliability in the Retrospective Assessment of Melanoma Risk. *American Journal of Epidemiology*, Vol 133, pp. 240–245, © 1991.

---

*In the paper by Weinstock et al.,[11] sensitivity and specificity of postdiagnosis responses on tanning ability were provided only for cases.

An example of both differential and nondifferential misclassification is given by a case-control study of childhood acute lymphoblastic leukemia conducted by Infante-Rivard and Jacques.[28] Four hundred and ninety-one cases and two sets of age-, sex- and broad geographical area-matched controls were chosen, one set from a population sample and the other from among hospital patients. For each individual in the study, the authors measured the actual distance between the residence and the nearest power line and compared this distance with the parent's answer to the question, "Within a radius of 1 km of your house, was there a high-voltage power line?" The authors classified cases into those living in a geographic area where people were concerned about an excess of the disease ("GA" cases) and "other" cases. When comparing GA cases with either population or hospital controls, substantial differential misclassification was detected, with a higher sensitivity, but lower specificity was seen for GA cases (Table 4-11). If—to calculate the odds ratio—analyses were limited to "other" cases versus hospital controls, however, nondifferential misclassification would have resulted, as their sensitivity and specificity values were found to be almost the same.

Effect of Misclassification of a Confounding Variable

Misclassification also affects the efficiency of adjustment for confounding effects. Whereas a nondifferential misclassification of a potential risk factor tends to bias the measure of association toward the null hypothesis, nondifferential misclassification of a confounding variable results in an imperfect adjustment when that variable is matched or controlled for in the analyses (see Chapters 5 and 7).[29] This imperfect adjustment results in residual confounding (see Sections 5.5.4 and 7.6).

Prevention of Misclassification

Misclassification has been extensively discussed in the epidemiological literature,[30–33] reflecting its importance in epidemiologic studies. As seen in the examples described in this section, misclassification may severely distort the magnitude of an association between a risk factor and a disease. If the true relative risk or odds ratio is close to 1.0, a nondifferential misclassification may completely mask the association. For example, for an exposure with a prevalence as high as 16% (i.e., in a range not unlike that of

TABLE 4-11 Sensitivity and specificity of response by parent of childhood (age 9 years or less) acute lymphoblastic leukemia cases to question, "Within a radius of 1 km (1000 m) of your house, was there a high-voltage power line?" Montreal Island, Quebec, Canada, 1980–1993.

	Sensitivity (%)*	Specificity (%)*
GA cases[†]	61.9	54.4
Other cases	34.9	90.6
Population controls	22.2	89.4
Hospital controls	35.8	90.2

*Gold standard: measured distance.
[†]Cases living in a geographic area where people were concerned about an excess of acute lymphoblastic leukemia cases.
Source: Data from C Infante-Rivera and L Jacques, Empirical Study of Parental Recall Bias. *American Journal of Epidemiology,* Vol 152, pp. 480–486, © 2000.

many risk factors), if the true odds ratio is approximately 1.3, the observed odds ratio may be virtually 1.0 if a nondifferential misclassification resulted from a measurement procedure with both sensitivity and specificity levels of approximately 70%. Differential misclassification of a confounding variable, on the other hand, may either dilute or strengthen an association, or even produce a spurious one. When the exposure is common, failing to demonstrate a real relationship or inferring that an association exists when it is spurious may have serious public health consequences (see Chapter 10).

Data are usually not available to allow a comparison between correctly classified and misclassified individuals in terms of available characteristics (e.g., educational level), but when they are, they may be informative. As seen in Table 4-10, of the 34 incident cases included in the case-control study on melanoma nested in the Nurses' Health Study cohort, 26 were correctly classified (8 true positives and 18 true negatives),[11] and 8 were misclassified (7 false positives and 1 false negative). A comparison could be made, for example, between the false positives and true negatives on the one hand (addressing the issue of specificity) and between the false negatives and true positives on the other (addressing the issue of sensitivity). In the Nurses' Health Study, the authors reported no important differences between the correctly and the incorrectly classified cases. (When studying tanning ability, it would not be unreasonable to postulate that recall of tanning ability could be influenced by factors such as family history of skin diseases or involvement in outdoor activities.) Similarity in pertinent characteristics of correctly classified and misclassified persons may perhaps indicate that recall bias is not a probable explanation for the misclassification and raises the possibility that the information bias originated from problems related to the instrument or the observer. Thus, the comparison between misclassified and nonmisclassified subjects need not be limited to respondent characteristics and should also include aspects of the data collection procedures. When interviews are taped, adherence to the protocol by interviewers can be compared. Additionally, information should be obtained on the reliability and validity of the instrument (e.g., a questionnaire), as discussed in Chapter 8.

A more general approach to assess information bias is based on the evaluation of the odds of "inaccurate self-reporting" as the outcome of interest (i.e., without specification of sensitivity or specificity). An example is given by a study of the validity of self-reported AIDS-specific diagnoses (such as esophageal candidiasis) vis-à-vis AIDS diagnoses documented by AIDS surveillance registries—with the latter used as the "gold standard."[34] In this study, when compared with former smoking and no smoking, current smoking was found to be strongly related to "inaccurate self-reporting" of any AIDS-specific diagnoses, as expressed by an odds ratio of 2.6 (95% confidence interval, 1.2, 5.6). On the other hand, the odds of inaccurate self-reporting in this study did not appear to be related to age, ethnic background, education, or time since the patient had first tested positive for the human immunodeficiency virus (HIV).

Prevention of misclassification of exposure and outcome is a function of the "state-of-the-art" measurement techniques that can be safely applied to the large number of subjects participating in epidemiologic studies. The use of objective (e.g., biological) markers of exposure and more accurate diagnostic techniques for ascertainment of outcomes, such as the use of ultrasound to diagnose asymptomatic atherosclerosis,[13] constitutes the most efficient approach for ameliorating the problems related to misclassification bias. In the meantime, if sensitivity and specificity of outcome or exposure measurements are known, it is possible to correct for misclassification; for example, in a case-control study, this can be done by using available formulas that estimate a "corrected odds ratio" as a function of the "observed odds ratio" and the estimated sensitivity and specificity of the exposure classification.[31–34,35] Furthermore, correction methods that can be applied to situations in which measurement errors affect both exposure variables and covariates (either categorical or continuous variables) have been described.[36] When misclassification parameters are unknown, sensitivity analysis could be used to obtain a range of plausible "corrected" estimates under different assumptions about the levels of misclassification (see Chapter 10, Section 10.3).

4.4 COMBINED SELECTION/INFORMATION BIASES

This section discusses biases that have both selection and information components. These include biases related to medical surveillance, cross-sectional studies, and evaluation of screening. The sections on cross-sectional and screening evaluation biases may seem somewhat repetitious vis-à-vis previous discussions on selection and information biases in this chapter. They have, however, been included here because they include examples specific to these areas and thus may be of special value to those especially interested in cross-sectional and screening intervention studies.

4.4.1 Medical Surveillance (or Detection) Bias

Medical surveillance bias occurs when a presumably medically relevant exposure leads to a closer surveillance for study outcomes that may result in a higher probability of detection in exposed individuals (i.e., when the identification of the outcome is not independent of the knowledge of the exposure). This type of bias is particularly likely when the exposure is a medical condition or therapy—such as diabetes or use of oral contraceptives—that leads to frequent and thorough checkups and the outcome is a disease that is characterized by a high proportion of subclinical cases and thus likely to be diagnosed during the frequent medical encounters resulting from the need to monitor the "exposure." For example, although there may be no basis to believe that oral contraceptive use can lead to renal failure, a spurious association would be observed if women taking oral contraceptives were more likely than other women to have medical checkups that included repeated measurements of serum creatinine concentration.

Depending on the study design, medical surveillance bias can be regarded as a type of either selection bias or information bias. In the context of a case-control study, medical surveillance bias can occur if cases are more likely to be identified (or selected into the study) if they are exposed (see Figure 4-2). In a cohort study, medical surveillance bias may be akin to information bias if, for example, the exposed individuals undergo a more thorough examination than the unexposed individuals.

Medical surveillance bias is more likely to occur when the outcome is ascertained through regular healthcare channels (e.g., electronic health records). Alternatively, *when the outcome is assessed systematically, regardless of exposure* in a concurrent cohort design, medical surveillance bias is less likely to occur.[3] Thus, meticulously standardized methods of outcome ascertainment are routinely used in most major cohort studies, such as the classic Framingham Study[37] or the Atherosclerosis Risk in Communities Study.[13] Another strategy to prevent medical surveillance bias that can be used when conducting cohort studies is to *mask exposure status when ascertaining the presence of the outcome.*

The strategies mentioned heretofore may not be feasible, however, when carrying out a case-control study in which the case diagnosis may have already been affected by the presence of the exposure. When this occurs, for analytical purposes, *information* should be obtained on the frequency, intensity, and quality of medical care received by study participants. For example, to assess the relationship between use of hormone replacement therapy and a given disease with a subclinical component (e.g., non–insulin-dependent diabetes) using a traditional case-control design, it is important to take into consideration medical care indicators, such as the frequency of medical visits in the past and whether the individual has medical insurance. Because education and socioeconomic status are usually related to availability and use of medical care, they too should be taken into consideration when trying to assess surveillance bias.

It is also possible to *obtain information on variables that indicate awareness of health problems*, such as compliance with screening exams and knowledge of subclinical disease or of results of blood measurements. For example, in a prospective study of the relationship of vasectomy to the risk of clinically diagnosed prostatic cancer (that is, not through systematic examination), the possibility of surveillance bias was assessed by examining variables that might reflect greater utilization of medical care.[38] In this study, no differences were found between subjects who had and those who had not had vasectomy with regard to their knowledge of their blood pressure or serum cholesterol levels. The proportions of study participants who had had screening sigmoidoscopy were also similar, leading the authors to conclude that vasectomized men were not under a greater degree of medical surveillance than those who had not been vasectomized. In addition, the frequency of digital rectal examinations was similar between the vasectomized (exposed) and the nonvasectomized (unexposed) groups, implying equal access to a procedure that may lead to the diagnosis of the study outcome (prostate cancer)

Finally, when medical surveillance bias occurs, the disease tends to be diagnosed earlier in exposed than in unexposed individuals; as a result, the proportion of less advanced disease in a cohort study is higher in the exposed group. In a case-control study, the bias is denoted by the fact that the association is found to be stronger or present only for the less advanced cases. In the cohort study discussed previously, Giovannucci et al.[38] found that the histologic severity staging of prostate cancer was similar for vasectomized and nonvasectomized men, a finding inconsistent with what would be expected if medical surveillance had been more intensive in the vasectomized group. *Stratification by disease severity at diagnosis* is thus an additional strategy to examine and take into consideration the possibility of surveillance bias.

4.4.2 Cross-Sectional Biases

Cross-sectional biases can be classified as incidence–prevalence bias and temporal bias. The former is a type of selection bias, whereas the latter can be regarded as an information bias.

Incidence–Prevalence Bias

Incidence–prevalence bias may result from the inclusion of prevalent cases in a study when the goal is to make inferences in relation to disease *risk*. As discussed in Chapter 3 (Section 3.3), the strength of an association is sometimes estimated using the prevalence rate ratio rather than the relative risk, as when analyzing data from a cross-sectional survey or when assessing cross-sectional associations at baseline in a cohort study. If the investigator is interested in assessing potentially causal associations, the use of the prevalence rate ratio as an estimate of the incidence ratio is subject to bias. Equation 2.3, described in Chapter 2 (Section 2.3), shows the dependence of the point prevalence odds [Prev/(1.0 − Prev)] on incidence (Inc) and disease duration (Dur), assuming that incidence and duration are approximately constant:

$$\frac{\text{Prev}}{1.0 - \text{Prev}} = \text{Inc} \times \text{Dur}$$

Equation 2.3 can be rewritten as Equation 2.4:

$$\text{Prev} = \text{Inc} \times \text{Dur} \times (1.0 - \text{Prev})$$

thus demonstrating that, in addition to incidence and duration, prevalence is a function of the term (1.0 − Prev) (which, in turn, obviously depends on the magnitude of the point prevalence rate).

As a corollary of Equation 2.4, the point prevalence rate ratio comparing exposed (denoted by subscript "+") and unexposed (denoted by subscript "−") individuals, obtained in cross-sectional studies, will be a function of (1) the relative risk, (2) the ratio of the disease duration in exposed individuals to that in unexposed individuals, and (3) the ratio of the term (1.0 − Prev) in exposed individuals to the same term in unexposed individuals. Ratios 2 and 3 represent two types of incidence–prevalence bias, that is, the *duration ratio bias* and the *point prevalence complement ratio bias*, respectively, when the prevalence rate ratio (PRR) is used to estimate the relative risk (see Section 3.3):

$$\text{PRR} = \left(\frac{q_+}{q_-}\right) \times \left(\frac{\text{Dur}_+}{\text{Dur}_-}\right) \times \left(\frac{1.0 - \text{Prev}_+}{1.0 - \text{Prev}_-}\right)$$

Where q_+ and q_- are the incidence values for exposed and unexposed individuals, respectively.

Duration Ratio Bias. This type of bias (which can be thought of as a type of selection bias) occurs when the prevalence rate ratio is used as a measure of association and the duration of the disease after its onset is different between exposed and unexposed persons. (Because duration of a chronic disease is so often related to survival, this type of bias may also be designated as *survival bias*.) For diseases of low prevalence, when the duration (or prognosis) of the disease is independent of the exposure (i.e., the same in exposed and unexposed), the prevalence rate ratio is a virtually unbiased estimate of the relative risk. On the other hand, when the exposure of interest affects the prognosis of the disease, bias will be present, as shown in the examples later in this chapter.

Point Prevalence Complement Ratio Bias. Even if duration is independent of exposure, regardless of the direction of the effect of the factor on the outcome, the prevalence rate ratio tends to underestimate the *strength* of the association between the exposure and the outcome (i.e., it biases the relative risk toward 1.0). The magnitude of this bias depends on both the prevalence rate ratio and the absolute magnitude of the point prevalence rates. When the point prevalence rate is higher in exposed than in unexposed individuals (prevalence rate ratio > 1.0), the point prevalence complement ratio [or $(1.0 - \text{Prev}_+)/(1.0 - \text{Prev}_-)$] is less than 1.0. It is close to 1.0 when the point prevalence rates are low in both exposed and unexposed, even if the prevalence rate ratio is relatively high. For example, if the prevalence of the disease in exposed subjects is 0.04 and that in unexposed subjects is 0.01, the prevalence rate ratio is high (0.04/0.01 = 4.0), but the bias resulting from the point prevalence complement ratio is merely 0.96/0.99 = 0.97; i.e., still < 1.0, but close enough to 1.0, so as to result in a practically negligible bias. On the other hand, when the prevalence is relatively high in exposed individuals, the point prevalence complement ratio can be markedly less than 1.0, thus resulting in important bias. For example, if the prevalence of the disease in exposed subjects is 0.40 and that in unexposed subjects is 0.10, the prevalence rate ratio is the same as in the previous example (4.0); however, the point prevalence complement ratio is 0.6/0.90 = 0.67 (i.e., the prevalence rate ratio underestimates the relative risk by 33%—even in the absence of duration ratio bias). The influence of the magnitude of prevalence is sometimes felt even for a low prevalence rate ratio. For example, if the point prevalence rates are 0.40 in exposed and 0.25 in unexposed subjects, the prevalence rate ratio is fairly small (1.6), but the bias factor is 0.80 (i.e., the prevalence rate ratio underestimates the relative risk by at least 20%—and more if there is also duration ratio bias). Obviously, the bias will be greatest when both the prevalence rate ratio and the prevalence rate in one of the groups (exposed or unexposed) are high. For studies of factors that decrease the prevalence of the disease (i.e., prevalence rate ratio < 1.0), the reciprocal reasoning applies; that is, $(1.0 - Prev_+)/(1 - Prev_-)$ will be greater than 1.0, and the magnitude of the bias will also be affected by the absolute rates.

Examples of Incidence–Prevalence Biases. In the examples that follow, it is assumed that the incidence and duration according to the exposure have remained stable over time.

- *Gender and acute myocardial infarction in US whites:* White US males have a much higher risk of myocardial infarction than white females. Some studies, however, have shown that, even after careful age adjustment, females have a shorter average survival than males.[39] Thus, the ratio ($Dur_{males}/Dur_{females}$) tends to be greater than 1.0, and as a consequence, the prevalence rate ratio expressing the relationship of sex to myocardial infarction overestimates the relative risk.
- *Current smoking and emphysema:* Smoking substantially increases the risk of emphysema. In addition, survival (and thus duration of the disease) in emphysema patients who continue to smoke after diagnosis is shorter than in those who quit smoking. As a result, prevalence rate ratios estimated in cross-sectional studies evaluating the association between current smoking and emphysema tend to underestimate the relative risk.
- *Tuberculin purified protein derivative (PPD) reaction and clinical tuberculosis:* In assessments of the relationship between the size of the PPD skin test reaction and clinical tuberculosis, prevalence rate ratios were shown to underestimate relative risks in a population-based study carried out by G Comstock et al. (unpublished observations) a few decades ago (Figure 4-5). This underestimation was likely due to the relatively high prevalence of clinical tuberculosis in this population at the time the study was carried out and thus to the occurrence of prevalence complement ratio bias.

Prevention of Incidence–Prevalence Bias. If the goal is to evaluate potential disease determinants, whenever possible, incident cases should be used in order to avoid incidence–prevalence bias. Incidence–prevalence bias, although more easily conceptualized by comparing incidence with prevalence (cross-sectional) rate ratio data, may also occur in case-control studies when prevalent rather than only newly developed (incident) cases are used. For example, if smoking decreases survival after diagnosis, thereby decreasing the disease's duration (as in myocardial infarction), a case-control study based on prevalent cases may include a higher proportion of nonsmoking cases (as smokers would have been selected out by death) than would a study based on incident cases, thus diluting the strength of the association (see Chapter 1, Figure 1-19).

Another problem in case-control studies is that newly *diagnosed* cases are used as proxies for newly *developed* cases. Thus, for diseases that may evolve subclinically for many years before diagnosis, such as chronic lymphocytic leukemia, diabetes, or renal insufficiency,

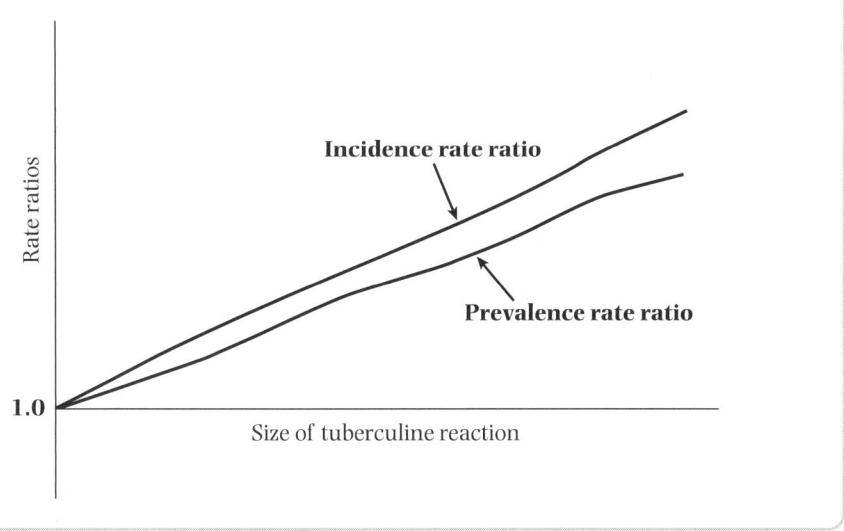

FIGURE 4-5 Schematic representation of the results of the study by Comstock et al. (unpublished) evaluating the relationship of size of PPD reaction to clinical tuberculosis. After an initial cross-sectional survey conducted in 1946, the cohort was followed over time for determination of incidence rates.

Source: Data from GW Comstock et al., personal communication.

presumed incident cases are, in fact, a mix of incident and prevalent cases, and incidence–prevalence bias may occur unbeknownst to the investigator. A cohort study efficiently prevents incidence–prevalence bias if its procedures include careful ascertainment and exclusion of all prevalent cases at baseline (clinical and subclinical) as well as a systematic and periodic search of newly developed clinical and subclinical outcomes.

Temporal Bias

In cross-sectional studies, the proper temporal sequence needed to establish causality, risk factor → disease, cannot be firmly established. In other words, it is difficult to know which came first, the exposure to the potential risk factor or the disease. *Temporal bias* occurs when the inference about the proper temporal sequence of cause and effect is erroneous. For example, results from a prevalence survey may establish a statistical association between high serum creatinine levels and the occurrence of high blood pressure. Because the time sequence cannot be established, however, a cross-sectional association between these variables may mean either that high serum creatinine (a marker of kidney failure) leads to hypertension or vice versa. A prospective study in which blood pressure levels are measured in persons with normal serum creatinine levels, who are then followed over time for ascertainment of hypercreatininemia can obviously identify the proper temporal sequence and thus lend support to the conclusion that high blood pressure predicts incipient renal insufficiency.[40]

Temporal bias may also occur in case-control studies—even those including only newly developed (incident) cases—when the suspected exposure is measured after disease diagnosis in cases. For example, because hepatitis B virus (HBV) is myelotoxic, it has been suggested that HBV may be an etiologic factor for the so-called idiopathic aplastic anemia (AA).[41] Temporal bias, however, could explain the relationship between HBV and AA in a case-control study if serum samples for determination of HBV antibody and antigen levels had been collected after AA onset, as individuals with AA may receive transfusions of blood contaminated with HBV even before a diagnosis is made. Thus, the erroneously inferred sequence is:

$$HBV \rightarrow AA,$$

but the true sequence is:

$$\text{undiagnosed AA} \rightarrow \text{blood transfusion} \rightarrow \text{diagnosed AA}.$$

An example of the reasoning underlying the possibility of temporal bias is given by the association between estrogen replacement therapy (ERT) in postmenopausal women and endometrial cancer.[42] Although the causal nature of this association is currently well established, it was initially disputed on the grounds that a higher likelihood of using ERT resulted from symptoms occurring as a consequence of incipient, undiagnosed endometrial cancer.[43] Thus, instead of the sequence:

$$ERT \rightarrow \text{endometrial cancer},$$

the true sequence would be:

$$\text{undiagnosed endometrial cancer} \rightarrow \text{symptoms} \rightarrow ERT \rightarrow \text{diagnosed endometrial cancer}.$$

Another example of temporal bias is given by a cross-sectional study of Dutch children, in which negative associations were found of pet ownership with allergy, respiratory symptoms, and asthma.[44] As aptly postulated by the study's investigators, these results may have resulted from the fact that families are likely to remove from the home (or not acquire) pets after such manifestations occur. This study also underscores why the term "reverse causality" is occasionally used in connection with a temporal bias of this sort.

A further example of this type of bias was suggested by Nieto et al.,[45] who found that the relationship of current smoking to prevalent clinical atherosclerosis (defined by self-reported physician-diagnosed heart attack or cardiac surgery) was much stronger when using longitudinal data than when using cross-sectional data (in contrast to the association between smoking and subclinical atherosclerosis, which was of similar strength for the longitudinal and the cross-sectional data). One possible explanation for these findings was that the occurrence of a heart attack (but not the presence of subclinical atherosclerosis) may lead to smoking cessation and thus to a dilution of the association when using prevalent cases.* This type of bias may occur even in prospective analyses when the outcome of interest is mortality. For example, the short-term mortality from lung cancer can be higher in individuals who stopped smoking recently than in current smokers because of the tendency of symptomatic individuals or those for whom a diagnosis has been made to quit smoking.[46] Epidemiologists usually handle this bias by excluding from the analysis the deaths that occur within a specified period after the beginning of the study.

To prevent temporal bias in a cross-sectional survey, it is occasionally possible to improve the information on temporality when obtaining data through questionnaires. Temporality pertaining to potential risk factors such as smoking, physical activity, and occupational exposures can be ascertained in cross-sectional samples by means of questions such as, "When were you first exposed to . . . ?" For some chronic diseases, such as angina pectoris, it is also possible to obtain information on the date of onset.

---

*Survival bias is, of course, another explanation, resulting from a poor prognosis of myocardial infarction in smokers.

The investigators can then establish the temporal sequence between risk factor and disease—assuming, of course, that the information from surveyed individuals is accurate. (Obviously, even if temporality can be established in a cross-sectional study, the investigator will still have the incidence–prevalence bias to contend with.) When the date of the beginning of the exposure is unknown, as in the example of viral hepatitis and AA the only solution is to use prospective data on exposure and outcome (a formidable challenge in this example, given the rarity of AA).

Finally, it may be possible to assess temporal bias occurring because the presumed exposure is a consequence of undiagnosed disease—as in the example of ERT and endometrial cancer mentioned previously in this chapter—by considering why the exposure occurred. In the study of Antunes et al.,[42] for instance, data can be stratified according to indication for ERT use, such as bleeding; if temporal bias is not a likely explanation for the relationship of estrogen to endometrial cancer, the association will be observed both for individuals who were prescribed estrogens because they were bleeding and for those who were given estrogens for other reasons (e.g., prevention of osteoporosis).

4.4.3 Biases Related to the Evaluation of Screening Interventions

Like any other epidemiologic study, studies of the evaluation of screening interventions are also prone to biases, of which five types are particularly relevant: selection bias, incidence–prevalence bias, length bias, lead time bias, and over diagnosis bias. (For a better understanding of these types of biases, the reader should review the concepts underlying the natural history of disease; see, e.g., Gordis.[10])

Selection Bias

Selection bias stems from the fact that when the evaluation of screening relies on an observational design, the screened group may differ substantially from the nonscreened group. Thus, for example, persons who attend a screening program may be of a higher socioeconomic status than those who do not and may therefore have a better prognosis regardless of the effectiveness of the screening program. *Prevention* of this type of selection bias is best carried out by using an experimental design (i.e., by randomly assigning screening status to study participants). While improving internal validity, however, experimental studies to evaluate screening programs are typically conducted in selected populations, thus potentially limiting their external validity.

Incidence–Prevalence Bias

Survival bias results from comparing prognosis in prevalent cases detected in the first screen, which is akin to a cross-sectional survey, with that in incident cases detected in subsequent screenings. This bias occurs because prevalent cases include long-term survivors, who have a better average survival than that of incident cases, in whom the full spectrum of severity is represented. This type of bias may occur in "pre–post" studies, as when comparing a screening strategy used in the first screening exam ("pre") that identifies prevalent cases with a different strategy used in subsequent screens identifying incident cases ("post").

A related bias is the so-called *length bias,* which occurs when a better prognosis for cases detected directly by the screening procedure (e.g., occult blood test for colorectal cancer) than for cases diagnosed between screening exams is used as evidence that the screening program is effective. To understand this type of bias, it is important to briefly review some key concepts related to the natural history of a disease and screening.

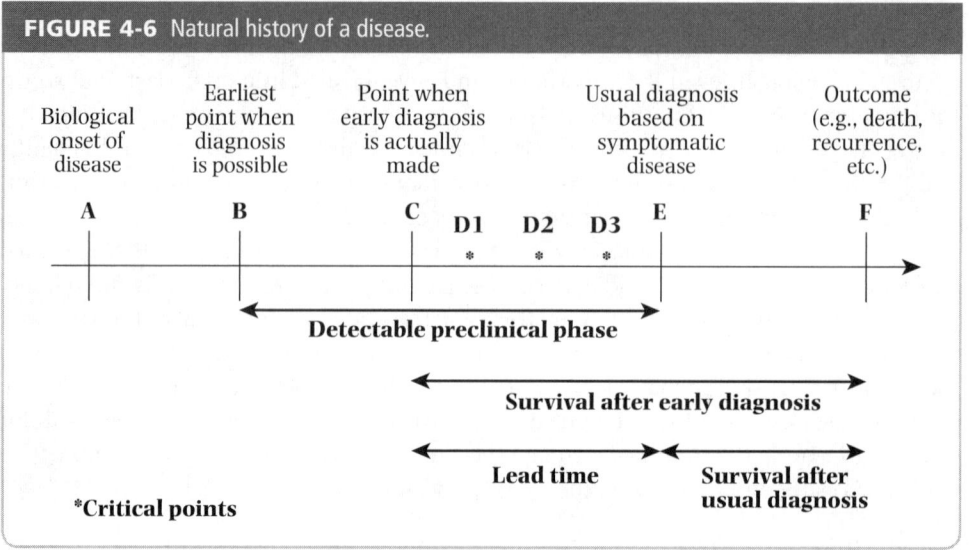

FIGURE 4-6 Natural history of a disease.

Source: Adapted from L Gordis, *Epidemiology*, © 2008, Elsevier Saunders.

The effectiveness of screening is positively related to the length of the detectable preclinical phase (DPCP; see Figure 4-6 and, for definitions, Table 4-12), which in turn reflects the rate at which the disease progresses. This means that for diseases with a rapid progression, it is difficult, if not outright impossible, to improve prognosis by means of early detection. For example, a short average DPCP and its attending poor survival characterize most cases of lung cancer, for which screening generally is not effective. On the other hand, the long DPCP of *in situ* cervical cancer (or high-grade squamous intraepithelial lesions) explains why treatment after an abnormal Pap smear is related to a cure rate of virtually 100%.

Even for the same disease, regardless of screening, it can be shown that patients whose disease has a longer DPCP have a better prognosis than those whose disease has a shorter DPCP (e.g., postmenopausal versus premenopausal breast cancer, respectively). For example, in the Health Insurance Plan Study of the effectiveness of screening for breast cancer, the so-called interval cases—that is, cases who were clinically diagnosed during the interval between the screening exams—had, on average, a higher case fatality rate than subclinical cases diagnosed as a result of the screening exam.[47] Although some of these cases may have been false negatives missed by the previous screening exam and therefore not true interval cases, many were probably characterized by rapidly growing tumors—that is, by a short DPCP (Figure 4-7). It follows that when evaluating a screening program, one must take into careful consideration the fact that cases detected by the screening procedure (e.g., mammography), which thus tend to have a longer DPCP, have an inherently better prognosis than the "interval" cases, *regardless of the effectiveness of screening*. Failure to do so results in *length bias*, which occurs when a better prognosis for "screening-detected" than for "interval" cases is used as evidence that the screening program is effective, when in reality it may be due to the longer DPCP of the former cases, reflecting a slower growing disease than that of interval cases.

Prevention of length bias can be accomplished by using an experimental approach and comparing the prognosis of *all* cases—which include cases with both short and long DPCPs—occurring in individuals randomly assigned to a screening program with that

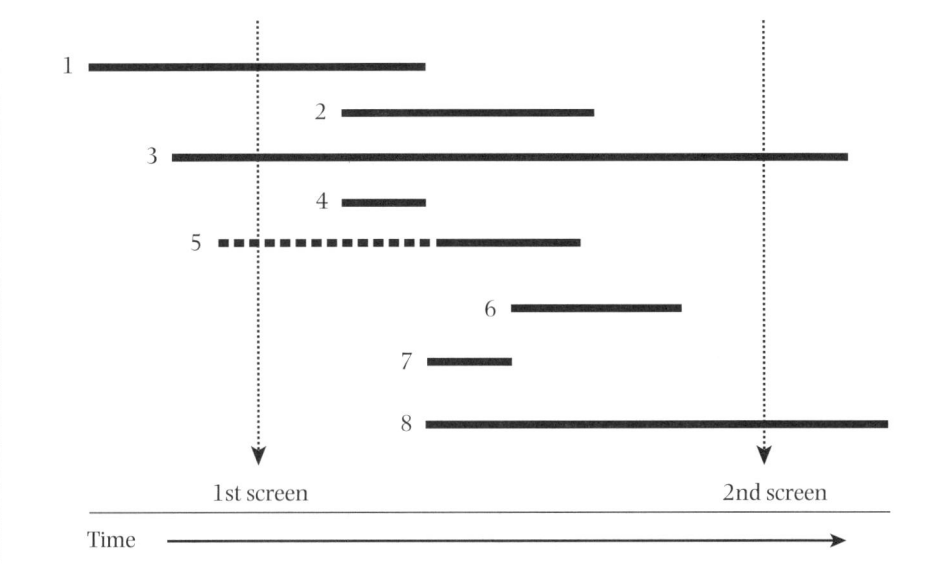

FIGURE 4-7 Schematic representation of the length of the detectable preclinical phase (DPCP) in cases occurring during a screening program. Cases with a longer DPCP (cases no. 1, 3, and 8) have a higher probability of identification at each screening exam. Cases with a shorter DPCP occurring between screening exams are the "interval" cases (cases no. 2, 4, 6, and 7). Case no. 5 is a false negative (missed by the first exam).

of *all* cases occurring in randomly assigned controls that do not undergo the screening exams. (The distribution of patients with long DPCPs versus those with short DPCPs is expected to be the same in the randomly assigned screening and control groups.)

Lead Time Bias

Lead time is the time by which diagnosis can be advanced by screening. It is the time between early diagnosis (Figure 4-6, point C) and the usual time when diagnosis would have been made if an early diagnostic test(s) had not been applied to the patient (Figure 4-6, point E; see also Table 4-12). The lead time, therefore, is contained within the DPCP.

When evaluating effectiveness of screening, lead time bias occurs when survival (or recurrence-free time) is counted from the point in time when early diagnosis was made. Thus, even if screening is ineffective, the early diagnosis adds lead time to the survival counted from the time of usual diagnosis. Survival may then be increased from time of early diagnosis but not from the biological onset of the disease (Figure 4-8).[48]

Lead time bias occurs only when estimating survival (or time-to-event) from time of diagnosis. Thus, lead time bias can be avoided by calculating the mortality risk or rate among all screened and control subjects rather than the cumulative probability of survival (or its complement, the cumulative case fatality probability) from diagnosis among cases.[10] If survival from diagnosis is chosen as the strategy to describe the results of the evaluation of a screening approach, the average duration of lead time must be estimated and taken into account when comparing survival after diagnosis between screened and nonscreened groups. For survival to be regarded as increased from the biological onset, it must be greater than the survival after usual diagnosis plus lead time (Figure 4-9). It is, thus, important to estimate average lead time.

TABLE 4-12 Natural history of a disease: definitions of components represented in Figure 4-6.

Component	Represented in Figure 4-6 as . . .	Definition
Detectable preclinical phase	The interval between points B and E	Phase that starts when early diagnosis becomes possible and ends with the point in time when usual diagnosis based on symptomatic disease would have been made.
Critical points	D1, D2, and D3	Points beyond which early detection and treatment are less and less effective vis-à-vis treatment following usual diagnosis. Treatment is totally ineffective after the last critical point (point D3 in the figure).
Lead time	The interval between points C and E	Period between the point in time when early diagnosis was made and the point in time when the usual diagnosis (based on symptoms) would have been made.

Source: Adapted from L. Gordis, *Epidemiology*, 4th Edition © 2008, Elsevier Saunders.

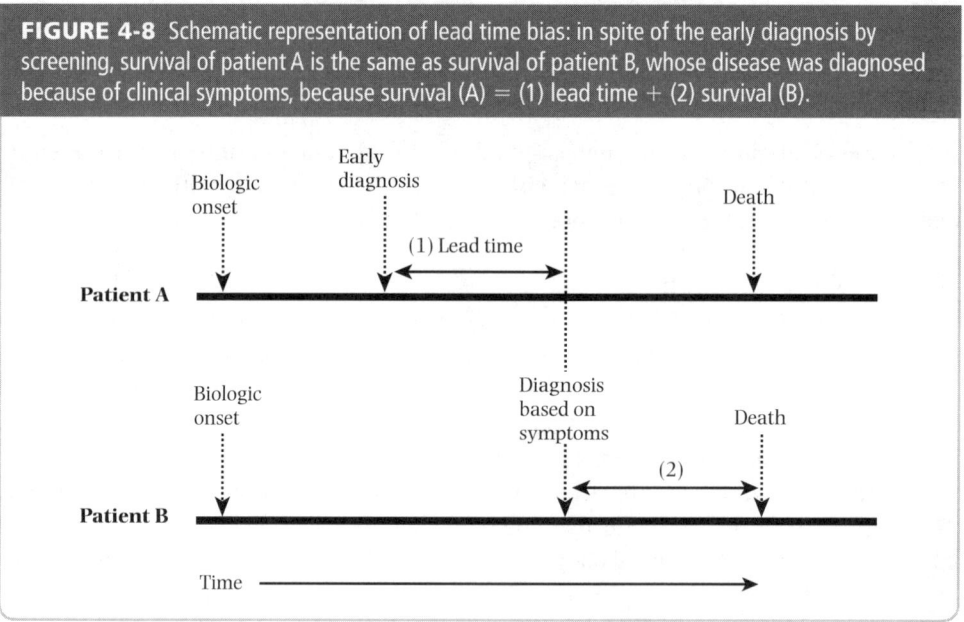

FIGURE 4-8 Schematic representation of lead time bias: in spite of the early diagnosis by screening, survival of patient A is the same as survival of patient B, whose disease was diagnosed because of clinical symptoms, because survival (A) = (1) lead time + (2) survival (B).

Source: Adapted from L Gordis, *Epidemiology*, © 2008, Elsevier Saunders.

If the disease for a given individual is identified through screening, it is impossible to know when "usual" diagnosis would have been made if screening had not been carried out. Thus, it is not possible to estimate the lead time for individual patients, only an average lead time. What follows is a simplified description of the basic approach used to estimate average lead time. A more detailed account of lead time estimation is beyond the scope of this intermediate methods text and can be found elsewhere.[48]

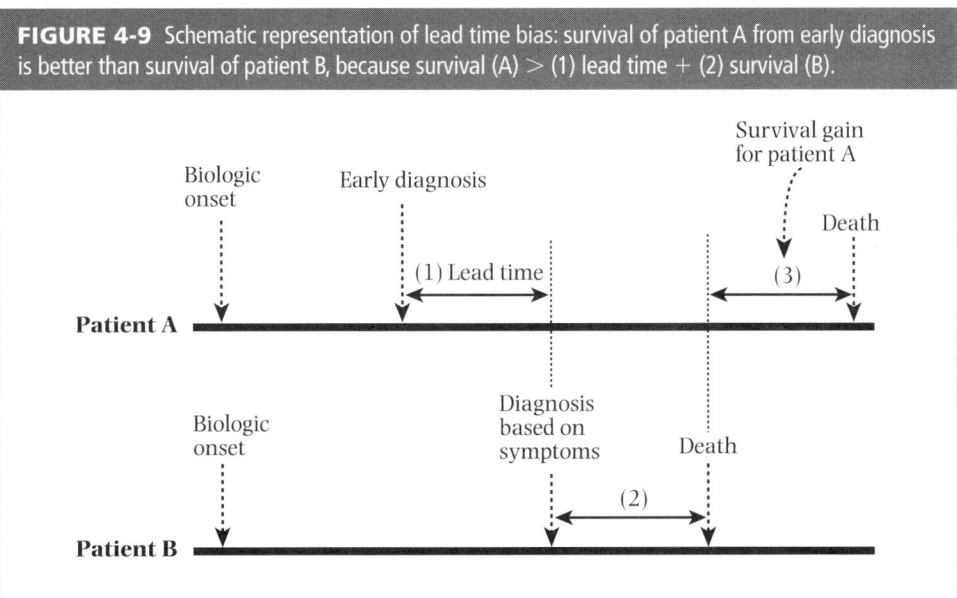

FIGURE 4-9 Schematic representation of lead time bias: survival of patient A from early diagnosis is better than survival of patient B, because survival (A) > (1) lead time + (2) survival (B).

Source: Adapted from L Gordis, *Epidemiology*, © 2008, Elsevier Saunders.

As mentioned previously, the lead time is a component of the DPCP. Thus, to estimate the average lead time, it is first necessary to estimate the average duration of the DPCP (Dur_{DPCP}) using the known relationship between prevalence ($Prev_{DPCP}$) and incidence (Inc_{DPCP}) of preclinical cases: that is, cases in the DPCP (see also Chapter 2, Section 2.3, Equation 2.4):

$$Prev_{DPCP} = Inc_{DPCP} \times Dur_{DPCP} \times (1.0 - Prev_{DPCP})$$

The duration of the DPCP can then be easily derived as

$$Dur_{DPCP} = \frac{Prev_{DPCP}}{Inc_{DPCP} \times (1.0 - Prev_{DPCP})}$$

If the prevalence of the disease is not too high (e.g., no greater than about 5%), $1.0 - Prev_{DPCP}$ will be close to 1.0, and thus, this equation can be simplified:

$$Dur_{DPCP} \approx \frac{Prev_{DPCP}}{Inc_{DPCP}}$$

To apply this formula, the $Prev_{DPCP}$ is estimated using data from the first screening exam of the target population, which is equivalent to a cross-sectional survey. The Inc_{DPCP} can be estimated in successive screening exams among screenees found to be disease-free at the time of the first screening. An alternative way to estimate Inc_{DPCP}, and one that does not require follow-up with the screenees, is to use the incidence of clinical disease in the reference population, if available. The rationale for this procedure, and an important assumption justifying screening, is that, if left untreated, preclinical cases would necessarily become clinical cases; thus, there should not be a difference between the incidence of clinical and that of preclinical disease. When using available clinical disease incidence (e.g., based on cancer registry data), however, it is important to adjust for differences in risk factor prevalence, expected to be higher in screenees than in the reference population from which clinical incidence is obtained. Thus, for example, a family history of breast cancer is likely to be more prevalent in individuals screened for breast cancer than in the female population at large.

Next, using the duration of the DPCP estimate, the estimation of the average lead time needs to take into account whether early diagnosis by screening is made at the first or in subsequent screening exams.

The estimation of the lead time of point prevalent preclinical cases detected at the first screening exam relies on certain assumptions regarding the distribution of times of early diagnosis during the DPCP. For example, if the distribution of early diagnosis by screening can be assumed to be homogeneous throughout the DPCP—that is, if the sensitivity of the screening test is independent of time within the DPCP (Figure 4-10A)—the lead time of point prevalent preclinical cases can be simply estimated as

$$\text{Lead time} = \frac{\text{DPCP}}{2}$$

The latter assumption, however, may not be justified in many situations. For most diseases amenable to screening (e.g., breast cancer), the sensitivity of the screening test, and thus the probability of early diagnosis, is likely to increase during the DPCP (Figure 4-10B) as a result of the progression of the disease as it gets closer to its symptomatic (clinical) phase. If this is the case, a more reasonable assumption would be that the average lead time is less than one-half of the DPCP. Obviously, the longer the DPCP, the longer the lead time under any distributional assumption. Also, because the DPCP and thus the average lead time are dependent on the validity of the screening exam, they become longer as more sensitive screening tests are developed.

FIGURE 4-10 Estimation of lead time as a function of the variability of the sensitivity of the screening exam during the detectable preclinical phase.

A. Sensitivity of screening exam is same throughout the detectable preclinical phase (DPCP): average lead time = ½ DPCP

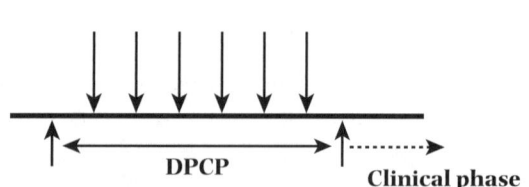

B. Sensitivity of screening exam increases during the detectable preclinical phase (DPCP) as a result of the progression of the disease: average lead time < ½ DPCP

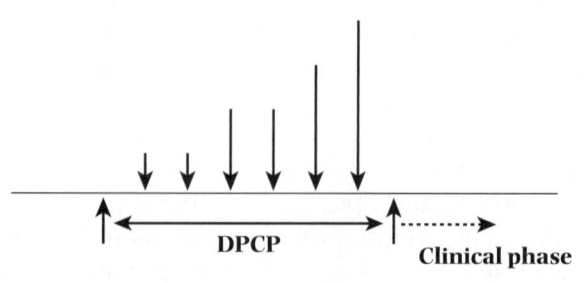

The duration of the lead time for *incident* preclinical cases identified in a program in which repeated screening exams are carried out is a function of how often the screenings are done (i.e., the length of the interval between successive screenings). The closer in time the screening exams are, the greater the probability that early diagnosis will occur closer to the onset of the DPCP—and thus, the more the lead time will approximate the DPCP.

Figure 4-11 schematically illustrates short and long between-screening intervals and their effects on the lead time. Assuming two persons with similar DPCPs whose diseases start soon after the previous screening, the person with the shorter between-screening interval (*a* to *b*, patient A) has his or her newly developed preclinical disease diagnosed nearer the beginning of the DPCP than the person with the longer between-screening interval (*a* to *c*, patient B). Thus, the duration of the lead time is closer to the duration of the DPCP for patient A than for patient B. The maximum lead time obviously cannot be longer than the DPCP.[49]

Over-Diagnosis bias

Over-diagnosis bias occurs when screening identifies patients whose early subclinical disease does not evolve to more advanced stages. Results of two recent trials of screening for prostate cancer with prostate-specific antigen (PSA) illustrate a potential over-diagnosis bias. In the US-based trial,[50] the cumulative hazards of death for individuals tested with PSA and for the control group were virtually the same for most of the

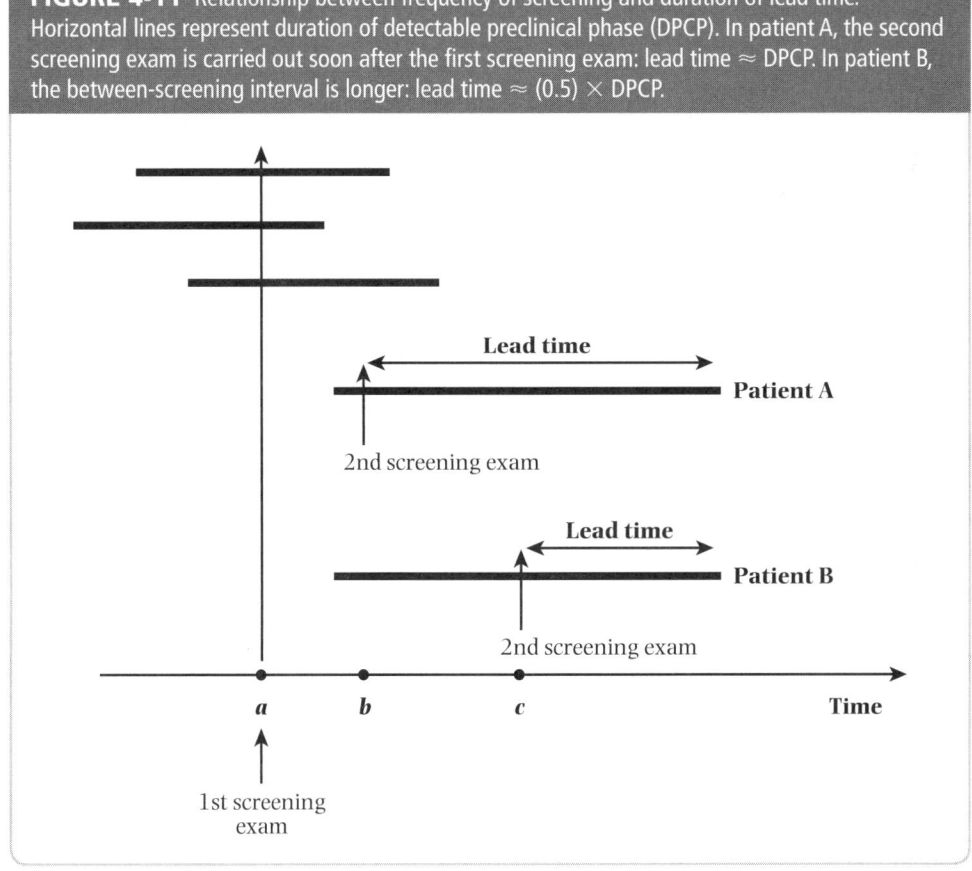

FIGURE 4-11 Relationship between frequency of screening and duration of lead time. Horizontal lines represent duration of detectable preclinical phase (DPCP). In patient A, the second screening exam is carried out soon after the first screening exam: lead time ≈ DPCP. In patient B, the between-screening interval is longer: lead time ≈ (0.5) × DPCP.

follow-up and at the end of the trial. In the European trial,[51] a significant difference in mortality could not be found between the screened and nonscreened groups. Because PSA is a reasonably sensitive test for the early diagnosis of prostate cancer, these results seem to be fairly surprising. A possible explanation for the results of these two studies is that as many as one-third of men younger than 70 years and between two-thirds to 100% of older men may have prostate cancer, but often in a microscopic, noninvasive form (see Table 4-13).[52] Thus, it is likely that many individuals—particularly as they age—die *with* prostate cancer, rather than *from* prostate cancer. Because it is not currently possible to identify cases that would not evolve to more invasive stages leading to death, if they represent a relative high proportion of all cases, the efficiency of screening would be diluted by their inclusion, when evaluating PSA. For example, in a population of 10,000, there are 2000 potential lethal cases that, without screening, would all die. With screening, and assuming that the effectiveness of the treatment is very high, 97.5%, only 50 deaths would occur. If the potentially lethal cases could be identified and screened, the number needed to screen to prevent one death would be 40 (i.e., 2000/50). On the other hand, if these potentially lethal cases could not be identified, the whole target population would have to be screened, and the number needed to screen to prevent one death would be 200 (i.e., 10,000/50). Thus, screening of only the "lethal" subgroup (those who would have died without screening) would be much more efficient than screening the whole target population.

Unfortunately, it is currently impossible to identify patients with prostate cancer who, if left unscreened, would result in death. A similar problem may exist with regard to *in situ* breast cancer.[53]

TABLE 4-13 Range of prevalence rates (%) of prostate cancer by age.

Age (years)	Prevalence ranges of prostate cancer (%)
50–59	10–42%
60–69	17–38%
70–79	25–66%
≥80	18–100%

Source: Adapted from: Franks, *J Pathol Bacteriol.* 1954;68:603–616; Bostwick et al., *Cancer.* 1992;70:291–301; Breslow et al., *Int J Cancer.* 1977;20:680–688; Baron & Angrist, *Arch Pathol.* 1941;32:787–793; Edwards et al., *Cancer.* 1953;6:531–554; Halpert & Schamlhorst, *Cancer.* 1966;695–698; Scott et al., *J Urol.* 1969;101:602–607.

REFERENCES

1. Sackett DL. Bias in analytical research. *J Chron Dis.* 1979;32:51–63.
2. Porta, M. *A Dictionary of Epidemiology.* 5th ed. New York, NY: Oxford University Press; 2008.
3. Lilienfeld DE, Stolley PD. *Foundations of Epidemiology,* 3rd ed. New York, NY: Oxford University Press; 1994.
4. Schlesselman J. *Case Control Studies: Design, Conduct, Analysis.* New York, NY: Oxford University Press; 1982.
5. Rothman K, Greenland S. *Modern Epidemiology,* 3rd ed. Philadelphia, PA: Wolters Kluwer Health/Lippincott; 2008.
6. Byrne C, Brinton LA, Haile RW, Schairer C. Heterogeneity of the effect of family history on breast cancer risk. *Epidemiology.* 1991;2:276–284.
7. MacMahon B, Yen S, et al. Coffee and cancer of the pancreas. *N Engl J Med.* 1981;304:630–633.
8. Hsieh CC, MacMahon B, Yen S, et al. Coffee and pancreatic cancer (Chapter 2). *N Engl J Med.* 1986;315:587–589.
9. Heederik K. Micro-epidemiology of the healthy worker effect? *Occup Environ Med.* 2006;63:83.
10. Gordis L. *Epidemiology,* 4th Ed. Philadelphia, PA: Elsevier Saunders; 2008.
11. Weinstock MA, Colditz GA, Willett WC, et al. Recall (report) bias and reliability in the retrospective assessment of melanoma risk. *Am J Epidemiol.* 1991;133:240–245.
12. Brinton LA, Hoover RN, Szklo M, Fraumeni JF Jr. Menopausal estrogen use and risk of breast cancer. *Cancer.* 1981;47:2517–2522.
13. Chambless LE, Heiss G, Folsom AR, et al. Association of coronary heart disease incidence with carotid arterial wall thickness and major risk factors: The Atherosclerosis Risk in Communities (ARIC) Study, 1987–1993. *Am J Epidemiol.* 1997;146:483–494.
14. Bild D, Bluemke DA, Burke GL, et al. Multi-ethnic Study of Atherosclerosis. *Am J Epidemiol.* 2002;156:871–881.
15. Mele A, Szklo M, Visani G, et al. Hair dye use and other risk factors for leukemia and pre-leukemia: A case-control study: Italian Leukemia Study Group. *Am J Epidemiol.* 1994;139:609–619.
16. Lilienfeld AM, Graham S. *J Natl Cancer Inst.* 1958;21:713–720.
17. Wei Q, Matanoski GM, Farmer ER, et al. DNA repair and susceptibility to basal cell carcinoma: A case-control study. *Am J Epidemiol.* 1994;140:598–607.
18. *The Health Effects of Passive Smoking.* Canberra: Australian Government Publishing Service. Commonwealth of Australia, National Health and Medical Research Council; November 1997.
19. Szklo M, Tonascia J, Gordis L. Psychosocial factors and the risk of myocardial infarctions in white women. *Am J Epidemiol.* 1976;103:312–320.
20. Doll R, Hill AB. Smoking and carcinoma of the lung; preliminary report. *Br Med J.* 1950;2:739–748.
21. Perneger TV, Whelton PK, Klag MJ, Rossiter KA. Diagnosis of hypertensive end-stage renal disease: Effect of patient's race. *Am J Epidemiol.* 1995;141:10–15.
22. Stewart WF, Linet MS, Celentano DD, et al. Age- and sex-specific incidence rates of migraine with and without visual aura. *Am J Epidemiol.* 1991;134:1111–1120.
23. Rose GA. Chest pain questionnaire. *Milbank Mem Fund Q.* 1965;43:32–39.
24. Bass EB, Follansbee WP, Orchard TJ. Comparison of a supplemented Rose Questionnaire to exercise thallium testing in men and women. *J Clin Epidemiol.* 1989;42:385–394.
25. Garber CE, Carleton RA, Heller GV. Comparison of "Rose Questionnaire Angina" to exercise thallium scintigraphy: Different findings in males and females. *J Clin Epidemiol.* 1992;45:715–720.

26. Sorlie PD, Cooper L, Schreiner PJ, et al. Repeatability and validity of the Rose questionnaire for angina pectoris in the Atherosclerosis Risk in Communities Study. *J Clin Epidemiol.* 1996;49:719–725.

27. Dosemeci M, Wacholder S, Lubin JH. Does nondifferential misclassification of exposure always bias a true effect toward the null value? *Am J Epidemiol.* 1990;132:746–748.

28. Infante-Rivard C, Jacques L. Empirical study of parental recall bias. *Am J Epidemiol.* 2000;152:480–486.

29. Greenland S. The effect of misclassification in the presence of covariates. *Am J Epidemiol.* 1980;112:564–569.

30. Wacholder S. When measurement errors correlate with truth: Surprising effects of nondifferential misclassification. *Epidemiology.* 1995;6:157–161.

31. Flegal KM, Brownie C, Haas JD. The effects of exposure misclassification on estimates of relative risk. *Am J Epidemiol.* 1986;123:736–751.

32. Flegal KM, Keyl PM, Nieto FJ. Differential misclassification arising from nondifferential errors in exposure measurement. *Am J Epidemiol.* 1991;134:1233–1244.

33. Willett W. An overview of issues related to the correction of non-differential exposure measurement error in epidemiologic studies. *Stat Med.* 1989;8:1031–1040; discussion 1071–1033.

34. Hessol NA, Schwarcz S, Ameli N, et al. Accuracy of self-reports of acquired immunodeficiency syndrome and acquired immunodeficiency syndrome-related conditions in women. *Am J Epidemiol.* 2001;153: 1128–1133.

35. Thomas D, Stram D, Dwyer J. Exposure measurement error: Influence on exposure-disease: Relationships and methods of correction. *Annu Rev Public Health.* 1993;14:69–93.

36. Armstrong BG. The effects of measurement errors on relative risk regressions. *Am J Epidemiol.* 1990;132:1176–1184.

37. Kannel WB. CHD risk factors: A Framingham study update. *Hosp Pract (Off Ed).* 1990;25:119–127, 130.

38. Giovannucci E, Ascherio A, Rimm EB, et al. A prospective cohort study of vasectomy and prostate cancer in US men. *J Am Med Assoc.* 1993;269:873–877.

39. Goldberg RJ, Gorak EJ, Yarzebski J, et al. A communitywide perspective of sex differences and temporal trends in the incidence and survival rates after acute myocardial infarction and out-of-hospital deaths caused by coronary heart disease. *Circulation.* 1993;87:1947–1953.

40. Perneger TV, Nieto FJ, Whelton PK, et al. A prospective study of blood pressure and serum creatinine: Results from the "Clue" Study and the ARIC Study. *J Am Med Assoc.* 1993;269:488–493.

41. Szklo M. Aplastic anemia. In: Lilienfeld AM, ed. *Reviews in Cancer Epidemiology*, vol 1. New York, NY: Elsevier North-Holland; 1980:115–119.

42. Antunes CM, Strolley PD, Rosenshein NB, et al. Endometrial cancer and estrogen use: Report of a large case-control study. *N Engl J Med.* 1979;300:9–13.

43. Horwitz RI, Feinstein AR. Estrogens and endometrial cancer: Responses to arguments and current status of an epidemiologic controversy. *Am J Med.* 1986;81:503–507.

44. Brunekreef B, Groot B, Hoek G. Pets, allergy and respiratory symptoms in children. *Int J Epidemiol.* 1992;21:338–342.

45. Nieto FJ, Diez-Roux A, Szklo M, et al. Short- and long-term prediction of clinical and subclinical atherosclerosis by traditional risk factors. *J Clin Epidemiol.* 1999;52:559–567.

46. Hammond EC, Horn D. Smoking and death rates; report on forty-four months of follow-up of 187,783 men: II: Death rates by cause. *J Am Med Assoc.* 1958;166:1294–1308.

47. Shapiro S, Venet W, Strax P, et al. Selection, follow-up, and analysis in the Health Insurance Plan Study: A randomized trial with breast cancer screening. *Natl Cancer Inst Monogr.* 1985;67:65–74.
48. Hutchison GB, Shapiro S. Lead time gained by diagnostic screening for breast cancer. *J Natl Cancer Inst.* 1968;41:665–681.
49. Morrison AS. *Screening in Chronic Disease.* New York, NY: Oxford University Press. Monographs in Epidemiology and Biostatistics, vol. 7; 1985.
50. Schroder FH, et al. Screening and prostate-cancer mortality in a randomized European study. *New Eng J Med.* 2009;360:1320–1328.
51. Andriole GL, et al. Mortality results from a randomized prostate-cancer screening trial. *New Eng J Med.* 2009;360:1310–1319.
52. Stamey et al. Biological determinants of cancer progression in men with prostate cancer. *J Am Med Assoc.* 1999;281:1395–1400.
53. Schonberg MA, Marcantonio ER, Ngo L, et al. Causes of death and relative survival of older women after a breast cancer diagnosis. *J Clin Oncol.* 2011;29:1570–1577.

EXERCISES

1. In a case-control study of risk factors of colon cancer, 430 cases were compared with 551 controls. The investigators used a questionnaire to obtain information about demographic variables, socioeconomic variables (e.g., education), weight, and height, among other variables. Using the self-reported weight and height information, body mass index [BMI, weight (kg)/height (m)^2] values were calculated. Participants with BMI $\geq$ 30 kg/m^2 were considered "obese." The association between obesity and colon cancer in this study is shown in the table.

	Cases	Controls
Obese	162	133
Nonobese	268	418

   a. Calculate the odds ratio relating obesity and colon cancer in this study.

   Subsequently, the investigators obtained additional funds to conduct a validation ancillary study of some of the information obtained from the participants' interviews. For the validation study, 100 participants (50 cases and 50 controls) were randomly selected and invited to attend a clinic, where diverse objective physical measurements and more extensive questionnaires were used in an attempt to estimate the validity of the self-reported information in the study. Despite intensive efforts for recruitment, only 60 of the 100 participants invited for the validation study agreed to the clinic visit. The participants who agreed to attend included a larger proportion of females and individuals of a higher educational level than those who declined.

   Using objectively measured weight and height, BMI was recalculated in the 60 individuals in the validation study. Among the individuals who were classified as obese using measured weight and height, 90% of the cases and 95% of the controls had also been classified as obese by the BMI based on self-reported information; 100% of those classified as nonobese using measured weight and height had been classified as such by the self-reported information.

   b. Assuming that weight and height values did not change between the times of the interviews and the validation study, calculate the "corrected" odds ratio based on the estimates obtained from the validation study. That is, estimate the odds ratio that would have been obtained if no misclassification of obese status based on self-reported weight and height information had occurred.
   c. How do you explain the difference between the observed and the "corrected" odds ratio obtained in this study?
   d. In addition to the need to assume no change in weight and height between interviews and validation assessment, what are, in your judgment, other important limitations of the use of the ancillary validation study (vis-à-vis the whole study) to estimate a "corrected" odds ratio, as you did in answer to Question 1b?

2. It is estimated that about one-third of prostate cancer cases can be present in men in their fourth or fifth decade of life without any clinical symptoms or signs.* Several observational studies (including cohort studies) have suggested that vasectomy may be related to prostate cancer risk. For example, in a meta-analysis of 5 cohort studies and 17 case-control studies, the pooled relative risk estimate was found to be 1.37 (95% confidence interval, 1.15, 1.62).[†] In these studies, prostate cancer was not systematically evaluated; rather, usual clinical diagnosis was the diagnostic strategy. Describe the possible threats to validity when inferring that this association is causal.

3. Two clinical trials have examined the association of PSA testing with mortality from prostate cancer[‡,§]. In one trial (Schröder et al.[‡]), the cumulative hazards of death for those tested for PSA and for the control groups were virtually the same for most of the follow-up and at the end of the trial. In the other trial (Andriole GL, et al.[§]), a significant difference could not be found between the groups. Why have the authors examined mortality rather than survival (or case fatality)?

4. A breast cancer screening program based on repeat free clinical breast examinations is implemented in a developing country for women aged 50–59 years. The program is open to all eligible women, but it is not compulsory.

   a. Do you expect the incidence among the women who take advantage of the program to be the same as for the total eligible population? Why?

   In women who choose to take advantage of the program, the average annual incidence of previously undetected breast cancer is found to be about 100 per 100,000 on follow-up. In the first exam, point prevalence is found to be approximately 200 per 100,000. Assume that, after cases are confirmed by biopsy, no false negatives go undetected.

   b. What is the average duration of the detectable preclinical phase in cases of breast cancer detected at the first exam?
   c. Define lead time bias in the context of evaluation of a screening program or procedure.
   d. How does lead time bias affect estimation of average survival time?
   e. Estimate the average lead time for prevalent cases in this example, and state the assumption underlying this estimation.
   f. As the interval between screening exams becomes shorter, what is the tendency of the average lead time value for incident cases that are detected after the initial screening?

---

*Stamey TA, McNeal JE, Yemoto CM, et al. Biological determinants of cancer progression in men with prostatic cancer. *J Am Med Assoc*. 1999;281:1395–1400.
[†]Dennis LK, Dawson DV, Resnick MI. Vasectomy and the risk of prostate cancer: A meta-analysis examining vasectomy status, age at vasectomy, and time since vasectomy. *Prostate Cancer Prostatic Dis*. 2002;5:193–203.
[‡]Schröder FH, et al. Screening and prostate-cancer mortality in a randomized European study. *New Engl J Med*. 2009;360:1320–1328.
[§]Andriole GL, et al. Mortality results from a randomized prostate-cancer screening trial. *New Engl J Med*. 2009;360:1310–1319.

Identifying Noncausal Associations: Confounding

CHAPTER 5

5.1 INTRODUCTION

The term *confounding* refers to a situation in which a noncausal association between a given exposure and an outcome is observed as a result of the influence of a third variable (or group of variables), usually designated as a *confounding variable*, or merely a *confounder*. As discussed later in this chapter, the confounding variable must be related to both the putative risk factor and the outcome under study. In an observational cohort study, for example, a confounding variable would differ between exposed and unexposed subjects and would also be associated with the outcome of interest. As shown in the examples that follow, this may result either in the appearance or strengthening of an association not due to direct causal effect or in the apparent absence or weakening of a true causal association.

From the epidemiologic standpoint, it is useful to conceptualize confounding as distinct from bias in that a confounded association, although not causal, is real (for further discussion of this concept, see Section 5.5.8). This distinction has obvious practical implications with respect to the relevance of exposures as *markers* of the presence or risk of disease for screening purposes (secondary prevention). If, on the other hand, the goal of the researcher is to carry out primary prevention, it becomes crucial to distinguish a causal from a noncausal association, the latter resulting from either bias or confounding. A number of statistical techniques are available to control for confounding; as described in detail in Chapter 7, the basic idea underlying adjustment is to use some *statistical model* to estimate what the association between the exposure and the outcome would be, given a constant value or level of the suspected confounding variable(s).

Confounding is more likely to occur in observational than in experimental epidemiology studies. In an experimental study (e.g., a clinical trial), the use of randomization reduces the likelihood that the groups under comparison (e.g., exposed/treated and unexposed/untreated) differ with regard to *both known and unknown* confounding variables. This is particularly true when large sample sizes are involved. Even if the randomization approach is unbiased and the samples are large, however, there may be random differences between the experimental (e.g., vaccinated) and the control (e.g., those receiving placebo) groups, possibly leading to confounding (Exhibit 5-1). In an observational prospective study, in addition to random differences between the comparison groups, factors related to the exposure may confound the association under study, as illustrated in the examples that follow and as further discussed in the next section.

- *Example 1.* The overall crude mortality rates in 1986 for six countries in the Americas[1] were as follows:

Costa Rica:	3.8 per 1000	Cuba:	6.7 per 1000
Venezuela:	4.4 per 1000	Canada:	7.3 per 1000
Mexico:	4.9 per 1000	United States:	8.7 per 1000

EXHIBIT 5-1 Confounding in experimental and nonexperimental epidemiologic studies.

Study design	Experimental: randomized clinical trial	Observational: prospective study
Approach	Random allocation ↙ ↘ A B	Nonrandom allocation ↙ ↘ A B
Example	A = vaccine B = placebo	A = smokers B = nonsmokers
Source of confounding (difference[s] between groups)	Random difference(s)	Random difference(s) and factors associated with the exposure of interest

Assuming that these crude mortality rates are accurate, the literal (and correct) interpretation of these data is that the United States and Canada had the highest rates of death during 1986. Although this interpretation of crude data is useful for public health planning purposes, it may be misleading when using mortality rates as indicators of health status, as it fails to take into consideration interpopulation age differences. In this example, the higher mortality rates in Canada and the United States reflect the fact that there is a much higher proportion of older individuals in these populations; because age is a very strong "risk factor" for mortality, these differences in age distribution result in these countries having the highest mortality rates. Inspection of age-specific mortality rates (see Chapter 7, Section 7.2) results in a very different picture, with the lowest mortality rates observed in Canada, the United States, and Costa Rica for every age group. With adjustment for age (e.g., using the direct method and the 1960 population of Latin America as the standard, see Chapter 7, Section 7.3.1), the relative rankings of the United States and Canada are reversed (mortality per 1000: Costa Rica: 3.7; Venezuela: 4.6; Mexico: 5.0; Cuba: 4.0; Canada: 3.2; United States: 3.6). Age is, therefore, a confounder of the observed association between country and mortality.

- *Example 2.* In a cohort study conducted in England,[2] participants who reported a higher frequency of sexual activity at baseline (as indicated by their reported frequency of orgasm) were found to have a decreased risk of 10-year mortality compared with those who reported lower sexual activity. Does sexual activity *cause* lower mortality? Or are people with higher levels of sexual activity (or capacity to have orgasms) healthier in general and thus, by definition, at lower risk of mortality? Although the authors of this study, aware of this problem, attempted to control for confounding by adjusting for a number of health-related surrogate variables (see Chapter 7), the possibility of a "residual confounding" effect remains open to question (see Section 5.5.4 and Chapter 7, Section 7.6).

- *Example 3.* It has been reported that certain medical or tertiary prevention interventions in patients with chronic obstructive pulmonary disease (COPD) are associated with unfavorable health outcomes.[3] For example, long-term oxygen therapy is associated with increased rates of readmission to a hospital; similarly, readmission rates are higher in patients taking anticholinergic drugs, given influenza vaccination, or undergoing respiratory rehabilitation. In evaluating these associations, however, it is important to consider the possibility of confounding by *severity*, as all of these interventions tend to be more often prescribed in the most severe COPD cases.[3] This phenomenon, known in the clinical epidemiology field as *confounding by severity* or *confounding by indication*,[4] frequently complicates the interpretation of results from observational studies of outcomes of clinical or pharmacologic interventions.
- *Example 4.* In a nested case-control study among Japanese-American men, low dietary vitamin C has been found to be related to colon cancer risk.[5] Although it is possible that this relationship is causal, an alternative explanation is that individuals who consume more vitamin C tend to have a healthier lifestyle in general and thus are exposed to true protective factors acting as confounders (e.g., other dietary items, physical exercise).

A way to explain confounding, which is found with increasing frequency in the epidemiology literature, is based on the *counterfactual model*.[6,7] This explanation relies on the notion that the attribution of causation to a particular exposure is based on the concept that the risk of the outcome observed among individuals exposed *would have been different in these same individuals had exposure been absent*. Because the latter group is, by definition, unobservable ("counterfactual"), epidemiologists are forced instead to use a different group (the unexposed) as comparison; thus, the essence of epidemiologic analysis rests on the assumption that a separate unexposed group is comparable to exposed individuals *if they had not been exposed*. Confounding is said to be present if this assumption is not correct; that is, if the risk in the unexposed group is not the same as that of the unobserved (counterfactual) exposed group had its members not been exposed. Using an alternative terminology, confounding is described as present when the exposed–unexposed groups are *nonexchangeable*.[8,9] Extending this concept to a case-control study, confounding will be present if controls are not equivalent with regard to exposure odds to a hypothetical (counterfactual) case-group where the disease of interest was absent.

Referring to the example on sexual activity and mortality described previously,[2] confounding is said to occur when the "low sexual activity" and the "high sexual activity" groups are "nonexchangeable"; that is, the former has a different mortality risk than the group with "high sexual activity" would have had if its members did not have such a high orgasm frequency (and vice versa).

To conceptualize confounding in terms of "nonexchangeability" has an intrinsic appeal in that it underscores the old notion that the groups under comparison should be selected from the same study base—a requirement that is optimally met in large trials with random allocation. This definition is also useful in the context of a formal mathematical modeling of confounding.[8] In view of its "counterfactual" nature, however, it is of limited practical value when analyzing epidemiologic data. Thus, the following paragraphs are based on the more traditional explanation of the confounding effect.

5.2 THE NATURE OF THE ASSOCIATION BETWEEN THE CONFOUNDER, THE EXPOSURE, AND THE OUTCOME

5.2.1 General Rule

The common theme with regard to confounding is that the association between an exposure and a given outcome is induced, strengthened, weakened, or eliminated by a third variable or group of variables (confounders). The essential nature of this phenomenon can be stated as follows:

> **The confounding variable is causally associated with the outcome**

and

> **noncausally or causally associated with the exposure**

but

> **is not an intermediate variable in the causal pathway between exposure and outcome**

This general rule is schematically represented in Figure 5-1. In this figure and throughout all of the figures in this chapter, the association of interest (i.e., whether a given exposure is causally related to the outcome) is represented by shaded boxes connected by a dotted arrow and a question mark; this arrow is pointing to the outcome, as the question of interest is whether the exposure *causes* the outcome. (An association between exposure and outcome can also occur because the "outcome" causes changes in "exposure": i.e., *reverse causality*, a situation that is discussed in Chapter 4, Section 4.4.2.)

Some exceptions to the previous general rule for the presence of confounding are discussed in Section 5.2.3; its components are dissected in the next section (5.2.2)

FIGURE 5-1 General definition of confounding. The confounder is causally associated with the outcome of interest and either causally or noncausally associated with the exposure; these associations may distort the association of interest: whether exposure causes the outcome. A unidirectional arrow indicates that the association is causal; a bidirectional arrow indicates a noncausal association.

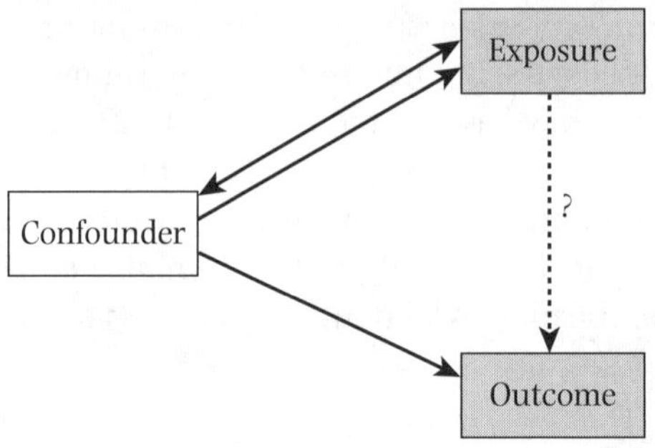

5.2 The Nature of the Association Between the Confounder, the Exposure, and the Outcome

using the previously discussed examples as illustrations (Figure 5-2). The confounding variables in Figure 5-2A and 5-2B are denoted as simple, and possibly oversimplified, characteristics ("age distribution" and "general health," respectively). In Figure 5-2C and Figure 5-2D, the postulated "confounding variables" are represented by more or less complex sets of variables. In Figure 5-2C, "severity" relates to the clinical status of the COPD patients; that is, disease stage, the presence of comorbidities, etc. In Figure 5-2D, the "confounder" is a constellation of variables related to general socioeconomic status (SES) and lifestyle characteristics that have their own interrelations. There is usually a trade-off in choosing simplicity over complexity in the characterization of these variables and in the conceptualization of their interrelations; this trade-off is directly relevant to the art of statistical "modeling" and is the core of the science of multivariate analysis, a key tool in analytical epidemiology (see Chapter 7, Sections 7.4 and 7.8).

5.2.2 Elements of the General Rule for Defining the Presence of Confounding

"The Confounding Variable Is Causally Associated with the Outcome"

In all of the examples illustrated in Figure 5-2, the confounding variables (age distribution, general health, severity of COPD, and SES/other lifestyle characteristics) determine the likelihood of the outcome (mortality rate, risk of death, readmission for COPD, and risk of colon cancer, respectively) to a certain degree.

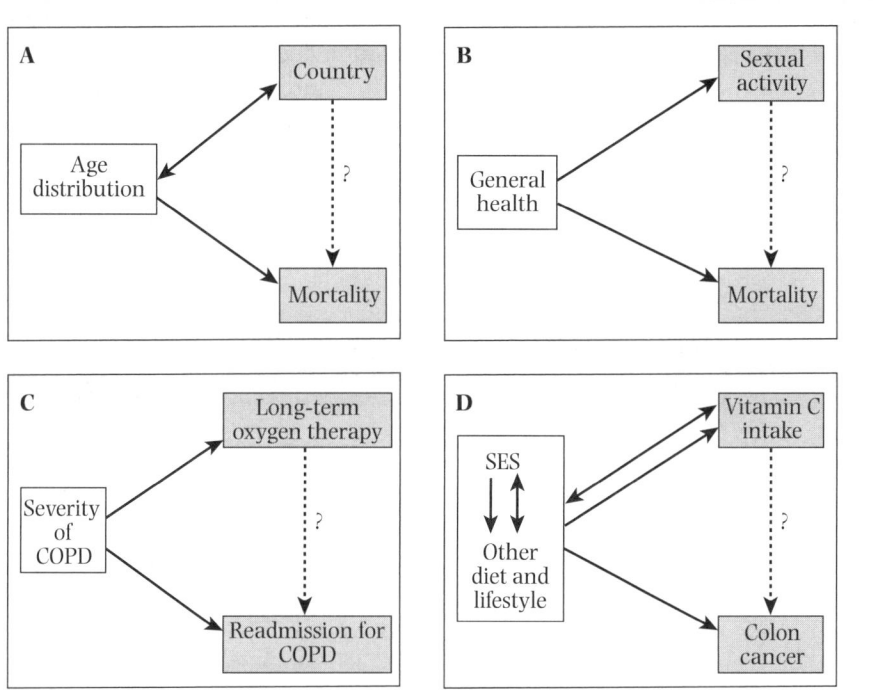

FIGURE 5-2 Schematic representation of the hypothetical relations of confounders, exposures of interest, and outcomes, based on the examples in the text. A unidirectional arrow indicates that the association is causal; a bidirectional arrow indicates a noncausal association. The main exposure and outcome are represented in shaded boxes; a dotted arrow with a question mark indicates the research question of interest.

Note: COPD: Chronic obstructive pulmonary disease; SES: Socioeconomic status

"And Noncausally or Causally Associated with the Exposure"

The examples in Figure 5-2 illustrate the different forms assumed by the relationships between the postulated confounders and the respective exposures of interest (country, sexual activity, long-term oxygen therapy, and vitamin C intake). For instance, in Figure 5-2A, in addition to a causal relationship with the outcome, the confounding variable (age) is related to the "exposure of interest" (country) in a noncausal fashion. In this example, the relationship between age distribution and country is postulated to be contextual rather than causal—that is, determined by a set of historical and social circumstances that are not unique to any given country.

The confounding variables may be also related to the exposure in a causal fashion, as in the case of the postulated relationship between "severity" and prescription of oxygen therapy in COPD patients (Figure 5-2C) and that of "good health" with sexual activity exemplified in Figure 5-2B. Finally, the example in Figure 5-2D shows the different types of relationship of the exposure of interest to the constellation of factors included in the "confounding complex": for example, lower SES may be causally related to vitamin C intake to the extent that it determines degree of access to food products that are rich in vitamin C. On the other hand, some other lifestyle characteristics related to SES (e.g., physical exercise) may be related to vitamin intake in a noncausal fashion.

An additional illustration of the rule that confounding may result when the confounding variable is causally related to the exposure of interest (not represented in Figure 5-2) is given by smoking and high-density lipoprotein (HDL) cholesterol in relationship to lung cancer. Smoking is known to *cause* a decrease in HDL levels,[10] thus explaining the apparent relationship of low HDL and lung cancer.

"But Is Not an Intermediate Variable in the Causal Pathway Between Exposure and Outcome"

The general rule defining a confounding variable excludes the situation in which the exposure determines the presence or level of the presumed confounder. In the previous examples, the assumption that this type of situation does not exist may not be entirely justified. For instance, in the example illustrated in Figure 5-2B, increased sexual activity may *cause* an improvement in general health (e.g., by leading to psychological well-being that may have an impact on physical health), which in turn results in a decrease in mortality (Figure 5-3). If this hypothesized mechanistic model is true, "general health" is the link in the causal pathway between sexual activity and mortality and should thus not be considered a confounder. Another example relates to the hypothesized causal

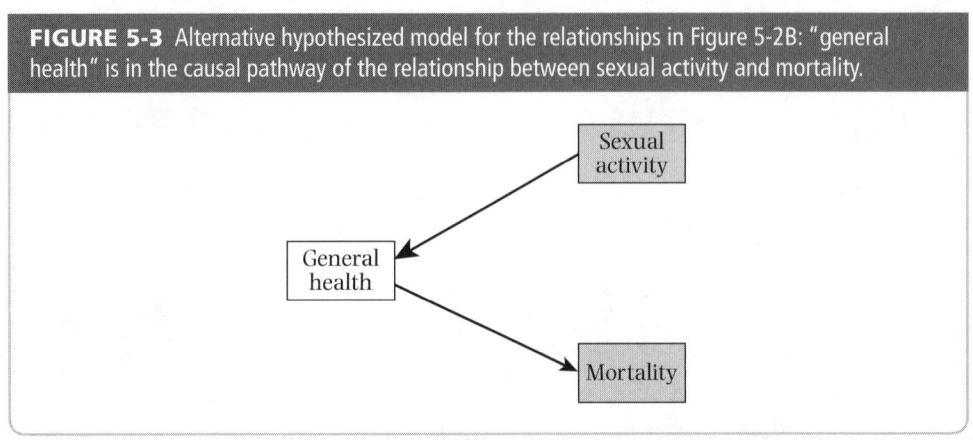

FIGURE 5-3 Alternative hypothesized model for the relationships in Figure 5-2B: "general health" is in the causal pathway of the relationship between sexual activity and mortality.

relationship between obesity and increased risk of mortality. Although it could be argued that this association is due to the "confounding" effect of hypertension, an alternative explanation is that hypertension is a *mediator* of the association between obesity and mortality rather than a confounder.[11]

5.2.3 Exceptions to the General Rule for the Presence of Confounding

"Confounding" Due to Random Associations

Although the general rule is that the confounding variable must be *causally* associated with the outcome (Figure 5-1), sometimes a random (statistical) association results in confounding. Thus, for example, in a case-control study, sampling (random) variability may create an imbalance between cases and controls with regard to a given variable related to the exposure, even though there is no such imbalance in the total reference population.

It is important to understand that this phenomenon is not exclusive to observational studies. The notion that randomized clinical trials are free of confounding is an *average* concept, akin to that of *unbiased designs* discussed in Chapter 4 (Section 4.1). Randomization *does not exclude* the possibility of confounding in a given clinical trial, as random differences with regard to important prognostic factors can also occur between randomly allocated groups, especially when the sample sizes are small. This is the reason why investigators analyzing results from randomized clinical trials assess imbalances in confounding factors between the study groups that, if present, are adjusted for using one of the available statistical techniques (see Chapter 7).

The "Confounder" Does Not Cause the Outcome but It Is a Marker of Another Unmeasured Causal Factor

Variables treated as confounders are occasionally surrogates of the true confounding variable(s). For example, *educational level* is often used as a surrogate for the considerably more complex SES construct (Figure 5-2D). Another example is *gender*; although sometimes treated as a confounder in the true sense of the word (i.e., as reflecting distinct sexual or hormonal differences that affect the risk of the outcome), it can be used as a marker of attitudes, behaviors, or exposures that are associated with gender due to contextual or cultural circumstances.

For further discussion of the importance of a solid theoretical foundation when considering complex relationships between risk factors, confounders, and their surrogates, see Section 5.3.

The "Confounder" as an Intermediate Variable in the Causal Pathway of the Relationship Between Exposure and Outcome

As discussed previously, the potential confounder should not be an intermediate variable in the causal pathway between the suspected risk factor and the outcome. It follows that it is inappropriate to adjust for such a variable. Although this rule is generally sound, exceptions to it occur when the investigator deliberately explores alternative mechanisms that could explain the association between the exposure and the outcome of interest.

The association of maternal smoking during the index pregnancy with an increased risk of perinatal death provides an example of a situation in which it may be appropriate to adjust for an intermediate variable. Low birth weight is known to be an important link in the causal chain between smoking and perinatal death (Figure 5-4). Thus, if the study question is, "Does smoking cause perinatal death?" (which does not address a specific mechanism, as may be the case when first examining a hypothesis), it is clearly inappropriate to adjust

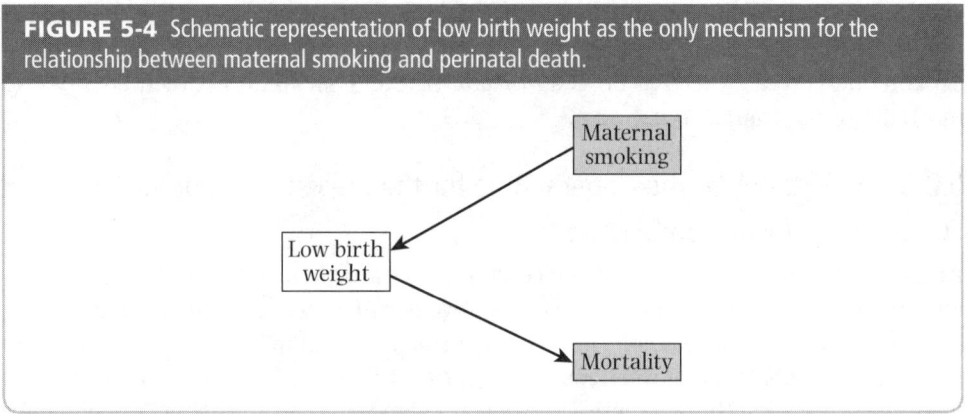

FIGURE 5-4 Schematic representation of low birth weight as the only mechanism for the relationship between maternal smoking and perinatal death.

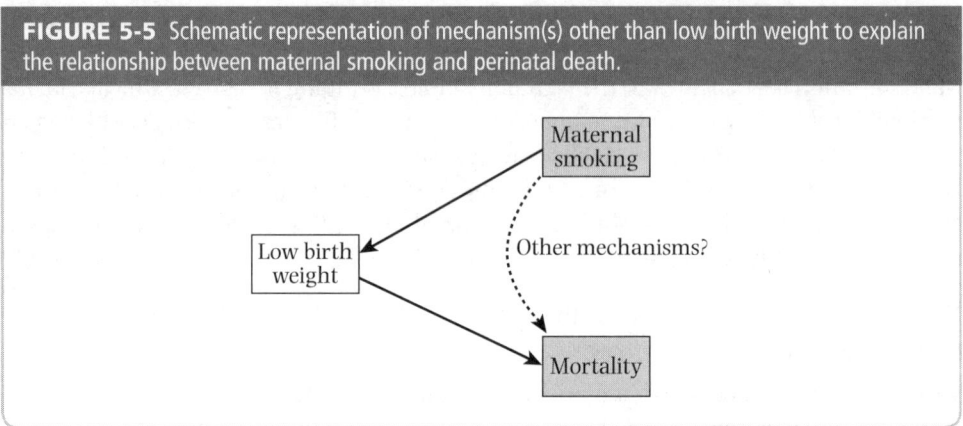

FIGURE 5-5 Schematic representation of mechanism(s) other than low birth weight to explain the relationship between maternal smoking and perinatal death.

for a possible mechanism, particularly a key mechanism such as low birth weight. After the principal link in the causality chain (low birth weight) is established, however, a different question may be asked: "Does smoking cause perinatal death through mechanism(s) *other than low birth weight?*" (Figure 5-5). In this situation, to treat birth weight as a "confounder" (at least in the sense of controlling for it) is appropriate; the presence of a residual (birth weight-adjusted) effect of smoking on perinatal mortality would indicate that, in addition to lowering birth weight, smoking may have a direct toxic effect.[12]

Similarly, in the previously mentioned obesity–hypertension example, even if the main mechanism whereby obesity increases mortality is an increase in blood pressure levels, it may be of interest to examine the blood pressure-adjusted association between obesity and mortality with the purpose of exploring the possibility that other mechanisms could explain the hypothesized relationship.

Another example is provided by a study of the causal pathways explaining why a genetic variation in the chemokine (C-C motif) receptor 5 (CCR5) is associated with slow progression of HIV infection among participants of the Multicenter AIDS Cohort Study.[13] The authors of this study examined the protective effect of CCR5 heterozygosity before and after controlling for CD4 count and viral load. Based on their findings, the authors concluded that "the protective effect [of CCR5 heterozygosity] on the occurrence of AIDS was completely mediated through an effect on the CD4 marker... Additional adjustment for the effect of an initial viral load measurement indicates that CCR5 heterozygosity did not have predictive value for either CD4 progression or the development of AIDS beyond its association with early viral load."[13(p.160)]

5.2 The Nature of the Association Between the Confounder, the Exposure, and the Outcome

The degree to which a given mechanism (or confounding variable) explains the relationship of interest is given by the comparison of adjusted (A) and unadjusted (U) measures of association (e.g., a relative risk [RR]). This comparison can be made using the ratio of the unadjusted to the adjusted relative risks, RR_U/RR_A, or the percentage excess risk explained by the variable(s) adjusted for*

$$\% \text{ Excess Risk Explained} = \frac{RR_U - RR_A}{RR_U - 1.0} \times 100 \quad \text{(Eq. 5.1)}$$

For example, in a study of the relationship between SES, health behaviors, and mortality in the Americans' Changing Lives longitudinal survey,[14] the age- and demographics-adjusted mortality rate ratio comparing those in the lowest income group with those in the highest income group was 3.2; trying to identify behavioral factors that might explain (mediate) the increased risk of mortality associated with low income, the authors further adjusted for smoking, alcohol drinking, sedentary lifestyle, and relative body weight, resulting in a reduction of the mortality rate ratio for low income to 2.8. Applying Equation 5.1, these data would suggest that these four behaviors explain approximately 18% of the predicted effect of income on mortality (i.e., [3.2 − 2.8]/[3.2 − 1]). Because the influence of major health risk behaviors explains only a "modest proportion of social inequalities in overall mortality," the authors concluded that "public health policies and interventions that exclusively focus on individual risk behaviors have limited potential for reducing socioeconomic disparities in mortality" and argued for the consideration of a "broader range of structural elements of inequality in our society."[14(pp.1707–1708)]

It is important to keep in mind, however, that if a residual association persists after a potentially intermediate variable is controlled for, this does not necessarily mean that there must be other causal pathways or mechanisms; the residual association may be due to *residual confounding* (see Section 5.5.4 and Chapter 7, Section 7.6). For example, even if hypertension were an important mechanism, a residual association between obesity and mortality could still be observed after controlling (adjusting) for blood pressure levels because of measurement error (e.g., random error due to within-individual variability in blood pressure). Under these circumstances, controlling for an imperfectly measured blood pressure will lead to incomplete adjustment and residual confounding. Likewise, when interpreting the results from the Americans' Changing Lives study on income, health behaviors, and mortality described previously here, Lantz

---

*Equation 5.1 examines the percentage excess risk explained in an *additive* scale. Alternatively, one may be interested in calculating the percentage excess risk explained in a *multiplicative scale* by using logarithmic transformations of the relative risks in the formula:

$$\% \text{ Excess multiplicative risk explained} = \frac{\log RR_U - \log RR_A}{\log RR_U} \times 100$$

$$= \left(1 - \frac{\log RR_A}{\log RR_U}\right) \times 100$$

The resulting percentage will be different from that obtained using Equation 5.1, reflecting the inherent difference in the two scales. One consideration when using the additive version of Equation 5.1 is that, because of the asymmetry of the relative risks in an additive scale, it cannot be applied in situations where the relative risks are below 1.0 (i.e., when the variable of interest is a protective factor). The recommended approach in this case is to calculate the "% excess risk explained" associated with the *absence of the protective factor*, i.e., using the inverted relative risks (e.g., $1/RR_U$ and $1/RR_A$) before applying Equation 5.1.

et al.[14] aptly acknowledged that errors in the reporting of these behaviors could have resulted in an underestimation of the mediating effects of individual behaviors on the income–mortality association.

It is also important to emphasize that any conclusion regarding direct and indirect effects based on the previous considerations should be based on solid theoretical understanding of the mechanisms underlying the associations under investigation. As discussed in more detail in the next section, the concept of proportion of effect explained by a putative mechanism (Equation 5.1) relies on the assumption that the relationship between the suspected intermediary variable and the outcome is free of confounding.[15,16] Because this assumption is often difficult to evaluate empirically, caution should be exercised when interpreting results of these analyses; at the very least, the proportion of risk estimated using Equation 5.1 should be interpreted as an approximate indication of the degree to which the hypothesized mechanism could explain the association of interest.

The importance of solid and explicit conceptual models when analyzing confounders and potential mechanisms cannot be overemphasized. These issues, as well as additional methodological tools that could help in the process of formulating such conceptual models, are discussed in the following section.

5.3 THEORETICAL AND GRAPHICAL AIDS TO FRAME CONFOUNDING

As suggested by the preceding discussion, confounding is a complex phenomenon; its proper conceptualization requires a clear understanding of the relationships between all variables involved as the basis for a well-defined theoretical model. The importance of selecting the proper statistical model when analyzing epidemiologic data is discussed in detail in Chapter 7 (Section 7.7). In this section, the issues are the *conceptual definition* of the variables involved as well as the *directionality* of the causal associations being investigated. For this purpose, some level of understanding (even if hypothetical) is necessary of the underlying pathophysiologic (or psychosocial) pathways representing the relationships between the suspected risk factor(s), confounder(s), and outcome(s). The more explicit this mechanistic model, the more straightforward the analytical approach and data interpretation will be.

A potentially useful analytical aid for this purpose is the directed acyclic graph (DAG). Originally developed in the field of artificial intelligence, this technique has been more recently used in the social science fields, including epidemiology.[15-18] The DAG (also known as a "causal diagram") is a formal and more elaborate extension of traditional graphs to represent confounding, such as shown in Figure 5-2; in these graphs, the direction of the association between the variables of interests and other unknown confounders is explicitly displayed to facilitate and guide the casual inference process. In DAG's jargon, the confounding effect is called a "backdoor path"; in the situation illustrated by the DAG in Figure 5-2B, for example, controlling for general health will effectively close the backdoor path that distorts the observed association between sexual activity and mortality.

DAGs can thus be used to make more explicit the relations between suspected risk factors and outcomes when confounding is suspected; they are particularly useful for the identification of pitfalls in the analyses of direct and indirect (confounded) effects discussed previously in this chapter, which could potentially lead to erroneous conclusions pertaining to the presence of causal relationships. Figures 5-6 and 5-7 show two examples, which have been used in previous publications, to illustrate the application of this technique.[16,17]

5.3 Theoretical and Graphical Aids to Frame Confounding 163

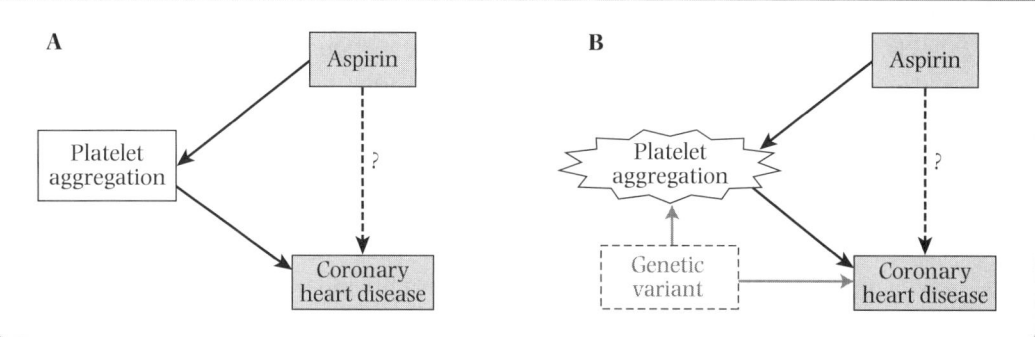

FIGURE 5-6 Directed acyclic graphs (DAGs) illustrating alternative hypothesis on the relationship between aspirin intake and risk of coronary heart disease (CHD). According to the DAG in (A), the association is mediated (at least partially) by platelet aggregation. In (B), platelet aggregation acts as a collider as its relationship with CHD is confounded by an unmeasured genetic variant (see text). The unmeasured variable is represented with faded font and in a dotted box.

Source: Based on an example from SE Cole and MA Hernán, Fallibility in Estimating Direct Effects. *International Journal of Epidemiology*, Vol 31, pp. 163–165, © 2002.

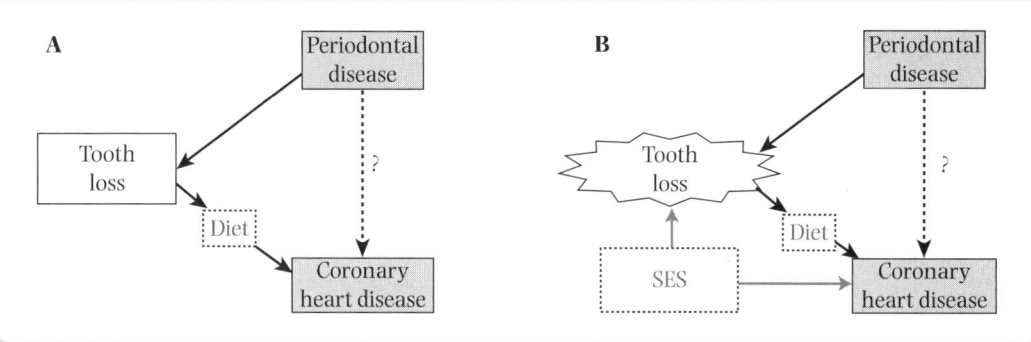

FIGURE 5-7 Directed acyclic graphs (DAGs) illustrating alternative hypothesis on the relationship between periodontal disease and risk of coronary heart disease (CHD). In (A), baseline periodontal disease and tooth loss (both observed variables in a study) are assumed to be caused by past periodontal disease. Through its relationship to diet, tooth loss is hypothesized to be an intermediary variable in the association between periodontal infection and risk of CHD. In (B), socioeconomic status (SES) is hypothesized to be a confounder of the association between tooth loss and CHD, thus making the latter a collider. Unmeasured variables are represented with faded font and in a dotted box.

Source: Based on an example from AT Merchant and W Pitiphat, Directed Acyclic Graphs (DAGs) An Aid to Assess Confounding in Dental Research. *Community Dentistry and Oral Epidemiology*, Vol 30, pp. 399–404, © 2002.

The DAG in Figure 5-6A illustrates the hypothesis that aspirin reduces the risk of coronary heart disease (CHD) through a decrease in platelet aggregation; based on this hypothesis, and in order to evaluate the mediating effect of platelet function and the possibility of additional mechanisms, the relationship between aspirin intake and CHD risk before and after controlling for platelet aggregation can be assessed by means of Equation 5.1. Alternatively, in the DAG in Figure 5-6B, an additional unidentified factor, a genetic variant, is hypothesized to be causally related to the suspected intermediate variable (platelet aggregation) and the outcome (CHD). In this situation, the relationship between the intermediate variable and the outcome is confounded by the genetic variant. Notably, the two causal pathways—[aspirin → platelet aggregation → CHD] and [genetic variant → platelet aggregation → CHD]—converge ("collide") at the suspected intermediary variable (platelet aggregation), that is said to be a *collider*. Using simulated data, Cole and Hernán[16] demonstrated that under certain assumptions regarding the strength and direction of the associations between the unknown genetic variant with CHD and platelet aggregation, adjusting for the latter *may introduce bias*; that is, may result in spurious estimates of the association between aspirin and CHD.

The example in Figure 5-7A and Figure 5-7B shows DAGs corresponding to alternative assumptions regarding mechanisms surrounding the putative relationship between periodontal disease and CHD. In a hypothetical cohort study, the association between periodontal disease and incidence of CHD is assessed.[17] Baseline periodontal disease is measured by clinical detachment loss, as a marker of lifetime periodontal disease; in addition, tooth loss is also recorded as a marker of past periodontal disease. Identification of a relationship between periodontal disease and CHD would support the infectious hypothesis of atherosclerosis;[19,20] on the other hand, this association could also be explained by the mediating effect of tooth loss (e.g., through its relationship with unhealthy diet). Thus, the investigator might study the relationship between periodontal disease and CHD incidence while controlling for tooth loss (and for diet, if information were available) (Figure 5-7A); however, the relationship between tooth loss/diet and CHD may be further confounded by another variable; for example, SES may be causally related to both CHD and to tooth loss (e.g., through poor dental care access; Figure 5-7B). In the latter situation, tooth loss acts as a collider, and controlling for it could result in spurious estimates of the "adjusted" periodontal disease–CHD association.

Additional examples of the application and interpretation of DAGs in the fields of neighborhood health effects and perinatal epidemiology have been provided by Fleisher and Diez Roux[18] and Hernán et al.,[21] respectively.

For the understanding of DAGs, the directionality of the arrows is critical. Those converging at platelet aggregation and tooth loss in Figures 5-6B and 5-7B, respectively, are unidirectional (i.e., they represent causal associations, defining these variables as colliders).

Of course, deciding which variables are involved and the directionality of their connections relies on knowledge of the subject matter and on the existence of a theoretical model. Framing confounding through the use of DAGs provides a foundation that facilitates the proper use of analytical tools described in the following section and in Chapter 7. For example, the application of this methodology for instrumental variable analysis is described in Section 7.5.

It is important to point out, however, that, although helpful, the use of DAGs is limited by their inability to handle effect modification and a large number of variables, among other limitations.[18]

5.4 ASSESSING THE PRESENCE OF CONFOUNDING

After properly framed, the existence of confounding can be assessed empirically. In an observational study, assessment of confounding effects is carried out for variables that are known or suspected confounders. The identification of potential confounders is usually based on *a priori* knowledge of the dual association of the possible confounder with the exposure and the outcome, the two poles of the study hypothesis. In addition

5.4 Assessing the Presence of Confounding

to the *a priori* knowledge about these associations, it is important to verify whether confounding is present in the study. There are several approaches to assess the presence of confounding, which are related to the following questions:

1. Is the confounding variable related to both the exposure and the outcome in the study?
2. Does the exposure–outcome association seen in the crude analysis have the same direction and similar magnitude as the associations seen within strata of the confounding variable?
3. Does the exposure–outcome association seen in the crude analysis have the same direction and similar magnitude as that seen after controlling (adjusting) for the confounding variable?

These different approaches to assess the presence and magnitude of confounding effects are illustrated using an example based on a hypothetical case-control study of male gender as a possible risk factor for malaria infection. The crude analysis shown in Exhibit 5-2 suggests that males are at a higher risk of malaria than females (odds ratio = 1.7; 95% confidence limits, 1.1–2.7). A "real" association between male gender and malaria can be inferred if these results are free of random (sampling) and systematic (bias) errors: that is, males do have a higher risk of malaria in this particular population setting. The next question is whether the association is *causal*—that is, whether there is something inherent to gender that would render males more susceptible to the disease than females (e.g., a hormonal factor). Alternatively, a characteristic that is associated with both gender and an increased risk of malaria may be responsible for the association. One such characteristic is work environment, in the sense that individuals who primarily work outdoors (e.g., in agriculture) are more likely to be exposed to the mosquito bite that results in the disease than those who work indoors (Figure 5-8). Thus, if the proportion of individuals with mostly outdoor occupations were higher in males than in females, working environment might explain the observed association between gender and malaria.

5.4.1 Is the Confounding Variable Related to Both the Exposure and the Outcome?

The associations of the confounder with both the exposure and work environment in this hypothetical example are shown in Exhibit 5-3, from which the following points should be highlighted.

- Compared with only 9% (13/144) of females, 43.6% (68/156) of males have mostly outdoor occupations, yielding an odds ratio of 7.8.
- Forty-two percent (63/150) of the malaria cases, but only 12% (18/150) of controls, have mostly outdoor occupations, yielding an odds ratio of 5.3.

EXHIBIT 5-2 Example of confounding: hypothetical study of male gender as a risk factor for malaria infection.

	Cases	Controls	Total	
Males	88	68	156	Odds ratio = 1.71
Females	62	82	144	
Total	150	150	300	

FIGURE 5-8 Work environment as a possible confounder of the association between male gender and malaria risk.

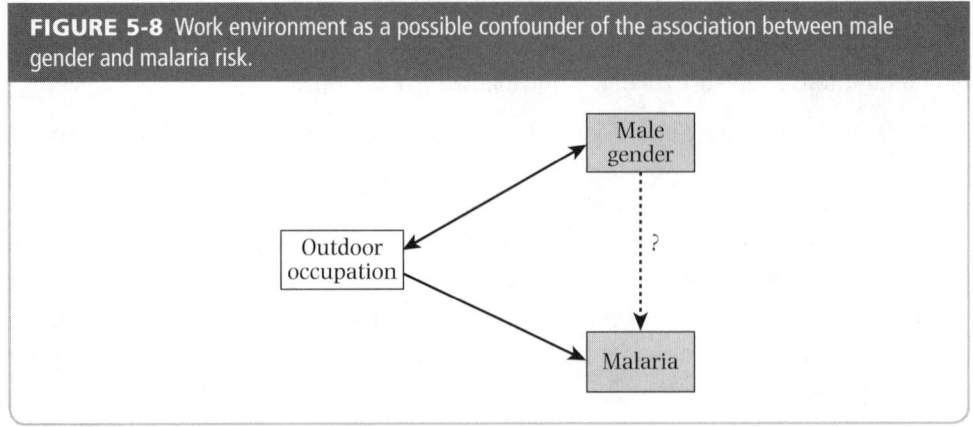

EXHIBIT 5-3 Association of the putative confounder (mostly outdoor occupation) with the exposure of interest (male gender) and the outcome (malaria) in the hypothetical study in Exhibit 5-2 and Figure 5-8.

Confounder versus exposure		Mostly outdoor	Mostly indoor	Total	
	Males	68	88	156	**Odds ratio = 7.8**
	Females	13	131	144	
				300	

Confounder versus outcome		Cases	Controls		
	Mostly outdoor	63	18		**Odds ratio = 5.3**
	Mostly indoor	87	132		
	Total	150	150	300	

The strong positive associations of the confounder (work environment) with both the risk factor of interest (male gender) and the outcome ("malaria status") suggest that work environment may indeed have a strong confounding effect.

5.4.2 Does the Exposure–Outcome Association Seen in the Crude Analysis Have the Same Direction and Similar Magnitude as Associations Seen Within Strata of the Confounding Variable?

Stratification according to the confounder represents one of the strategies to *control for* its effect (see Chapter 7, Section 7.2). When there is a confounding effect, the associations seen across strata of the potentially confounding variable are of similar magnitude to each other but are all different from the crude estimate. In the previous example, the data can be stratified by the confounder (work environment) to verify whether the association between the exposure (male gender) and the outcome (malaria) is present *within* the relevant strata (mostly outdoors or mostly indoors). As shown in Exhibit 5-4, the estimated odds ratios in both strata are very close to one and are different from the crude value (1.71), thus suggesting that work environment is a confounder

EXHIBIT 5-4 Stratified analyses of the association between gender and malaria (from Exhibit 5-2), according to whether individuals work mainly outdoors or indoors.

Mostly outdoor occupation

	Cases	Controls	
Males	53	15	Odds ratio = 1.06
Females	10	3	
Total	63	18	

Mostly indoor occupation

	Cases	Controls	
Males	35	53	Odds ratio = 1.00
Females	52	79	
Total	87	132	

that explains virtually all of the associations between male gender and the presence of malaria. If the association seen in the unadjusted analysis had persisted within strata of the suspected confounder, it would have been appropriate to conclude that a confounding effect of work environment did not explain the association observed between male gender and malaria.

With regard to using stratification as a means to verify presence of confounding, it must be emphasized that, as demonstrated by Miettinen and Cook[22] for odds ratios (and subsequently by Greenland[23] for rate ratios and absolute differences between rates), the crude odds ratio is sometimes different from the stratum-specific odds ratios *even if confounding is absent*. Because of the occasional "noncollapsibility" of stratum-specific estimates, the strategy of comparing stratum-specific odds ratios with the crude (pooled/unadjusted) odds ratio for the assessment of confounding should be confirmed through the use of the previous strategy and that which follows.

5.4.3 Does the Exposure–Outcome Association Seen in the Crude Analysis Have the Same Direction and Magnitude as That Seen after Controlling (Adjusting) for the Confounding Variable?

Perhaps the most persuasive approach to determine whether there is a confounding effect is the comparison between adjusted and crude associations. The gender-malaria infection example is also used in Chapter 7, Section 7.3.3, to illustrate the use of the Mantel-Haenszel approach to calculate an adjusted odds ratio. As described in that section, the Mantel-Haenszel adjusted odds ratio in this example is 1.01. (This odds ratio is merely a weighted average of the stratum-specific odds ratios shown in Exhibit 5-4.) The comparison between the crude (1.71) and the work environment–adjusted (1.01) odds ratios is consistent with and confirms the inference based on the previous strategies illustrated in Exhibits 5-3 and 5-4 that the increased risk of malaria in males (odds increased by 71%) resulted from their being more likely to work outdoors.

As another example of the comparison between crude and adjusted associations, Table 5-1 shows results from the same cohort study that served as the basis for the example described in Section 5.1 (Figure 5-2C). In this study, the presence of confounding by indication was assessed as a way to explain the adverse outcomes

TABLE 5-1 Association between medical interventions and risk of readmission to a hospital in chronic COPD patients: estimating the proportion of risk explained by markers of COPD severity (FEV_1, PO_2, and previous admission to a hospital).

	Crude hazard ratio	Adjusted hazard ratio*	Excess risk explained by covariates[†]
Long-term oxygen therapy	2.36[‡]	1.38	72%
Respiratory rehabilitation	1.77[‡]	1.28	64%
Anticholinergics	3.52[‡]	2.10[‡]	56%
Under the care of pulmonologist[§]	2.16[‡]	1.73[‡]	37%

*Adjusted for FEV_1, PO_2, and previous admission, using Cox Proportional Hazards Regression (see Chapter 7, Section 7.4.4).
[†]Calculated using Equation 5.1 (see text).
[‡]$p < 0.05$
[§]versus internist
Source: Data from García-Aymerich et al., Paradoxical Results in the Study of Risk Factors of Chronic Obstructive Pulmonary Disease (COPD) Re-admission. *Respiratory Medicine*, Vol 98, pp. 851–857, © 2004.

of long-term oxygen therapy and other medical interventions in chronic obstructive pulmonary disease (COPD) patients.[3] The authors of this study used Equation 5.1* to estimate that three markers of disease severity (forced expiratory volume in 1 second [FEV_1], partial pressure of oxygen [PO_2], and previous admission) *explained* about 72% ([2.36 − 1.38]/[2.36 − 1]) of the excess risk associated with long-term oxygen therapy in these patients; as shown in Table 5-1, the paradoxical detrimental effects of other medical interventions (respiratory rehabilitation, treatment with anticholinergics) and being under the care of a pulmonologist could also be partially explained by disease severity.

A further example serves to illustrate the different approaches to assess confounding in a cohort study of employed middle-aged men (Western Electric Company study) that examined the relationship of vitamin C and beta carotene intakes to risk of death.[24] For the tables that follow, the suspected risk factor is defined on the basis of a summary index that takes both vitamin C and beta carotene intakes into consideration. For simplification purposes, this intake index defining the exposure of interest is classified as "low," "moderate," or "high." The potential confounder for these examples is current smoking, categorized as absent or present. In this example, the question of interest is whether there is an inverse relationship between intake index and the outcome, all-cause death rate, and if so, whether it can be partly or totally explained by the confounding effect of smoking.

The first approach to assess whether confounding can explain the graded unadjusted relationship found in this study (Table 5-2)—that is, whether the confounder is associated with both exposure and outcome—is illustrated in Tables 5-3 and 5-4. An inverse relationship between current smoking and the exposure, intake index, was

---

*Equation 5.1 was presented as a tool to evaluate the proportion of the association explained by a potentially mediating variable. As this example illustrates, however, it may also be used to assess the proportion of the association explained by confounding; as with the previous application, the importance of a proper theoretical basis and required assumptions need to be carefully considered (see Sections 5.3 and 5.4).

TABLE 5-2 Unadjusted mortality rates and corresponding rate ratios in the Western Electric Company Study population according to intake index.

Intake index	No. of person-years of observation	No. of deaths	Mortality/1000 person-years	Rate ratio
Low	10,707	195	18.2	1.00
Moderate	10,852	163	15.0	0.82
High	11,376	164	14.4	0.79

Source: Data from DK Pandey et al., Dietary Vitamin C and β-Carotene and Risk of Death in Middle-Aged Men, The Western Electric Study. *American Journal of Epidemiology*, Vol 142, pp. 1269–1278, © 1995.

TABLE 5-3 Percentage distribution of person-years of observation in the Western Electric Company Study population, according to vitamin C/beta carotene intake index and current smoking.

			Percentage distribution		
			Intake index		
Current smoking	No. of individuals	Person-years	Low	Moderate	High
No	657	14,534 (100.0%)	29.3	35.3	35.4
Yes	899	18,401 (100.0%)	35.0	31.1	33.9

Source: Data from DK Pandey et al., Dietary Vitamin C and β-Carotene and Risk of Death in Middle-Aged Men, The Western Electric Study. *American Journal of Epidemiology*, Vol 142, pp. 1269–1278, © 1995.

TABLE 5-4 Mortality rates and corresponding rate ratios in the Western Electric Company Study population by current smoking.

Current smoking	No. of person-years	No. of deaths	Mortality/1000 person-years	Rate ratio
No	14,534	165	11.3	1.00
Yes	18,401	357	19.4	1.72

Source: Data from DK Pandey et al., Dietary Vitamin C and β-Carotene and Risk of Death in Middle-Aged Men, The Western Electric Study. *American Journal of Epidemiology*, Vol 142, pp. 1269–1278, © 1995.

observed in this study, with a higher percentage of the low-intake and a slightly lower percentage of the high-intake categories seen in current smokers than in nonsmokers (Table 5-3). Current smoking was also found to be associated with a 72% increase in all-cause mortality (Table 5-4). Because of its dual association with both intake index (exposure) and mortality (outcome), smoking can be regarded as a potential confounder of the association of the composite vitamin C-beta carotene intake index with all-cause mortality.

The second approach to examine confounding (stratification according to categories of the suspected confounder) is illustrated in Table 5-5, which shows that the rate ratios in the strata formed by current smoking categories are similar to the unadjusted rate ratios. The results of the third approach (adjustment) are presented in Table 5-6, which show the rate ratios adjusted using the direct method (see Chapter 7, Section 7.3.1). Although slightly weakened, the inverse graded relationship of intake index with all-cause mortality remained after adjustment for current smoking. Thus, it can be concluded that although current smoking (categorized dichotomously as "no" or "yes") fulfilled strategy 1 criteria needed to define it as a confounder (Tables 5-3 and 5-4), it acted only as an extremely weak confounder in this study. This weak confounding effect may be explained by the relatively weak relationship

TABLE 5-5 Mortality rates and corresponding rate ratios associated with vitamin C/beta carotene intake index, according to current smoking, Western Electric Company Study.

Current smoking	Vitamin C/beta carotene intake index	No. of person-years	Mortality/1000 person-years	Rate ratio
No	Low	4260	13.4	1.0
	Moderate	5131	10.7	0.80
	High	5143	10.3	0.77
Yes	Low	6447	21.4	1.0
	Moderate	5721	18.9	0.88
	High	6233	17.8	0.83
Total (unadjusted)	Low	10,707	18.2	1.0
	Moderate	10,852	15.0	0.82
	High	11,376	14.4	0.79

Source: Data from DK Pandey et al., Dietary Vitamin C and β-Carotene and Risk of Death in Middle-Aged Men. The Western Electric Study. *American Journal of Epidemiology*, Vol 142, pp. 1269–1278, © 1995.

TABLE 5-6 Unadjusted and smoking-adjusted all-cause mortality ratios rate in the Western Electric Company Study.

Rate ratios	Vitamin C/beta carotene intake index rate ratios		
	Low	Moderate	High
Unadjusted	1.00	0.82	0.79
Adjusted*	1.00	0.85	0.81

*Adjusted using the direct method and the total cohort (sum of the person-years of observation for the three intake index categories) as standard population (see Chapter 7, Section 7.3.1).
Source: Data from DK Pandey et al., Dietary Vitamin C and β-Carotene and Risk of Death in Middle-Aged Men. The Western Electric Study. *American Journal of Epidemiology*, Vol 142, pp. 1269–1278, © 1995.

between smoking and intake index (Table 5-3) coupled with a total mortality rate ratio for the current smoking category of only 1.72 (Table 5-4). This may be due in part to the lack of specificity of the outcome, which included both smoking-related and nonsmoking-related deaths. (It could also be argued that adjustment for only two categories of smoking, which does not take into account either duration or amount of smoking, leaves room for substantial residual confounding; see Section 5.5.4.)

5.5 ADDITIONAL ISSUES RELATED TO CONFOUNDING

5.5.1 The Importance of Using Different Strategies to Assess Confounding

Although, as discussed previously in this chapter, the most persuasive evidence supporting presence of confounding is the demonstration that the crude and the adjusted estimates differ, it is useful to consider the other strategies discussed to evaluate confounding. For example, observation of the directions of the associations of the confounder with the exposure and the outcome permits an *a priori* expectation as to whether removal of confounding would lead to an increase or a decrease in the strength of the association (see Section 5.5.5). Should the adjusted estimate be inconsistent with the expectation, the adjustment procedure must be verified for a possible error. For example, in a case-control study in which cases are younger than controls and age is directly (positively) related to the exposure of interest, confounding is expected to result in an unadjusted relative risk estimate closer to 1.0. Thus, it would be against expectation and consequently requiring verification if the unadjusted estimate was found to be further away from the null hypothesis than the adjusted estimate.

Stratification is also a useful step when analyzing epidemiologic data, as it also allows the formulation of an *a priori* expectation of the effects of confounding on the association, and thus of the effects of adjustment on the association (notwithstanding the noncollapsibility caveat, previously referred to, that even when confounding is absent the pooled measure of association may be different from the stratum-specific ones). For example, when the estimates in the strata formed by the confounder are closer to the null hypothesis than the pooled unadjusted value, the relative risk should be closer to 1.0 after adjustment. (Exceptions include certain situations in which multiple variables confound each other.) Another reason why stratification is a useful analytical strategy is that, in addition to assessing confounding, it allows the examination of the presence of interaction, as discussed in more detail in Chapters 6 and 7.

5.5.2 Confounding Is Not an "All-or-None" Phenomenon

In the example illustrated in Exhibits 5-2 through 5-4, the confounding variable (work environment) appears to be responsible for the entirety of the relationship between the exposure of interest (male gender) and the outcome (malaria). Likewise, the relationship between long-term oxygen therapy or respiratory rehabilitation and risk of readmission among COPD patients could be almost entirely explained by the confounding effect of severity (Table 5-1).[3] In other instances, however, the confounding effect is only partial. In the example shown in Table 5-1, the increased risk of readmission associated with anticholinergic therapy or being under the care of a pulmonologist diminished somewhat after controlling for markers of severity; however, a relatively strong and statistically significant relative risk was still observed—which, in addition to resulting from residual confounding, could also mean that these markers confound part, but not all, of the entirety of the observed associations. Similarly, in the example shown in Tables 5-2 through 5-6, adjustment for smoking had only a slight effect on the association between vitamin C/beta carotene intake index and mortality.

5.5.3 Excessive Correlation Between the Confounder and the Exposure of Interest

Although, by definition, a confounding variable is correlated with the exposure of interest (Figure 5-1), on occasion, the correlation is so strong that adjustment becomes difficult, if not impossible. This is a problem analogous to the situation known in biostatistics as *collinearity*. Consider, for example, the exposure "air pollution" and the suspected confounder "area of residence." Given the high degree of correlation between these variables, it would be difficult (if not impossible) to control for the effect of residence when assessing the effect of air pollution on respiratory symptoms. Figure 5-9 schematically represents a perfect correlation between dichotomous exposure and confounding variables, which makes adjustment for the confounder impossible. The ideal situation for effective control of confounding is that in which there is a clear-cut correlation between exposure and confounder but the variability is sufficient to allow adequate representation of all cross-tabulated cells shown in Figure 5-10.

An example of the difficulty posed by excessive correlations among variables is given by the assessment of the role of dietary components as risk factors. When examining the observational association between dietary animal protein intake and a given outcome, it may be difficult to control for the possible confounding role of dietary fat, given the strong correlation between animal protein and fat intake.[25] Other examples of collinearity include education-income, serum HDL cholesterol-triglycerides, and race-SES. A similar situation occurs when components of the same exposure variable are strongly correlated, making it difficult to adjust for one while looking at the "independent" contribution of the other. For example, it may be difficult, if not impossible, to examine smoking duration while simultaneously and finely controlling for age of smoking initiation.

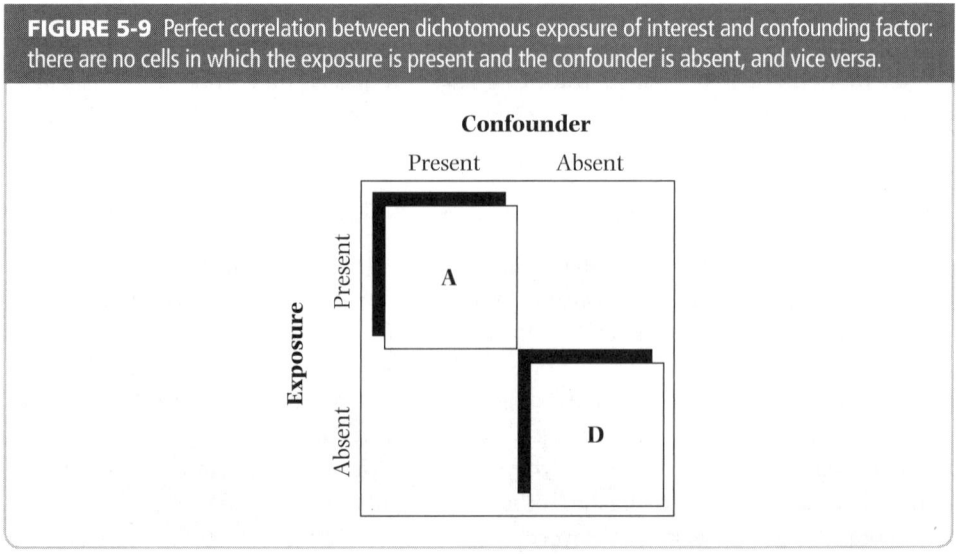

FIGURE 5-9 Perfect correlation between dichotomous exposure of interest and confounding factor: there are no cells in which the exposure is present and the confounder is absent, and vice versa.

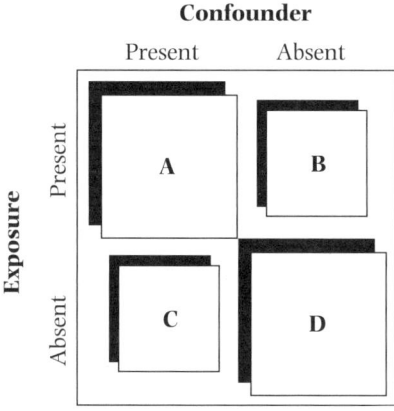

FIGURE 5-10 Correlation between an exposure of interest and a confounding factor: all four cells for a cross-tabulation of dichotomous categories are represented. In this schematic representation, the larger sizes of cells A and D denote the magnitude of the positive correlation between the exposure and the confounder.

As a corollary of the preceding discussion, it is important to underscore that it is only possible to adjust for a confounder while examining the relationship between exposure and outcome when levels of the confounder and those of the exposure overlap, a situation not always encountered in observational epidemiology studies. For example, it would be impossible to adjust for age if there were no overlap in ages between exposed and unexposed individuals (e.g., if all of those exposed were over 45 years old and all of those unexposed were less than 45 years old).

A related issue is *over-adjustment* (*or overmatching*), which occurs when adjustment (or matching, see Chapter 1, Section 1.4.5) is carried out for a variable so closely related to the variable of interest that no variability in the latter remains (see Chapter 7, Section 7.7). For example, in a case-control study, making the case and control groups very similar or identical regarding the confounder may result in their also being very similar or identical regarding the exposure, thereby resulting in an apparent null association. In general, it must be kept in mind that when adjustment is carried out for a given confounding variable, it is also carried out for all variables related to it. For example, when adjusting for area of residence, adjustment is also carried out to a greater or lesser extent for factors related to residence, such as ethnic background, income, religion, and dietary habits.

5.5.4 Residual Confounding

Residual confounding, which is discussed in more detail in Chapter 7 (Section 7.6), occurs when either the categories of the confounder controlled for are too broad, resulting in an imperfect adjustment, or when some confounding variables remain unaccounted for. Thus, in one of the examples discussed previously (Table 5-6), the use of only two categories of smoking ("present" or "absent") may explain the similarity between the crude and the smoking-adjusted relative risks expressing the relationship between vitamin C/beta carotene intake index and mortality. If the confounding effect of smoking were a function of other exposure components, such as amount, duration, or time since quitting, marked residual confounding might have remained after adjusting for only two smoking categories.

Another example is the study of the association between sexual activity and mortality discussed previously.[2] Aware of the possibility of confounding, the authors of this study used multiple logistic regression (see Chapter 7, Section 7.4.3) to adjust for several health-related variables. Data on these variables were collected at the baseline examination, including presence of prevalent coronary heart disease, total serum cholesterol, smoking, systolic blood pressure, and occupation (manual vs nonmanual). The lower mortality of study participants with a higher frequency of sexual intercourse persisted when these variables were adjusted for. The authors, nevertheless, aptly concluded that "despite this, confounding may well account for our findings," pointing out that in an observational study, variables unaccounted for may confound the observed association even after adjustment has been attempted. For example, in this study, other diseases affecting both sexual activity and mortality (e.g., diabetes, psychiatric conditions) were not taken into account. Furthermore, subtle health status differences that are not captured by the presence or absence of known diseases and risk factors (e.g., psychological profile or general "well-being") remained unaccounted for, thus underscoring the difficulties of fully taking into consideration the confounding effects of general health status in observational epidemiologic studies.

Another type of residual confounding occurs when the construct validity of the variable used for adjustment is not ideal; that is, the variable is an imperfect marker of the true variable one wishes to adjust for. Thus, the appropriateness of educational level as a proxy for social class has been questioned, particularly when comparing whites and blacks in the United States.[26] Likewise, in the COPD readmission example, the relative risk estimates after controlling for FEV_1, PO_2, and previous hospital admission, might be still subject to residual confounding by indication if these variables are imperfect markers of COPD severity, as suggested by the authors when they stated that "possible explanations for residual confounding in our study are: the existence of other confounders in the associations between medical care related factors and COPD re-admission, measurement error in questionnaires and lung function testing, and the lack of information on longitudinal changes of the relevant variables."[3(p.855)]

The different causes of residual confounding are discussed in more detail in Chapter 7, Section 7.6.

5.5.5 Types of Confounding Effects: Negative, Positive, and "Qualitative" Confounding

Confounding may lead to an overestimation of the true strength of the association (*positive confounding*) or its underestimation (*negative confounding*). In other words, in positive confounding, the magnitude of the unadjusted (vis-à-vis the adjusted) association is exaggerated; in negative confounding, it is attenuated. The terms *overestimation* and *underestimation* are used in reference to the null hypothesis. Thus, for example, an adjusted odds ratio of 0.7 is (in absolute terms) "greater" than an unadjusted odds ratio of 0.3; however, the fact that the former is closer than the latter to the odds ratio denoting lack of association (1.0) defines the confounding effect as "positive."

In Table 5-7, hypothetical examples showing relative risk estimates illustrate the effect of confounding. The first three examples show unadjusted associations, which either disappear or become weaker when confounding is adjusted for. Examples of positive confounding are abundant, including most of the examples used previously in this chapter (e.g., gender/malaria vis-à-vis occupation, which would be analogous to example 1 in Table 5-7 or the example of vitamin C intake/colon cancer vis-à-vis healthy lifestyle, possibly comparable to example 3 in Table 5-7).

Examples 4 through 6 in Table 5-7 show the reverse situation—namely, negative confounding, in which the unadjusted is an "underestimate" of the adjusted relative risk (vis-à-vis the null hypothesis). Adjustment reveals or strengthens an association that was rendered either absent (example 4) or weakened (examples 5 and 6) because of confounding. An example of negative confounding, in which the adjusted relative risk is further away from 1.0 when compared with the unadjusted value, is a study by Barefoot et al.[27] Using the Cook-Medley Hostility scale, a subscale of the widely used Minnesota Multiphasic Personality Inventory to measure psychological constructs, the authors examined the relationship of hostility to the incidence of acute myocardial infarction. Although the completely unadjusted results were not given, the relative risk was reported to change from 1.2 when only age and sex were adjusted for to about 1.5 when systolic blood pressure, smoking, triglycerides, sedentary work, and sedentary leisure were also included in the Cox proportional hazard regression model (see Chapter 7, Section 7.4.4). Thus, it can be concluded that one or more of these additional covariates (blood pressure, smoking, triglycerides, sedentary lifestyle) were negative confounders of the association between hostility and myocardial infarction incidence.

An extreme case of confounding is when the confounding effect results in an inversion of the direction of the association (Table 5-7, examples 7 and 8), a phenomenon that can be properly designated as *qualitative confounding*. For instance, in example 1 in Section 5.1, the US/Venezuela ratio of crude mortality rates is 8.7/4.4 = 1.98; however, when the age-adjusted rates are used, it becomes 3.6/4.6 = 0.78. The opposite patterns of the adjusted and crude rate ratios can be explained by the striking difference in the age distribution between these two countries.

TABLE 5-7 Hypothetical examples of unadjusted and adjusted relative risks according to type of confounding (positive or negative).

Example no.	Type of confounding	Unadjusted relative risk	Adjusted relative risk
1	Positive	3.5	1.0
2	Positive	3.5	2.1
3	Positive	0.3	0.7
4	Negative	1.0	3.2
5	Negative	1.5	3.2
6	Negative	0.8	0.2
7	Qualitative	2.0	0.7
8	Qualitative	0.6	1.8

176 CHAPTER 5 | Identifying Noncausal Associations: Confounding

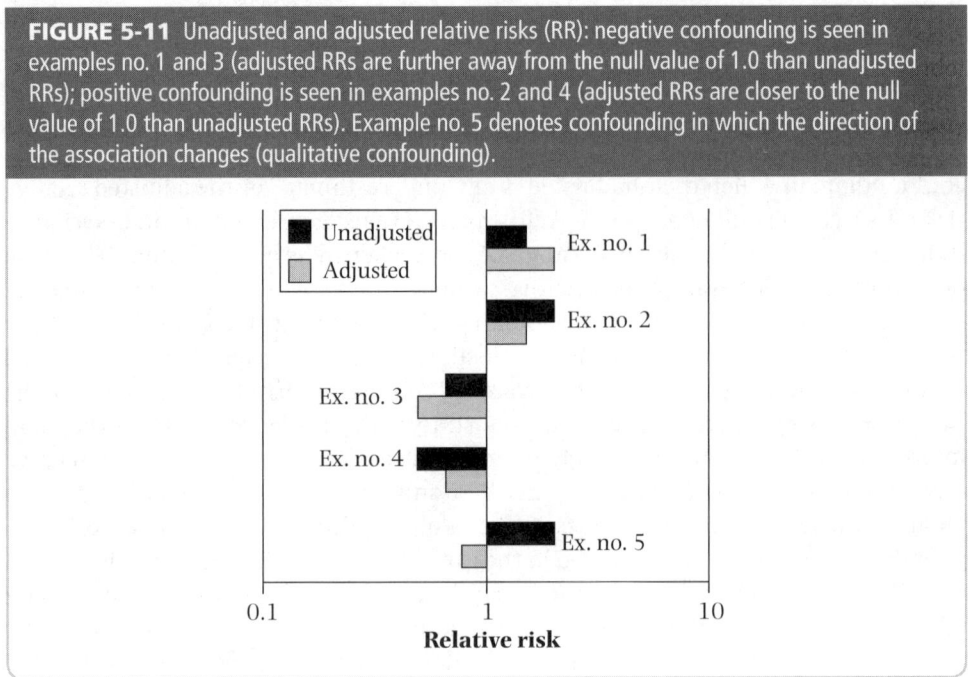

FIGURE 5-11 Unadjusted and adjusted relative risks (RR): negative confounding is seen in examples no. 1 and 3 (adjusted RRs are further away from the null value of 1.0 than unadjusted RRs); positive confounding is seen in examples no. 2 and 4 (adjusted RRs are closer to the null value of 1.0 than unadjusted RRs). Example no. 5 denotes confounding in which the direction of the association changes (qualitative confounding).

As a summary, Figure 5-11 shows schematic representations of negative, positive, and qualitative confounding effects.

The direction of the confounding effect (positive or negative) can be inferred from the directions of the associations of the confounder with exposure and outcome, if known. The expectations of the changes brought about by the adjustment, resulting from the directions of these associations are summarized in Table 5-8. Thus, positive confounding is to be expected when the confounder–exposure association is in the same direction as the confounder–outcome association. When these associations are in divergent directions, there will be negative confounding (or qualitative confounding in extreme cases). (Not shown in Table 5-8, when exposure and disease are *inversely* associated,[28] negative confounding will be expected if the associations of confounder is in the same direction for both exposure and outcome and positive when these go in divergent directions.)

5.5.6 Statistical Significance in Assessing Confounding

It is inappropriate to rely on statistical significance to identify confounding, especially when either the exposure (in case-control studies) or the outcome (in cohort studies) varies markedly according to the confounding variable. For example, in a hypothetical case-control study examining the relationship of the occurrence of menopause to disease Y in women aged 45 to 54 years old, small, statistically nonsignificant differences in age between cases and controls may cause an important confounding effect in view of the strong relationship between age and presence of menopause in this age range. Thus, even if there is no association whatsoever between occurrence of menopause and disease, if for each year of age the odds of menopause hypothetically increased from 1:1 to 1.5:1 (e.g., for an increase in menopause prevalence from 50% to 60%), a case-control age difference as small as 1 year (which might not be statistically significant if the study sample were not large) would result in an age-unadjusted menopause relative odds of 1.5.

TABLE 5-8 Directions of the associations of the confounder with the exposure and the outcome, and expectation of change of estimate with adjustment (assume a direct relationship between exposure and outcome, i.e., for exposed/unexposed, relative risk, or odds ratio > 1.0).

Association of confounder with exposure is	Association of confounder with outcome is	Type of confounding	Expectation of change from unadjusted to adjusted estimate
Direct*	Direct*	Positive‡	Unadjusted > Adjusted
Direct*	Inverse†	Negative§	Unadjusted < Adjusted
Inverse†	Inverse†	Positive‡	Unadjusted > Adjusted
Inverse†	Direct*	Negative§	Unadjusted < Adjusted

*Direct association: presence of the confounder is related to an increased probability of the exposure or the outcome.
†Inverse association: presence of the confounder is related to a decreased probability of the exposure or the outcome.
‡Positive confounding: when the confounding effect results in an unadjusted measure of association (e.g., relative risk) further away from the null hypothesis than the adjusted estimate.
§Negative confounding: when the confounding effect results in an unadjusted measure of association closer to the null hypothesis than the adjusted estimate.

For those who insist on using the *p* value as a criterion to identify confounding, it may be wiser to use more "lenient" (conservative) *p* values as a guide to identify possible confounders—for example, 0.20. Doing so decreases the beta error and, thus, increases the probability of accepting the presence of confounding even when there are small differences between cases and controls in case-control studies or between exposed and unexposed subjects in cohort studies. This strategy, however, should not replace the investigator's consideration of the *strength* of the associations of the suspected confounder(s) with the exposure and outcome as a means to identify confounding.

5.5.7 Conditional Confounding

A presumed confounding variable may be confounded by other variables. Thus, univariate evaluation may suggest that a given variable Z is a confounder, but the same variable may not act as a confounder when other variables are adjusted for. Similarly, Z may not appear to be a confounder univariately because it is negatively confounded by other variables, in which case a confounding effect of Z may become evident only after adjustment.

5.5.8 Confounding and Bias

Should confounding be regarded as a type of selection bias? Some epidemiology textbooks suggest that confounding is one more type of bias (e.g., Rothman and Greenland[29]), essentially because a confounded association can be considered as a "biased estimate" of the causal association (that which is expressed by the adjusted estimate—assuming that the adjustment procedure is appropriate and not subject to residual confounding). In contrast, other textbooks (e.g., Lilienfeld and Stolley[30] and Gordis[31]) differentiate between "spurious" associations due to bias and "indirect" (or "statistical") associations due to confounding, thus suggesting that confounding is distinct from bias.

The rationale for keeping confounding conceptually distinct from bias can be described as follows. Assuming no random variability, schematic representations of confounding and bias are shown in Figure 5-12A and Figure 5-12B, respectively. In

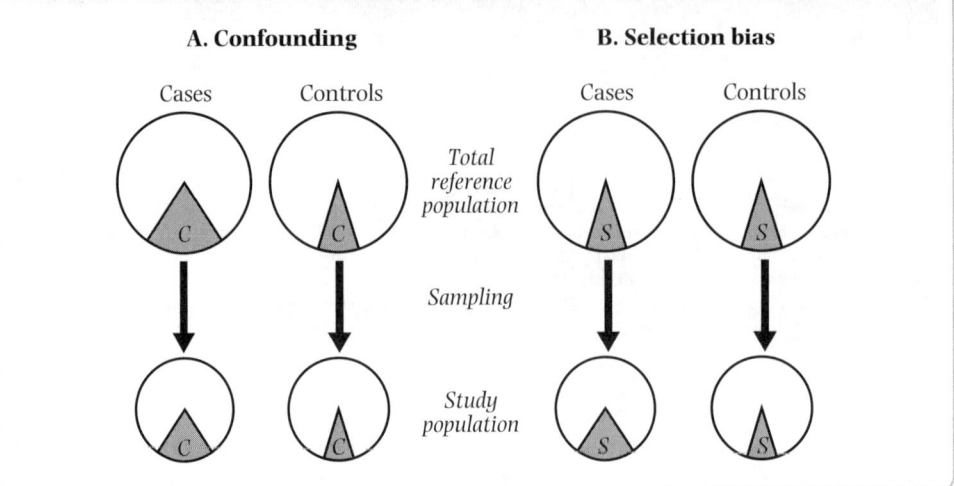

FIGURE 5-12 Schematic representation of positive confounding and selection bias. In the total reference population, confounding factor C is more common in cases than in controls; assuming no random variability, the study samples of cases and controls reflect the higher frequency of C in cases than in controls (A). In selection bias (B), the frequency of factor S is the same in cases and controls; however, through the selection process, it becomes more common in cases than in controls. Thus, confounding exists "in nature," whereas selection bias is a result of the sampling process.

these figures, circles represent cases or controls, with larger and smaller circles denoting the reference population and study sample subsets, respectively. In Figure 5-12A, representing confounding, the proportion of confounder C (e.g., smoking) in the reference population is truly greater in cases than in controls; thus, any factors related to C (e.g., alcohol intake) are more frequent in cases. Assuming no random variability, in confounding, the study samples accurately reflect the fact that C is more common in cases than in controls. On the other hand, in Figure 5-12B, the proportion of cases and controls in whom a certain selection factor S is present is the same in the reference population; however, in the study samples, selection bias has resulted in cases having a (spuriously) higher proportion of S than controls. Consider, for example, a case-control study in which cases are ascertained in hospitals that preferentially admit upper SES patients; on the other hand, controls are sampled from noncases from the population at large. As a result of this type of selection bias, positive associations will be observed in this study for exposures related to high SES.

This conceptual distinction between confounding and bias may be of only intellectual interest when assessing causal relationships (because for accepting a relationship as causal, both confounding and bias must be deemed unlikely explanations). However, it becomes important when epidemiologic findings are considered in the context of public health practice. Whether confounding is labeled as a bias or not, there is a clear-cut role for true, yet confounded associations, as they allow identification of markers that may be useful to define high-risk groups for secondary prevention.

As summarized in Exhibit 5–5, for primary prevention purposes, a causal association between the risk factor and the disease outcome must exist; otherwise, modification of the former will not lead to a reduction of the risk of the latter. However, a (true) statistical association between a confounding factor and the disease allows the identification

EXHIBIT 5-5 The relationship between type of evidence needed in epidemiologic studies and type of prevention carried out (primary or secondary).

Goal	Type of evidence needed
Primary prevention: prevention or cessation of risk factor exposure (eg, saturated fat intake and atherosclerosis).	Causal association *must* be present; otherwise, intervention on risk factor will not affect disease outcome. For example, if fat did not cause atherosclerosis, a lower fat intake would not affect atherosclerosis risk.
Secondary prevention: early diagnosis via selective screening of "high-risk" subjects (e.g., identification of individuals with high triglyceride levels).	Association may be *either* causal or statistical (the latter must not be biased): that is, the association may be *confounded*. For example, even if hypertriglyceridemic individuals had a higher probability of developing atherosclerotic disease because of the confounding effect of low high-density lipoprotein levels, atherosclerosis is *truly* more common in these individuals.

of *high-risk groups*, which should be the main focus of secondary prevention (screening) and of primary prevention based on established causes, if known and if amenable to intervention. An example is given by the known fact that, in the United States, African Americans have a much greater risk of hypertension than whites. This association is almost certainly not causal (due to a genetic factor predominantly found in African Americans, for example); on the other hand, it is clearly confounded by poverty-related lifestyle risk factors for hypertension, such as obesity and an unhealthy diet, known to be more common in African Americans. Such a *confounded relationship*—referred to by Lilienfeld and Stolley as *indirect*[30]—nevertheless serves to identify African Americans as a high-risk group for hypertension, in whom both screening for hypertension and intervention on known hypertension risk factors (e.g., obesity) should be pursued vigorously. Thus, unlike a spurious relationship resulting from bias, a confounded, yet true statistical relationship allows identification of individuals with a higher likelihood of disease occurrence and is therefore useful for public health purposes.

5.6 CONCLUSION

Confounding, along with bias, constitutes a formidable threat to the evaluation of causal relationships. In this chapter, issues related to the definition of confounding effects as well as some approaches to verify the presence of confounding were discussed. The assessment of confounding being done before carrying out statistical adjustment was underscored as a means of predicting the magnitude and direction of possible changes (if any) in the measure of association brought about by adjustment. The concept of residual confounding (which is also discussed in Chapter 7) was introduced in this chapter, as was the notion that statistical significance testing should not be used as a criterion to evaluate confounding. Finally, the rationale for not classifying confounding as a type of bias was discussed in the context of the public health usefulness of confounded, yet true associations, as a way to identify high-risk groups.

REFERENCES

1. *Las condiciones de salud en las Americas*. Washington, DC: OPS/PAHO: Organizacion Panamericana de las Salud/Pan American Health Organization; 1990. Publicacion Cientifica no. 524.
2. Davey Smith G, Frankel S, Yarnell J. Sex and death: Are they related? Findings from the Caerphilly Cohort Study. *Br Med J.* 1997;315:1641–1644.
3. Garcia-Aymerich J, Marrades RM, Monso E, et al. Paradoxical results in the study of risk factors of chronic obstructive pulmonary disease (COPD) re-admission. *Respir Med.* 2004;98:851–857.
4. Salas M, Hofman A, Stricker BH. Confounding by indication: An example of variation in the use of epidemiologic terminology. *Am J Epidemiol.* 1999;149:981–983.
5. Heilbrun LK, Nomura A, Hankin JH, Stemmermann GN. Diet and colorectal cancer with special reference to fiber intake. *Int J Cancer.* 1989;44:1–6.
6. Greenland S, Robins JM. Identifiability, exchangeability, and epidemiological confounding. *Int J Epidemiol.* 1986;15:413–419.
7. Savitz DA. *Interpreting Epidemiologic Evidence: Strategies for Study Design and Analysis*. New York, NY: Oxford University Press; 2003.
8. Greenland S. Confounding. In: Gail MH, Benichou J, eds. *Encyclopedia of Epidemiologic Methods*. Chichester, NY: John Wiley & Sons; 2000:254–261.
9. Pearce N, Greenland, S. Confounding and interaction. In: Ahrens W, Pigeot I, eds. *Handbook of Epidemiology*. Leipzig, Germany: Springer-Verlag Berlin Heidelberg; 2005:371–397.
10. Broda G, Davis CE, Pajak A, et al. Poland and United States Collaborative Study on Cardiovascular Epidemiology: A comparison of HDL cholesterol and its subfractions in populations covered by the United States Atherosclerosis Risk in Communities Study and the Pol-MONICA Project. *Arterioscler Thromb Vasc Biol.* 1996;16:339–349.
11. Manson JE, Stampfer MJ, Hennekens CH, Willett WC. Body weight and longevity: A reassessment. *J Am Med Assoc.* 1987;257:353–358.
12. Rush D. A correction by the author: "Maternal smoking: A reassessment of the association with perinatal mortality." *Am J Epidemiol.* 1973;97:425.
13. Taylor JM, Wang Y, Ahdieh L, et al. Causal pathways for CCR5 genotype and HIV progression. *J Acquir Immune Defic Syndr.* 2000;23:160–171.
14. Lantz PM, House JS, Lepkowski JM, et al. Socioeconomic factors, health behaviors, and mortality: Results from a nationally representative prospective study of US adults. *J Am Med Assoc.* 1998;279:1703–1708.
15. Greenland S, Pearl J, Robins JM. Causal diagrams for epidemiologic research. *Epidemiology.* 1999; 10:37–48.
16. Cole SR, Hernán MA. Fallibility in estimating direct effects. *Int J Epidemiol.* 2002;31:163–165.
17. Merchant AT, Pitiphat W. Directed acyclic graphs (DAGs): An aid to assess confounding in dental research. *Community Dent Oral Epidemiol.* 2002;30:399–404.
18. Fleischer NL, Diez Roux AV. Using directed acyclic graphs to guide analyses of neighborhood health effects: an introduction. *J Epidemiol Community Health.* 2008;62:842–846.
19. Muhlestein JB, Anderson JL. Chronic infection and coronary artery disease. *Cardiol Clin.* 2003;21: 333–362.
20. Nieto FJ. Infections and atherosclerosis: New clues from an old hypothesis? *Am J Epidemiol.* 1998; 148:937–948.
21. Hernán MA, Hernández-Diaz S, Werler MM, Mitchell AA. Causal knowledge as a prerequisite for confounding evaluation: An application to birth defects epidemiology. *Am J Epidemiol.* 2002;155:176–184.

22. Miettinen OS, Cook EF. Confounding: Essence and detection. *Am J Epidemiol*. 1981;114:593–603.
23. Greenland S. Absence of confounding does not correspond to collapsibility of the rate ratio or rate difference. *Epidemiology*. 1996;7:498–501.
24. Pandey DK, Shekelle R, Selwyn BJ, et al. Dietary vitamin C and beta-carotene and risk of death in middle-aged men: The Western Electric Study. *Am J Epidemiol*. 1995;142:1269–1278.
25. Shimakawa T, Sorlie P, Carpenter MA, et al. Dietary intake patterns and sociodemographic factors in the atherosclerosis risk in communities study: ARIC Study Investigators. *Prev Med*. 1994;23:769–780.
26. Krieger N, Williams DR, Moss NE. Measuring social class in US public health research: Concepts, methodologies, and guidelines. *Annu Rev Public Health*. 1997;18:341–378.
27. Barefoot JC, Larsen S, von der Lieth L, et al. Hostility, incidence of acute myocardial infarction, and mortality in a sample of older Danish men and women. *Am J Epidemiol*. 1995;142:477–484.
28. Mehio-Sibai A, Feinleib M, Sibai TA, Armenian HK. A positive or a negative confounding variable? A simple teaching aid for clinicians and students. *Ann Epidemiol*. 2005;15:421–423.
29. Rothman K, Greenland S. *Modern Epidemiology*, 3rd ed. Philadelphia, PA: Wolters Kluwer Health/Lippincott; 2008.
30. Lilienfeld DE, Stolley PD. *Foundations of Epidemiology*, 3rd ed. New York, NY: Oxford University Press; 1994.
31. Gordis L. *Epidemiology*, 4th ed. Philadelphia, PA: Elsevier Saunders; 2008.

EXERCISES

1. A case-control study was carried out to examine the relationship between alcohol drinking and lung cancer.
   a. In general, which conditions must be met for a variable to be a confounding variable?
   b. Indicate with a blank 2 × 2 table (or tables) how the possible confounding effect of smoking in this study can be assessed in a straightforward manner (assume that both alcohol drinking and smoking are defined as binary, yes/no variables).

2. In a study of serum dioxin levels and risk of diabetes among Air Force veterans,[*] the odds ratio of diabetes comparing those with high serum dioxin with those with low serum dioxin levels was found to be 1.71. After adjustment for serum triglyceride levels, however, the estimated odds ratio for high serum dioxin decreased to 1.56.
   a. Assuming that triglyceride levels are not in the causal pathway of the suspected dioxin → diabetes association and that there is no random or measurement error, what is the best explanation for this finding?
   b. Assuming, instead, that triglyceride level is in the causal pathway of the dioxin → diabetes association, how do you explain the fact that the association remained positive even after adjustment for triglyceride levels? To answer this question, assume that there is no random or measurement error.

3. By examining the exhibit below, indicate whether, in a case control study, positive or negative confounding has occurred:

Situation no.	Confounder associated with exposure	Confounder more common in cases	Confounder more common in controls
1	Positively	Yes	
2	Negatively	Yes	
3	Positively		Yes
4	Negatively		Yes

---

[*] Longnecker MP, Michalek JE. Serum dioxin level in relation to diabetes mellitus among Air Force veterans with background levels of exposure, *Epidemiology* 2000: 11(1): 44–48.

4. Severe restrictions on the transfer of mentally disturbed prisoners to psychiatric hospitals were introduced in Auckland in 1983, whereas the policy in other parts of New Zealand remained unchanged.[†] The data to support the contention that this policy resulted in an increase in suicides are shown here.

	Auckland		Other areas in New Zealand	
	1973–1982	1983–1987	1973–1982	1983–1987
Number of suicides	2	18	5	6
Number of prisoner-years	5396	3277	20,059	9815
	Suicide rates (per 100,000)			
Crude	37.1	549.3	24.9	61.1
Adjusted for sentence length*	26.8	367.9	27.1	54.4

*Because longer sentences (years to be spent in prison) are associated with an increased risk of suicide, the suicide rates were adjusted for the effect of sentence length.

a. In areas of New Zealand other than Auckland, adjustments for sentence length caused only a small increase in the rate for 1973–1982 but a marked decrease in the rate for 1983–1987. What do these data tell you about what happened to average length of sentences from the earlier to the later period?

b. What else would you like to know before inferring that the temporal difference in the Auckland suicide rates resulted from the changes in policy?

5. In a hypothetical case-control study examining the relationship of exposure X to disease Y, the unadjusted odds ratio was found to be 1.5 ($p < 0.05$). The authors examined the possibility that current smoking could be a confounding factor. The percentages of current smokers were found to be 32% in cases and 37% in controls ($p = 0.25$). The relative risk for the association of smoking with the exposure in this study was found to be very strong (OR = 20.0, $p < 0.001$). Based on the small difference in current smoking percentage between cases and controls, would you conclude that current smoking is not a confounder? Why?

[†] Skegg K, Cox B. Impact of psychiatric services on prison suicide. Lancet 1991, Dec 7; 338(8780): 1436–1438.

Defining and Assessing Heterogeneity of Effects: Interaction

CHAPTER 6

6.1 INTRODUCTION

The term *interaction* is used in epidemiology to describe a situation in which two or more risk factors modify the effect of each other with regard to the occurrence or level of a given outcome. This phenomenon is also known as *effect modification* and needs to be distinguished from the phenomenon of confounding. As discussed in detail in Chapter 5, *confounding* refers to a situation in which a variable that is associated with both the exposure and the outcome of interest is responsible for the entirety or part of the statistical association between the exposure and the outcome. Interaction between a given variable (*effect modifier*) and a given exposure is a different phenomenon, as detailed in the following sections. The clear distinction between confounding and interaction notwithstanding, it is important to recognize that, as discussed later in this chapter, under certain circumstances, interaction might cause confounding (see Section 6.8) and the presence of confounding might cause the appearance of an interaction effect (Section 6.10.2).

For dichotomous variables, *interaction* means that the effect of the exposure on the outcome differs depending on whether or not another variable (the effect modifier) is present. If interaction exists and the presence of the effect modifier strengthens (accentuates) the effect of the exposure of interest, this variable and the exposure are said to be *synergistic* (*positive interaction*); if the presence of the effect modifier diminishes or eliminates the effect of the exposure of interest, it can be said that the effect modifier and the exposure are *antagonistic* (*negative interaction*). Likewise, in the case of continuous variables, interaction means that the effect of exposure on outcome (e.g., expressed by the regression coefficient; see Chapter 7, Section 7.4.1) depends on the *level* of another variable (rather than on its presence/absence).

A minimum of three factors is needed for the phenomenon of interaction to occur. For this chapter, the main putative risk factor is designated as factor A, the outcome variable as Y, and the third factor (potential effect modifier) as Z. In addition, although it is recognized that there are differences between absolute or relative differences in risk, rate, and odds, the generic terms *risk, attributable risk,* and *relative risk* are mostly used. In this chapter, the term *homogeneity* indicates that the effects of a risk factor A are homogeneous or similar in strata formed by factor Z. *Heterogeneity* of effects, therefore, implies that these effects are dissimilar.

The discussion that follows is largely based on the simplest situation involving interaction between two independent variables with two categories each and a discrete outcome (e.g., disease present or absent). Other types of interaction, which can be assessed but are not discussed in detail in this textbook, include those based on more than two "independent" variables, or on continuous variables.

Interaction can be defined in two different yet compatible ways. Each definition leads to a specific strategy for the evaluation of interaction, both of which are discussed in detail in the following section.

1. *Definition based on homogeneity or heterogeneity of effects:* Interaction occurs when the effect of a risk factor A on the risk of an outcome Y is not homogeneous in strata formed by a third variable Z. When this definition is used, variable Z is often referred to as an *effect modifier.*
2. *Definition based on the comparison between observed and expected joint effects of risk factor A and third variable Z:* Interaction occurs when the observed joint effect of A and Z differs from that expected on the basis of their independent effects.

6.2 DEFINING AND MEASURING EFFECT

As discussed by Petitti,[1] the term "effect" needs to be used with caution when inferring etiologic relationships from observational studies. A more appropriate term to define interaction would be perhaps "association modification," but as the expression "effect modification" is widely used in the literature regardless of the soundness of the causal inference, we use it in a somewhat nonspecific sense, i.e., expressing both causal and noncausal interactions.

An important issue in the evaluation of interaction is how to measure "effect." Effect can be measured either by the attributable risk (*additive model*) or by a relative difference—for example, the relative risk (*multiplicative model*). The conceptual basis for the evaluation of interaction is the same for both models.

6.3 STRATEGIES TO EVALUATE INTERACTION

6.3.1 Assessment of Homogeneity of Effects

Variability in susceptibility to an outcome given exposure to a risk factor is reflected by the between-individual heterogeneity of the effect of the risk factor. This is virtually a universal phenomenon for both infectious and noninfectious diseases. For example, even for a strong association, such as that between smoking and lung cancer, not every exposed person develops the disease. Assuming that chance does not play a role in determining which smokers develop lung cancer, this suggests that smoking by itself is not a sufficient cause. Thus, smokers who develop lung cancer are likely to differ from smokers who do not, in that another component cause[2] must be present in smokers who develop lung cancer. This component risk factor may act by either completing the multicausal constellation needed to cause lung cancer or by increasing susceptibility to smoking-induced lung cancer (see also Chapter 10, section 10.2.1). In the latter situation, this component cause can be thought of generically as a susceptibility factor, which could be either genetically or environmentally determined.

A simplistic representation of the conceptual framework for interaction defined as heterogeneity of effects is shown in Figure 6-1. After it is observed that a statistical association exists between a risk factor A and a disease outcome Y, and it is reasonably certain that the association is not due to confounding, bias, or chance, the key question in evaluating interaction is this: Does the magnitude or direction of the effect of A on Y vary according to the occurrence of some other variable Z in the study population? A positive answer suggests the presence of interaction. For example, because diabetes is a stronger risk factor for coronary heart disease (CHD) in women than in men, it can be concluded that there is interaction (i.e., that gender modifies the effect of diabetes on CHD risk).[3]

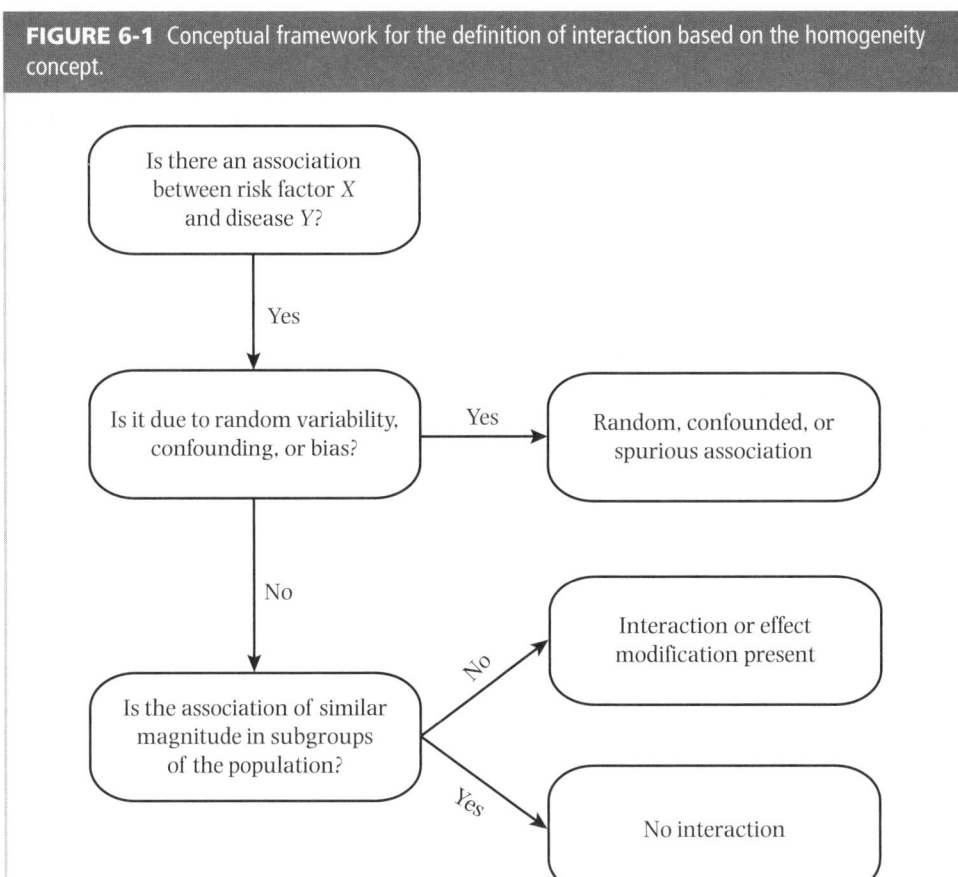

FIGURE 6-1 Conceptual framework for the definition of interaction based on the homogeneity concept.

The conceptualization of interaction as the occurrence of heterogeneous effects of A (e.g., asbestos exposure) according to the presence or absence of Z (e.g., smoking) explains why the expression "effect modification" is used as a synonym for *interaction*. For example, appropriate language when describing the interaction between smoking and asbestos in regard to the risk of respiratory cancer is that "the *effect* of asbestos exposure on respiratory cancer risk is modified by cigarette smoking in that it is stronger in smokers than in nonsmokers." The expression *effect modifier* suggests that the investigator has decided to consider A as the "main" variable of interest, and Z as the effect modifier. From the preventive standpoint, the variable not amenable to intervention (e.g., a gene) is usually regarded as the effect modifier, in contrast to an exposure that can be prevented or eliminated. Thus, for example, in a prospective study conducted in Eastern Finland, apolipoprotein e4 was shown to modify the effect of frequent drinking on dementia, in that a strong positive association was only present for carriers of the e4 allele.[4] Another example is that recessive mutant alleles can be said to modify the effect of dietary phenylalanine on risk of clinical hyperphenylalaninemias, as diet-induced disease will only occur if these alleles are present. In both these examples, the choice of which variables are the effect modifiers (apolipoprotein e4 allele, recessive mutant alleles for hyperphenylalaninemia), although somewhat arbitrary, underscores the fact that these modifiers are immutable, whereas, on the other hand, both frequent drinking and diet can be altered. Another common strategy is to choose a variable with a known effect on the outcome as effect modifier and a novel potential risk factor as the independent variable of interest.

188 CHAPTER 6 | Defining and Assessing Heterogeneity of Effects: Interaction

As mentioned previously, a key issue in the evaluation of interaction is that it involves at least three variables: the main factor of interest A (e.g., diabetes), the potential effect modifier Z (e.g., gender), and a given outcome Y (e.g., coronary heart disease). There may, however, be more than two interacting independent variables—e.g., if diabetes were a more important risk factor for women than for men only among older subjects. In this hypothetical example, the simultaneous presence of two variables would be needed to modify the effect of diabetes: gender and age.

Detection of Additive Interaction: The Absolute Difference or Attributable Risk Model

Additive interaction is considered to be present when the attributable risk in those exposed to factor A (AR_{exp}, i.e., the absolute difference in risks between those exposed and those not exposed to A; see Chapter 3, Equation 3.4) varies (is heterogeneous) as a function of a third variable Z.

The easiest way to evaluate interaction in this instance is to calculate the attributable risks for those exposed to risk factor A for each stratum defined by levels of the potential effect modifier Z. Hypothetical examples of this strategy to evaluate additive interaction are shown in Tables 6-1 and 6-2. In Table 6-1, the absolute excess risks of Y attributable to A do not differ according to exposure to Z. In Table 6-2, the attributable risk for A is larger for those exposed than for those not exposed to Z, denoting heterogeneity of the absolute effects of A. In these tables, there are two different reference categories for the attributable risks associated with A: for the stratum in which Z is absent, the reference category is Z absent, A absent; for the stratum in which Z is present, the reference category is Z present, A absent.

The patterns shown in Tables 6-1 and 6-2 can be examined graphically (Figure 6-2A). A graph using an arithmetic scale to plot risks is used to assess additive interaction. The risks or rates for each category of the risk factor A are plotted separately for individuals

TABLE 6-1 Hypothetical example of absence of additive interaction.

Z	A	Incidence rate (per 1000)	Attributable risk (per 1000)*
No	No	10.0	0
	Yes	20.0	10.0
Yes	No	30.0	0
	Yes	40.0	10.0

*Attributable risk for A within strata of Z.

TABLE 6-2 Hypothetical example of presence of additive interaction.

Z	A	Incidence rate (per 1000)	Attributable risk (per 1000)*
No	No	5.0	0
	Yes	10.0	5.0
Yes	No	10.0	0
	Yes	30.0	20.0

*Attributable risk for A within strata of Z.

exposed and those not exposed to the third variable Z. In this type of graph (with an arithmetic scale in the ordinate), the steepness of the slopes is a function of the absolute differences. Thus, when the absolute difference in risk of the outcome according to A (attributable risk in those exposed to A) is the same regardless of exposure to Z, the two lines are parallel. When the absolute differences differ, denoting additive interaction, the lines are not parallel.

Detection of Multiplicative Interaction: The Relative Difference or Ratio Model

Multiplicative interaction is considered to be present when the relative difference (ratio) in the risk of an outcome Y between subjects exposed and those not exposed to a putative risk factor A differs (is heterogeneous) as a function of a third variable Z. Hypothetical examples of the evaluation of multiplicative interaction are shown

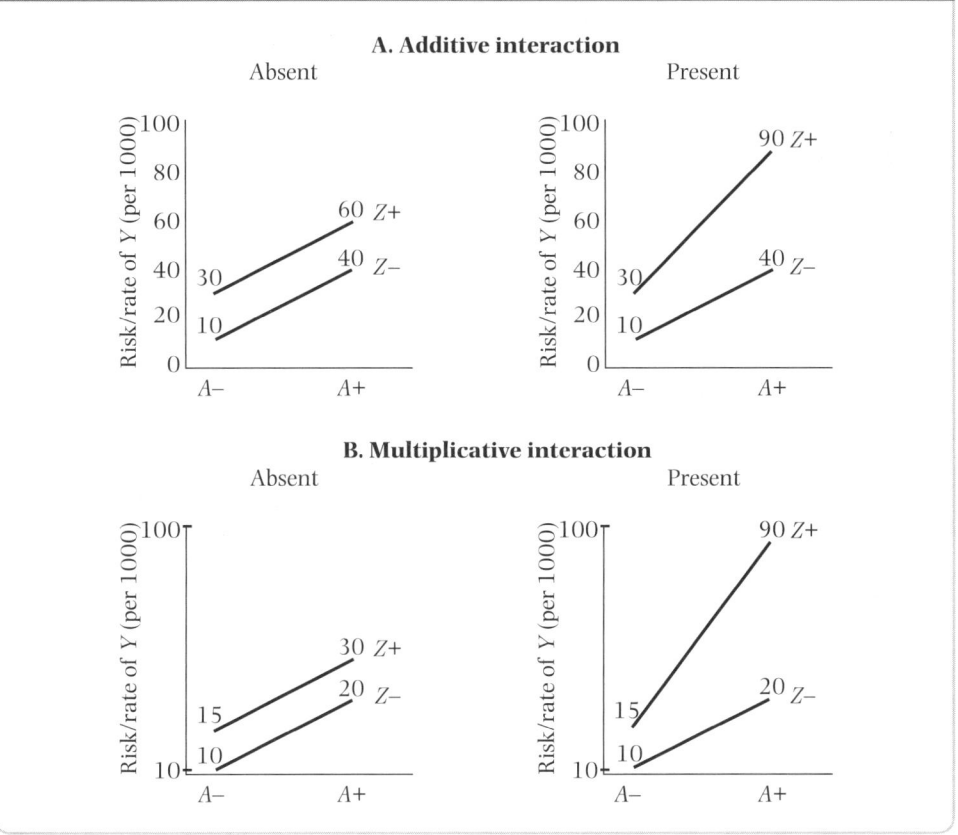

FIGURE 6-2 Assessment of interaction by means of graphs. For additive interaction (A), an arithmetic scale should be used on the ordinate (slopes represent absolute differences). Interaction is absent on the left panel because the absolute difference between A+ and A− is the same regardless of the presence of Z (60 − 30 = 40 − 10 = 30 per 1000). Interaction is present on the right panel because the absolute difference between A+ and A− is greater when Z is present (90 − 30 = 60 per 1000) than when Z is absent (40 − 10 = 30 per 1000). For multiplicative interaction (B), a logarithmic scale should be used on the ordinate (slopes represent relative differences). Interaction is absent on the left panel because the relative difference between A+ and A− is the same regardless of the presence of Z (30/15 = 20/10 = 2). Interaction is present on the right panel because the relative difference between A+ and A− is higher when Z is present (90/15 = 6) than when Z is absent (20/10 = 2).

in Tables 6-3 and 6-4. (Consistent with Tables 6-1 and 6-2, there are two different reference categories for the relative risks associated with A: for the stratum in which Z is absent, the reference category is Z absent, A absent; for the stratum in which Z is present, the reference category is Z present, A absent.) In Table 6-3, the relative risk for A is the same for those exposed and those not exposed to Z. In Table 6-4, the relative risk for A is larger for those exposed than for those not exposed to Z, indicating that the effects of A measured by the relative risk are heterogeneous according to Z.

As for additive interaction, multiplicative interaction can be evaluated graphically by plotting the rates for each category of A according to the strata defined by Z (Figure 6-2B). For multiplicative interaction assessment, however, a log scale is used in the ordinate. Thus, the steepness of the slopes is a function of the relative differences: when the risk ratios for A are the same in those exposed and in those not exposed to Z, the Z-specific curves are parallel, indicating absence of multiplicative interaction. Nonparallel lines suggest the presence of multiplicative interaction.

6.3.2 Comparing Observed and Expected Joint Effects

As discussed previously, an alternative definition of interaction is when the *observed joint effect* of A and Z differs from the *expected joint effect*. The expected joint effect can be estimated by assuming that the effects of A and Z are independent. Thus, to compare observed and expected joint effects of A and Z, it is first necessary to estimate their independent effects.

As in the evaluation of homogeneity, the strategy of comparing the observed with the expected joint effects is based on a common conceptual framework for both additive and multiplicative models; the only difference between these models is whether absolute or relative differences are used in the evaluation of interaction.

TABLE 6-3 Hypothetical example of absence of multiplicative interaction.

Z	A	Incidence rate (per 1000)	Relative risk (per 1000)*
No	No	10.0	1.0
	Yes	20.0	2.0
Yes	No	25.0	1.0
	Yes	50.0	2.0

*Relative risk for A within strata of Z.

TABLE 6-4 Hypothetical example of multiplicative interaction.

Z	A	Incidence rate (per 1000)	Relative risk (per 1000)*
No	No	10.0	1.0
	Yes	20.0	2.0
Yes	No	25.0	1.0
	Yes	125.0	5.0

*Relative risk for A within strata of Z.

The conceptual framework underlying this strategy is shown schematically in Exhibit 6-1. In the exhibit, the areas of the rectangles designated A and Z represent the independent effects of the potential risk factor A and effect modifier Z. If there is no interaction, when exposure occurs to both these factors, the observed joint effect is expected to be merely the sum of their independent effects, as denoted by the area of the rectangle $A + Z$ in Exhibit 6-1A. (The term *sum* is not used here in the context of a simple [arithmetic] sum, which would make it limited to the additive model; rather, it implies the *combined* effects of A and Z either in absolute or in relative terms.) In Exhibit 6-1B, the observed joint effect exceeds the expected joint effect. The area to the right of the dotted line represents the excess caused by interaction. As the observed joint effect is greater than expected, there is positive interaction or synergism. If the observed joint effect of A and Z is smaller than that expected, however, there is negative interaction or antagonism (Exhibit 6-1C).

Detection of Additive Interaction: The Absolute Difference or Attributable Risk Model

When evaluating the presence of additive interaction by comparing observed and expected joint effects, the joint effect of A and Z is estimated as the arithmetic sum of the independent effects measured by the attributable risks in exposed individuals (AR_{exp}). Exhibit 6-2 presents two hypothetical examples showing the absence (A) and presence (B) of additive interaction. The first step is to calculate incidence rates for each of the four table cells defined by the two factors A and Z. The cell representing the absence of both exposures (−/−) is designated as the single reference category. The observed attributable risks in Exhibit 6-2 represent the observed absolute incidence differences between each category and the reference category. In this manner, it is possible to separate the observed independent effects of A and Z and thus to estimate their joint effect. The meanings of the different categories in Exhibit 6-2 are described in Table 6-5.

Estimation of the expected (Expd) joint effect of A and Z measured by the attributable risk is carried out by a simple sum of their independent observed (Obs) attributable risks, as follows:

$$\text{Expd } AR_{A+Z+} = \text{Obs } AR_{A+Z-} + \text{Obs } AR_{A-Z+} \quad \text{(Eq. 6.1)}$$

Thus, the expected joint attributable risk in the example shown in Exhibit 6-2A is $(20.0 + 10.0 = 30.0)/1000$. This expected joint effect is identical to the observed joint effect, thus indicating the absence of additive interaction. On the other hand, the observed joint attributable risk shown in Exhibit 6-2B of $50.0/1000$ is higher than the expected joint AR of $30.0/1000$, denoting positive additive interaction.

The expected joint effect can also be estimated by an expected (Expd) joint incidence (Inc), as follows:

$$\begin{aligned}\text{Expd Inc}_{A+Z+} &= \text{Obs Inc}_{A-Z-} + (\text{Obs Inc}_{A+Z-} - \text{Obs Inc}_{A-Z-}) \\ &\quad + (\text{Obs Inc}_{A-Z+} - \text{Obs Inc}_{A-Z-}) \\ &= \text{Obs Inc}_{A-Z-} + \text{Obs } AR_{A+Z+} - \text{Obs } AR_{A-Z+}) \quad \text{(Eq. 6.2)}\end{aligned}$$

For example, for Exhibit 6-2B,

$$\text{Expd Inc}_{A+Z+} = [10.0 + (30.0 - 10.0) + (20.0 - 10.0) = 40.0]/1000$$

which is less than the observed joint incidence of $60.0/1000$, thus again denoting positive additive interaction.

EXHIBIT 6-1 Conceptual framework of the definition of interaction based on comparing expected and observed joint effects.

A. When there is *no* interaction, the *observed* joint effect of risk factors A and Z equals the sum of their independent effects:

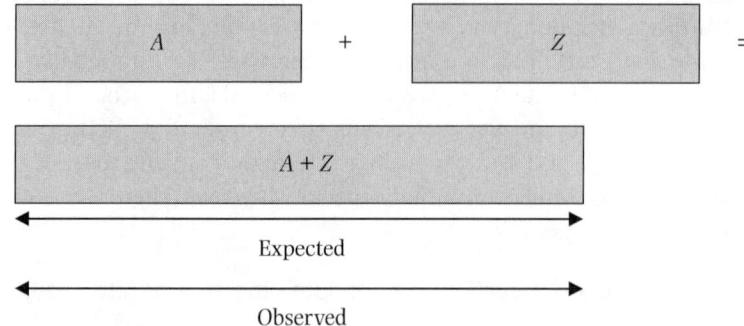

B. When there is *positive* interaction (*synergism*), the *observed* joint effect of risk factors A and Z is *greater* than the *expected* on the basis of summing their independent effects:

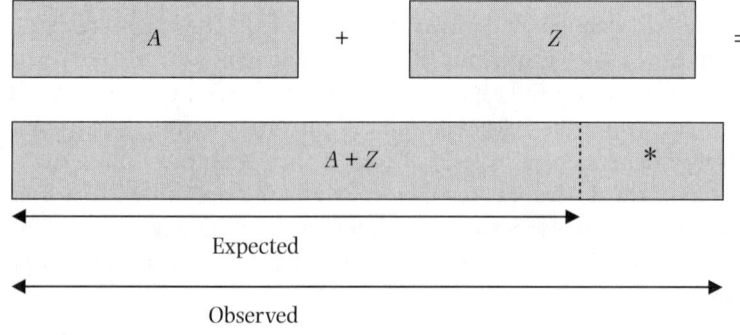

* Excess due to positive interaction

C. When there is *negative* interaction (*antagonism*), the *observed* joint effect of risk factors A and Z is *smaller* than the *expected* on the basis of summing their independent effects:

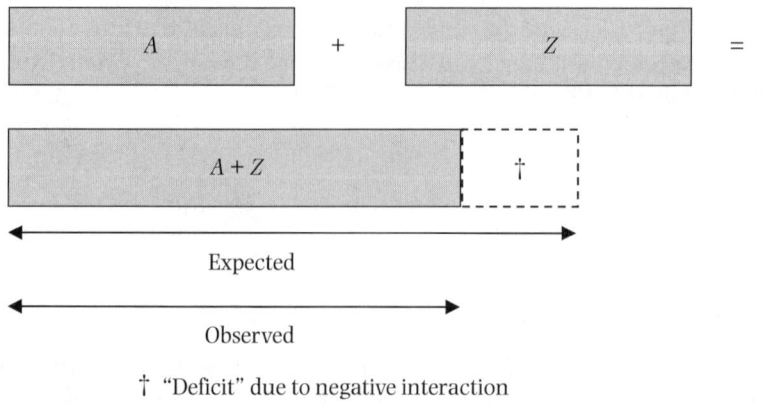

† "Deficit" due to negative interaction

Note: The rectangle areas denote the magnitude of the effects.

EXHIBIT 6-2 Detection of interaction through the comparison of expected and observed joint effects: additive interaction.

A. No additive interaction

Observed incidence rates/1000

Z	A –	A +
–	10.0	30.0
+	20.0	40.0

Observed attributable risks*/1000

Z	A –	A +
–	0.0	20.0
+	10.0	30.0

Joint expected AR = 10.0 + 20.0 = 30.0
Joint observed AR = 30.0

B. Additive interaction present

Observed incidence rates/1000

Z	A –	A +
–	10.0	30.0
+	20.0	60.0

Observed attributable risks*/1000

Z	A –	A +
–	0.0	20.0
+	10.0	50.0

Joint expected AR = 10.0 + 20.0 = 30.0
Joint observed AR = 50.0

*In the exposed.

TABLE 6-5 Assessment of interaction: additive model.

Factor Z	Factor A	Observed attributable risks represent
Absent	Absent	Reference category = 0.0
Absent	Present	Independent effect of A (i.e., in the absence of Z) (e.g., in Exhibit 6-2A, 30.0 − 10.0 = 20.0)
Present	Absent	Independent effect of Z (i.e., in the absence of A) (e.g., in Exhibit 6-2A, 20.0 − 10.0 = 10.0)
Present	Present	Joint effect of A and Z (e.g., in Exhibit 6-2A, 40.0 − 10.0 = 30.0

Detection of Multiplicative Interaction: The Relative Difference or Ratio Model

The strategy for detecting multiplicative interaction is analogous to that for detecting additive interaction; however, in the evaluation of multiplicative interaction, the expected joint effect is estimated by multiplying the independent relative effects of A and Z:

$$\text{Expd RR}_{A+Z+} = \text{Obs RR}_{A+Z-} \times \text{Obs}_{A-Z+} \qquad \text{(Eq. 6.3)}$$

Independent and joint effects expressed by relative risks are shown in Exhibit 6-3, with interpretations akin to those for additive interaction based on Exhibit 6-2. In Exhibit 6-3A, the expected (3.0 × 2.0 = 6.0) and the observed joint effects are equal, suggesting no multiplicative interaction. In Exhibit 6-3B, the expected joint relative risk is also 6.0, but the observed joint relative risk is 9.0, denoting positive multiplicative interaction.

6.3.3 Examples of Interaction Assessment in a Cohort Study

Data from a cohort study conducted in Washington County, Maryland, allow evaluation of additive and multiplicative interactions between father's educational level and maternal smoking on the risks of neonatal and postneonatal deaths[5] (Tables 6-6 and 6-7). As shown in Table 6-6A, both the relative risks and the attributable risks for the maternal smoking/neonatal mortality associations are heterogeneous according to the educational level of the father, thus denoting both multiplicative and additive interactions, which express the magnification of the smoking effect on neonatal mortality when father's educational level is low. (The heterogeneity in Table 6-6, however, may be due to residual confounding resulting from the use of broad educational and smoking categories; see Chapter 5, Section 5.4.3 and Chapter 7, Section 7.6. For the purposes of this example, however, it is assumed that the heterogeneity is not due to residual confounding.) The interaction on both scales is confirmed when the

EXHIBIT 6-3 Detection of interaction through the comparison of expected and observed joint effects: multiplicative interaction.

A. No multiplicative interaction

	Observed incidence rates/1000			Observed relative risks	
	A			A	
Z	−	+	Z	−	+
−	10.0	30.0	−	1.0	3.0
+	20.0	60.0	+	2.0	6.0

Joint expected RR = 2.0 × 3.0 = 6.0
Joint observed RR = 6.0

B. Multiplicative interaction present

	Observed incidence rates/1000			Observed relative risks	
	A			A	
Z	−	+	Z	−	+
−	10.0	30.0	−	1.0	3.0
+	20.0	90.0	+	2.0	9.0

Joint expected RR = 2.0 × 3.0 = 6.0
Joint observed RR = 9.0

6.3 Strategies to Evaluate Interaction

TABLE 6-6 Neonatal death rates per 1000 live births according to smoking status of the mother and education of the father, Washington County, MD, 1953–1963.

A. Homogeneity strategy

Father's education	Mother's smoking	Estimated no. of live births	Rate/1000 live births	AR†/1000 live births	RR*
9+ grades	No	5967	14.9	0	1.0
	Yes	3833	17.1	2.2	1.1
0–8 grades	No	1967	16.4	0	1.0
	Yes	767	46.1	29.7	2.8

B. Comparison of joint observed and expected effects

	Incidence/1000 live births mother's smoking		AR*/1000 live births mother's smoking		RR† mother's smoking	
Father's education	No	Yes	No	Yes	No	Yes
9+ grades (unexposed)	14.9	17.1	0	2.2	1.0	1.1
0–8 grades (exposed)	16.4	46.1	1.5	31.2	1.1	3.1

Expected joint effects:
  Additive → AR = 1.5 + 2.2 = 3.7/1000 live births
  Multiplicative → RR = 1.1 × 1.1 = 1.2

Observed joint effects:
  Additive → AR = 31.2/1000 live births
  Multiplicative → RR = 3.1

*Attributable risk in the exposed.
†Relative risk.
Source: Data from GW Comstock and FE Lundin, Parental Smoking and Perinatal Mortality. *American Journal of Obstetrics and Gynecology,* Vol 98, pp. 708–718, © 1967.

joint observed and expected effects are compared in Table 6-6B. For the additive model, the observed joint attributable risk is 31.2/1000 live births, whereas the expected is only 3.7/1000 (i.e., 1.5 + 2.2). For the multiplicative model, observed and expected joint relative risks are 3.1 and 1.2, respectively. Little or no interaction on either scale is apparent when assessing the association of maternal smoking and father's education with *post*neonatal mortality (Tables 6-7A and 6-7B). The small differences between observed and expected joint effects (or the slight heterogeneity of effects) are probably due to random variability.

The study by Ndrepepa et al.[6] on the interaction between gender and diabetes in the prognosis of 4460 patients who underwent coronary stenting for stable or unstable angina is another example of how to assess interaction in a cohort (prognostic) study. The 1-year mortality after the procedure is shown in Table 6-8. In those exposed to diabetes, both the attributable risk and the relative risk are much higher in women than in men. When comparing the joint observed with the joint expected measures of association (Table 6-8B), the former is higher than the latter in both models, thus confirming the heterogeneity seen in Table 6-8A.

TABLE 6-7 Postneonatal death rates per 1000 live births according to smoking status of the mother and education of the father, Washington County, MD, 1953–1963.

A. Homogeneity strategy

Father's education	Mother's smoking	Estimated no. of live births	Rate/1000 live births	AR†/1000 live births	RR*
9+ grades	No	5967	6.1	0	1.0
	Yes	3833	11.1	5.0	1.8
0–8 grades	No	1967	12.3	0	1.0
	Yes	767	19.8	7.5	1.6

B. Comparison of joint observed and expected effects

Father's education	Incidence/1000 live births mother's smoking		AR*/1000 live births mother's smoking		RR† mother's smoking	
	No	Yes	No	Yes	No	Yes
9+ grades (unexposed)	6.1	11.1	0	5.0	1.0	1.8
0–8 grades (exposed)	12.3	19.8	6.2	13.7	2.0	3.2

Expected joint effects:
    Additive → AR = 6.2 + 5.0 = 11.2/1000 live births
    Multiplicative → RR = 2.0 × 1.8 = 3.6

Observed joint effects:
    Additive → AR = 13.7/1000 live births
    Multiplicative → RR = 3.2

*Attributable risk in the exposed.
†Relative risk.
Source: Data from GW Comstock and FE Lundin, Parental Smoking and Perinatal Mortality. *American Journal of Obstetrics and Gynecology*, Vol 98, pp. 708–718, © 1967.

6.4 ASSESSMENT OF INTERACTION IN CASE-CONTROL STUDIES

The preceding discussion of the assessment of interaction has relied on absolute and relative measures of risk (incidence rates, attributable risks, and relative risks) obtained in cohort studies. What follows is a discussion of the same concepts and strategies applied to the analysis of case-control data. Because case-control studies provide an efficient approach to frame and analyze cohort data (see Chapter 1, Section 1.4.2), the concept of interaction does not have a distinct or special meaning in these studies. Thus, the discussion that follows merely aims at facilitating the application of the concept of interaction to the analysis of case-control data. The formulas presented in the following section are equally applicable to cohort and case-control studies.

6.4.1 Assessment of Homogeneity of Effects

In a case-control study, the homogeneity strategy can be used only to assess multiplicative interaction. The reason for this is that absolute measures of disease risk are usually

6.4 Assessment of Interaction In Case-Control Studies

TABLE 6-8 Mortality rate per 100 patients after one year following coronary stenting for stable or unstable angina, according to gender and presence of diabetes, January 1995–July 2000.

A. Homogeneity strategy

Gender	Diabetes	Mortality/100 patients	AR†/100	RR*
Men	Absent	4.1	0	1.0
	Present	6.1	2.0	1.5
Women	Absent	3.4	0	1.0
	Present	10.3	6.9	3.0

B. Comparison of joint observed and expected effects

Gender	Mortality/100 patients		AR*/100		RR†	
	Diabetes absent	Diabetes present	Diabetes absent	Diabetes present	Diabetes absent	Diabetes present
Men ("unexposed")	4.1	6.1	0	2.0	1.0	1.5
Women ("exposed")	3.4	10.3	−0.7	6.2	0.83	2.5

Expected joint effects:
  Additive → AR = −0.7 + 2.0 = 1.3/100 patients
  Multiplicative → RR = 0.83 × 1.5 = 1.2

Observed joint effects:
  Additive → AR = 6.2/100 patients
  Multiplicative → RR = 2.5

*Attributable risk in the exposed.
†Relative risk.
Source: Data from G Ndrepepa, J Mehilli, H Bollwein, et al., Sex-Associated Differences in Clinical Outcomes after Coronary Stenting in Patients with Diabetes Mellitus. *American Journal of Medicine*, Vol 117, pp. 830–836, © 2004.

not available in case-control studies; thus, it is not possible to measure the absolute difference between exposed and unexposed—that is, the attributable risk (absolute excess risk) in those exposed to the main risk factor. As a result, the homogeneity of attributable risks (in exposed subjects) in strata formed by the potential effect modifier Z cannot be assessed in case-control studies. As shown in the next section, however, it is possible to assess additive interaction in a case-control study by using the strategy of comparing observed and expected joint effects.

In case-control studies, the assessment of the homogeneity of effects is typically based on the odds ratio. This assessment, as illustrated in Table 6-9, is analogous to the assessment of the homogeneity of relative risks. In Table 6-9, cases and controls are stratified according to categories of both the putative risk factor of interest, A, and the potential effect modifier, Z. Different reference categories are used for the comparison of the odds ratios associated with A in the strata formed by Z: when Z is absent, the reference category—denoted by an odds ratio of 1.0—is that in which A is also absent. On the other hand, for the individuals exposed to Z, the reference category with an odds ratio of 1.0 is formed by subjects exposed to Z but unexposed to A. Thus, each odds ratio derived in Table 6-9 refers to the effect of A, first in the absence (upper half) and then in the presence (lower half) of Z.

TABLE 6-9 Outline of table illustrating the homogeneity strategy for assessing multiplicative interaction in case-control studies.

	Exposed to A?	Cases	Controls	Odds ratio	What does it mean?
Z absent	No			1.0	Reference category =
	Yes				Effect of A in the absence of Z
Z present	No			1.0	Reference category =
	Yes				Effect of A in the presence of Z

It is important to emphasize that the independent effect of Z cannot be estimated when this strategy is used. This point should be kept in mind when contrasting this strategy with that described in the section that follows, of comparing observed and expected joint effects.

The interpretation of results in Table 6-9 is straightforward: when multiplicative interaction is present, odds ratios will be dissimilar; when absent, they will be similar. For example, in the study by Shapiro et al.[7] examining the interaction between use of oral contraceptives and heavy smoking on the odds of myocardial infarction (Table 6-10), the odds ratios were only somewhat heterogeneous (4.5 vs 5.6), indicating that multiplicative interaction, if present, was not strong. (Shapiro et al. examined three smoking categories: none, 1 to 24 cigarettes/day, and ≥ 25 cigarettes/day. For simplification purposes, however, only the nonsmoking and heavy smoking categories are discussed in this and subsequent sections.) In contrast, in the study by Coughlin[8] on the relationship between asthma and idiopathic dilated cardiomyopathy (Table 6-11), notwithstanding small numbers, the odds ratios appeared to be fairly heterogeneous according to the presence of hypertension, thus suggesting the presence of multiplicative interaction.

Another example of multiplicative interaction comes from the study by Honein et al.[9] of the relationships of isolated clubfoot in the offspring with maternal smoking and a family history of clubfoot (Table 6-12). In this study, the odds ratio related to maternal smoking was higher if a family history of clubfoot was also present than if it was absent.

It has been pointed out by Morabia et al.[10] that the odds ratios may be heterogeneous when relative risks are not, a phenomenon that these authors designated as *interaction fallacy*. Morabia et al. argued that although the likelihood of this "fallacy" is usually negligible in most real-life instances in chronic disease epidemiology, it may increase when the risk of the outcome is expected to be high (e.g., in an acute epidemic situation, or when studying population groups in which there is a strong genetic susceptibility to the risk factor-induced disease).

6.4.2 Comparing Observed and Expected Joint Effects

The strategy of comparing observed and expected joint effects in case-control studies is similar to the technique used when incidence data are available. That is, the independent effects of A and Z are estimated in order to compute the expected joint effect, which is then compared with the observed joint effect. When the expected and observed joint effects differ, interaction is said to be present.

Table 6-13 shows schematically how assessment of both additive and multiplicative interactions can be carried out in case-control studies using this strategy. In Table 6-13,

6.4 Assessment of Interaction In Case-Control Studies

TABLE 6-10 The relationship of smoking and oral contraceptive (OC) use to the odds of myocardial infarction in women.

Heavy smoking*	OC use	Odds ratio	What does it mean?
No	No	1.0	Reference category
	Yes	4.5	Effect of OC in nonsmokers
Yes	No	1.0	Reference category
	Yes	5.6	Effect of OC in heavy smokers

*$\geq$ 25 cigarettes/day.
Source: Data from S Shapiro et al., Oral-Contraceptive Use in Relation to Myocardial Infarction. *Lancet*, Vol 1, pp. 743–747, © 1979.

TABLE 6-11 Relationship of hypertension and asthma to idiopathic dilated cardiomyopathy.

Hypertension	Asthma	Odds ratio	What does it mean?
No	No	1.0	Reference category
	Yes	2.4	Effect of asthma in normotensives
Yes	No	1.0	Reference category
	Yes	13.4	Effect of asthma in hypertensives

Source: Data from SS Coughlin, *A Case-Control Study of Dilated Cardiomyopathy*. Doctoral Dissertation, p. 109, © 1987.

TABLE 6-12 Odds ratios for the association between maternal smoking and isolated clubfoot, according to family history of clubfoot.

Family history of clubfoot	Maternal smoking	Cases (no.)	Controls (no.)	Odds ratio
Absent	Absent	203	2143	1.00
	Present	118	859	1.45
Present	Absent	11	20	1.00
	Present	14	7	3.64

Source: MA Honein, LJ Paulozzi, CA Moore, Family History, Maternal Smoking, and Clubfoot: An Indication of a Gene-Environment Interaction. *American Journal of Epidemiology*, Vol 152, pp. 658–665, © 2000.

independent effects (measured by odds ratios) of A and Z can be estimated by using a single reference category formed by individuals unexposed to both A and Z. The effect of A alone (i.e., the independent effect of A in absence of Z) is estimated by the odds of the category $A+Z-$ relative to that of the reference category, $A-Z-$. Similarly, the independent effect of Z is estimated by the ratio of the odds of the category $A-Z+$ to that of the reference category.

Detection of Additive Interaction

As mentioned previously, in case-control studies it is not possible to use Equations 6.1 or 6.2 (Section 6.3.2), as they require incidence data that are usually not available when using this design. Thus, it is important to rewrite these equations in terms of relative risks or odds ratios so that they can be applied to the case-control data shown

TABLE 6-13 Outline of table to assess both additive and multiplicative interaction in case-control studies using the strategy of comparing expected and observed joint effects.

What is measured	Exp. to Z?	Exp. to A?	Cases	Controls	Odds ratio
Reference category	No	No			$OR_{A-Z-} = 1.0$
Indep. effect of A	No	Yes			OR_{A+Z-}
Indep. effect of Z	Yes	No			OR_{A-Z+}
Observed joint effect	Yes	Yes			OR_{A+Z+}

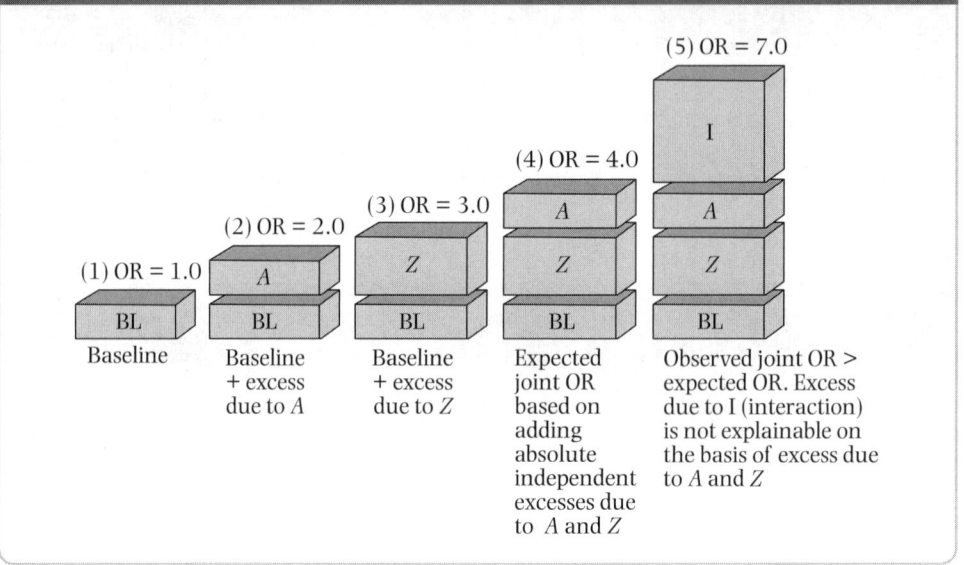

FIGURE 6-3 Schematic representation of the meaning of the formula, Expected OR_{A+Z+} = Observed OR_{A+Z-} + Observed OR_{A-Z+} − 1.0. Note that when the independent relative odds for A and Z are added, the baseline is added twice; thus it is necessary to subtract 1.0 from the expected joint OR: that is, Expected OR_{A+Z+} = (Excess due to A + baseline) + (Excess due to Z + baseline) − baseline = OR_{A+Z-} + OR_{A-Z+} − 1.0.

schematically in Table 6-13. Figure 6-3 allows an intuitive derivation of a formula based on odds ratios that is equivalent to Equations 6.1 and 6.2.* In the figure, the baseline value (odds ratio = 1.0) shown in column 1 represents the odds for individuals unexposed to both A and Z. The absolute excesses due to A (column 2) and Z (column 3) are depicted by the parts of the columns above the baseline. The expected joint effect (column 4) is then the baseline odds ratio plus the independent excess due to A plus the independent excess due to Z, as follows:

$$\text{Expd OR}_{A+Z+} = 1.0 + (\text{Obs OR}_{A+Z-} - 1.0) + (\text{Obs OR}_{A-Z+} - 1.0) \qquad (\text{Eq. 6.4})$$

$$= \text{Obs OR}_{A+Z-} + \text{Obs OR}_{A-Z+} - 1.0$$

---

*It is inappropriate to use an arithmetic scale on the ordinate as well as a baseline of zero to plot odds ratios when evaluating multiplicative interaction (see Chapter 9, Section 9.3.5). Figure 6-3 uses an arithmetic (additive) scale in order to facilitate an intuitive understanding of the formula for estimating the expected joint odds ratios when assessing additive interaction.

Because two baselines are added up in the equation, it is necessary to subtract 1.0 from the sum of the independent odds ratios. The formal derivation of Equation 6.4 is demonstrated as follows. Starting with Equation 6.2, in which Expd Inc and Obs Inc denote expected incidence and observed incidence, respectively (Section 6.3.2),

$$\text{Expd Inc}_{A+Z+} = \text{Obs Inc}_{A-Z-} + (\text{Obs Inc}_{A+Z-} - \text{Obs Inc}_{A-Z-})$$
$$+ (\text{Obs Inc}_{A-Z+} - \text{Obs Inc}_{A-Z-})$$

and dividing every term by Inc_{A-Z-}, this equation can be expressed in terms of relative risk as

$$\text{Expd RR}_{A+Z+} = 1.0 + (\text{Obs RR}_{A+Z-} - 1.0) + (\text{Obs RR}_{A-Z+} - 1.0)$$

and thus,

$$\text{Expd RR}_{A+Z+} = \text{Obs RR}_{A+Z-} + \text{Obs RR}_{A-Z+} - 1.0 \qquad \text{(Eq. 6.5)}$$

In a typical case-control study, the relative risks are estimated by the odds ratios, and thus, in Equation 6.5, relative risks can be replaced with odds ratios. Equations 6.4 and 6.5, although using odds ratio or relative risks, are based on absolute excesses (attributable risks in exposed) and thus estimate expected joint *additive* effects. An example is shown in Table 6-14, based on the same study used as an example in Table 6-10. The data in the table suggest that there is a strong additive interaction, as Obs $\text{OR}_{A+Z+} = 39.0$ and Expd $\text{OR}_{A+Z+} = 10.5$.

Similarly, using the example shown in Table 6-12, when setting the odds ratio for the combined category of absent family history and absent maternal smoking at 1.0, the independent effects of these variables on isolated clubfoot in the offspring are expressed by odds ratios of 5.81 and 1.45, respectively (see Table 6-15). Thus, the expected joint odds ratio is estimated at $5.81 + 1.45 - 1.0 = 6.26$. As the observed joint odds ratio is 21.1, it can be concluded that strong additive interaction is present.

Note that Equation 6.5 cannot be used to assess additive interaction when one of the variables (A or Z) has been matched for, as its odds ratio has been set at 1.0 by design (see Chapter 1, Section 1.4.5); in other words, the independent effect of a variable for which cases and controls have been matched cannot be determined. Because the homogeneity strategy cannot be used to examine additive interaction in case-control studies either, it follows that it is not possible to evaluate additive interaction between a matched factor and other factors in (matched) case-control studies.

Detection of Multiplicative Interaction

In case-control studies, the evaluation of multiplicative interaction based on comparing observed and expected joint effects is analogous to the strategy used in the context of a cohort study. Evaluation of multiplicative interaction comparing expected and observed joint effects is based on the same type of table as that used for assessing additive interaction (e.g., Table 6-14). The expected joint odds ratio is estimated as merely the product of the multiplication of the independent odds ratios.

$$\text{Expd OR}_{A+Z+} = \text{Obs OR}_{A+Z-} \times \text{Obs OR}_{A-Z+} \qquad \text{(Eq. 6.6)}$$

which is the analogue of Equation 6.3. (These equations also can be used to assess multiplicative interaction when the odds ratio/relative risks are below 1.0.) Using Table 6-14's findings, it is possible to estimate the expected joint odds ratio as

TABLE 6-14 Example of how to assess interaction on both scales in a case-control study using the formulas Expd OR_{A+Z+} = Obs OR_{A+Z-} + Obs OR_{A-Z+} − 1.0 (additive) and Expd Obs OR_{A+Z+} = Obs OR_{A+Z-} × Obs OR_{A-Z+} (multiplicative): the relationship of heavy smoking and oral contraceptive (OC) use to the odds of myocardial infarction in women.

Heavy smoking (Z)*	OC use (A)	Odds ratio
No	No	1.0
No	Yes	4.5
Yes	No	7.0
Yes	Yes	**39.0**

Observed OR_{A+Z+}: 39.0
Expected OR_{A+Z+}:
  Additive model: 4.5 + 7.0 − 1.0 = 10.5
  Multiplicative model: 4.5 × 7.0 = 31.5

*≥ 25 cigarettes/day.
Source: Data from S Shapiro et al., Oral-Contraceptive Use in Relation to Myocardial Infarction. Lancet, Vol 1 (8119) pp. 743–747, © 1979.

TABLE 6-15 Odds ratios for the association between maternal smoking and isolated clubfoot, according to family history of clubfoot.

Family history of clubfoot	Maternal smoking	Cases (no.)	Controls (no.)	Odds ratio
Absent	Absent	203	2143	1.0
	Present	118	859	(118/203) ÷ (859/2143) = 1.45
Present	Absent	11	20	(11/203) ÷ (20/2143) = 5.81
	Present	14	7	(14/203) ÷ (7/2143) = 21.11

Source: MA Honein, LJ Paulozzi, CA Moore, Family History, Maternal Smoking, and Clubfoot: An Indication of a Gene-Environment Interaction. American Journal of Epidemiology, Vol 152, pp. 658–665, © 2000.

Expd OR_{A+Z+} = 4.5 × 7.0 = 31.5. As the expected joint odds ratio (31.5) is fairly close to the observed (39.0), interaction, if present, is weak on the multiplicative scale, which is the same conclusion derived previously from using the homogeneity strategy (Section 6.4.1, Table 6-10). On the other hand, multiplication of the independent odds ratios in the family history of clubfoot/maternal smoking example results in a joint expected odds ratio of 8.42 (5.81 × 1.45)—which is much lower than the joint observed odds ratio of 21.1 (Table 6-15). Thus, in addition to a strong additive interaction, there is also a strong multiplicative interaction of these variables with regard to the outcome, isolated clubfoot in the offspring—a finding that is consistent with the heterogeneity seen in Table 6-12.

As for additive interaction, this strategy cannot be used to evaluate multiplicative interaction between a matched variable and another factor, as the independent effect of the former cannot be measured. The homogeneity strategy, however, can be applied to assess multiplicative interaction in matched case-control studies. This is done by stratifying the matched sets according to the levels of the matched variables and

6.5 More on the Interchangeability of the Definitions of Interaction

TABLE 6-16 Hypothetical example of evaluation of interaction in a case-control study between smoking and alcohol use, in which cases and controls are matched by current smoking ("yes" versus "no")

Pair no.	Smoking	Cases	Control	Odds ratio for alcohol use by smoking*
1	No	+	−	
2	No	−	+	
3	No	−	−	$OR_{alc\|nonsmok} = 2/1 = 2.0$
4	No	+	−	
5	No	+	+	
6	Yes	+	−	
7	Yes	+	−	
8	Yes	−	+	$OR_{alc\|smok} = 4/1 = 4.0$
9	Yes	+	−	
10	Yes	+	−	

Note: The signs (+) and (−) denote alcohol users and nonusers, respectively.
*Using the ratio of discrepant pairs.

evaluating homogeneity of the odds ratios across the strata. Thus, in the schematic example shown in Table 6-16, the heterogeneity of odds ratios for alcohol use (based on discrepant case-control pairs; see Chapter 3, Section 3.4.1) in strata formed by the matched variable, smoking (yes vs no), suggests the presence of multiplicative interaction. A summary of the issues related to the evaluation of interaction between the matched variable and another factor in matched case-control studies is given in Table 6-17.

As stated at the beginning of this section, Equations 6.5 and 6.6 can also be used when assessing interaction in cohort studies. For example, using the relative risks from Table 6-6, it is possible to construct a table similar to Table 6-13 (that is, Table 6-18). In Tables 6-6 and 6-18, the father's educational level of 0 to 8 grades was categorized as "exposed." The expected joint effects are expressed by relative risks of $(1.1 + 1.1 − 1.0) = 1.2$ in an additive scale and $(1.1 \times 1.1) = 1.2$ in a multiplicative scale. The difference between these expected values and the observed joint relative risk of 3.1 leads to the same conclusion reached previously using incidence rates to calculate attributable risks and relative risks (Table 6-6): that there is interaction in both scales.

6.5 MORE ON THE INTERCHANGEABILITY OF THE DEFINITIONS OF INTERACTION

It can be easily shown mathematically that the two definitions of interaction (i.e., based on homogeneity of effects or on the comparison between observed and expected joint effects) are completely interchangeable: that is, if the effects are heterogeneous, then the observed is different from the expected joint effect and vice versa. Consider, for example,

TABLE 6-17 Summary of issues related to the evaluation of interaction in matched case-control studies using as an example smoking as the matched variable and alcohol as the exposure of interest.

Scale	Strategy	Information needed	Is this strategy feasible?	Why?
Additive	Homogeneity of effects	ARs for alcohol use according to smoking	No	Because incidence rates for alcohol according to smoking are unavailable in case-control studies.
Additive	Observed vs expected joint effects	ORs expressing independent effects of smoking and of alcohol use	No	The OR expressing the independent effect of smoking is unavailable because cases and controls have been matched for smoking.
Multiplicative	Homogeneity of effects	ORs for alcohol use according to smoking	Yes	ORs for alcohol use are available for case-control pairs according to smoking.
Multiplicative	Observed vs expected joint effects	ORs expressing independent effects of smoking and alcohol use	No	The OR expressing the independent effect of smoking is unavailable because cases and controls have been matched for smoking.

Note: AR: attributable risks in exposed subjects; OR: odds ratio.

two variables, A and Z, and their potential effects with regard to a given outcome. To evaluate joint additive effects, under the hypothesis of no interaction:

$$\text{Expd RR}_{A+Z+} = \text{Obs RR}_{A+Z+} = \text{Obs RR}_{A+Z-} + \text{Obs RR}_{A-Z+} - 1.0 \quad \text{(Eq. 6.7)}$$

The equation can be rewritten as

$$\text{Obs RR}_{A+Z+} - \text{Obs RR}_{A-Z+} = \text{Obs RR}_{A+Z-} - 1.0 \quad \text{(Eq. 6.8)}$$

As shown previously (Section 6.4.2), to derive relative risks from the formula for assessing the expected joint additive effect, all incidence terms in the equation are divided by the incidence when both factors are absent (i.e., Inc_{A-Z-}). Working backward, the incidence when both factors are absent times the relative risk for a given exposed category equals the incidence in that exposed category (e.g., $\text{Inc}_{A+Z-} = \text{Inc}_{A-Z-} \times \text{RR}_{A+Z-}$). Thus, Equation 6.8 is equivalent to

$$\text{Inc}_{A+Z+} - \text{Inc}_{A-Z+} = \text{Inc}_{A+Z-} - \text{Inc}_{A-Z-} \quad \text{(Eq. 6.9)}$$

Therefore, when the observed joint additive effect of A and Z is the same as the expected effect (Equation 6.7), the effect of A in the presence of Z will be the same as the effect of A in the absence of Z (Equation 6.9). Alternatively, when the observed joint effects are different from the expected joint effects (i.e., interaction is present), the effects of A will vary according to the presence or absence of Z.

The same reasoning applies to the assessment of multiplicative interaction. For example, under the assumption of no interaction on a multiplicative scale,

$$\text{Expd RR}_{A+Z+} = \text{Obs RR}_{A+Z+} = \text{Obs RR}_{A+Z-} \times \text{Obs RR}_{A-Z+} \quad \text{(Eq. 6.10)}$$

TABLE 6-18 Neonatal death rates per 1000 live births according to smoking status of the mother and education of the father, Washington County, MD, 1953–1963.

Father's education (grades)	Mother's smoking	Rate/1000 live births	Relative risk
Higher (9+) (unexposed)	No	14.9	1.0
Higher (9+) (unexposed)	Yes	17.1	1.1
Lower (0–8) (exposed)	No	16.4	1.1
Lower (0–8) (exposed)	Yes	46.1	3.1

Source: Data from GW Comstock and FE Lundin, Parental Smoking and Perinatal Mortality. *American Journal of Obstetrics and Gynecology*, Vol 98, pp. 708–718, © 1967.

Equation 6.10 can be rewritten as

$$\frac{\text{Obs RR}_{A+Z+}}{\text{Obs RR}_{A-Z+}} = \frac{\text{Obs RR}_{A+Z-}}{1.0} \quad \text{(Eq. 6.11)}$$

The equivalence of Equations 6.10 and 6.11 means that when the observed joint effects are equal to the multiplication of the independent effects (Equation 6.10), then the relative risk for one factor does not vary as a function of the level of the other factor (Equation 6.11) and vice versa.

6.6 WHICH IS THE RELEVANT MODEL? ADDITIVE VERSUS MULTIPLICATIVE INTERACTION

The popularity of the Mantel-Haenszel adjustment approach (Chapter 7, Section 7.3.3) and of multiple regression methods based on multiplicative models (Chapter 7, Sections 7.4.3 through 7.4.6) has often led to equating interaction almost exclusively with multiplicative interaction when studying dichotomous outcomes. If the odds ratios or relative risks are homogeneous across strata of a potential effect modifier, it may be erroneously concluded that there is no interaction in general, even though this conclusion applies exclusively to multiplicative interaction. Yet, as discussed later in this chapter, additive interaction may be of greater interest if disease prevention is being contemplated. Thus, even when using the odds ratio or the relative risk to describe study data, it is often important to also explore the presence of additive interaction. Evaluation of additive interaction can be carried out even in the context of inherently multiplicative models, such as the logistic regression and Cox models.[11,12]

In the biological sciences, the notion of interaction has been closely related to the mechanisms underlying a causal relationship. A discussion of the limits of inferring biologic mechanisms from the observation of interactions in epidemiologic studies can be found in the literature[13] and is beyond the scope of this textbook. Thompson[14] has pointed out that epidemiology can detect mostly macro associations and that its sensitivity to identify intermediate variables tends to be limited, thus making it difficult to interpret interactions using results of epidemiologic research. Usually, interaction detected in epidemiologic studies may merely represent the joint effect of exposures occurring within a short period before the development of clinical disease (Figure 6-4). An interaction detected by epidemiologic observation often does not take into account the usually long causal chain that characterizes chronic disease processes such as atherosclerosis or neoplasms. This chain could be characterized by either multiplicative or additive joint effects of other causal components, which are needed to create causal constellations[2] responsible for the earlier progression of the disease from one phase (e.g., metabolically altered cells) to another (e.g., abnormal cell multiplication). The inability to identify and describe the physiologic and anatomic cell abnormalities in the pathogenetic sequence leading to the disease endpoint severely limits epidemiology's ability to select the best model(s) for interaction. As a consequence, choice of a model by epidemiologists is usually dictated by pragmatism—for example, when selecting the statistical model for adjustment purposes or when considering the possible application of findings in setting up public health policy (see also Chapter 10).

From the viewpoint of translating epidemiologic findings into public health practice, presence of additive interaction is important, even if multiplicative interaction is absent.[15] A hypothetical example is given in Table 6-19, which examines the relationship of familial history of disease Y and smoking to the incidence of Y. Although relative risks describing the relationship between smoking and incidence are homogeneous in those with and without a family history, the attributable risks differ markedly according to family history: 20/100 in those with and only 5/100 in those without a positive family history. Thus, there is strong additive interaction but no multiplicative interaction. Depending on the prevalence of the combination of family history and smoking in the target population,

TABLE 6-19 Hypothetical example of additive interaction (public health interaction) without multiplicative interaction: incidence of disease Y by smoking and family history of Y.

Family history	Smoking	Incidence/100	Attributable risk (exposed)	Relative risk
Absent	No	5.0	Reference	1.0
	Yes	10.0	5.0	2.0
Present	No	20.0	Reference	1.0
	Yes	40.0	20.0	2.0

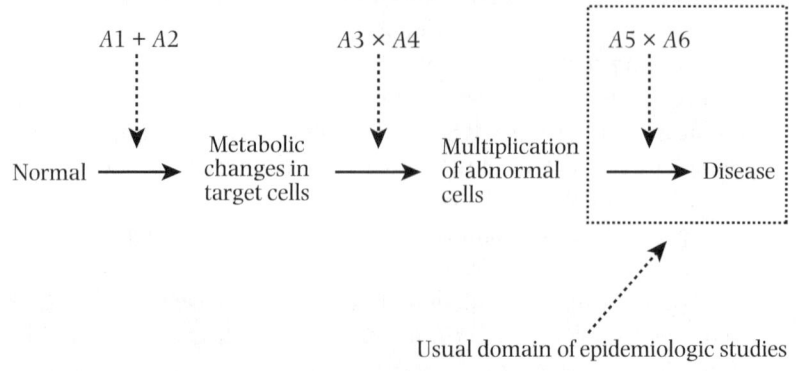

FIGURE 6-4 Schematic representation of a causal chain in which both additive and multiplicative interactive effects occur. Causal components $A1$ and $A2$ interact in an additive fashion to produce metabolic changes in the target cells. For multiplication of abnormal cells and progression to clinical disease, additional causal components are required ($A3$ and $A4$, $A5$ and $A6$, respectively), which interact in a multiplicative fashion.

prevention or elimination of smoking in those with a positive, compared with those with a negative, family history could lead to a greater reduction in the number of incident cases in the reference population.* Positive additive interaction may even occur in the presence of negative multiplicative interaction (Table 6-20) and takes precedence over the latter in terms of defining high-risk groups which should be the target of preventive action.

6.7 THE NATURE AND RECIPROCITY OF INTERACTION

6.7.1 Quantitative Versus Qualitative Interaction

When the association between factor A and outcome Y exists and is of the same direction in each stratum formed by Z, but the strength of the association varies across strata, *quantitative* interaction is said to exist. On the other hand, *qualitative* interaction is regarded as present either when the effects of A on the outcome Y are in opposite directions (*crossover*) according to the presence of the third variable Z or when there is an association in one of the strata formed by Z but not in the other (Figure 6-5). In other words, the *nature* of A is dependent on the presence of the effect modifier Z.

An example of qualitative interaction is given in a study by Stanton and Gray.[16] To examine the effects of caffeine consumption on waiting time to conception, the authors obtained information retrospectively on pregnancies occurring from 1980 through 1990 in 1430 noncontracepting women who had been pregnant at least once. The main exposure of interest was daily caffeine intake, estimated from the consumption of caffeinated beverages during the first month of pregnancy. Whereas relative risks of delayed conception (> 1 year) were below 1 for caffeine consumption among smoking women, an increase in delayed conception risk was seen in nonsmoking women with a high ($\geq$ 300 mg/day) caffeine consumption (Table 6-21). According to the authors, the qualitative interaction found in their study supports the notion that smoking increases the rate of caffeine clearance and that, in contrast, cessation of smoking results in slower caffeine elimination.

In the example shown in Table 6-21, the point estimates of the effects of high caffeine consumption appear to cross over as a function of smoking (i.e., there is a positive association of high caffeine intake with delayed conception in nonsmokers and a negative association in smokers). Qualitative interaction can be expressed either by this type of crossover (Figure 6-5A) or by an association between the factor of interest and

TABLE 6-20 Hypothetical example of negative multiplicative and positive additive interactions: incidence of disease Y by family history of Y and smoking.

Family history	Smoking	Incidence/100	Attributable risk (exposed)	Relative risk
Absent	No	10	Reference	1.0
	Yes	40	30/100	4.0
Present	No	40	Reference	1.0
	Yes	100	60/100	2.5

---

*The impact of the elimination of smoking in those with a family history is best estimated by means of the population attributable risk, which takes into account the strength of the association between smoking and disease in each stratum of family history, as well as the prevalence of the joint presence of these factors (see Chapter 3, Section 3.2.2).

the outcome in the presence but not in the absence of an effect modifier (or vice versa) (Figure 6-5B). Examples of the latter type of qualitative interaction are as follows:

- The results of the Health Insurance Plan randomized clinical trial of the effectiveness of mammography showed that menopausal status seemed to modify the effect of mammography.[17] Specifically, in this study a lower breast cancer death rate in the group undergoing mammography compared with the control group was seen only in postmenopausal women. In premenopausal women, no difference in rates was found between the experimental and the control groups.
- In a large population-based cohort study conducted in Sweden on the relationship of paternal age to schizophrenia,[18] the hazard ratio was found to be 1.60 for individuals without a family history and close to 1.0 for those with a family history (p for interaction = 0.04; see section 6.9). (The authors interpreted this finding as supportive of the notion that accumulating *de novo* mutations in germ cells of older fathers might result in an increased risk of schizophrenia in their offspring.)
- In a study by Williams et al.,[19] although high anger proneness score was associated with an increased coronary heart disease (CHD) risk in normotensive individuals, no association was seen for hypertensive patients (Figure 6-6). This pattern, if true, denotes a *negative* interaction; that is, antagonism between hypertension and high anger score with regard to the outcome.
- In a cohort study conducted by Shanmugham JR et al.,[20] a strong heterogeneity was seen for the association of alcohol and oral cancer across strata formed by folate intake in women: the relative risk for alcohol intake equal to ≥ 30 g/day in those with a low folate intake (< 350 µg/day) was 3.36, but it was only 0.98 for those with a high folate intake (≥ 350 µg/day).

These examples underscore the notion that when qualitative interaction is present it is always present in both the additive and the multiplicative models and is thus independent of the measurement scale (Figure 6-5). Consider, for example, the data shown in Table 6-21: because the relative risk in nonsmoking women with a caffeine

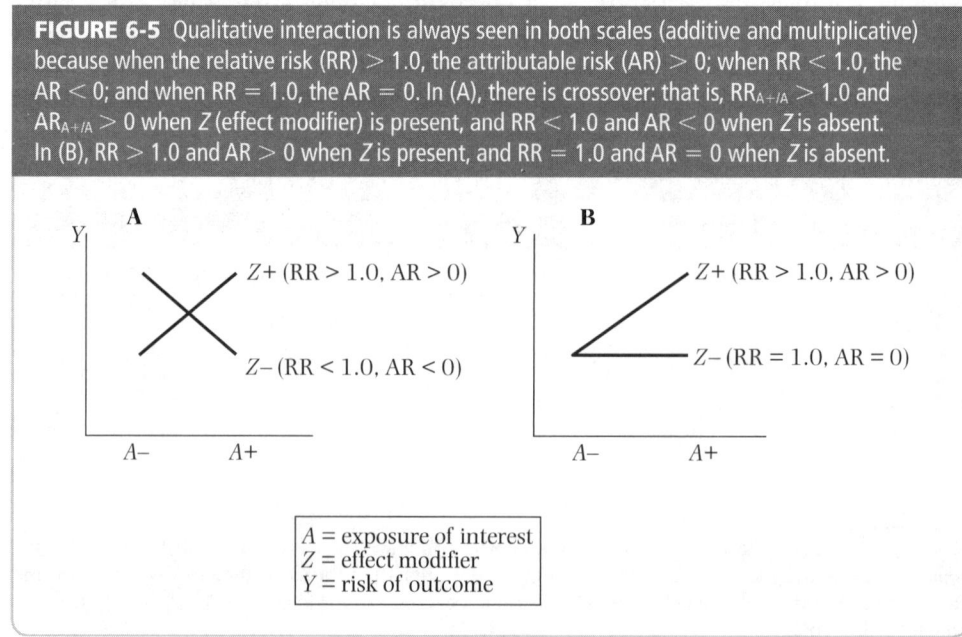

FIGURE 6-5 Qualitative interaction is always seen in both scales (additive and multiplicative) because when the relative risk (RR) > 1.0, the attributable risk (AR) > 0; when RR < 1.0, the AR < 0; and when RR = 1.0, the AR = 0. In (A), there is crossover: that is, $RR_{A+/A}$ > 1.0 and $AR_{A+/A}$ > 0 when Z (effect modifier) is present, and RR < 1.0 and AR < 0 when Z is absent. In (B), RR > 1.0 and AR > 0 when Z is present, and RR = 1.0 and AR = 0 when Z is absent.

TABLE 6-21 Relationship between caffeine consumption and risk of delayed conception (> 1 year) according to smoking among 2465 pregnancies occurring in noncontracepting women between 1980 and 1990.

Caffeine consumption (mg/Day)	Nonsmoking women			Smoking women		
	Pregnancies	Delayed conception	RR	Pregnancies	Delayed conception	RR
None	575	47	1.0	76	15	1.0
1–150	975	69	0.9	233	33	0.7
151–300	290	26	1.1	166	18	0.5
≥ 300	89	17	2.3	83	11	0.7

Note: RR: Relative risk.
Source: Data from CK Stanton and RH Gray, The Effects of Caffeine Consumption on Delayed Conception. *American Journal of Epidemiology*, Vol 142, pp. 1322–1329, © 1995.

consumption of ≥ 300 mg/day is greater than 1.0, the attributable risk by definition must be greater than 0; in smokers, on the other hand, the relative risk for caffeine consumption of ≥ 300 mg/day is less than 1.0; thus, by definition, the attributable risk has to be less than 0. Although Table 6-21 presents only relative risks and therefore, on a first glance, may be regarded as particularly suitable for assessing multiplicative interaction, the occurrence of qualitative interaction indicates that interaction is present in both scales; in other words, when there is qualitative interaction, the scale does not need to be specified. A similar inference can be drawn from the study of paternal age and schizophrenia mentioned previously: as the relative risk in those without a family history is 1.60, the attributable risk by definition has to be greater than zero. On the other hand, as the relative risk in those with a family history is close to 1.0, the attributable risk will be close to zero. Similarly, because it is based on absolute differences in cumulative incidence (or event-free survival)—denoted by the fact that the scale on the ordinate is arithmetic—the data in Figure 6-6 imply the presence of an *additive* interaction between hypertension status and anger proneness in relation to risk of CHD; however, because this interaction is *qualitative* (a difference was shown in normotensives but *not* among hypertensives), it must also be present in a multiplicative scale; indeed, the age-adjusted relative hazard comparing individuals with high and low anger scores reported by Williams et al.[18] was 2.97 among normotensives and 1.05 among hypertensives.

6.7.2 Reciprocity of Interaction

Interaction is completely reciprocal, in that if Z modifies the effect of A, then A modifies the effect of Z. As mentioned previously, the choice of A as the suspected risk factor of interest and Z as the potential effect modifier is arbitrary and a function of the hypothesis being evaluated. For example, because the effect of cigarette smoking on lung cancer is strong and has been firmly established, it may be of interest to explore its role as an effect modifier when assessing other potential lung cancer risk factors. Factors that cannot be modified (e.g., genes, gender) are often treated as effect modifiers.

The concept of interaction reciprocity is illustrated in Table 6-22, which rearranges the data from Table 6-21 such that smoking becomes the risk factor of interest and caffeine consumption becomes the effect modifier (for simplification purposes, only two

210 CHAPTER 6 | Defining and Assessing Heterogeneity of Effects: Interaction

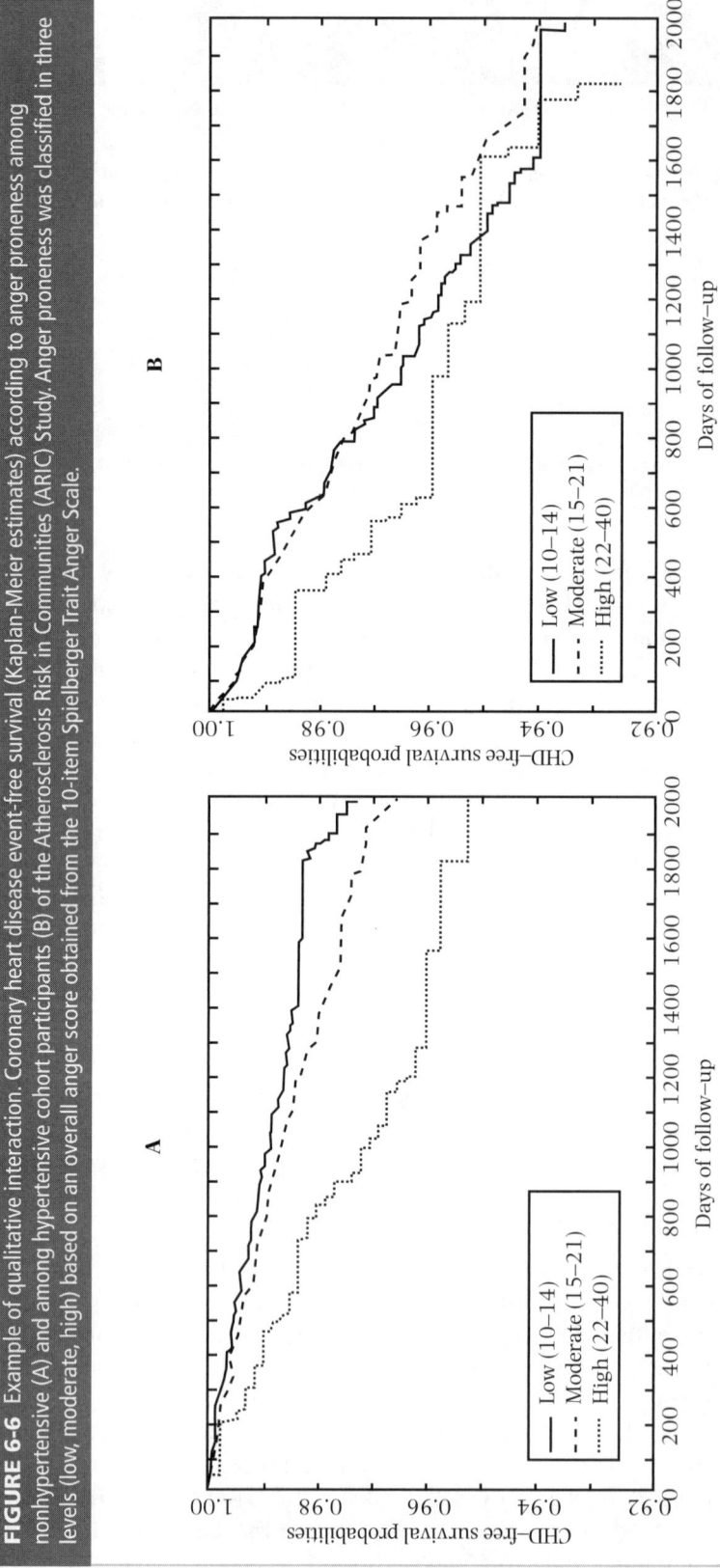

FIGURE 6-6 Example of qualitative interaction. Coronary heart disease event-free survival (Kaplan-Meier estimates) according to anger proneness among nonhypertensive (A) and among hypertensive cohort participants (B) of the Atherosclerosis Risk in Communities (ARIC) Study. Anger proneness was classified in three levels (low, moderate, high) based on an overall anger score obtained from the 10-item Spielberger Trait Anger Scale.

Source: JE Williams, CC Paton, IC Siegler, ML Eigenbrodt, FJ Nieto, HA Tyroler. Anger Proneness Predicts Coronary Heart Disease Risk: Prospective Analysis from the Atherosclerosis Risk in Communities (ARIC) Study, *Circulation*, Vol 101, pp. 2034–2039, © 2000.

caffeine consumption categories are used). As seen, smoking is positively associated with delayed conception in mothers who consume no caffeine, but it seems to be a protective factor in those with a high level of consumption. This pattern is the mirror image of the pattern shown in Table 6-21, again emphasizing that there is no intrinsic hierarchical value when deciding which variable should be treated as the effect modifier and which as the factor of primary interest.

6.8 INTERACTION, CONFOUNDING EFFECT, AND ADJUSTMENT

Although on occasion the same variable may be both a confounder and an effect modifier, confounding and interaction are generally distinct phenomena. Confounding effects are undesirable, as they make it difficult to evaluate whether a statistical association is also causal. Interaction, on the other hand, if true, is part of the web of causation[21] and may have important implications for prevention, as in the example of anger and CHD shown in Figure 6-6.

When a variable is found to be both a confounding variable and an effect modifier, adjustment for this variable is contraindicated. When additive interaction is found, it is not appropriate to adjust for the effect modifier to obtain an adjusted attributable risk, and when there is multiplicative interaction, it is inappropriate to obtain an effect modifier-adjusted relative risk or odds ratio. This is because when there is interaction the notion of an overall adjusted (weighted) mean value (main effect) makes little sense. For example, if odds ratios are found to be 2.0 for men and 25.0 for women, an "average" that summarizes the increase in odds for all individuals regardless of gender is meaningless. This notion is even more important in qualitative interaction; if the odds ratios for a given exposure are 0.3 for men and 3.5 for women, an "average, gender-adjusted" odds ratio may denote no association whatsoever—an illogical inference given that strong associations, albeit in opposite directions, exist in both sexes (for additional examples, see Chapter 7, Section 7.3.1).

Because some heterogeneity is usually found, the epidemiologist is often faced with the dilemma as to whether to adjust for the possible effect modifier. One solution is to carry out statistical testing and not to adjust if the homogeneity null hypothesis is rejected (see Section 6.9 and Appendix C). If, for example, the two odds ratios are 2.3 and 2.6, however, it is probably appropriate to adjust and obtain an average adjusted effect, regardless of the p value. (If the sample size is very large, a small degree of heterogeneity may be statistically significant even if devoid of medical or public health significance.)

TABLE 6-22 Relationship between maternal smoking and risk of delayed conception (> 1 year) according to heavy caffeine consumption ($\geq$ 300 mg/day) among 824 pregnancies occurring in noncontracepting women between 1980 and 1990.

	No caffeine consumption			Caffeine consumption $\geq$ 300 mg/day		
Smoking	Pregnancies	Delayed conception	RR	Pregnancies	Delayed conception	RR
No	575	47	1.0	90	17	1.0
Yes	76	15	2.4	83	11	0.7

Note: RR: Relative risk.
Source: Data from CK Stanton and RH Gray, The Effects of Caffeine Consumption on Delayed Conception, *American Journal of Epidemiology*, Vol 142, pp. 1322–1329, © 1995.

On the other hand, if the odds ratios are 12.0 and 1.5, even if the heterogeneity is not found to be statistically significant, adjustment may be contraindicated. Although no clear-cut rule exists regarding whether to adjust in the presence of heterogeneity, consideration of the following question may be helpful: "Given heterogeneity of this magnitude, am I willing to report an average (adjusted) effect that is reasonably representative of all strata of the study population formed on the basis of the suspected effect modifier?" Some examples and possible answers to this question are shown in Table 6-23 and may help in the pragmatic evaluation of this issue. Regardless of whether a "Z-adjusted" effect is reported, it is often informative to report the stratum-specific values as well.

6.8.1 Joint Presence of Two Factors that Interact as a Confounding Variable

When there is interaction, the *joint presence* of variables that interact may produce a confounding effect, even if each individual variable is not identified as a confounder. In the interaction example shown in Table 6-24, the incidence of the outcome is the same in individuals exposed and unexposed to factor *A* when data are stratified by factors *B* and *C* and their joint presence. However, because the prevalence of the joint presence of *B* and *C* is higher in those exposed to *A and* because, in addition, there is strong interaction between *B* and *C*, the crude incidence is greater in the individuals exposed to *A* than in the unexposed. Note that the risk factor distributions are the same in exposed and unexposed when their joint presence is ignored. Thus, the joint presence of interacting risk factors should always be considered when evaluating confounding effects.

6.9   STATISTICAL MODELING AND STATISTICAL TESTS FOR INTERACTION

The examples given in this chapter refer to risk of disease as the outcome, but interaction may be studied in relationship to any outcome (e.g., the mean value of a physiologic variable such as glucose level). As mentioned previously, it is also possible to examine interaction for continuous variables, as when assessing homogeneity of effects of continuous blood pressure levels on stroke between men and women or between blacks and whites. In this situation, the investigator often uses more complex statistical approaches to evaluate interaction—for example, by including "interaction terms" in the regression equation (see Chapter 7, Section 7.4.2). These models can also be used to evaluate interaction between categorical variables as an alternative to the stratification methods presented in the previous sections.

Another question with important practical implications is whether the observed heterogeneity is produced by chance. When using regression models to evaluate interaction, the answer to this question is simply indicated by the statistical significance of the interaction term in the regression equation (see Chapter 7, Section 7.4.8, and Appendix A, Section A.9). When evaluating interaction using the stratification techniques described in the previous sections, formal statistical tests are available to assess whether an observed heterogeneity is statistically significant. These tests, including tests for additive interaction in case-control studies, have been described in detail in other textbooks (see, e.g., Schlesselman[22] or Selvin[23]) and are illustrated in Appendix C.

It should be emphasized again that statistical tests of homogeneity, although helpful, are not sufficient to evaluate interaction fully. When sample sizes are large, as in multicenter studies, even a slight heterogeneity of no practical value or biologic importance may be statistically significant. On the other hand, although not

TABLE 6-23 Relative risks (RR) for factor A in relation to outcome Y, stratified by potential effect modifier Z.

Suspected effect modifier (Z)		Given a heterogeneity of this magnitude, should a weighted average (Z-adjusted) effect that applies to all Z strata of the study population be reported?
Absent	Present	
2.3	2.6	Yes. Even if the difference in RRs is statistically significant, it makes sense to say that, on the average—that is regardless of Z—the relative risk has a value somewhere between 2.3 and 2.6.
2.0	20.0	Even if this difference is not statistically significant, presentation of a Z-adjusted, "average" RR may not be appropriate in view of the great difference in the magnitude of the RRs. It is recommended that Z-specific RRs be presented.
0.5	3.0	No. When there is a suggestion of qualitative interaction, Z-specific RRs should be presented.
3.0	4.5	Perhaps. Although this quantitative interaction may be of interest, effects are in the same direction, and it *may* be appropriate to present a Z-adjusted RR. In addition, it is wise to present Z-specific RRs as well.

TABLE 6-24 Hypothetical example of interaction as a confounding variable. Assume the incidence of the outcome in the absence of factors B and C to be zero in both individuals exposed to A and those unexposed to A. When stratified by the isolated presence of each factor (B and C) and by the interaction term, there is no association between B and C or their interaction term with the incidence of the outcome. However, as the interaction term is related to a higher incidence and is more common in the exposed group, the total incidence in the exposed group is substantially greater than that in the unexposed group.

Factor	Prevalence of factor among exposed and among unexposed to A (%)	Incidence of outcome (per 1000)
Exposed to factor A		
B alone	18	10
C alone	20	15
B + C present	15	50
Unexposed to factor A		
B alone	18	10
C alone	20	15
B + C present	3	50

Total incidence in exposed to A =
$[(0.010 \times 0.18) + (0.015 \times 0.20) + (0.050 \times 0.15)] \times 1000 = 12.3$ (per 1,000)
Total incidence in unexposed to A =
$[(0.010 \times 0.18) + (0.015 \times 0.20) + (0.050 \times 0.03)] \times 1000 = 6.3$ (per 1,000)

statistically significant, relative risk point estimates that are markedly different from each other suggest the possibility of true heterogeneity. Ideally, such nonstatistically significant, yet marked, heterogeneity should be confirmed by a study with sufficient statistical power to detect it.

6.10 INTERPRETING INTERACTION

There are many reasons why an observed effect of an exposure may differ according to the level or the presence of a third variable. The apparent heterogeneity may be due to chance, selective confounding, or bias. It could, in addition, result from a heterogeneous exposure dose (often unbeknownst to the investigator). Differential susceptibility at different levels in the pathogenesis of the disease in question is yet another explanation for heterogeneity of effects. A succinct practical guide to the main issues involved in interpreting an observed interaction follows.

6.10.1 Heterogeneity Due to Random Variability

Heterogeneity may result from random variability produced by the stratification by a suspected effect modifier. Random variability may occur in spite of an *a priori* specification of interaction in the context of the hypothesis to be evaluated. A more common situation, however, is when interaction is not specified *a priori* but the investigator decides to carry out subgroup analysis. The decision to examine subgroups is often motivated by overall null study findings. The investigator may decide to pursue more specific hypotheses once the original postulated association was not observed. Post hoc questions posed by the frustrated epidemiologist may, for example, include the following: "Since I cannot find an association when studying all study participants, will I be able to find it in men only? In older men? In older men with a high educational level?" And so on.

Sample size inevitably decreases as more strata are created in subgroup analysis, making it likely that heterogeneity would occur by chance alone. Thus, subgroup analysis should be regarded as an exploratory strategy. The detection of heterogeneity should be assessed vis-à-vis its plausibility. An example is provided by the Multiple Risk Factor Intervention Trial study, a randomized clinical trial that assessed the effectiveness of multiple cardiovascular risk factor cessation strategies. An increased mortality was found in hypertensive participants with electrocardiographic changes undergoing the experimental interventions.[24] Although not predicted when the study was planned, the harmful effect of the intervention limited to this subset of study participants led to the biologically plausible hypothesis that potassium-depleting drugs may be contraindicated in hypertensive patients with cardiac abnormalities. After observed by means of subgroup analysis, interaction has to be confirmed in a study especially designed to evaluate it.

6.10.2 Heterogeneity Due to Confounding

When associations between *A* and *Y* in strata formed by *Z* are being explored, differential confounding effects across strata may be responsible for the heterogeneity of effects. As a hypothetical example, consider a case-control study assessing the relationship between coffee intake and cancer *Y* (Table 6-25). The investigator wishes to assess gender as an effect modifier and accordingly stratifies cases and controls by gender and coffee intake (yes/no). In this hypothetical example, smoking is a cause of cancer *Y*, female cases and controls include only nonsmokers, smoking is associated with coffee drinking, and male cases include a higher proportion of smokers than controls. As smoking is related to coffee intake and cancer *Y*, it acts as a positive confounder in males. Assuming that coffee intake is not causally related to cancer *Y*, in females (who are all nonsmokers) a relative odds of 1.0 is found. The confounding effect of smoking in males, on the other hand, results in male cases having a higher odds of coffee intake than controls, and as

TABLE 6-25 Apparent interaction due to confounding (hypothetical example).

Gender/smoking	Coffee intake	Cases	Controls	Odds ratio
Female/nonsmoker	Yes	10	10	
	No	90	90	1.0
	Total	100	100	
Male/total	Yes	38	22	
	No	62	78	2.2
	Total	100	100	
Male/smoker	Yes	35	15	
	No	35	15	1.0
	Total	70	30	
Male/nonsmoker	Yes	3	7	
	No	27	63	1.0
	Total	30	70	

Note: Assume that smoking causes cancer Y; 50% of smokers but only 10% of nonsmokers drink coffee; coffee intake is not independently related to cancer Y; all females are nonsmokers; and 70% of male cases and 30% of male controls are smokers.

a consequence, the relative odds are found to be markedly higher than 1.0. There is, therefore, heterogeneity due to confounding by smoking limited to males.

The possibility that interaction may be explained partially or entirely by a confounding effect makes it essential to adjust for potential confounders when assessing interaction. In the example shown in Table 6-25, the confounding effect of smoking explains the entire apparent gender heterogeneity of the relationship of coffee intake to cancer Y. In most real-life instances, confounding may either exaggerate or decrease heterogeneity. An example is given by Yu et al.,[25] who examined the interaction of cigarette smoking and alcohol drinking in chronic hepatitis B surface antigen (HBsAg) carriers with regard to the risk of liver cirrhosis (Table 6-26). An unadjusted heterogeneity for smoking according to drinking could be detected, which became more marked for heavy smokers ($\geq$ 20 cigarettes/day) versus nonsmokers (but less so for moderate smokers) when the relative risk was simultaneously adjusted for confounding factors using a Cox proportional hazards model (see Chapter 7, Section 7.4.4).

6.10.3 Heterogeneity Due to Bias

As for confounding, the observed heterogeneity may also result from differential bias across strata. For example, in a study of the incidence of medically treated miscarriage in a county in North Carolina, Savitz et al.[26] found that, overall, blacks appeared to have a lower risk of miscarriage than whites. The authors interpreted this finding as probably resulting from bias due to underascertainment of miscarriage among blacks. As shown in Table 6-27, when stratification according to educational status was undertaken, the apparent decreased risk of miscarriage in blacks was seen only in the lower educational strata. This pattern of an apparent modification of the race effect by educational level is probably due to the underascertainment bias operating only in less educated blacks.

Another example of possible misclassification resulting in apparent interaction is given by Bryson et al.'s[27] population-based case-control study of the relationship of gestational diabetes to eclampsia or severe preeclampsia. As seen in Table 6-28, these authors found a marked heterogeneity when the data on the association of gestational

TABLE 6-26 Relative risks of liver cirrhosis according to alcohol drinking and cigarette smoking in chronic HBsAg carriers.

			Relative risk	
Variable	Total no.	No. of incident cases	Without adjustment	With multivariate adjustment*
Nondrinker				
Nonsmoker	744	31	1.0	1.0
< 20 cigarettes/day	267	19	1.7	1.5
≥ 20 cigarettes/day	167	14	2.0	1.9
Drinker				
Nonsmoker	111	1	1.0	1.0
< 20 cigarettes/day	100	6	6.7	3.9
≥ 20 cigarettes/day	105	7	7.4	9.3

*Simultaneously adjusted for age, HBsAg carrier status at recruitment, elevation of serum aminotransferase concentration for at least 6 months, educational level, and blood type, using a Cox proportional hazards model (see Chapter 7, Section 7.4.4).

Source: Data from MW Yu et al., A Prospective Study of Liver Cirrhosis in Asymptomatic Chronic Hepatitis B Virus Carriers. *American Journal of Epidemiology*, Vol 145, pp. 1039–1047, © 1997.

TABLE 6-27 Risk of miscarriage per 100 pregnancies, corrected for induced abortions in relation to maternal years of education: Alamance County, North Carolina, 1988–1991.

	White		Black		Black/white ratio
	No.	Risk/100	No.	Risk/100	
Total	325	7.7	93	5.5	0.7
Mother's years of education:					
< 9	12	10.4	0	–	–
10–11	52	8.0	15	4.5	0.6
12	111	6.3	44	4.7	0.7
≥ 13	150	9.2	33	9.5	1.0

Source: Data from DA Savitz et al., Medically Treated Miscarriage in Alamance County, North Carolina, 1988–1991. *American Journal of Epidemiology*, Vol 139, pp. 1100–1106, © 1994.

diabetes with eclampsia were stratified by level of prenatal care, as ascertained by using a dichotomized Kotelchuck index.[28] In this study, the difference in odds ratios by level of care seemed to occur mainly for severe eclampsia (test for interaction, $p = 0.02$). As expected, an earlier, aggressive treatment of preeclampsia in those with "high" prenatal care may be the explanation for the lesser increase in gestational diabetes-related odds of severe eclampsia; on the other hand, the authors also suggested that, in those with a low level of care, preexisting diabetes may have been misclassified as gestational, which may have artificially increased the strength of the association in these individuals.

TABLE 6-28 Odds ratios for the association of gestational diabetes to eclampsia stratified by level of prenatal care.

	Level of care		p value for interaction
	High*	Low*	
Case status	Odds ratio (95% confidence interval)		
Eclampsia	0.61 (0.15, 2.49)	4.16 (1.24, 13.96)	0.07
Severe eclampsia	1.25 (0.88, 1.79)	3.13 (1.76, 5.52)	0.02
Mild preeclampsia	1.45 (1.22, 1.73)	1.72 (1.20, 2.44)	NS
Gestational hypertension	1.35 (1.17, 1.55)	1.61 (1.20, 2.15)	NS

* "High" and "Low" correspond to "adequate/adequate plus," and "inadequate/intermediate" in the dichotomized Kotelchuck index.
Source: CL Bryson, GN Iannou, SJ Rulyak, et al. Association Between Gestational Diabetes and Pregnancy-Induced Hypertension. *American Journal of Epidemiology*, Vol 158, pp. 1148–1153, © 2003.

An illustration of how information bias can result in an apparent heterogeneity of effects is presented in Figure 6-7, which shows results of a hypothetical case-control study on the potential effect modification of the relationship between overweight and disease Y by smoking. In this study, the misclassification of overweight *within* each stratum formed by smokers or nonsmokers is nondifferential–that is, the levels of sensitivity and specificity are the same for cases and controls. However, these validity levels differ between smokers and nonsmokers. Even though the true odds ratios for overweight are the same for smokers and nonsmokers (2.25), different levels of sensitivity and specificity levels across strata result in an apparent heterogeneity (see Chapter 4, Section 4.3.3, and Figure 4-4 and Exhibits 4-3 and 4-4 for similar calculations).

6.10.4 Heterogeneity Due to Differential Intensity of Exposure

An apparent interaction can occur when there is heterogeneity in the levels of exposure to the risk factor of interest according to the alleged effect modifier. For example, in a study of epidemic asthma in New Orleans, White et al.[29] investigated the role of airborne soy dust originating from vessel cargo from the New Orleans harbor. The association was stronger when the maximum wind speed was below 12 miles per hour (relative odds = 4.4) than when wind speeds were higher (relative odds = 1.7). This heterogeneity was probably due to a heavier exposure to soy dust resulting from slower wind speeds and would thus not represent "true" interaction using the narrow criterion of differential biological susceptibility to the same environmental exposure level. For practical purposes, however, there may be important public health implications of identifying this kind of heterogeneity. Another example is the potential effect modification by gender of the relationship of smoking to respiratory diseases, which may be created or exaggerated by the fact that the level of exposure to smoking is higher in men than in women.

6.10.5 Interaction and Host Factors

Facilitation and, ultimately, level of exposure are also the result of anatomical or pathophysiological characteristics of the host. For example, a qualitative interaction has been found in a case-control study by Reif et al.[30] between the shape of the skull in pet dogs

FIGURE 6-7 Apparent interaction between smoking and overweight in a case-control study. Within each stratum (smokers or nonsmokers), the levels of misclassification of overweight are the same in cases and controls; however, levels of nondifferential misclassification are different across strata formed by smoking.

True odds ratios showing no heterogeneity

Smoking status	BMI status	Cases	Controls	Odds ratio$_{TRUE}$
Smokers	Overweight	200	100	2.25
	Not overweight	800	900	
Nonsmokers	Overweight	200	100	2.25
	Not overweight	800	900	

Sensitivity and specificity of information on overweight

		Cases	Controls
Smokers:	Sensitivity	0.80	0.80
	Specificity	0.85	0.85
Nonsmokers:	Sensitivity	0.95	0.95
	Specificity	0.98	0.98

Values of indices of validity are different between smokers and nonsmokers, although within each stratum they are the same for cases and controls (nondifferential misclassification within each stratum)

Misclassified odds ratios

	Smokers				Nonsmokers		
Overweight	Cases	Controls	OR$_{MISCL}$	Overweight	Cases	Controls	OR$_{MISCL}$
Yes	280	215	1.4	Yes	206	113	2.0
No	720	785		No	794	887	

and passive smoking in relationship to lung cancer: the increase in odds of lung cancer was limited to dogs with a short nose (brachycephalic and mesocephalic), presumably because of the absence of a mechanical barrier to carcinogenic particles represented by the ciliae of the long-nosed (dolichocephalic) dogs. (An alternative explanation is that there are genetic differences in susceptibility to smoking-induced lung cancer between these types of dogs.) In a subsequent study by the same authors, a qualitative interaction was again found between passive smoking and skull shape with regard to nasal cancer, except that a higher odds of cancer was found for the long-nosed than for the shorter-nosed dogs,[31] leading the authors to speculate that "an increased risk of nasal cancer among long-nosed dogs may be explained by enhanced filtration, and impaction of particles in the mucosa."

These examples underscore the importance of considering the intensity and/or facilitation of exposure when attempting to explain heterogeneity of effects. Effective exposure dose is obviously a function of the net result of the amount of "exposure" in the individual's environment (the example of soy dust), the dose absorbed into the organism, and the dose that reaches the cellular levels (the examples of canine lung and nasal cancers).

From the host viewpoint, effect modifiers can act on different portals of entry (skin, gastrointestinal, respiratory). For example, it is well known that exposure to the same intensity of a skin pathogen (e.g., streptococcus) is related to a higher probability of infection in individuals with an existing skin rash than in those with a normal skin. Thus, factors that produce skin lesions (e.g., skin allergens, mechanical trauma) interact with infectious agents in increasing risk of infection.

The biological mechanism of effect modification can also vary at the metabolic or cellular level. Interaction between metabolic pathways and exposure to risk factors is exemplified by genetic disorders such as phenylketonuria. In this disorder, the inability to oxidize a metabolic product of phenylalanine found in many food items may result in severe mental deficiency. Another example is that, judging from experiments in mice, it is possible that humans, too, have a differential genetic susceptibility to salt-induced hypertension.[32] At the immunological level, the interactions between certain drugs (e.g., steroids, immunosuppressants) and infectious agents in relationship to risk and/or severity of infections are well known. The relatively low risk of coronary heart disease in white women at similar levels of exposure to traditional cardiovascular risk factors as men in the United States suggests that endogenous hormones may play a role in modifying the effects of these risk factors,[33] notwithstanding the lack of a protective effect of estrogen therapy shown in recent clinical trials.[34,35]

6.11 INTERACTION AND SEARCH FOR NEW RISK FACTORS IN LOW-RISK GROUPS

The strength of an association measured by a relative difference (e.g., a relative risk) is a function of the relative prevalence of other risk factors.[22,36] This concept seems to have been first recognized by Cornfield et al.,[37(p.194)] who stated this:

> If two uncorrelated agents, A and B, each increases the risk of a disease, and if the risk of the disease in the absence of either agent is small ... then the apparent relative risk for A ... is less than the (relative) risk for A in the absence of B.

This notion is readily understood when considering a situation in which a risk factor is strongly associated with the disease, as in the case of smoking and lung cancer: to examine the role of a weaker factor A, it would be intuitively logical to study nonsmokers, as otherwise the vast majority of cases would be explained by smoking. In other words, a magnification of the relative risk for A in those unexposed to smoking (vis-à-vis smokers) is expected (i.e., a negative multiplicative interaction).[22] The tendency toward a negative multiplicative interaction when examining the joint effect of a strong risk factor Z and a weak risk factor A can be intuitively understood by considering two facts: (1) the maximum absolute risk associated with the exposure to any risk factor cannot surpass 100%, and (2) the higher the independent relative risk associated with exposure to Z, the more the risk in those exposed to Z approximates 100%.

For illustration purposes, let us assume a simple hypothetical example involving risk factors Z and A, shown in Table 6-29, in which the baseline incidence of the disease (i.e., the incidence in those unexposed to both risk factors) is about 10% and the independent relative risk for Z (i.e., in the absence of A) is 9.0 (reflecting an incidence in those unexposed to A but exposed to Z of 90%). As the incidence in those exposed to A in the stratum exposed to Z cannot surpass the 100% mark, the maximum possible relative risk for A if Z is present is 100% ÷ 90% = 1.1. A similar absolute difference in incidence of 10% due to exposure to A in those unexposed to Z would result in a relative risk of 20% ÷ 10% = 2.0. A similar reasoning can be applied to a situation in which Z is a constellation of risk factors, rather than a single variable: for example, when studying cardiovascular disease outcomes, Z can be defined as the simultaneous presence of the traditional cardiovascular risk factors (hypertension, hypercholesterolemia, smoking, and diabetes).

An example is given by the known gender difference with regard to the prevalence of gallstones. It is estimated that in the population at large, 80% of women and 8% of men have gallbladder disease.[38] Thus, the relative risks for risk factors other than gender would have a tendency to be larger in men than in women.

Because of its intuitive appeal, the idea of studying "emergent" risk factors in individuals with no known risk factors is on occasion considered in the design of a study. For example, in a study of the putative protective effect of antibiotics on CHD, Meier et al.[39] compared prior antibiotic use (obtained from pharmacy records) in CHD cases and controls; in selecting these groups, the authors excluded all individuals with a known prior history of CHD or other cardiovascular diseases, as well as individuals with evidence of hypertension, hypercholesterolemia, or diabetes. It is important to realize, however, that the use of this strategy may limit the generalizability of the study findings to the general population, which includes both low- and high-risk individuals. Furthermore, associations that rely on synergism between risk factors may be missed altogether. For example, if infections are neither sufficient nor necessary causes for atherosclerosis but rather are involved in atherogenesis because of their synergism with other cardiovascular risk

TABLE 6-29 Example of negative interaction between a stronger and a weaker risk factor.

Factor Z	Factor A	Population size	Incidence /100	Attributable risk for A/100	Relative risk for A	Relative risk for Z
Absent	Absent	1000	10.0	0	1.0	1.0
	Present	1000	20.0	10.0	2.0	1.0
Present	Absent	1000	90.0	0	1.0	9.0*
	Present	1000	100.0	10.0	1.1	5.0†

*Relative risk of Z in persons unexposed to A.
†Relative risk of Z in persons exposed to A.

factors (e.g., hypercholesterolemia, diabetes), as suggested elsewhere,[40] the "low-risk" approach may underestimate the potential impact of infections (or, by analogy, antibiotics) on atherosclerosis.

6.12 INTERACTION AND "REPRESENTATIVENESS" OF ASSOCIATIONS

An important assumption when generalizing results from a study is that the study population should have an "average" susceptibility to the exposure under study with regard to a given outcome. When susceptibility is unusual, results cannot be easily generalized. For example, results of a study on the effectiveness of a vaccine in African children may not be applicable to Swiss children, as inadequate nutrition in the former may significantly alter the immune system and thus the production of antibodies to the killed or inactivated agent.

Consider, for example, the findings in Table 6-11, with regard to the influence of interaction on the ability to generalize. Assuming that hypertensive individuals are indeed more susceptible to asthma-induced cardiomyopathy than normotensives, the large odds ratio (13.4) found in hypertensives is obviously not generalizable to nonhypertensives, whose odds ratio for asthma pertaining to cardiomyopathy is much smaller (2.4). It follows that the so-called average effect of asthma on cardiomyopathy is a function of the prevalence of hypertension in the population to which one wishes to generalize results. Assuming that the relative odds from Coughlin's study[8] (Table 6-11) represented the true estimates, in populations in which most individuals are hypertensive, the odds ratio would approximate 13.4; on the other hand, in populations with a low proportion of hypertensives the relative odds would be closer to 2.4. Whereas the example of hypertension and asthma is based on an easily measurable effect modifier (hypertension), differences in the strength of an association from population to population may also be due to between-population differences in the prevalence of unmeasured environmental or genetic effect modifiers.

Although it is difficult to establish to which extent the susceptibility of a given study population differs from an "average" susceptibility, the assessment of its epidemiological profile (based on well-known risk factors) may indicate how "usual" or "unusual" that population is. Thus, in studies of breast cancer, assuming no bias, a study population in which the well-known association with age at first pregnancy were not found would suggest that it might not be a population of "average" susceptibility. This strategy, however, is limited because level of susceptibility to a known risk factor may not be representative of the level of susceptibility regarding the exposure under study (see also Chapter 10, Section 10.2.4).

REFERENCES

1. Petitti DB. Associations are not effects. *Am J Epidemiol*. 1991;133:101–102.
2. Rothman K, Greenland S. *Modern Epidemiology*, 3rd ed. Philadelphia, PA: Wolters Kluwer Health/Lippincott; 2008.
3. Kannel WB. Lipids, diabetes, and coronary heart disease: Insights from the Framingham Study. *Am Heart J*. 1985;110:1100–1107.
4. Anttila T, Helkala EL, Viitanen M, et al. Alcohol drinking in middle age and subsequent risk of mild cognitive impairment and dementia in old age: A prospective population based study. *Br Med J*. 2004;329:539.
5. Comstock GW, Lundin FE, Jr. Parental smoking and perinatal mortality. *Am J Obstet Gynecol*. 1967;98:708–718.
6. Ndrepepa G, Mehilli J, Bollwein H, et al. Sex-associated differences in clinical outcomes after coronary stenting in patients with diabetes mellitus. *Am J Med*. 2004;117:830–836.
7. Shapiro S, Slone D, Rosenberg L, et al. Oral-contraceptive use in relation to myocardial infarction. *Lancet*. 1979;1:743–747.
8. Coughlin S. *A Case-Control Study of Dilated Cardiomyopathy* [Doctoral Dissertation]. Baltimore, MD: The Johns Hopkins Bloomberg School of Public Health; 1987.
9. Honein MA, Paulozzi LJ, Moore CA. Family history, maternal smoking, and clubfoot: An indication of a gene-environment interaction. *Am J Epidemiol*. 2000;152:658–665.
10. Morabia A, Ten Have T, Landis JR. Interaction fallacy. *J Clin Epidemiol*. 1997;50:809–812.
11. Thompson WD. Statistical analysis of case-control studies. *Epidemiol Rev*. 1994;16:33–50.
12. Cox D. Regression models and life table (with discussion). *J Roy Stat Soc [B]*. 1972;34:187–20.
13. Darroch J. Biologic synergism and parallelism. *Am J Epidemiol*. 1997;145:661–668.
14. Thompson WD. Effect modification and the limits of biological inference from epidemiologic data. *J Clin Epidemiol*. 1991;44:221–232.
15. Rothman KJ, Greenland S, Walker AM. Concepts of interaction. *Am J Epidemiol*. 1980;112:467–470.
16. Stanton CK, Gray RH. Effects of caffeine consumption on delayed conception. *Am J Epidemiol*. 1995;142:1322–1329.
17. Shapiro S, Venet W, Strax P, et al. Selection, follow-up, and analysis in the Health Insurance Plan Study: A randomized trial with breast cancer screening. *Natl Cancer Inst Monogr*. 1985;67:65–74.
18. Sipos A, Rasmussen F, Harrison G, et al. Paternal age and schizophrenia: A population based cohort study. *Br Med J*. 2004;329:1070.
19. Williams JE, Paton CC, Siegler IC, et al. Anger proneness predicts coronary heart disease risk: Prospective analysis from the Atherosclerosis Risk in Communities (ARIC) Study. *Circulation*. 2000;101:2034–2039.
20. Shanmugham JR, Zavras AI, Rosner B, et al. Alcohol-folate interactions in the risk of oral cancer in women: A prospective cohort study. *Cancer Epidemiol Biomarkers Prev*. 2010;19:2516–2524.
21. MacMahon B, Pugh TF. *Epidemiology: Principles and Methods*. Boston, MA: Little, Brown and Co.; 1970.
22. Schlesselman J. *Case Control Studies: Design, Conduct, Analysis*. New York, NY: Oxford University Press; 1982.
23. Selvin S. *Statistical Analysis of Epidemiologic Data*. New York, NY: Oxford University Press; 1991.
24. Cohen JD. Abnormal electrocardiograms and cardiovascular risk: Role of silent myocardial ischemia: Evidence from MRFIT. *Am J Cardiol*. 1992;70:14F–18F.

25. Yu MW, Hsu FC, Sheen IS, et al. Prospective study of hepatocellular carcinoma and liver cirrhosis in asymptomatic chronic hepatitis B virus carriers. *Am J Epidemiol.* 1997;145:1039–1047.

26. Savitz DA, Brett KM, Evans LE, Bowes W. Medically treated miscarriage in Alamance County, North Carolina, 1988–1991. *Am J Epidemiol.* 1994;139:1100–1106.

27. Bryson CL, Ioannou GN, Rulyak SJ, Critchlow C. Association between gestational diabetes and pregnancy-induced hypertension. *Am J Epidemiol.* 2003;158:1148–1153.

28. Kotelchuck M. An evaluation of the Kessner Adequacy of Prenatal Care Index and a proposed Adequacy of Prenatal Care Utilization Index. *Am J Public Health.* 1994;84:1414–1420.

29. White MC, Etzel RA, Olson DR, Goldstein IF. Reexamination of epidemic asthma in New Orleans, Louisiana, in relation to the presence of soy at the harbor. *Am J Epidemiol.* 1997;145:432–438.

30. Reif JS, Dunn K, Ogilvie GK, Harris CK. Passive smoking and canine lung cancer risk. *Am J Epidemiol.* 1992;135:234–239.

31. Reif JS, Bruns C, Lower KS. Cancer of the nasal cavity and paranasal sinuses and exposure to environmental tobacco smoke in pet dogs. *Am J Epidemiol.* 1998;147:488–492.

32. Szklo M. Epidemiologic patterns of blood pressure in children. *Epidemiol Rev.* 1979;1:143–169.

33. Szklo M. Epidemiology of coronary heart disease in women. In: Gold E, ed. *The Changing Risk of Disease in Women.* Lexington, MA: Collamore Press; 1984:233–241.

34. Anderson GL, Limacher M, Assaf AR, et al. Effects of conjugated equine estrogen in postmenopausal women with hysterectomy: The Women's Health Initiative randomized controlled trial. *J Am Med Assoc.* 2004;291:1701–1712.

35. Hulley S, Grady D, Bush T, et al. Randomized trial of estrogen plus progestin for secondary prevention of coronary heart disease in postmenopausal women: Heart and Estrogen/progestin Replacement Study (HERS) Research Group. *J Am Med Assoc.* 1998;280:605–613.

36. Rothman KJ, Poole C. A strengthening programme for weak associations. *Int J Epidemiol.* 1988; 17:955–959.

37. Cornfield J, Haenszel W, Hammond EC, et al. Smoking and lung cancer: Recent evidence and a discussion of some questions. *J Natl Cancer Inst.* 1959;22:173–203.

38. Greenberger N, Isselbacher KJ. Diseases of the gallbladder and bile ducts. In: Isselbacher K, Braunwald E, Wilson JD, et al., eds. *Harrison's Principles of Internal Medicine,* 13th ed. New York, NY: McGraw-Hill; 1994:1504–1516.

39. Meier CR, Derby LE, Jick SS, et al. Antibiotics and risk of subsequent first-time acute myocardial infarction. *J Am Med Assoc.* 1999;281:427–431.

40. Nieto FJ. Infections and atherosclerosis: New clues from an old hypothesis? *Am J Epidemiol.* 1998;148:937–948.

EXERCISES

1. In a prospective study of the relationship of hepatitis B and C viruses to newly developed hepatocellular carcinoma, the authors examined the interaction between alcohol and hepatitis C virus (HCV). The following table is based on this study's results:

Alcohol drinking	Anti-HCV*	Number of persons	Incidence rates/100,000
Absent	Negative	8968	78.7
Absent	Positive	2352	127.1
Present	Negative	461	309.7
Present	Positive	90	384.9

*Anti-HCV: antibodies against hepatitis C virus.

   a. Using the category "absent–negative" as the reference, calculate the relative risks and the attributable risks (in the exposed) for those with positive antibodies to HCV only, for those exposed to alcohol only, and for those exposed to both.
   b. Calculate the expected joint relative risk (multiplicative model) and the expected joint attributable risk in the exposed (additive model).
   c. Assuming no random variability, is there multiplicative or additive interaction? If so, is it positive or negative?
   d. Using the homogeneity strategy and alcohol as the effect modifier, confirm your answers to the previous questions.

2. Haffner et al. examined coronary heart disease risk according to presence of type 2 diabetes, stratified by whether individuals had had a prior myocardial infarction.* The results of the study are shown in the table.

Cumulative incidence (%), relative risks, and exposure attributable risks (%) of myocardial infarction (MI) during a 7-year follow-up, according to previous myocardial infarction history and presence of type 2 diabetes.

Diabetes	Previous MI	Incidence (%)*	Relative risk	Attributable risk in those with previous MI (%)
Present	Yes	45.0	2.2	24.8
	No	20.2	1.0	Reference
Absent	Yes	18.8	5.4	15.3
	No	3.5	1.0	Reference

*In those with a previous MI, incidence refers to incidence of a recurrent MI.

   a. What types of interaction can be inferred by inspection of the table?
   b. Is it appropriate to merely show a diabetes-adjusted measure of association? Why?
   c. Can you speculate as to why the relative risk for a previous MI is closer to one in the stratum with diabetes present than in the stratum with diabetes absent?

---

*Haffner SM, Lehto S, Ronnemaa T, et al. Mortality from coronary heart disease in subjects with type 2 diabetes and in nondiabetic subjects with and without prior myocardial infarction. *N Engl J Med* 1998;339:229–234.

3. A case-control study was conducted by Gustavsson et al.[†] to examine the joint associations of asbestos exposure and smoking with lung cancer odds. Results are shown in the table for exposure to asbestos of ≥ 2.5 fiber-years and smoking of more than 20 cigarettes.

Odds ratios* of lung cancer according to exposure to asbestos for 2.5 fiber-years or more and smoking of more than 20 cigarettes/day.

	Never smokers	Smoking > 20 cigarettes/day
Unexposed to asbestos	1.0	45.4
≥ 2.5 fiber-years	10.2	80.6

*Odd ratios adjusted for age, inclusion year, residential radon, environmental nitrogen oxide, diesel exhaust, and combustion products.

a. What is the value of the odds ratio expressing the independent association of smoking > 20 cigarettes/day with lung cancer?

b. What is the value of the odds ratio expressing the independent association of exposure of ≥ 2.5 fiber-years of asbestos with lung cancer?

c. What is the joint expected odds ratio for each of the two models (additive and multiplicative)?

d. Assuming no bias or confounding, what are your conclusions resulting from the comparison of the joint expected with the joint observed odds ratios?

4. Using a case-control design, the interaction between urine pH and cigarette smoking was examined by Alguacil et al., with regard to bladder cancer odds.[‡] Results of this study are shown in the table. (In the original table, data for a category of former smokers are also shown. For simplification purposes, results are only shown for nonsmokers and current smokers.)

Distribution of cases and controls according to ph of the urine and smoking status.

Smoking status	Urine pH	Number of cases	Number of controls	Unadjusted odds ratio	Adjusted odds ratio (95% CI)*
Nonsmokers	> 6.0	67	114	1.0	1.0
	≤ 6.0	39	67	1.0	1.0 (0.6, 1.8)
Current smokers	> 6.0	144	84	1.0	1.0
	≤ 6.0	158	54	1.6	2.1 (1.3, 3.2)

*Adjusted for age (5 categories), study region, gender, cigarettes per day and duration of smoking.

[†]Gustavsson P, Nyberg F, Pershagen G, et al. Low-dose exposure to asbestos and lung cancer: dose-response relations and interaction with smoking in a population-based case-referent study in Stockholm, Sweden. Am J Epidemiol. 2002;155:1016–1022
[‡]Alguacil J, Kogevinas M, Silverman D, et al. Urinary pH, cigarette smoking and bladder cancer risk. Carcinogenesis 2011;32;843–7.

a. The heterogeneity of the odds ratios across strata of the potential effect modifier (presence or absence of current smoking) suggests the presence of interaction. Assuming no random error or bias, is the interaction additive or multiplicative?

b. With adjustment, the odds ratio for the pH-bladder cancer association in the stratum of nonsmokers did not change. However, for smokers, the odds ratio increased from 1.6 to 2.1. What do these findings suggest?

PART FOUR
Dealing with Threats to Validity

CHAPTER 7 Stratification and Adjustment: Multivariate Analysis in Epidemiology 229

CHAPTER 8 Quality Assurance and Control 313

Stratification and Adjustment: Multivariate Analysis in Epidemiology

CHAPTER 7

7.1 INTRODUCTION

Analytic epidemiologic studies are designed to evaluate the association between environmental exposures or other subject characteristics (e.g., demographic variables, genetic polymorphisms) and disease risk. Even if the epidemiologist's interest is focused on a single exposure, there are usually several other factors that need to be considered in the analysis, either because they may distort (confound) the exposure–disease relationship (see Chapter 5) or because the magnitude of the association between exposure and disease may vary across levels of these variables (effect modification; see Chapter 6). *Stratification* and *multivariate analysis* (*modeling*) are the analytical tools that are used to control for confounding effects, to assess effect modification, and to summarize the associations of several predictor variables with disease risk in an efficient fashion.

The simplest method to analyze the possible presence of confounding is *stratification*, which is frequently a very informative method because: (1) it allows a straightforward and simultaneous examination of the possible presence of both confounding and effect modification; and (2) because examining stratified results is often useful when choosing the appropriate statistical technique for adjustment.

Multivariate analysis refers to a series of analytical techniques, each based on a more or less complex mathematical model, which are used to carry out *statistical adjustment*—that is, the estimation of a certain measure of association between an exposure and an outcome while controlling for one or more possible confounding variables. Effect modification can also be assessed in the context of multivariate analysis. The next section presents an example to illustrate the basic idea of stratification and adjustment as two often-complementary alternatives to discern and control for confounding variables. The following sections discuss in more detail some of the adjustment techniques frequently used in epidemiology. Because it can be seen as both an "adjustment" technique and a study design feature, *matching* (including individual and frequency matching) has been previously addressed in Chapter 1 of this book, in which the main observational design strategies were discussed (Section 1.4.5). In this chapter, the issue of individual matching is taken up again, but only insofar as it relates to the application of this strategy in adjusting for follow-up length in cohort studies (Section 7.4.6), and to demonstrate its analytic convergence with the Mantel-Haenszel approach when matched sets are treated as strata for the adjustment of the odds ratio (Section 7.3.3).

The chapter ends with a section describing alternative approaches to stratification and adjustment that might be useful to control for confounding in specific circumstances: propensity scores, instrumental variables, and Mendelian randomization.

7.2 STRATIFICATION AND ADJUSTMENT TECHNIQUES TO DISENTANGLE CONFOUNDING

Table 7-1 shows a hypothetical example of a case-control study of male gender as a possible risk factor for malaria infection. This example was used in Chapter 5 to illustrate how to assess whether a variable is a confounder (Section 5.4). The crude analysis shown at the top of the table suggests that males are at higher risk of malaria (odds ratio = 1.71). If random and systematic errors (bias) are deemed to be unlikely explanations for the observed association, the possibility of confounding needs to be considered (i.e., whether the association may be explained by characteristics related to both gender and increased odds of malaria). One such characteristic is occupation: individuals who work mostly outdoors (e.g., agricultural workers) are more likely to be exposed to mosquito bites than those who work indoors and are therefore at a higher risk of malaria. Thus, the observed association could be explained if the likelihood of working outdoors differed between genders. In Section 5.4.1, occupation was shown to be related to both gender (the "exposure") and malaria (the "outcome") (strategy 1 for the assessment of confounding; see Exhibit 5-3); it was also shown that when the data were stratified by type of occupation (strategy 2 to assess confounding), the stratified estimates were different from the pooled (crude) estimate. These results are presented in the lower part of Table 7-1. By stratifying the study results according to the potential

TABLE 7-1 Example of stratified analysis: hypothetical study of male gender as a risk factor for malaria infection.

Crude analysis

	All cases and controls			
	Cases	Controls	Total	
Males	88	68	156	OR = 1.71
Females	62	82	144	
Total	150	150	300	

Stratified analysis by occupation

	Cases and controls with mostly outdoor occupations			
	Cases	Controls	Total	
Males	53	15	68	OR = 1.06
Females	10	3	13	
Total	63	18	81	

	Cases and controls with mostly indoor occupations			
	Cases	Controls	Total	
Males	35	53	88	OR = 1.00
Females	52	79	131	
Total	87	132	219	

confounder, it is possible to *control for* its effect; that is, it is possible to assess the association between the risk factor of interest (male gender) and the disease (malaria) separately for those whose work is mostly outdoors (odds ratio = 1.06) and for those who work mostly indoors (odds ratio = 1.00). Because these stratum-specific odds ratios are similar to each other and fairly different from the crude estimate (odds ratio = 1.71), it can be concluded that occupation is a confounder of the association between male gender and the presence of malaria. The fact that the stratified odds ratios are very close to 1.0 suggests that, after occupation is taken into account, there is *no* association between gender and the presence of malaria—in other words, that the crude association can be "explained" by the confounding effect of occupation. (As discussed in Chapter 5, Section 5.5.1, unadjusted odds ratios, rate ratios, and absolute differences can be different from the stratum-specific estimates even if confounding is not present.[1,2] Thus, the assessment of potential confounding effects by means of stratification must be confirmed by the use of the other strategies discussed in Chapter 5 and in this chapter.)

The stratified data shown in the two-by-two tables in the lower part of Table 7-1 allow a closer examination of why occupation is a confounder in this hypothetical example: (1) 43.6% (68 of 156) of males have mostly outdoor occupations, compared with only 9% (13 of 144) of females (odds ratio = 7.8) and (2) 42% (63 of 150) of the malaria cases have mostly outdoor occupations compared with 12% (18 of 150) of controls (odds ratio = 5.3). The strong positive associations of the confounder (occupation) with both the risk factor of interest (male gender) and case-control status explain the (positive) confounding effect.

The stratified analysis also allows the assessment of the possible presence of interaction (see Chapter 6). In the previous example (Table 7-1), the fact that stratum-specific odds ratios are very similar (homogeneous) indicates that no interaction is present, and thus, an overall occupation-adjusted odds ratio can be calculated. As described later in this chapter, this can be done by calculating a *weighted average* of the stratum-specific estimates, for example, using the Mantel-Haenszel weighted odds ratio, OR_{MH}, which turns out to be 1.01 in this particular example (see Section 7.3.3). Compared with the examination of the stratum-specific results, the calculation of this weighted average (i.e., the "adjusted" odds ratio) requires the assumption that the association is *homogeneous* across strata. On the other hand, when the odds ratios are not too similar (e.g., 1.4 and 2.0), it may be difficult to decide whether the observed heterogeneity is real—that is, whether there is actual effect modification, as opposed to its being the result of random variability caused by the small size of the strata (see Chapter 6, Section 6.10.1), in which case it can be ignored. In other words, the issue is whether presence of interaction should be accepted by the investigator. As discussed in Chapter 6, Section 6.9, in addition to the statistical significance of the observed heterogeneity, its magnitude should be considered when deciding whether interaction is present; thus, stratum-specific odds ratios of 1.4 and 20.0 are more likely to reflect a true interaction than odds ratios of 1.4 and 2.0. Other factors that should be considered are whether the interaction is quantitative (e.g., stratum-specific odds ratios of 1.4 and 2.0) or qualitative (e.g., odds ratios of 1.4 and 0.3) and, most importantly, its perceived biological plausibility.

If interaction is judged to be present, adjustment (e.g., obtaining a combined odds ratio) is unwarranted, for in this case, the "adjusted" odds ratio has no relevance, as it will be a weighted average of heterogeneous stratum-specific odds ratios. Consider, for example, the study by Reif et al.,[3] cited in Chapter 6, showing that an association between environmental tobacco smoke and lung cancer in pet dogs was present in short-nosed dogs (odds ratio = 2.4) and virtually absent (odds ratio = 0.9) in long-nosed dogs.

The biological plausibility of this possible qualitative interaction was discussed in Section 6.10.5. Assuming that this interaction is real, adjustment for skull shape (nose length) is obviously not warranted, as an adjusted odds ratio, representing the weighted average of the stratum-specific odds ratios of 2.4 and 0.9, has no useful interpretation.

Another example is provided in Table 7-2, which summarizes the results from a case-control study of oral contraceptive use as a possible risk factor for myocardial infarction among women of reproductive ages.[4] As shown in the upper part of Table 7-2, the odds of disease among women who used oral contraceptives was estimated to be about 70% higher than the odds in those who did not use oral contraceptives. The possibility of confounding by age, however, was considered by the authors of this study. Because age was known to be directly related to the outcome (risk of myocardial infarction) and inversely related to the exposure (increased oral contraceptive use among younger women), it could act as a *negative* confounder (see Chapter 5, Section 5.5.5).

In a stratified analysis by age, also shown in Table 7-2, all but one of the strata had estimated odds ratios further away from 1.0 than the overall crude estimate, confirming the expectation of negative confounding (i.e., age driving the estimated crude association

TABLE 7-2 Example of stratified analysis: Case-control study of oral contraceptives (OC) and myocardial infarction in women.

Crude analysis

All cases and controls

	Cases	Controls	
OC	29	135	OR = 1.7
No OC	205	1607	
	234	1742	

Stratified by analysis: by age

Age 25–29

	Cases	Controls	
OC	4	62	OR = 7.2
No OC	2	224	

Age 30–34

	Cases	Controls	
OC	9	33	OR = 8.9
No OC	12	390	

Age 35–39

	Cases	Controls	
OC	4	26	OR = 1.5
No OC	33	330	

Age 40–44

	Cases	Controls	
OC	6	9	OR = 3.7
No OC	65	362	

Age 45–49

	Cases	Controls	
OC	6	5	OR = 3.9
No OC	93	301	

Source: Data from S Shapiro et al., Oral-Contraceptive Use in Relation to Myocardial Infarction. *Lancet*, Vol 1 pp. 743–747, © 1979.

toward the null). The adjusted odds ratio (see Section 7.3.3) for the data in Table 7-2 was found to be 3.97, thus more than twice the crude estimate. As mentioned previously, implicit when calculating any average, this adjusted odds ratio estimate requires assuming that the associations are homogeneous (i.e., that the observed between-strata differences in odds ratios result from random variation). In this example, this assumption is probably reasonable, given the small number of cases in some of the cells and the fact that all odds ratios are in the same direction (denoting absence of qualitative interaction; see Chapter 6, Section 6.7.1). On the other hand, it could be argued that the quantitative differences among odds ratios in Table 7-2 are too large and thus that the estimation of a single average (adjusted) estimate supposedly "representative" of all age strata is not warranted. For example, one could argue that the association seems to be stronger in women younger than 35 years (odds ratios of 7.2 and 8.9) than in older women (odds ratios ranging from 1.5 to 3.9). Acceptance of this heterogeneity of the values of odds ratios suggests an alternative approach that consists of calculating two age-adjusted odds ratios: one for women 25 to 34 years old (i.e., the weighted average odds ratio for the two younger groups) and another for women 35 to 49 years old (i.e., the weighted average odds ratio for the three older groups). (These calculations yield OR_{MH} values of 8.3 and 2.7, respectively; see Section 7.3.3.) This example illustrates the advantages of stratification for assessing the presence of confounding and/or interaction and for deciding when adjustment is appropriate and how it should be carried out. It also illustrates a common situation in epidemiologic analysis: the exposure of interest seems to have heterogeneous effects according to a certain grouping of a third variable, sometimes not considered before the analysis of the data. Given the large number of possibilities for grouping variables when conducting stratified analysis and the potential random variability of apparent subgroup effects (Section 6.10.1), this type of analysis, if not based on biologically plausible a priori hypotheses, should be considered as exploratory.

Because the previous examples were based on the assessment of stratified odds ratios, they were used to illustrate the evaluation of multiplicative interaction. It is, however, important to bear in mind that if the measure of association of interest is the attributable risk (Section 3.2.2), it is additive interaction that should be considered (see Section 6.6), as discussed in the context of the direct method of adjustment in Section 7.3.1.

7.2.1 Stratification and Adjustment: Assumptions

Compared with adjustment, stratification is virtually (but not completely) assumption free. Note that stratification is akin to frequency matching (discussed in Chapter 1, Section 1.4.5) in that it requires assuming that the strata are meaningful and properly defined. This means that there should be homogeneity *within* each stratum. For example, for the strata in Table 7-1, it must be implicitly assumed that there is uniformity regarding the association of gender with malaria in each of the two occupational strata (mostly outdoors or mostly indoors); similarly, in Table 7-2, it is assumed that the association of oral contraceptives with myocardial infarction is homogeneous within each 5-year age group. If this assumption were not appropriate in each of these examples, other more precisely defined categories (e.g., more specific occupational categories, or finer age intervals, respectively) would have to be chosen for the stratified analysis. This assumption is equivalent to the assumption of *lack of residual confounding*, described later in this chapter (Section 7.6)

For adjustment, further assumptions must be met. As described in the next section, all adjustment techniques are based on assuming some kind of *statistical model* that summarizes the association between the variables under investigation. Sometimes the statistical model is a simple one, as in the case of *adjustment methods based on stratification*, namely direct and indirect adjustment (Sections 7.3.1 and 7.3.2) or the Mantel-Haenszel method (Section 7.3.3). As discussed previously, for the calculation of a (weighted) mean of a number of stratum-specific odds ratios, it is assumed that these are homogeneous across strata (i.e., that there is no [multiplicative] interaction). These simpler stratification-based adjustment methods are most often used when controlling for a limited number of potential confounders that are categorical or that can be categorized (see Section 7.3.4). On the other hand, more mathematically complex models are the basis for *multivariate adjustment methods based on regression methods*.* As described more extensively in Section 7.4, these more complex models are used as tools for epidemiologic inferences about the relationships between a number of factors and a disease, while simultaneously controlling (or adjusting) for the potentially mutual confounding effects of all these factors. These multiple-regression methods can also handle continuous covariates.

In the following paragraphs, some of the most frequently used techniques for adjustment and multivariate analysis of epidemiologic data are briefly described. Sections 7.3 and 7.4 describe the techniques based on stratification and those based on multiple-regression methods, respectively. Section 7.5 describes alternative methods to control for confounding that are applicable in certain situations. Each of these analytical techniques is based on both a conceptual and a mathematical model (i.e., something we could refer to as a "statistical model"). Sections 7.6 and 7.7 discuss some potential limitations of multivariate adjustment (residual confounding and overadjustment), and the final section of this chapter (Section 7.7) presents a summary and overview of common uses of multivariate statistical modeling techniques in epidemiologic practice.

7.3 ADJUSTMENT METHODS BASED ON STRATIFICATION

7.3.1 Direct Adjustment

Direct adjustment has been traditionally used for age adjustment when comparing morbidity and mortality rates across countries or regions or across different time periods, although age adjustment is by no means its only application. The popularity of more mathematically sophisticated statistical methods (such as those presented in the following sections) has limited the use of direct adjustment in epidemiology research in recent years, but the method remains a straightforward technique that is particularly useful to illustrate the basic principles of statistical adjustment.

The direct method is described in most introductory epidemiologic textbooks (e.g., Gordis[5]). Table 7-3 outlines the procedure when comparing incidence rates between two groups, A and B (e.g., exposed and unexposed), stratified according to the suspected confounding variable (strata $i = 1$ to k).

---

*The term *multivariate analysis*, commonly used in the epidemiology literature, is in contrast with "crude" analysis, which assesses the relationship between one variable and one outcome. Most often, the term *multivariate* is used when simultaneously controlling for more than one variable (in contrast to *bivariate analysis*). It is, however, used in a different way in the field of biostatistics, where *multivariate analysis* usually refers to the multiple-regression techniques involving more than one *dependent* variable.

TABLE 7-3 Direct adjustment for comparison of incidence (I) in two study groups.

Suspected confounding variable (1)	Study group A				Study group B				Standard population		
	No. (2)	Cases (3)	Incidence (4) = (3)/(2)		No. (5)	Cases (6)	Incidence (7) = (6)/(5)		No. (8)	Expected cases using I of A (9) = (4) × (8)	Expected cases using I of B (10) = (7) × (8)
Stratum 1	n_{A1}	x_{A1}	I_{A1}		n_{B1}	x_{B1}	I_{B1}		W_1	$I_{A1} \times W_1$	$I_{B1} \times W_1$
Stratum 2	n_{A2}	x_{A2}	I_{A2}		n_{B2}	x_{B2}	I_{B2}		W_2	$I_{A2} \times W_2$	$I_{B2} \times W_2$
Stratum 3	n_{A3}	x_{A3}	I_{A3}		n_{B3}	x_{B3}	I_{B3}		W_3	$I_{A3} \times W_3$	$I_{B3} \times W_3$
—	—	—	—		—	—	—		—	—	—
Stratum k	n_{Ak}	x_{Ak}	I_{Ak}		n_{Bk}	x_{Bk}	I_{Bk}		W_k	$I_{Ak} \times W_k$	$I_{Bk} \times W_k$
Total	N_A	X_A	I_A		N_B	X_B	I_B		$\sum_i W_i$	$\sum_i [I_{Ai} \times W_i]$	$\sum_i [I_{Bi} \times W_i]$

Adjusted incidence

$$I_A^* = \frac{\sum_i [I_{Ai} \times W_i]}{\sum_i W_i} \qquad I_B^* = \frac{\sum_i [I_{Bi} \times W_i]}{\sum_i W_i}$$

Briefly:

1. For each stratum of the suspected confounding variable, the incidence is calculated in the two study groups (columns 4 and 7).
2. A standard population with a specific number of individuals in each stratum is identified (column 8).
3. The *expected* number of cases in each stratum of the standard population (expected under the assumption that the age-specific incidence rates in the standard population are equal to those of either study group A or B, respectively) is calculated by multiplying each of the corresponding stratum-specific rates observed in study group A (column 9) and in study group B (column 10) times the number of subjects in the equivalent standard population stratum.
4. The overall sums of expected cases in the standard population (based on the rates of A and B) divided by the total number of individuals in the standard population are the *adjusted* or *standardized* incidence rates I_A^* and I_B^* —that is, the incidence rates that would be observed in groups A and B if these populations had exactly the same age distribution as the standard population or, conversely, the incidence that would be observed in the standard population if it had the stratum-specific rates of study group A or the stratum-specific rates of study group B.

It should be evident from looking at the formula for the calculation of the adjusted rates that these are *weighted averages* of the stratum-specific rates in each study group, using as weights the corresponding number of subjects in each stratum of the standard population. The fact that both averages are calculated using the same weights allows their comparison. The resulting adjusted rates can then be used to calculate either the adjusted attributable risk (AR) in those exposed (for standard error of this estimate, see Appendix A, Section A.6) or the relative risk (RR):

$$\text{Adjusted AR} = I_A^* - I_B^*$$

$$\text{Adjusted RR} = \frac{I_A^*}{I_B^*}$$

As discussed in the previous section, the main assumption implicit in the calculation of adjusted attributable risks or relative risks obtained by direct adjustment is that these measures of association are *homogeneous* across the strata of the confounding variable(s)—that is, if an overall summary measure of association across strata of a given variable is calculated, it is assumed that this *average* is reasonably representative of each and all the involved strata. Further specification of this assumption is necessary, namely whether the homogeneity refers to an absolute scale (additive model) or a relative scale (multiplicative model). This concept is simplistically illustrated by the hypothetical situations shown in Tables 7-4 and 7-5, in which there is strong confounding by age: that is, the outcome is more frequent in older than in younger subjects, and the study groups are quite different with regard to their age distributions.

In Table 7-4, the attributable risks are homogeneous across the two age strata (stratum-specific attributable risks = 10%), and both are different from the crude overall attributable risk (20%), denoting a confounding effect by age. Because the stratum-specific attributable risks are homogeneous (identical in this hypothetical example), the weighted average of these differences (i.e., the adjusted attributable risk) does not vary with the choice of the standard population (lower half of Table 7-4). The same is

TABLE 7-4 Hypothetical example of direct adjustment when stratum-specific absolute differences (attributable risks) are homogeneous.

Age (yrs)	Study group A			Study group B			AR (%)	RR
	N	Cases	Rate (%)	N	Cases	Rate (%)		
< 40	100	20	20	400	40	10	**10**	2.00
≥ 40	200	100	50	200	80	40	**10**	1.25
Total	300	120	40	600	120	20	20	2.00

Calculation of the adjusted estimates:

	Younger standard population			Older standard population		
Age (yrs)	N	Expected cases if A rates	Expected cases if B rates	N	Expected cases if A rates	Expected cases if B rates
< 40	500	100	50	100	20	10
≥ 40	100	50	40	500	250	200
Total	600	150	90	600	270	210
Adjusted rate (%)		25	15		45	35
AR		**10%**			**10%**	
RR		1.67			1.29	

Note: AR: attributable risk; RR: relative risk.

not true, however, when calculating an adjusted relative risk in this example: because relative risks vary by age, the adjusted relative risk (i.e., the weighted average of the non-homogeneous age-specific relative risks) depends on which stratum is given more weight when choosing the standard population. For example, because the relative risk is higher in the younger (2.0) than in the older (1.25) stratum, the use of a younger standard population results in a higher age-adjusted relative risk (1.67) than that obtained when using an older standard population (1.29). In conclusion, because there is homogeneity of attributable risks (i.e., no additive interaction), it is appropriate to use directly adjusted rates for the purpose of calculating an age-adjusted attributable risk. Given the heterogeneity of relative risks by age, however, it is not appropriate to estimate an age-adjusted relative risk in this case. In this situation, the adjusted relative risk may vary depending on the standard chosen. This is a matter of special concern in situations in which there is qualitative or strong quantitative interaction.

A situation opposite to that depicted in Table 7-4 is shown in Table 7-5. In the hypothetical example given in Table 7-5, the stratum-specific relative risks are homogeneous; however, the same is not true for the attributable risks. Thus, the adjusted relative risks are identical regardless of the choice of the standard population, but the value of the adjusted attributable risk estimate depends on which stratum is given more weight. For instance, the older standard population yields a higher adjusted attributable risk because the attributable risk is greater for the older (15%) than for the younger (3%) stratum. Thus, given the heterogeneity of stratum-specific attributable risks, it is not appropriate

TABLE 7-5 Hypothetical example of direct adjustment when stratum-specific relative differences (relative risks) are homogeneous.

Age (yrs)	Study group A			Study group B			AR (%)	RR
	N	Cases	Rate (%)	N	Cases	Rate (%)		
< 40	100	6	6	400	12	3	3	**2.00**
≥ 40	200	60	30	200	30	15	15	**2.00**
Total	300	66	22	600	42	7	15	3.14

Calculation of the adjusted estimates:

Age (yrs)	Younger standard population			Older standard population		
	N	Expected cases if A rates	Expected cases if B rates	N	Expected cases if A rates	Expected cases if B rates
< 40	500	30	15	100	6	3
≥ 40	100	30	15	500	150	75
Total	600	60	30	600	156	78
Adjusted rate (%)		10	5		26	13
AR		5%			13%	
RR		**2.00**			**2.00**	

Note: AR: attributable risk; RR: relative risk.

to calculate an age-adjusted attributable risk. On the other hand, an age-adjusted relative risk accurately reflects the homogeneity of multiplicative effects by age when comparing groups *A* and *B*.

Other practical considerations about the direct method of adjustment are as follows:

- This method is used for the *comparison* of rates in two or more study groups; the *absolute* value of an adjusted rate is usually not the main focus because it depends on the choice of the standard population, which is often arbitrary.
- Several options are available for the choice of the standard population, including the following:
  1. An entirely artificial population (e.g., 1000 subjects in each stratum).
  2. One of the study groups. This will make calculations simpler and save time, for the observed rate in the group chosen to be the standard population is, by definition, "standardized." When one of the study groups is particularly small, it should be used as the standard so as to minimize random variability. This is because when the smaller group is used as the standard, there is no need to use its statistically unstable stratum-specific rates to estimate expected numbers of events, as its total observed rate *is* the adjusted rate. The more precise age-specific rates of the other (larger) group(s) produce a more stable expected number of events and thus more precise adjusted rate(s).
  3. The sum of the study populations or groups.

4. A population that may be either a reference population or the population from which the study groups originate (e.g. the population of the state, province or country where the study is conducted—or the whole world when the focus is on comparing several countries). When comparing occupational groups in residents of a metropolitan area, for example, it would be reasonable to select the total metropolitan area working population as the standard. Although this choice is still arbitrary, the resulting adjusted rates will be at least somewhat representative of the "true" study group rates.

5. The so-called *minimum-variance* standard population, which produces the most statistically stable adjusted estimates and is thus particularly useful when sample sizes are small. When two groups are compared using the same notation as in Table 7-3, for each stratum (i), the stratum-specific minimum-variance standard population is calculated as

$$W_i = \frac{1}{\frac{1}{n_{Ai}} + \frac{1}{n_{Bi}}} = \frac{n_{Ai} \times n_{Bi}}{n_{Ai} + n_{Bi}} \quad \text{(Eq. 7.1)}$$

For the example shown in Table 7-4, the minimum-variance standard population would therefore be

Stratum age under 40 years:

$$\text{Standard population} = \frac{100 \times 400}{100 + 400} = 80$$

Stratum age greater than or equal to 40 years:

$$\text{Standard population} = \frac{200 \times 200}{200 + 200} = 100$$

If one of the groups (e.g., population A) is much smaller than the other—that is, if $n_{Ai} \ll n_{Bi}$—then $(1/n_{Ai}) \gg (1/n_{Bi})$, and thus, Equation 7.1 reduces to $W_i \approx n_{Ai}$, which formally supports the recommendation mentioned previously that when one of the groups is small, it should be used as the standard.

- As mentioned previously, although the direct method of adjustment has been traditionally used for age-adjusted comparisons of mortality and morbidity rates by time or place, it is an appropriate method to carry out adjustment for any categorical variables. It can also be used to simultaneously adjust for more than one variable (see layout in Table 7-6). Obviously, the latter application will be limited if there are too many strata and data are sparse.
- The direct method can be used for the adjustment of any rate or proportion (mortality, case fatality rate, incidence per person–time, prevalence). Thus, this method can also be used in the context of a case-control study to obtain the *adjusted* proportions of exposed cases and controls, which in turn could be used to calculate an adjusted odds ratio.

7.3.2 Indirect Adjustment

Like the direct adjustment method, indirect adjustment has been traditionally used for age adjustment of mortality and morbidity data. In the indirect method of adjustment, which has been particularly popular in the field of occupational epidemiology, the expected

TABLE 7-6 Example of layout for using the direct method for simultaneous adjustment for gender, race, and education (categorically defined).

Gender	Race	Education (yrs)	Stratum (i)	Study group A rate	Study group B rate	Standard population (weights)
Male	Black	< 12	1	–	–	–
		≥ 12	2	–	–	–
	White	< 12	3	–	–	–
		≥ 12	4	–	–	–
Female	Black	< 12	5	–	–	–
		≥ 12	6	–	–	–
	White	< 12	7	–	–	–
		≥ 12	8	–	–	–

number of events (e.g., deaths) in a study group (e.g., an occupational cohort) is calculated by applying reference rates ("standard" rates) to the number of individuals in each stratum of the study group(s). For each study group, the ratio of the total number of observed events to the number of expected events (if the rates in the study group were the "standard" rates) provides an estimate of the factor-adjusted relative risk or rate ratio *comparing the study group with the population that served as the source of the reference rates* (Table 7-7). When used in the context of mortality data, this ratio is known as the *standardized mortality ratio* (*SMR*), with similar terms used for morbidity data, such as *standardized incidence ratio* (*SIR*) and *standardized prevalence ratio* (*SPR*). For simplification purposes, the remaining discussion will use the acronym, SMR, even though it also applies to SIR and SPR.

The so-called indirect method is considered to be particularly useful either when stratum-specific risks or rates are missing in one of the groups under comparison or when the study group(s) is (are) small so that the stratum-specific rates are too unstable, thus resulting in statistically unreliable expected numbers when using the direct method (columns 9 and 10 in Table 7-3).

When carrying out indirect adjustment, it is not appropriate to define the population serving as the source of the rates as a "standard population," the reason being that the true standard population is actually the study group(s) to which the external reference ("standard") rates are applied. The calculation of the SMRs is based on applying the rates of a reference population to each study group's distribution. Thus, *when comparing more than one study group to the source of reference rates*, the SMRs are in fact adjusted to different standards (i.e., the study groups themselves). As a corollary, the comparison of SMRs for different study groups may be inappropriate, as illustrated in the hypothetical example in Table 7-8. In this example, the two study groups have identical age-specific rates; however, because of their different age distributions, crude overall rates are different (18.3% and 11.7%). Application of the "standard" (reference) rates to each of these study groups results in expected numbers that are unevenly weighted and, consequently, in different SMRs (0.42 and 0.64). As discussed in detail by Armstrong,[6] this situation arises when the ratios of rates in study groups and in the reference population are not homogeneous across strata.

Thus, although the use of SMRs to compare study groups is a relatively common practice in the epidemiologic literature, it is not always appropriate. SMRs are obviously

7.3 Adjustment Methods Based on Stratification

TABLE 7-7 Indirect adjustment: comparing the observed mortality in a study population with that of an external reference population.

	Study population A		Reference population	
Suspected confounding variable (1)	No. (2)	Observed deaths (3)	Mortality rate (4)	Expected deaths in A if it had rates of reference population (5) = (4) × (2)
Stratum 1	n_{A1}	x_{A1}	M_1	$M_1 \times n_{A1}$
Stratum 2	n_{A2}	x_{A2}	M_2	$M_2 \times n_{A2}$
Stratum 3	n_{A3}	x_{A3}	M_3	$M_3 \times n_{A3}$
...	...	...	...	...
Stratum k	n_{Ak}	x_{Ak}	M_k	$M_k \times n_{Ak}$
Total		$\sum_i x_{Ai}$		$\sum_i [M_i \times n_{Ai}]$

Standardized mortality ratio

$$\text{SMR} = \frac{\text{Observed deaths}}{\text{Expected deaths}} = \frac{\sum_i x_{Ai}}{\sum_i [M_i \times n_{Ai}]}$$

TABLE 7-8 Hypothetical example of two study groups with identical age-specific rates but different age distributions: use of the indirect method using external reference rates results in different SMRs.

	Study group A			Study group B			External reference rates
Age (yrs)	N	Deaths	Rate	N	Deaths	Rate	
< 40	100	10	**10%**	500	50	**10%**	12%
≥ 40	500	100	**20%**	100	20	**20%**	50%
Total	600	**110**	18.3%	600	**70**	11.7%	

	Expected no. of deaths obtained by applying the reference rates to groups A and B	
Age (yrs)	Study group A	Study group B
< 40	12% × 100 = 12	12% × 500 = 60
≥ 40	50% × 500 = 250	50% × 100 = 50
Total number expected	262	110
SMR (observed/expected)	110/262 = **0.42**	70/110 = **0.64**

appropriate when the comparison of interest is that between each study group and the reference population. It is interesting to note that when the goal is to compare two populations (e.g., an occupational group vs the total area population serving as the source of "standard" rates, or any study group vs a reference population), the direct and indirect methods converge: in this situation, the calculation of the SMR can also

FIGURE 7-1 When only two populations are compared, the direct and indirect methods converge. The approach can be regarded as a direct method in which one of the populations (*A*) is the standard or as an indirect method using the other population (*B*) as the source of the reference ("standard") rates.

Suspected confounding variable	Population *A* distribution	Stratum-specific rates in population *B*
Stratum 1	n_{A1}	M_1
Stratum 2	n_{A2}	M_2
Stratum 3	n_{A3}	M_3
.	.	.
.	.	.
.	.	.
Stratum *k*	n_{Ak}	M_k

be thought of as a direct method, with one of the groups under comparison (e.g., an occupational group) serving as the "standard population" (Figure 7-1).

7.3.3 Mantel-Haenszel Method for Estimating an Adjusted Measure of Association

When the measure of association of interest is the odds ratio (e.g., when one is analyzing results of a case-control study), the method described by Mantel and Haenszel[7] to calculate an overall adjusted odds ratio is frequently used for adjusting for one or more categorically defined potential confounders. Table 7-9 shows the notation for the formulation of the Mantel-Haenszel adjusted odds ratio for data stratified into *k* strata:

$$\text{OR}_{\text{MH}} = \frac{\sum_i \frac{a_i d_i}{N_i}}{\sum_i \frac{b_i c_i}{N_i}}$$

which is equivalent to a *weighted average of the stratum-specific odds ratios*.* For standard error and confidence interval estimate, see Appendix A, Section A.8.

The calculation of the OR_{MH} is straightforward, as illustrated by the following examples. In Table 7-1 the crude association between the presence of malaria and gender

---

* This formula is algebraically identical to the following formula:

$$\text{OR}_{\text{MH}} = \frac{\sum_i \left(\frac{b_i c_i}{N_i} \times \frac{a_i d_i}{b_i c_i} \right)}{\sum_i \frac{b_i c_i}{N_i}} = \frac{\sum_i w_i \text{OR}_i}{\sum_i w_i}$$

Thus, the OR_{MH} is a weighted average of the stratum-specific odds ratio (OR_i), with weights equal to each stratum's ($b_i c_i / N_i$).

TABLE 7-9 Notation for the calculation of the Mantel-Haenszel adjusted odds ratio in a case-control study, stratified according to a potential confounding variable.

Stratum i	Cases	Controls	Total
Exposed	a_i	b_i	m_{1i}
Unexposed	c_i	d_i	m_{2i}
Total	n_{1i}	n_{2i}	N_i

suggested that males were at a higher odds of the disease; however, when the association was examined by strata of occupation, no association with gender was observed in either occupational category. In addition to inspecting the occupation-specific odds ratios, a summary odds ratio can be calculated, expressing the occupation-adjusted association between gender and malaria. The adjusted OR_{MH} (the weighted average of the occupational stratum-specific odds ratio) is calculated as follows:

$$OR_{MH} = \frac{\sum_i \frac{a_i d_i}{N_i}}{\sum_i \frac{b_i c_i}{N_i}} = \frac{\frac{53 \times 3}{81} + \frac{35 \times 79}{219}}{\frac{10 \times 15}{81} + \frac{52 \times 53}{219}} = 1.01$$

The estimate of OR_{MH} lies between the stratum-specific estimates (1.06 and 1.00). It is, however, closer to the stratum "mostly indoor occupation" because of the larger sample size in that stratum, for which the estimate is consequently given more "weight" ($b_i c_i / N_i$) when calculating the average adjusted OR_{MH}.

In the example in Table 7-2, the age-adjusted estimate of the OR_{MH} is

$$OR_{MH} = \frac{\sum_i \frac{a_i d_i}{N_i}}{\sum_i \frac{b_i c_i}{N_i}} = \frac{\frac{4 \times 224}{292} + \frac{9 \times 390}{444} + \frac{4 \times 330}{393} + \frac{6 \times 362}{442} + \frac{6 \times 301}{405}}{\frac{2 \times 62}{292} + \frac{12 \times 33}{444} + \frac{33 \times 26}{393} + \frac{65 \times 9}{442} + \frac{93 \times 5}{405}} = 3.97$$

The assumption implicit in the Mantel-Haenszel procedure for the calculation of an adjusted odds ratio is that there is homogeneity of effects (expressed by odds ratios in this case) across the categories of the stratifying variable. In other words, it is assumed that there is no multiplicative interaction between the exposure and the stratifying variable (see Section 6.3.1). For example, when calculating an overall adjusted odds ratio for the data shown in Table 7-2, it is implicitly assumed that the odds ratio of myocardial infarction in relation to oral contraceptive use is approximately 4 (the calculated weighted average being 3.97) for *all* age strata. As discussed previously (Section 7.2), in this example, the observed differences in the stratum-specific odds ratio values are assumed to result from random variation; if the observed heterogeneity is considered excessive, an option is to calculate separate age-adjusted odds ratios for younger and older women, as follows:

$$OR_{MH, 25-34\,y} = \frac{\frac{4 \times 224}{292} + \frac{9 \times 390}{444}}{\frac{2 \times 62}{292} + \frac{12 \times 33}{444}} = 8.3$$

$$\text{OR}_{\text{MH, 35-49 y}} = \frac{\dfrac{4 \times 330}{393} + \dfrac{6 \times 362}{442} + \dfrac{6 \times 301}{405}}{\dfrac{33 \times 26}{393} + \dfrac{65 \times 9}{442} + \dfrac{93 \times 5}{405}} = 2.7$$

Mantel-Haenszel Adjusted Rate Ratio

The Mantel-Haenszel method has been extended to the calculation of an adjusted rate ratio in the context of a cohort study with incidence data based on person-time.[7(pp.219–221)] Table 7-10 shows the general layout of the data from each of the stratum-specific tables. Based on the notation in this table, the Mantel-Haenszel estimate of the adjusted rate ratio is calculated as

$$\text{RR}_{\text{MH}} = \frac{\sum_i \dfrac{a_{1i} y_{0i}}{T_i}}{\sum_i \dfrac{a_{0i} y_{1i}}{T_i}}$$

An example of the application of this formula is presented in Table 7-11, based on data[8] from one of the examples used in Chapter 5 to illustrate the techniques for the assessment of confounding (Section 5.4). The estimated RR_{MH} comparing "high" versus "low" vitamin index intake obtained in Table 7-11 is identical to the corresponding smoking status-adjusted rate ratio when using the direct method of adjustment based on data presented in Table 5-5.

Mantel-Haenszel Method and the Odds Ratio for Paired Case-Control Data

As presented in basic textbooks (e.g., Gordis[5]) and briefly discussed in Section 3.4.1, in matched paired case-control studies, the odds ratio is calculated by dividing the number of pairs in which the case is exposed and the control is not by the number of pairs in which the case is unexposed and the control is exposed. In Table 7-12, each cell represents the number of pairs for the corresponding category defined by case-control and exposure status. Thus, in the two-by-two cross-tabulation shown on the left-hand side of Table 7-12, the odds ratio is estimated as the ratio of discordant pairs, b/c. An example is provided on the right-hand side of the table, from a report from the Atherosclerosis Risk in Communities (ARIC) study on the association between chronic cytomegalovirus (CMV) infection and carotid atherosclerosis (measured by B-mode ultrasound).[9] In this study, atherosclerosis cases and controls were individually matched by age, sex, ethnicity, field center, and date of examination; the paired odds ratio (i.e., the odds ratio controlling for all matching variables) is estimated as $65/42 = 1.55$. The rationale for

TABLE 7-10 Notation for the calculation of the Mantel-Haenszel adjusted rate ratio in a prospective study based on person-time incidence rates stratified according to a potential confounding variable.

Stratum i	Cases	Person-time
Exposed	a_{1i}	y_{1i}
Unexposed	a_{0i}	y_{0i}
Total		T_i

TABLE 7-11 Example for the calculation of the Mantel-Haenszel adjusted rate ratio (RR_{MH}): data on mortality in individuals with high and low vitamin C/beta-carotene intake index, by smoking status, Western Electric Company Study.

	Vitamin C/beta carotene intake index	No. of deaths	Person-years	Stratified RRs
Nonsmokers	High	53	5143	RR = 0.77
	Low	57	4260	
	Total		9403	
smokers	High	111	6233	RR = 0.83
	Low	138	6447	
	Total		12,680	

$$RR_{MH} = \frac{\sum_i \frac{a_{1i} y_{0i}}{T_i}}{\sum_i \frac{a_{0i} y_{1i}}{T_i}} = \frac{\frac{53 \times 4260}{9403} + \frac{111 \times 6447}{12,680}}{\frac{57 \times 5143}{9403} + \frac{138 \times 6233}{12,680}} = 0.81$$

Note: The "moderate" vitamin intake index category in Table 5-4 has been omitted for simplicity. All rates ratios in the table compare those with "high" with those with "low" vitamin intake index.
Source: Data from DK Pandey et al., Dietary Vitamin C and β-Carotene and Risk of Death in Middle-Aged Men, The Western Electric Study. *American Journal of Epidemiology*, Vol 142, pp. 1269–1278, © 1995.

TABLE 7-12 Layout of a two-by-two table for the calculation of a paired odds ratio and an example.

		Notation				Example*	
		Controls				Controls	
		Exposed	Unexposed			CMV+	CMV−
Cases	Exposed	a	b	Cases	CMV+	214	65
	Unexposed	c	d		CMV−	42	19
	Paired OR $= \frac{b}{c}$				Paired OR $= \frac{65}{42} = 1.55$		

Note: Each cell represents the number of pairs for each category defined by case-control and exposure status.
*Cases represent individuals with carotid atherosclerosis defined by B-mode ultrasound; controls are individuals without atherosclerosis, individually match-paired to cases by age group, sex, ethnicity, field center, and date of examination. Cytomegalovirus (CMV) infection status is defined according to the presence or absence of IgG serum antibodies.
Source: Data from PD Sorlie et al., Cytomegalovirus/Herpesvirus and Carotid Atherosclerosis: The ARIC Study. *Journal of Medical Virology*, Vol 42, pp. 33–37, © 1994.

estimating the odds ratio as the ratio of discordant pairs in a matched case-control study is readily grasped by the application of the Mantel-Haenszel method for averaging stratified odds ratios.

The data in Table 7-12 can be rearranged as in Table 7-13, where each of the 340 pairs in this study is now a stratum with a size n of 2. The resulting 340 two-by-two tables can be arranged as in Table 7-13 because the pairs can only be one of four possible types (each of the cells in Table 7-12): for example, for the first type of pair in which both case and control are CMV+ (cell "a" on the left panel of Table 7-12), there

TABLE 7-13 Calculation of the paired odds ratio for the data in Table 7-12, based on the Mantel-Haenszel estimation approach.

Four possible pair types:	Exp	Case	Cont	Total	No. of pairs in Table 7-12	Each pair contributes to OR_{MH} Numerator $\left(\dfrac{a \times d}{N}\right)$	Denominator $\left(\dfrac{b \times c}{N}\right)$
Type 1 Concordant	+	1	1				
	−	0	0	2	$a = 214$	0	0
Type 2 Discordant	+	1	0				
	−	0	1	2	$b = 65$	½	0
Type 3 Discordant	+	0	1				
	−	1	0	2	$c = 42$	0	½
Type 4 Concordant	+	0	0				
	−	1	1	2	$d = 19$	0	0

$$OR_{MH} = \frac{(214 \times 0) + (65 \times 1/2) + (42 \times 0) + (19 \times 0)}{(214 \times 0) + (65 \times 0) + (42 \times 1/2) + (19 \times 0)} = \frac{65 \times 1/2}{42 \times 1/2} = \frac{65}{42} = \frac{b}{c}$$

Note: Exp: exposure status; Cont: controls; OR: odds ratio.

would be a total of 214 identical tables; for the second type (the "b" cell, discordant, with case exposed and control unexposed), there would be 65 tables; and so on. In the last two columns of Table 7-13, the contribution to the numerator and denominator of the OR_{MH} of each of the 340 pairs is indicated. The contribution (to either the numerator or the denominator) from all the strata based on concordant pairs is always 0, whereas the discordant pairs contribute to either the numerator ("b"-type pairs) or the denominator ("c"-type pairs). All of these contributions, which are always ½—that is, $(1 \times 1)/2$—cancel out, with the actual number of discordant pairs in the numerator and the denominator resulting in the well-known formula $OR_{MH} = b/c$. Thus, this formula represents a *weighted average odds ratio for stratified data (using the Mantel-Haenszel weighing approach), where the strata are defined on the basis of matched pairs.*

When there is more than one control per case, the ratio of discrepant pairs, by definition, cannot be used, but the use of the Mantel-Haenszel approach allows the estimation of the odds ratio, adjusted for the matching variables. Table 7-14 shows a hypothetical example of the application of this approach in a case-control study with two controls individually matched to each case.

7.3.4 Limitations of Stratification-Based Methods of Adjustment

The techniques described in the previous sections (direct and indirect adjustment, Mantel-Haenszel odds ratio or rate ratio) can be used for multivariate analysis; that is, for simultaneously controlling for more than one covariate. This can be done simply by constructing the strata based on all possible combinations of the adjustment variables (e.g., see Table 7-6). These stratification-based methods, however, have practical limitations for multivariate adjustment, as follows:

TABLE 7-14 Example of the use of the Mantel-Haenszel approach in a matched case-control study with two controls per case.

Exposed	Case	Control	Total	No. of Pairs	Numerator $\left(\dfrac{a \times d}{N}\right)$	Denominator $\left(\dfrac{b \times c}{N}\right)$
Yes	1	0				
No	0	2	3	200	0.67	0
Yes	1	1				
No	0	1	3	100	0.33	0
Yes	0	1				
No	1	1	3	50	0	0.33
Yes	0	2				
No	1	0	3	30	0	0.67
Yes	0	0				
No	1	2	3	120	0	0
Yes	1	2				
No	0	0	3	40	0	0

Above: "Each pair contributes to OR$_{MH}$"

$$\text{OR}_{MH} = \frac{(200 \times 0.67) + (100 \times 0.33) + (50 \times 0) + (30 \times 0) + (120 \times 0) + (40 \times 0)}{(200 \times 0) + (100 \times 0) + (50 \times 0.33) + (30 \times 0.67) + (120 \times 0) + (40 \times 0)} = \frac{167.0}{36.6} = 4.56$$

Note: OR: odds ratio.

1. Although they can be used to adjust for several covariates simultaneously, adjustment is carried out only for the association between one independent variable and an outcome at a time. For example, to assess the association of oral contraceptives with myocardial infarction while controlling for age and educational level, it would be necessary to create one two-by-two table for oral contraceptives vis-à-vis myocardial infarction for each stratum defined by combining age groups and educational levels. If the exposure of interest were educational level and the covariates to be adjusted for were age and oral contraceptive use, however, a new set of two-by-two tables would have to be created (representing education vs myocardial infarction for each stratum defined by categories of age and oral contraceptive use).

2. These methods allow adjustment only for categorical covariates (e.g., gender); continuous covariates need to be categorized, as age was in the example shown in Table 7-2. Residual differences within these more or less arbitrarily defined categories may in turn result in residual confounding (Section 7.6 and Chapter 5, Section 5.5.4).

3. Finally, data become sparse when the strata are too numerous. For the direct method, for example, if the sample size of a given stratum is 0, no corresponding stratum-specific rate is available for application to the standard population in that stratum; as a result, the adjusted rate becomes undefined.

Thus, in practice, stratification methods are usually limited to simultaneous adjustment for few categorical confounders (usually one or two), with a small number of categories each. When simultaneous adjustment for multiple covariates (including continuous variables) is needed, methods based on multiple-regression techniques are typically used.

7.4 MULTIPLE REGRESSION TECHNIQUES FOR ADJUSTMENT

Multiple-regression techniques are better suited to address the limitations of the simpler techniques discussed heretofore, as they allow the examination of the effects of all exposure variables reciprocally and simultaneously adjusting for all the other variables in the model. In addition, they allow adjusting for continuous covariates, and within reasonable limits, they are generally more efficient than stratification-based methods when data are sparse. Moreover, in addition to multivariate *adjustment*, multiple-regression techniques are useful for *prediction* (that is, for estimating the predicted value of a certain outcome as a function of given values of independent variables, as in the case of the prediction equations of coronary risk that were developed from the Framingham study using logistic regression)[10] (see Section 7.4.3).

The sections that follow describe four of the most frequently used regression models for multivariate adjustment in epidemiology: (1) linear regression, used when the outcome is continuous (e.g., blood pressure); (2) logistic regression, preferentially used when the outcome is categorical (cumulative incidence, prevalence); (3) proportional hazards (Cox) regression, used in survival analysis; and (4) Poisson regression, used when incidence rate (based on person-time) is the outcome of interest. It is beyond the scope of this chapter to discuss these techniques in detail; for this, the reader is referred to a general statistics textbook (e.g., Armitage et al.[11]) and to the specific references given in each section. Instead, the discussion focuses on the applied aspects of multiple regression.

In spite of their different applications and even though only one of the models is specifically defined as "linear," the fundamental underpinning of all regression techniques discussed in this chapter is a *linear function*. This can be clearly seen in Table 7-15, in which the right-hand side of all models is exactly the same $(b_0 + b_1x_1 + b_2x_2 + \ldots + b_kx_k)$, thus explaining why they are collectively termed *generalized linear models*. The models listed in the table differ only with regard to the

TABLE 7-15 Multiple regression models and interpretation of the regression coefficients.

	Model	Interpretation of b_1
Linear	$y = b_0 + b_1x_1 + b_2x_2 + \ldots + b_kx_k$	Increase in outcome y mean value (continuous variable) per unit increase in x_1, adjusted for all other variables in the model
Logistic	$\log(\text{odds}) = b_0 + b_1x_1 + b_2x_2 + \ldots + b_kx_k$	Increase in the log odds of the outcome per unit increase in x_1, adjusted for all other variables in the model
Cox	$\log(\text{hazard}) = b_0 + b_1x_1 + b_2x_2 + \ldots + b_kx_k$	Increase in the log hazard of the outcome per unit increase in x_1, adjusted for all other variables in the model
Poisson	$\log(\text{rate}) = b_0 + b_1x_1 + b_2x_2 + \ldots + b_kx_k$	Increase in the log rate of the outcome per unit increase in x_1, adjusted for all other variables in the model

type of dependent variable or outcome postulated to be related to predictors in a linear fashion. Consequently, and as underscored in the sections that follow, the interpretation of the multiple-regression coefficients is similar for all these models, varying only with regard to the outcome variable.

In the next section, the concept of linear regression is reviewed in the context of the simplest situation, namely that involving only one predictor variable (one x). The four sections that follow briefly review the basic features of the regression models listed in Table 7-15. Finally, Sections 7.4.6 to 7.4.8 cover issues regarding the application of these models to matched and nested studies and to situations when a "linear" model is not reasonable, as well as issues related to statistical inference based on the parameter estimates.

7.4.1 Linear Regression: General Concepts

Simple linear regression is a statistical technique usually employed to assess the association between two continuous variables. Figure 7-2, for example, shows a plot of the cross-sectional values of systolic blood pressure (SBP) and the carotid intimal-medial thickness (IMT), a measure of atherosclerosis obtained by B-mode ultrasound imaging, in a subset of 1410 participants from the ARIC study.[12] Each dot in the scatter of points represents an individual, with corresponding SBP and IMT values in the abscissa and ordinate, respectively. It can be seen that although there is a wide scatter, there is a tendency for the IMT values to be higher when SBP is also higher, and vice versa. This pattern warrants the assessment of whether SBP and IMT are *linearly* associated. The hypothesis regarding a possible linear association between these two continuous variables can be expressed as the following questions:

1. Is the average increase in IMT levels associated with a given increase in SBP approximately constant throughout the entire range of SBP values?

2. Can the association between SBP and IMT be assumed to follow a straight-line pattern (the statistical *model*) with the scatter around the line being the consequence of random error?

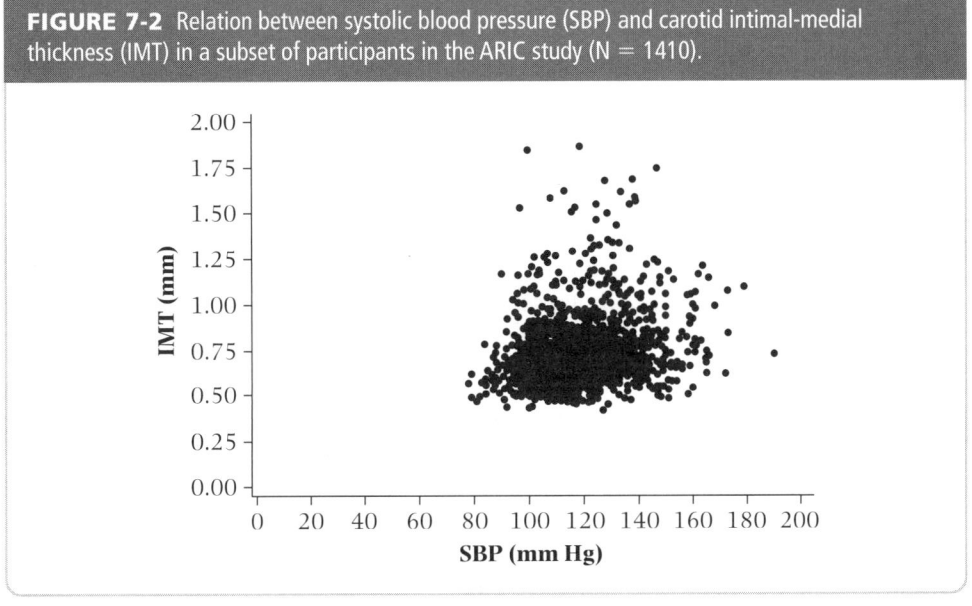

FIGURE 7-2 Relation between systolic blood pressure (SBP) and carotid intimal-medial thickness (IMT) in a subset of participants in the ARIC study (N = 1410).

Note: IMT: intimal-medial thickness; SBP: systolic blood pressure.

In addition to inspecting the scatter plot visually (e.g., Figure 7-2), assessing whether the relationship between two continuous variables (e.g., SBP and IMT) is *statistically compatible* with a perfect straight line can be done by calculating the *Pearson linear correlation coefficient* (r) (see, e.g., Armitage et al.,[11(pp195–197)] as well as an application in Chapter 8, Section 8.4.2). The correlation coefficient values range from −1.0 (when there is a perfect negative correlation—i.e., when all the points form a perfect straight line with a negative slope) to +1.0 (when there is a perfect positive correlation—i.e., when the points form a straight line with a positive slope). A value of 0 indicates no linear correlation. In the example in Figure 7-2, the value of the Pearson correlation coefficient is 0.21, with a corresponding *p* value of 0.0001. The small *p* value in this example suggests that there is some kind of linear correlation between SBP and IMT not likely to be explained by chance, even though the magnitude of the coefficient implies that the correlation is only moderate. This conclusion fits the graphical display in Figure 7-2: although there is an average tendency for higher SBP values to be associated with higher IMT values, there is a substantial dispersion of values around this hypothetical linear relationship.

The correlation coefficient value contains no information about the *strength* of the association between the two variables that is represented by the slope of the hypothetical line, such as the amount of increase to be expected in IMT per unit increase in SBP. To estimate the strength of the linear association, it is necessary to find the formula for the regression line that best fits the observed data. This line can be formulated in terms of two parameters (β_0 and β_1), which relate the mean (expected) value of the *dependent variable* (conventionally noted as $E(y)$ and placed in the ordinate of the plot) as a function of the *independent* or *predictor variable* (conventionally noted as x, in the abscissa). The general formula for the regression line is

$$E(y) = \beta_0 + \beta_1 x$$

"$E(y)$" is also known as the "predicted" value of y as a function of x. Heretofore, it is denoted as "y" to simplify the notation.

Figure 7-3 shows the graphic representation of this general regression line. Inspection of this formula and the figure underscores the straightforward interpretation of the two parameters, β_0 and β_1 as follows:

- β_0 is the *intercept*—that is, the estimated value of y when $x = 0$.
- β_1 is the *regression coefficient*—that is, the estimated increase in the dependent variable (y) per unit increase in the predictor variable (x). Thus, when $x = 1$, then $y = \beta_0 + \beta_1$; for $x = \square 2$, then $y = \beta_0 + \beta_1 \times 2$, and so on. This regression coefficient corresponds to the slope of the regression line; it reflects the *strength* of the association between the two variables—that is, how much increase (or decrease, in the case of a descending line) in y is to be expected (or predicted) as x increases. The absolute value of β_1 depends on the units of measurement for both x and y.

After this *statistical model* is formulated, the practical question is how to estimate the regression line that *best* fits a given set of data, such as the data in Figure 7-2. (In linear regression, the method often used to estimate the values of the regression coefficients [or "parameters"] is the *least-squares method*. This consists in finding the parameter values that minimize the sum of the squares of the vertical distances between each of the observed points and the line. (For details on the methods to estimate the regression line, see any general statistics textbook, e.g., Armitage et al.[11] or Kleinbaum et al.,[13] or a more

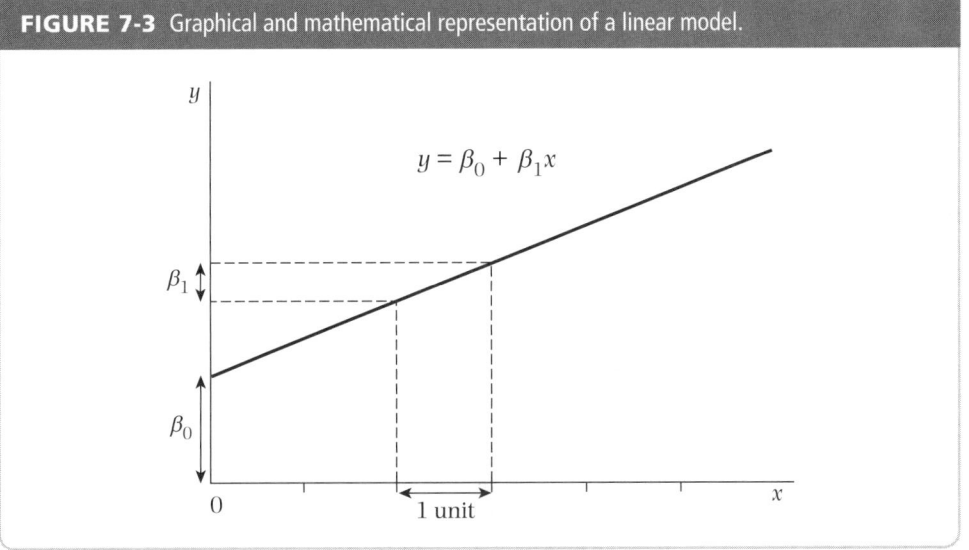

FIGURE 7-3 Graphical and mathematical representation of a linear model.

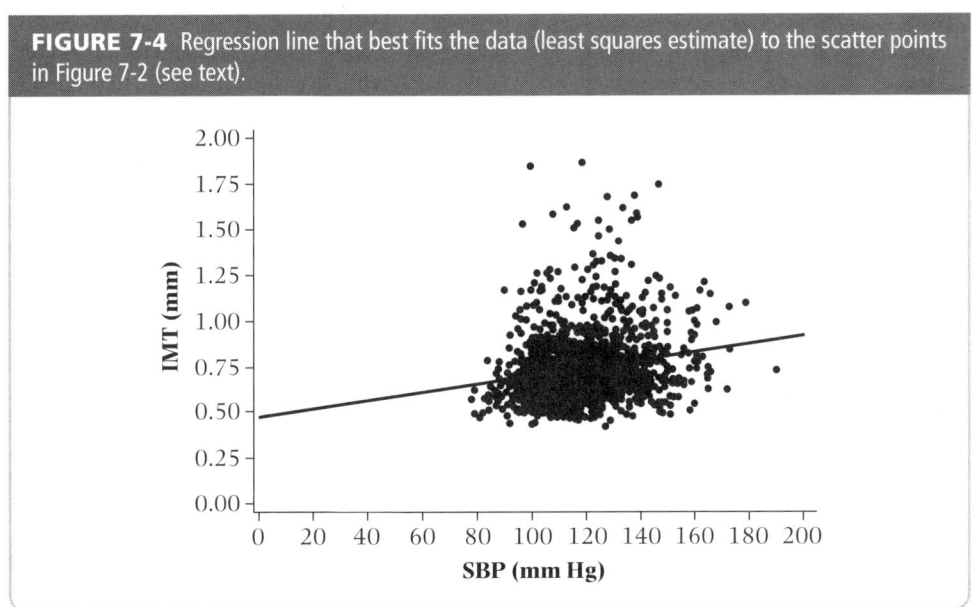

FIGURE 7-4 Regression line that best fits the data (least squares estimate) to the scatter points in Figure 7-2 (see text).

Note: IMT: intimal-medial thickness; SBP: systolic blood pressure.

specialized text, e.g., Draper and Smith.[14]). For example, Figure 7-4 shows the regression line that best fits the observed data shown in Figure 7-2. The notation traditionally used to represent the estimated linear regression line is as follows:

$$y = b_0 + b_1 x + e$$

That is, the symbols for the parameters denoted by the Greek letter beta (β) are replaced by the letter b to denote that these are *estimates*. The error term, e, represents the difference between each observed y value and the corresponding predicted value (e.g., the vertical distance between each point in the scatter in Figure 7-4 and the y value at the line). (For the sake of simplicity, the error term will be omitted from the remaining formulas in this chapter.) Returning to Figure 7-4, the mathematical formula for the estimated regression line shown in the figure is

$$\text{IMT (mm)} = 0.4533 + 0.0025 \times \text{SBP (mm Hg)} \qquad \text{(Eq. 7.2)}$$

The value of the intercept (0.4533 mm in this example) is purely theoretical; it does not have any real biological relevance in this case. It corresponds to the estimated IMT when SBP = 0 (i.e., when the previous equation reduces to IMT [mm] = 0.4533). The fact that the intercept is biologically meaningless is a common occurrence in many applications of linear regression in biomedical research because the value of 0 for many variables is not biologically viable or has no practical relevance. This is illustrated in Figure 7-4 and schematically in Figure 7-5, which shows how the intercept value is often a mere extrapolation of the regression line to meet the ordinate (y axis), well beyond the range of biologically plausible values.*

More relevant in most circumstances is the value of the regression coefficient. In the previous example, the estimate of the regression coefficient for SBP implies that, in these cross-sectional data, an SBP increase of 1 mm Hg is associated with an average IMT increase of 0.0025 mm. This regression coefficient is the slope of the line in Figure 7-4, expressing the *strength* of the association between SBP and IMT, in contrast with the

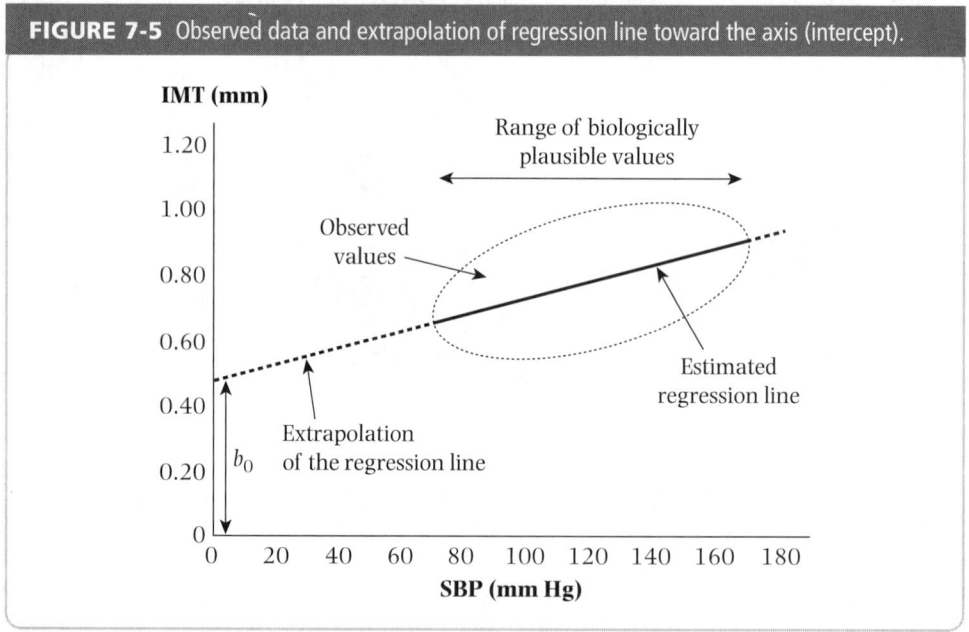

FIGURE 7-5 Observed data and extrapolation of regression line toward the axis (intercept).

Note: IMT: intimal-medial thickness; SBP: systolic blood pressure.

---

*The value of the intercept is useful if the investigator's intention is to use the regression results to predict the expected value of the dependent variable, given certain characteristics. To solve the equation, one needs to use the values of all the coefficients, including the intercept (see examples in the context of logistic regression in Section 7.4.3).

There are ways to improve the interpretability of the intercept by using transformations of the original continuous variables in the regression. For example, the mean systolic blood pressure could be subtracted from each individual's blood pressure value in the study population in Figure 7-4. This new variable (i.e., the difference between each individual's blood pressure and the mean) could then be used in the regression, instead of the actual blood pressure value. In this case, even though the intercept is still defined as the estimated IMT for an individual with a value of 0 for the independent variables (x), it can be interpreted as the estimated IMT for an individual with the *average* blood pressure value in the study population.

correlation coefficient, which only evaluates the degree to which a given set of quantitative data fits a straight line.

The previous model assumes that the increase is *linear* (i.e., that the increase in IMT as a function of the increase in SBP is constant). This assumption is obviously implicit in the fact that one single regression coefficient was given in the previous equation (0.0025 mm increase in IMT per mm Hg increase in SBP), which is assumed to apply to the entire range of SBP values. Whether this simple model is appropriate will depend on each particular circumstance, as discussed in more detail in Section 7.4.7.

Another important issue when interpreting the "slope" (regression coefficient) of a regression function is the unit to which it corresponds. For example, it may be expressed as the increase in IMT per 5 mm Hg increase in SBP, rather than per 1 mm Hg, which would then be translated as a value of $5 \times 0.0025 = 0.0125$ mm in this example. The importance of specifying the units of variables x and y when reporting and interpreting the magnitude of the regression coefficient (slope) cannot be sufficiently emphasized.

It is important to keep in mind, however, that comparison of the strength of the association between different variables (particularly continuous variables) based on the size of the regression coefficients should generally be avoided. This is related to the general problem of comparing the strength of the associations across different variables that was discussed in Chapter 3 (Section 3.5); further discussion of this issue is presented in Chapter 9, Section 9.3.4.

The regression coefficient (b_1) estimates the average increase in the dependent variable (e.g., IMT) per unit increase in the independent variable (e.g., SBP), and like any other statistical estimate, it is subject to uncertainty and random error. Thus, it is important to estimate the standard error of the regression coefficient to evaluate its statistical significance and to calculate the confidence limits around its point estimate (see Section 7.4.8 and Appendix A). The standard error (SE) estimate is readily provided by most statistical packages performing linear regression; for the regression coefficient $b_1 = 0.0025$ in the previous example, it was estimated as $SE(b_1) = 0.00032$.

Both the line in Figure 7-4 and the corresponding mathematical formula (Equation 7.2) can be seen as a way to summarize data (a sort of "sketch") that tries to capture the "essence" of the relationship of interest, while avoiding unnecessary and cumbersome details subject to random variability and measurement error (see Section 7.8). The attractiveness of the model proposed in the example—that the relationship between SBP and IMT is linear—lies in its simplicity and the fact that the regression coefficient has a very straightforward and easy interpretation: it is the slope of the regression function, or the average increase in IMT (in mm) per mm Hg increase in SBP. This model, however, may not be either appropriate or the best to describe the data. It is, for example, possible that additional parameters describing more complex relationships (e.g., a curve) may better describe the data. Adding new parameters to the model (e.g., a square term to take into account a curvilinear relationship) may improve its predictive capabilities (see Section 7.4.7); however, this often results in a more complex interpretation of the regression coefficient(s). There is usually a trade-off between simplicity (interpretability) and completeness (predictive power, statistical fit) of any statistical model. In the last section of this chapter (Section 7.8), conceptual issues related to the art and science of statistical modeling are briefly discussed.

An additional example of the use of linear regression is based on the ecological analysis discussed in Chapter 1. Figure 1-10 displays the death rates for coronary heart disease (CHD) in men from 16 cohorts included in the Seven Countries Study vs an estimate of the mean fat intake in each study site.[15] That figure also shows the value of the correlation coefficient ($r = 0.84$), which indicates to which extent the scatter of points fits a straight line; the corresponding regression equation is

$$y = -83 + (25.1 \times x)$$

where y is the 10-year rate of coronary mortality (per 10,000) and x is the percentage of calories from fat in the diet. The regression estimates can be interpreted as follows:

- The intercept (–83) has a basically meaningless "real-life" interpretation, as it represents the theoretical rate in a country where there is no consumption of fat whatsoever. Its negative value underscores its merely theoretical interpretation.
- The regression coefficient (25.1) represents the estimated average increase in the 10-year coronary mortality (per 10,000) associated with a 1% increase in the proportion of calories from fat in the diet. In other words, according to this model, an increment of 1% in the proportion of calories from fat is related to an increase of 0.00251 (or 2.51 per thousand) in coronary mortality over 10 years. (Obviously, any causal inference from data such as these must take into consideration the possibility of ecologic fallacy or other biases.) As in the preceding example, the previous model also assumes that the increase is *linear*: i.e., that the increase in mortality as a function of the increase in dietary fat is constant so that it is as harmful for the level of fat in the diet to change from 10% to 11% as it is to change from 40% to 41%. On the other hand, careful inspection of the data in the figure suggests that the increase in mortality may be *nonlinear*: that the relationship may be curvilinear, with sharper increases in mortality at higher than at lower levels of dietary fat intake. To examine this alternative hypothesis, it would be necessary to test nonlinear models by including quadratic terms or dummy variables (see Section 7.4.7).
- Finally, it is beyond the scope of this text to discuss statistical properties and assumptions related to the use of linear regression. Detailed discussions of these topics can be found in general statistics textbooks (e.g., Armitage et al.[11]) as well as more specialized textbooks (e.g., Draper and Smith[14]).

7.4.2 Multiple Linear Regression

The extension of the simple linear regression model (see previous section) to a multivariate situation is based on the so-called multiple-linear regression models. Multiple-linear regression models are typically used for adjustment when the outcome (the y or dependent variable) is a continuous variable, although an application for a binary outcome is briefly discussed at the end of this section. The question is whether a given variable (x_1) is *linearly* associated with the outcome (y), after controlling for a number of other covariates (e.g., x_2 and x_3). The corresponding linear regression model is written as follows:

$$y = \beta_0 + \beta_1 x_1 + \beta_2 x_2 + \beta_3 x_3$$

The postulated risk factors (x's or independent variables) can be either continuous or categorical (e.g., dichotomous), as shown in the example later. Categorical variables can have multiple levels, which can be either treated as ordinal or transformed in a set of binary (indicator) variables (see Section 7.4.7).

As an example of the use of multiple linear regression, it may be of interest to know whether SBP is linearly associated with carotid IMT (as a proxy for atherosclerosis) and whether this association is independent of age, gender, and body weight. The results of a series of multiple regression analyses to answer this question, using the subset of individuals from the ARIC study that was used in the example in the preceding section are shown in Table 7-16.

The first model is based on the same example discussed previously and includes only SBP as the independent variable (Figure 7-4 and Equation 7.2). Model 2 adds the variable age and can be written as follows:

$$\text{IMT(mm)} = \beta_0 + \beta_1 \times \text{SBP(mm Hg)} + \beta_2 \times \text{Age (years)}$$

The estimated values of the regression coefficients, obtained by the least squares method (see previous section), are displayed in Table 7-16 (model 2). Using these values, the equation can be rewritten as a function of the estimates: that is, b_0, b_1, and b_2 (again omitting the error term, e, for simplicity):

$$\text{IMT(mm)} = -0.0080 + 0.0016 \times \text{SBP(mm Hg)} + 0.0104 \times \text{Age (years)} \quad \text{(Eq. 7.3)}$$

To represent this model graphically, a three-dimensional plot is needed: one dimension for SBP, one for age, and one for IMT. The scatter of points will be a three-dimensional *cloud* of points in this three-axis space and the model in Equation 7.3 expresses the formula of a *plane* that is supposed to fit this three-dimensional scatter (i.e., of the linear relations between the three variables). Each of the regression coefficients in model 2 can be interpreted as follows:

- The intercept ($b_0 = -0.008$) corresponds to the estimated IMT of a 0-year-old individual with SBP = 0 mm Hg; as in the preceding example, this represents an extrapolation with no practical use or meaningful interpretation (see Section 7.4.1).
- The regression coefficient for SBP ($b_1 = 0.0016$ mm) represents the estimated average increase in IMT per mm Hg increase in SBP *while controlling for age effects* (i.e., after the associations of age with both SBP and IMT have been removed).
- Similarly, the regression coefficient for age ($b_2 = 0.0104$ mm) represents the estimated average increase in IMT per year increase in age *while controlling for SBP* (i.e., after removing the associations of SBP with both age and IMT).

TABLE 7-16 Multiple-linear regression analyses of the cross-sectional association between systolic blood pressure and carotid IMT (mm) in a subset of participants of the Washington County cohort of the Atherosclerosis Risk in Communities (ARIC) Study, ages 45–64 years, 1987–1989.

	Linear regression coefficient			
	Model 1	Model 2	Model 3	Model 4
Intercept	0.4533	−0.0080	0.0107	−0.0680
Systolic blood pressure (1 mm Hg)	0.0025	0.0016	0.0014	0.0012
Age (1 yr)	Not included	0.0104	0.0096	0.0099
Gender (1 = male, 0 = female)	Not included	Not included	0.0970	0.0981
Body mass index (1 kg/m²)	Not included	Not included	Not included	0.0033

Note: IMT: intimal-medial thickness of the carotid arteries (measured in millimeters): average of B-mode ultrasound measurements taken at six sites of the carotid arteries in both sides of the neck.

(For a succinct derivation and additional interpretation of the adjusted regression coefficients in multiple linear regression, the reader should consult Kahn and Sempos.[16] More detailed discussions of multiple regression can be found in the statistical textbooks referred to previously.)

The estimated coefficient for SBP (b_1 = 0.0016 mm) in model 2 is smaller than the corresponding coefficient in model 1 (0.0025 mm). This is because age is a confounder of the relationship between SBP and IMT. In other words, some of the apparent relationship between SBP and IMT observed in the crude analysis (model 1) appears to be due to the fact that people with higher SBP tend to be older, and older people tend to have a higher degree of atherosclerosis. In model 2, the strength of the association between SBP and IMT is reduced because the (positive) confounding effect of age is removed, at least partially (see Section 7.6).

An important assumption in the model represented in Equation 7.3 is that there is *no interaction between SBP and age*, the two variables included in the model. In other words, implicit in the formulation of this statistical model ($y = \beta_0 = \beta_1 x_1 + \beta_2 x_2$) is the fact that the change in y associated with a unit change in x_1 is assumed to be constant for the entire range of x_2, and vice versa. In the previous example, the increase in IMT per unit increase in SBP, the estimate b_1 = 0.0016 mm, is not only adjusted for age but also should be applicable to individuals of all ages (and the converse is true for b_2). If interaction is present—that is, for example, if the association of SBP with IMT is deemed to be different between older and younger individuals—the previous model (Equation 7.3) will not be appropriate. As discussed in Chapter 6, when a given factor (in this example, age) modifies the effect of the variable of interest (in this example, SBP), it is recommended that the association between the variable of interest and the outcome be assessed in strata formed by the effect modifier categories. Thus, rather than age adjustment, age-stratified models (i.e., separate models for each age group) should be used, a situation that is analogous to the examples discussed in Section 7.2. An alternative analytical technique to deal with interaction in the context of multiple-regression analyses is to include *interaction terms* (also known as *product terms*) in the regression equation. For instance, in the present example, if an interaction between SBP and age is suspected, the following model can be used:

$$\text{IMT} = \beta_0 + (\beta_1 \times \text{SBP}) + (\beta_2 \times \text{age}) + [\beta_3 \times (\text{SBP} \times \text{age})] \quad \text{(Eq. 7.4)}$$

where (SBP × age) represents a new variable that is obtained by multiplying the values of SBP and age in each individual. If SBP and age were binary variables, the previous model would be analogous to stratified models. In comparison with stratified analyses, the use of interaction terms increases the statistical efficiency and has the advantage of allowing the evaluation of interaction between continuous variables. The interaction term can be conceptualized as the excess change not explained by the sum of the individual independent effects of two independent (x) variables; it is schematically represented in Figure 6-3 of Chapter 6 (Interaction) by the excess, "I," on the joint-effect column (right-hand side). If interaction is present, the inclusion of the interaction term in the model is important for prediction, as it increases the amount of the variability in the outcome explained by the full model vis-à-vis the sum of the isolated effects of the individual predictors in the model.

When two variables x_2 and x_3 interact and the effect of another variable x_1 is of interest, it is important to adjust x_1 for x_2, x_3 *and* the interaction term ($x_2 \times x_3$). Adjusting for the interaction term is important because the distributions of x_2 or x_3 (when examined individually) may be the same for the different categories of x_1 (say, exposed vs unexposed), but the distributions of the *joint* presence of x_2 and x_3 ($x_2 \times x_3$) may be different, and thus the interaction term may act as a confounding variable. (See Chapter 6, Section 6.8, and Table 6-24) In addition, as interaction itself is amenable to confounding effects (see Chapter 6, Section 6.10.2), it is obviously important to adjust the interaction term for the other variables in the model. For more details, refer to biostatistics textbooks (e.g., Armitage et al.[11])

Model 3 in Table 7-16 adds a new variable, gender. This is a dichotomous variable, arbitrarily assigned a value of 1 for males and 0 for females. As with any other variable, the coefficient $b_3 = 0.097$ is interpreted as the adjusted increase in IMT (mm) per "unit increase in gender," only that what this actually means in this case is the average difference in IMT between males and females, adjusted for the other variables in the model (SBP and age) (Figure 7-6). (If the variable gender had been coded as 1 for females and 0 for males, the results would have been identical to those shown in Table 7-16, except that the sign of the coefficient would have been negative—i.e., $b_3 = -0.097$, representing the difference, females minus males, in IMT.)

The interpretation of the coefficients in model 4, shown in Table 7-16, is consistent with that of models 2 and 3, except that there is additional adjustment for body mass index (BMI). As seen in the table, the magnitude of the coefficient for SBP decreased in models 3 and 4, thus implying that not only age but also gender and BMI were (positive) confounders of the observed relationship between SBP and IMT. The increase in IMT per mm Hg increase in SBP after simultaneously controlling for age, gender, and BMI (model 4; 0.0012 mm) is about one-half of the estimated value when none of these variables was adjusted for (model 1; 0.0025 mm). For inferential purposes, it is important to consider

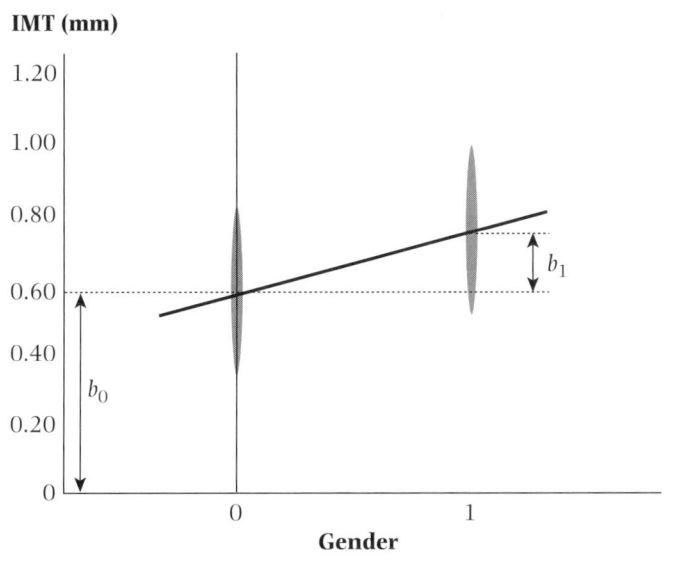

FIGURE 7-6 Graphical interpretation of the regression coefficient for a dichotomous variable, such as gender (as in models 3 and 4 in Table 7-16). For analogy with the regression situation with a continuous independent variable (e.g., Figure 7-4), the regression line is plotted between the two clusters, even though no values are possible between $x = 0$ and $x = 1$. Note that intercept (b_0) corresponds to the mean IMT value in females ($x = 0$), while the regression coefficient (b_1) represents the average difference between males and females.

Note: IMT: intimal-medial thickness.

the possibility that confounders not included in the model and residual confounding due, for example, to misclassification of covariates such as BMI, may be responsible for at least part of the apparent residual "effect" of SBP, denoted by a regression coefficient of 0.0012 mm (see Section 7.6).

As indicated in Figure 7-4, a model with one independent variable (model 1) can be easily represented in a graph; so can model 2, although it would require a three-dimensional graph. In contrast, models 3 and 4 (i.e., regression models with more than three dimensions—with one y variable and more than two x variables) cannot be represented in a simple graph; however, the interpretation of the regression coefficients of models 3 and 4 remains analogous to that of models 1 and 2: these coefficients still represent the average estimated increase in the y variable per unit increase in the corresponding x variable, simultaneously adjusted for all other x variables in the model. As an extension of the previous discussion regarding model 2, the formulations for models 3 and 4 also imply *lack of interaction between the independent variables* included in the model: in other words, the effect of each variable (each estimated b) is assumed to be constant across all levels of the other variables. The presence of interactions would require conducting stratified analysis or including "interaction terms" in the model as previously described.

A further example of multiple-linear regression results taken from a study assessing correlates of leukocyte count in middle-aged adults[17] is shown in Table 7-17. In interpreting the findings in the table, the following points must be emphasized: (1) all coefficients refer to units of the dependent variable (i.e., 1000 leukocytes/mm^3), and (2) each linear regression coefficient represents the expected change in the mean leukocyte count for a given unit change of the independent variable, while simultaneously adjusting for all other variables included in the regression model. To be interpretable, the units of the regression coefficients must be specified (e.g., for age, a 5-year increment) (see Section 7.4.1). The negative sign of a coefficient means that, on average, the leukocyte count *decreases* as the corresponding x variable increases.

TABLE 7-17 Multiple-linear regression analysis of demographic and constitutional correlates of leukocyte count (in thousands per mm^3) among never-smokers ($n = 5,392$) in the Atherosclerosis Risk in Communities (ARIC) Study cohort, 1987–1989.

Variable (increment for b)	Linear regression coefficient*	Standard error of b
Age (5 years)	−0.066	0.019
Sex (1 = male, 0 = female)	0.478	0.065
Race (1 = white, 0 = black)	0.495	0.122
Work activity score (1 unit)	−0.065	0.021
Subscapular skinfold (10 mm)	0.232	0.018
Systolic blood pressure (10 mm Hg)	0.040	0.011
FEV$_1$ (1 L)	−0.208	0.047
Heart rate (10 beats/min)	0.206	0.020

*All regression coefficients are statistically significant (Wald statistic; see Section 7.4.8), $P < 0.01$.
Source: Data from FJ Nieto et al., Leukocyte Count Correlates in Middle-Aged Adults: The Atherosclerosis Risk in Communities (ARIC) Study. *American Journal of Epidemiology*, Vol 136, pp. 525–537, © 1992.

Examples of how to interpret data from Table 7-17 are as follows:

- The mean leukocyte count decreases by $(0.066 \times 1000)/mm^3$ (or 66 cells/mm^3) per unit increase in age (i.e., 5 years), after controlling for the other variables in the table. This is equivalent to an average adjusted decrease of 13.2 cells/mm^3 per year of age (i.e., 66/5 years), or 132 cells/mm^3 per 10 years of age, and so on.
- Because the variable sex is categorical, the "unit increase" actually represents the average difference between males and females. The regression coefficient estimate ($b = 0.478$) can thus be interpreted as males having on average 478 more leukocytes per cubic millimeter than females, after adjusting for the other variables listed in the table.

The value of the intercept was omitted from Table 7-17, as it has no practical value or meaningful interpretation in this example. (Its interpretation would be the expected leukocyte count value for a person with a 0 value in all the independent variables—i.e., a newborn black woman, with zero systolic blood pressure (SBP), zero FEV_1, no heartbeat, etc.)

In this and the previous sections, linear regression methods have been described in the context of their usual application (i.e., the assessment of predictors of a continuous outcome variable) (e.g., intimal-medial thickness). It is, however, possible to extend this method to the evaluation of binary (dichotomous) variables, such as the presence of carotid atherosclerosis defined as a categorical variable (present or absent), or the occurrence of an incident event (e.g., disease, death), using the approach proposed by Feldstein.[18] In Feldstein's model, the regression coefficients are interpreted as the *predicted increase in the probability (prevalence or incidence) of the outcome* of interest in relationship to a given increase or change in the value of the independent variable(s), while simultaneously adjusting for all the other variables in the model.[16(pp144–147)] One theoretical caveat of this method relates to the violation of some of the basic assumptions of linear regression (e.g., that the errors *e* are normally distributed; see Armitage et al.[11]). Another important problem is related to extrapolations to extreme values, which can, at least theoretically, result in absurd estimates of the predicted probability (e.g., < 0 or > 1). As a consequence of these problems, Feldstein's binary linear regression model has fallen into disuse, particularly in the presence of alternatives resulting from the increasing availability and power of computational resources, such as the logistic regression model and related methods (see the following sections). The approach, however, tends to provide adjusted estimates in line with those obtained by other regression strategies.

7.4.3 Multiple Logistic Regression

For binary outcome variables such as the occurrence of death, disease, or recovery, the logistic regression model offers a more robust alternative to binary multiple linear regression. The logistic regression model assumes that the relationship between a given value of a variable *x* and the probability of a binary outcome follows the so-called logistic function:

$$P(y|x) = \frac{1}{1 + e^{-(b_0 + b_1 x)}} \quad \text{(Eq. 7.5)}$$

where $P(y|x)$ denotes the probability (*P*) of the binary outcome (*y*) for a given value of *x*. The outcome of this equation, a probability, is constrained to values within the 0 to 1 range.

Figure 7-7A shows a graphical depiction of this function in the case of a continuous variable x. It is noteworthy to point out that this function's shape seems to be biologically plausible for the kinds of dose–response relationships observed in toxicology and risk assessment—that is, situations where low doses of x induce a weak response up to a certain threshold, after which the response increases markedly up to a certain level of x; beyond that level, a saturation effect occurs (when the probability of the outcome becomes close to 1). Biological plausibility, however, is not the main reason for the popularity of the logistic regression for the multivariate analysis of predictors of a binary outcome. Rather, the reasons why this is one of the most popular methods for multivariate analysis of epidemiologic data are the convenience and interpretability of its regression estimates, which are easily translated into odds ratio estimates; this is readily apparent when Equation 7.5 is expressed in the following mathematically equivalent form:

$$\log\left(\frac{P}{1-P}\right) = \log(\text{odds}) = b_0 + b_1 x \quad \text{(Eq. 7.6)}$$

where P is the short notation for $P(y|x)$ in Equation 7.5.

This expression is analogous to the simple linear regression function (Section 7.4.1), except that the ordinate is now the logarithm of the odds (log odds, also known as *logit*), rather than the usual mean value of a continuous variable. Thus, if the relationship between exposure (x) and the occurrence of the outcome is assumed to fit the logistic regression model, that implies that the log odds of the outcome increases linearly with x (Figure 7-7B).

In the context of a *cohort study* (in which data on the incidence of the outcome are obtained), the interpretation of the parameters from the logistic regression equation is analogous to that of the parameters of the linear regression model (Section 7.4.1), as follows:

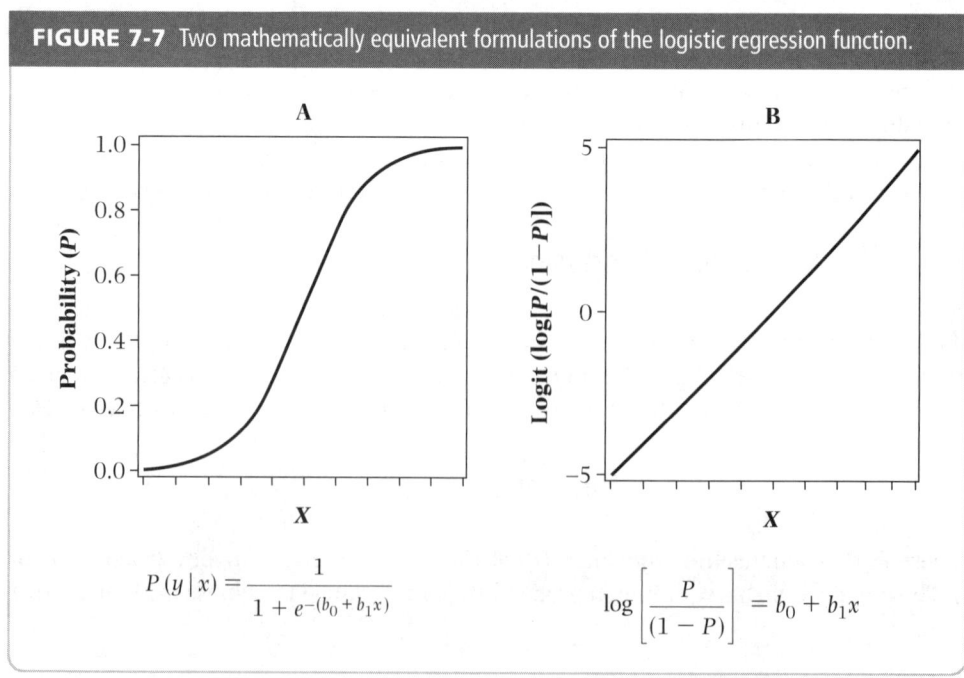

FIGURE 7-7 Two mathematically equivalent formulations of the logistic regression function.

- The intercept (b_0) is an estimate of the log odds of the outcome when $x = 0$. As in linear regression, this value may not have a useful interpretation in itself if $x = 0$ is a mere extrapolation of the realistic (possible) range of the exposure values.
- The logistic regression coefficient (b_1) is the estimated increase in the log odds of the outcome per unit increase in the value of x; or, in other words, $e^{(b_1)}$ is the odds ratio associated with a one-unit increase in x.

As an illustration of the meaning of b_1 in a logistic function, consider a situation where x is the dichotomous variable, sex, for which values of 1 and 0 are assigned to males and females, respectively. After the value of the regression coefficient is estimated, the predicted logistic regression equations can be formulated for each gender as follows:

$$\text{For males: } \log(\text{odds})_{\text{males}} = b_0 + b_1 \times 1 = b_0 + b_1$$

$$\text{For females: } \log(\text{odds})_{\text{females}} = b_0 + b_1 \times 0 = b_0$$

Thus, b_1 is the difference in log odds between males and females, which, as a result of the arithmetic properties of logarithms, is also the log odds ratio comparing males and females:

$$b_1 = \log(\text{odds})_{\text{males}} - \log(\text{odds})_{\text{females}} = \log\left[\frac{(\text{odds})^{\text{males}}}{(\text{odds})^{\text{females}}}\right] = \log(OR)$$

Similarly, if the variable x in Equation 7.6 is continuous, the regression coefficient, b_1, representing the increase in log odds per unit increase in x, can be translated into the log odds ratio when comparing any value of x with a value $(x - 1)$.

It follows that the odds ratio corresponding to a unit increase in the independent variable (e.g., when comparing males to females in the example above) is the antilogarithm (i.e., the exponential function) of the regression coefficient, b_1:

$$OR = e^{b_1}$$

For example, Table 7-18 shows the logistic regression coefficients corresponding to the associations between several risk factors and coronary heart disease (CHD) incidence in a subset of participants from the ARIC study.[19] These analyses are based on the cumulative incidence of CHD between the baseline examination (1987–1989)

TABLE 7-18 Results from a logistic regression analysis of binary and continuous predictors of coronary heart disease (CHD) incidence in the Washington County cohort of the Atherosclerosis Risk in Communities (ARIC) Study, ages 45–64 years at baseline, 1987–1994.

Variable	Logistic regression coefficient	Odds ratio
Intercept	−8.9502	—
Gender (male = 1, female = 0)	1.3075	3.70
Smoking (yes = 1, no = 0)	0.7413	2.10
Age (1 yr)	0.0114	1.011
Systolic blood pressure (1 mm Hg)	0.0167	1.017
Serum cholesterol (1 mg/dL)	0.0074	1.007
Body mass index (1 kg/m²)	0.0240	1.024

and December 1994, among 3597 Washington County participants who were free of clinical CHD at baseline. A total of 171 incident CHD events (myocardial infarction, CHD death, or coronary bypass surgery) were identified by the end of the follow-up. (For more details on methods and results from the follow-up study in the full ARIC cohort, see Chambless et al.[20]) The column labeled "Logistic Regression Coefficient" in Table 7-18 presents the intercept as well as the adjusted regression coefficients for each assessed independent variable. Each regression coefficient shown in Table 7-18 is adjusted for all the other variables in the model (listed in the table) and can be converted to an adjusted odds ratio (shown in the last column). For example, for gender, the adjusted odds ratio of incident CHD comparing males to females is

$$OR_{males/females} = e^{1.3075} = 3.70$$

Taking an example of a continuous variable, SBP, the adjusted odds ratio for a one-unit increase (1 mm Hg) is

$$OR_{1 \text{ mm Hg SBP}} = e^{0.0167} = 1.017$$

The odds ratio for SBP is very small because it is calculated for a very small increase in the independent variable (1 mm Hg). An odds ratio related to a more clinically meaningful SBP unit, such as a 10-mm Hg increase, can, however, be easily obtained by transforming the value of the coefficient into this SBP unit and then recalculating the corresponding odds ratio:

$$OR_{10 \text{ mm Hg SBP}} = e^{10 \times 0.0167} = 1.18$$

The odds ratios for age, serum cholesterol, and body mass index in Table 7-18 also correspond to small changes (1 year, 1 mg/dL, and 1 kg/m², respectively) and can similarly be converted to more meaningful units. For serum cholesterol, for example, the odds ratio corresponding to a 20-mg/dL increase in serum cholesterol is

$$OR_{20 \text{ mg/dL chol}} = e^{20 \times 0.0074} = 1.16$$

For age, the odds ratio corresponding to a 5-year increase in age is

$$OR_{5 \text{ years age}} = e^{5 \times 0.0114} = 1.06$$

The validity of these calculations depends on one of the main assumptions underlying the use of continuous variables in multiple-regression methods (see also Sections 7.4.1 and 7.4.7): that the relationships are linear (in the log odds scale, in this particular case) across the entire range of the data (e.g., for age, that the increase in the log odds of CHD incidence associated with an age unit increase is the same throughout the age range of study participants). This assumption, however, will not apply if continuous variables are categorized into binary exposure variables, such as, "older" versus "younger" age categories, or "hypertension present" versus "hypertension absent," as illustrated in Table 7-19.

It is interesting to compare the values of the estimates shown in Table 7-19 with those in Table 7-18. The definitions of gender and smoking did not change, but because those of the adjusting covariates (all the other variables) did, the "adjusted" regression coefficients and corresponding odds ratios for gender and smoking are slightly different; however, the estimates for the other predictors obviously changed more markedly, as a result of their transformation from continuous (Table 7-18) to categorical (Table 7-19) variables. For example, the adjusted odds ratio for hypertension (1.67) in Table 7-19 is interpreted as the ratio of the CHD incidence odds for individuals meeting

TABLE 7-19 Results from a logistic regression analysis of binary predictors of coronary heart disease (CHD) incidence in the Washington County cohort of the Atherosclerosis Risk in Communities (ARIC) Study, ages 45–64 years at baseline, 1987–1994.

Variable	Logistic regression coefficient	Odds ratio
Intercept	−4.5670	—
Gender (male = 1, female = 0)	1.3106	3.71
Current smoking (yes = 1, no = 0)	0.7030	2.02
Older age* (yes = 1, no = 0)	0.1444	1.16
Hypertension† (yes = 1, no = 0)	0.5103	1.67
Hypercholesterolemia‡ (yes = 1, no = 0)	0.4916	1.63
Obesity§ (yes = 1, no = 0)	0.1916	1.21

*Age ≥ 55 yr.
†Blood pressure ≥ 140 mm Hg systolic or ≥ 90 mm Hg diastolic or antihypertensive therapy.
‡Total serum cholesterol ≥ 240 mg/dL or lipid-lowering treatment.
§Body mass index ≥ 27.8 kg/m² in males and ≥ 27.3 kg/m² in females.

the criteria used to define hypertension (blood pressure ≥ 140 mm Hg systolic or ≥ 90mm Hg diastolic or antihypertensive therapy) to the odds of those not meeting any of these hypertension criteria. This is very different from the estimate for SBP in Table 7-18, both in value and in interpretation. It is important to recognize that the dichotomous definition of hypertension (or that of any other intrinsically continuous variable), while avoiding the assumption of linearity inherent to the continuous definition, is not assumption free, as it implies that the risk of CHD is homogeneous *within* categories of hypertension. If there is a gradient of risk within the hypertension categories, this information is lost in the model and this loss of information may result in residual confounding (Section 7.6). Consider, for example, the assessment of the association between smoking and CHD odds, with adjustment for hypertension (and other variables), as depicted in Table 7-19: because the relationship between blood pressure and CHD follows a dose–response (graded) pattern, residual confounding may have occurred if hypertensives among smokers had higher blood pressure values than hypertensives among nonsmokers. Notwithstanding the possible loss of information, unlike some of the examples discussed previously, the use of dichotomous variables as shown in Table 7-19 allows an interpretation of the *intercept* in logistic regression that may be useful in a couple of ways.

First, in the context of data from a prospective study and on the basis of Equation 7.6, the intercept can be interpreted as the log (odds) for individuals with values of 0 for all the independent variables. For example, according to the results presented in Table 7-19, the intercept represents the log (odds) of incident CHD for nonsmoking females who are aged 45 to 54 years, nonhypertensive, nonhypercholesterolemic, and nonobese. This value is calculated as $-4.567 + 0$, or, transformed to the corresponding value in an arithmetic scale, odds = $e^{-4.567} = 0.0104$.

For predictive purposes, this result can be translated into the more readily interpretable cumulative incidence (probability, p) estimate (see Chapter 2, Section 2.4) as follows:

$$P = \frac{\text{Odds}}{1 + \text{Odds}} = \frac{0.0104}{1 + 0.0104} = 0.0103, \text{ or } 1.03\%$$

This example underscores the utility of the intercept when the assigned values of 0 fall within biologically plausible ranges of values of the independent variables. In contrast, interpretation of the intercept per se is meaningless when using results such as those from Table 7-18.

Second, as for regression models in general, the intercept is needed in logistic regression for obtaining the predicted probability (cumulative incidence) of the outcome for an individual with a given set of characteristics. For example, based on the results in Table 7-19, the probability of CHD for a male smoker who is younger than 55 years, hypertensive, nonhypercholesterolemic, and obese can be estimated simply by substituting the values of each x variable in an equation of the form shown in Equation 7.5, as follows:

$$P = \frac{1}{1 + e^{-[-4.567+(1.3106 \times 1)+(0.703 \times 1)+(0.1444 \times 0)+(0.5103 \times 1)+(0.4916 \times 0)+(0.1916 \times 1)]}}$$

$$= \frac{1}{1 + e^{-(-4.567+1.3106+0.703+0.5103+0.1916)}} = 0.1357 = 13.57\%$$

Similarly, the results from Table 7-18 can be used to estimate the probability of CHD in an individual with specific values of each of the physiologic parameters measured. This could be done for an individual with average values for all the covariates. For example, the average values of the covariates presented in Table 7-18 for the individuals in this ARIC cohort were as follows (the average value of dichotomous covariates is the *proportion* of individuals with the value that was coded as 1): male gender = 0.469; smoking = 0.229; age = 54.7 years; SBP = 119.1 mm Hg; cholesterol = 217.7 mg/dL; BMI = 27.8 kg/m². Thus, using the results from Table 7-18, the predicted probability of incident CHD for an "average individual" in the cohort will be

$$P = \frac{1}{1+e^{-[-8.9502+(1.3075 \times 0.469)+(0.7413 \times 0.229)+(0.0114 \times 54.7)+(0.0167 \times 119.1)+(0.0074 \times 217.7)+(0.024 \times 27.8)]}}$$

$$= \frac{1}{1+e^{-(-3.27649948)}}$$

$$= 0.0364 = 3.63\%$$

(The concept of an "average individual" is an abstract one, particularly with respect to the average of binary variables. For example, in this case, it means an individual who is "0.469 male" and "0.229 smoker" and who has the mean value of all the other continuous covariates.)

As another example of the application of the logistic model for prediction, Framingham study investigators produced the so-called Framingham multiple-logistic risk equation, which can be used to estimate the risk of cardiovascular disease over time for a person with a given set of values for a number of relevant variables (gender, age, serum cholesterol, systolic blood pressure, cigarette smoking, left ventricular hypertrophy by electrocardiogram, and glucose intolerance).[10]

The use of these models for prediction purposes assumes, of course, that the model fits the data reasonably well. Furthermore, the previous discussion about the interpretation of the intercept and the calculation of predicted probabilities of the event is relevant when the data are prospective. The use of the logistic regression model for the analyses of cohort data, however, is limited in that the model uses cumulative incidence data and therefore has to rely on two important assumptions: that follow-up of study participants is complete and that consideration of time to event is not important. These assumptions, however, are often not met because of staggered entries in many cohort studies in which recruitment is carried out over a more or less extended time period, subsequent losses of follow-up, and because of the variability of latency periods for most outcomes of interest (see Chapter 2, Section 2.2). For the analysis of cohort data with incomplete follow-up for some observations, more appropriate multivariate analysis tools are available, as discussed in the following two sections.

The most frequent application of the logistic regression model is in the context of case-control studies, where it constitutes the primary analytical tool for multivariate analyses.[21,22] In a *case-control study*, the interpretation of regression coefficients is identical to that of the cohort study (i.e., the log of the odds ratio), as shown in the following examples. On the other hand, when the data come from a case-control study, the intercept is not readily interpretable, as the sampling fractions for cases and controls are arbitrarily selected by the investigator (for a more technical discussion of this issue, see Schlesselman[22]).

An example of the use of multiple regression in a case-control study is based on a study of the seroprevalence of hepatitis B virus in health care workers in Boston in the late 1970s and early 1980s (i.e., before the introduction of the hepatitis B virus vaccine).[23] Some findings of this study are presented in Table 7-20, which shows the results of a multiple-logistic regression analysis aimed at identifying variables associated with the odds of positivity for hepatitis B serum antibodies. Table 7-20 shows both the logistic regression coefficients and the corresponding odds ratios (as well as their 95% confidence interval; see Section 7.4.8 and Appendix A, Section A.9). The intercept was omitted because of its irrelevance (discussed previously). The first three variables are dichotomous; thus, the regression coefficient for each of these variables represents the difference in the log odds between the two corresponding categories (in other words, the antilog of the regression coefficient represents the odds ratio comparing the "exposure" category—coded as 1—with the reference category—coded as 0). For example, for the variable "recent needlestick," the value 0.8459 is the estimated difference in the log odds of positive antibodies to hepatitis B between those with and those without a history of a recent needlestick, after adjusting for all the other variables in the table. Consequently, the odds ratio associated with recent needlestick is estimated as $e^{0.8459} = 2.33$. The two bottom variables in Table 7-20 (age and years in occupation) were entered in the model

TABLE 7-20 Multivariate logistic regression analysis in a case-control study of risk factors for the presence of hepatitis B virus serum antibodies in health workers, Boston, Massachusetts, 1977–1982.

Characteristics	Logistic regression coefficient	Odds ratio (95% confidence interval)
Occupational/blood exposure (yes/no)	0.7747	2.17 (1.31–3.58)
Recent needlestick (yes/no)	0.8459	2.33 (1.19–4.57)
Hepatitis A virus positive serology (yes/no)	0.6931	2.00 (1.13–3.54)
Age (1 yr)	0.0296	1.03 (0.99–1.06)
Years in occupation (1 yr)	0.0198	1.02 (0.97–1.08)

Source: Data from A Gibas et al., Prevalence and Incidence of Viral Hepatitis in Health Workers in the Prehepatitis B Vaccination Era. *American Journal of Epidemiology.* Vol 136, pp. 603–610, © 1992.

as continuous, and the regression coefficients and corresponding odds ratios are given for increments of 1 year. For example, for "Years in Occupation," the value 0.0198 represents the adjusted estimated increase in log odds of positive antibodies per year increase in length of employment as a health worker. In other words, the adjusted odds ratio corresponding to an increase in 1 year of occupation is estimated as $e^{0.0198} = 1.02$.

It should be reemphasized that the logistic regression model is a *linear model in the log odds scale*, as was seen in Equation 7.6. What this means in practical terms is that when a continuous variable is entered as such, the resulting coefficient (and corresponding odds ratio) is assumed to represent the linear increase in log odds (or the exponential increase in odds) per unit increase in the independent variable *across the entire range of x values*. For example, the estimated increase in the odds of positive hepatitis B antibodies per year of occupation (i.e., odds ratio = 1.02) shown in Table 7-20 is assumed to be the same when comparing 3 with 2 years as it is when comparing 40 with 39 years of occupation. Again, as discussed in Sections 7.4.1 and 7.4.7, if this assumption is not justified (e.g., if the increase in the odds of infection associated with a 1-year change in the occupation is higher in more recently hired, less experienced workers), the previous model will be incorrect, and alternative models using categorical definitions of the variable (dummy variables) or other forms of parameterization (e.g., quadratic terms) must be used.

Finally, a word of caution is necessary on the use (*or abuse*) of the logistic regression model for the analysis of cohort or cross-sectional data. The adjusted odds ratio resulting from the exponentiation of the logistic regression coefficient obtained in these studies is often used as a surrogate of the relative risk or prevalence rate ratio, respectively. As discussed in detail in Chapter 3, this interpretation is justified only for the analyses of rare outcomes, but when the frequency of the outcome of interest is high (e.g., 10% or 20%), the odds ratio is a *biased* estimate of the relative risk (or the prevalence rate ratio) as it tends to exaggerate the magnitude of the association. The investigator choosing to use logistic regression in these types of studies (often because of its ease and convenient features) should always keep in mind the *built-in* bias associated with the odds ratio as an estimate of the incidence or prevalence rate ratio when the outcome is common (see Chapter 3, Section 3.4.1). Alternatively, investigators might consider using other regression procedures, such as the *log-binomial regression model*, which result in direct estimates of the incidence or prevalence rate ratio.[24]

7.4.4 Cox Proportional Hazards Model

When the analysis is based on time-to-event (or survival) data, one of the options is to model the data using the hazard (or instantaneous force of morbidity or mortality) scale (see Chapter 2, Section 2.2.4). The assumption underlying this approach is that exposure to a certain risk factor (or the presence of a certain characteristic) is associated with a fixed relative increase in the instantaneous risk of the outcome of interest compared with a baseline or reference hazard (e.g., the hazard in the unexposed). In other words, it is assumed that at any given time (t), the hazard in those exposed to a certain risk factor [$h_1(t)$] is a multiple of some underlying hazard [$h_0(t)$]. Figure 7-8 illustrates this model, which can be mathematically formulated as follows:

$$h_1(t) = h_0(t) \times B \qquad \text{(Eq. 7.7)}$$

That is, at any given point in time, the hazard among those exposed to the risk factor of interest is the hazard among those not exposed to it, multiplied by a constant factor (B). The hazards in both the exposed and the reference groups may be approximately constant

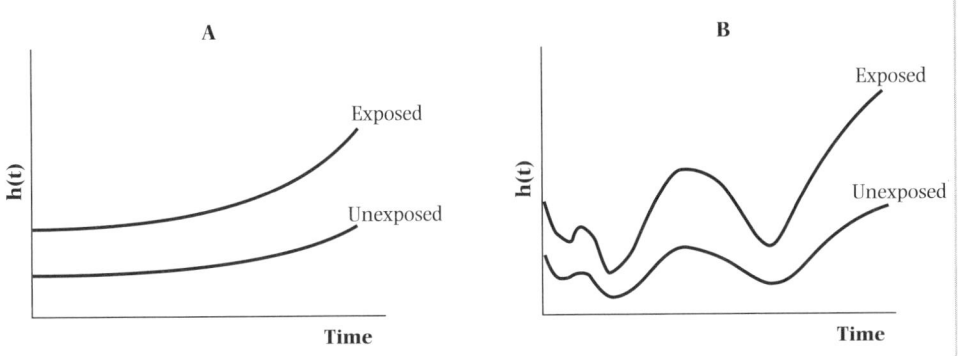

FIGURE 7-8 Hazard over time in two hypothetical situations in which exposed individuals have twice the hazard of those unexposed. A represents a situation with a relatively stable hazard that slowly increases over time, such as hazard of death as adult individuals age; B represents a situation in which the hazard fluctuates with time, such as the hazard of a car accident that increases or decreases as a function of the car's velocity at any given point in time, with the presence of the exposure (e.g., having worn-out tires) doubling the risk of having an accident, compared with its absence (having new tires).

or may increase over time (see Figure 7-8A; e.g., the instantaneous risk of mortality as individuals age) or fluctuate over time (see the hypothetical example in Figure 7-8B; e.g., the risk of an accident as the driving speed changes). In both examples in Figure 7-8, it is assumed that at any given point in time, the hazard among those exposed (e.g., car wearing old tires) is multiplied by 2 regardless of the baseline hazard (e.g., wearing new tires); in other words, that the hazard ratio (or relative hazard) comparing exposed and unexposed is constant throughout the observation period.

For estimating B—that is, the constant multiplication factor in Equation 7.7—it is convenient to define it in terms of an exponential function: $B = e^b$, i.e., by reformulating Equation 7.7 as

$$h_1(t) = h_0(t) \times e^b \quad \text{(Eq. 7.8)}$$

If $h_0(t)$ represents the hazard in the unexposed group at any given point in time, then the hazard ratio (HR) comparing the exposed and the unexposed is

$$\text{HR} = \frac{h_1(t)}{h_0(t)} = e^b$$

Or taking logarithms

$$\log(\text{HR}) = b$$

Like the odds ratio, the hazard ratio is a multiplicative measure of association; consequently, many of the issues related to the logistic regression coefficients (log odds ratio) apply as well to the regression coefficients from the Cox model (log hazard ratio). Thus, for example, the issues related to the type of independent variable included in the model (continuous, ordinal, categorical) are similar in the Cox and logistic regression models.

Table 7-21 shows the results of two alternative analyses using Cox proportional regression (models 1 and 2) to assess predictors of incident CHD in the Washington County cohort of the ARIC study. In Table 7-21, the independent variables included as predictors are the same as those used previously to illustrate the logistic regression

TABLE 7-21 Results of Cox proportional regression analysis of binary and continuous predictors of coronary heart disease (CHD) incidence in the Washington County cohort of the Atherosclerosis Risk in Communities (ARIC) Study, ages 45–64 years at baseline, 1987–1994.

Model	Variable	Cox regression coefficient	Hazard ratio
1	Gender (male = 1, female = 0)	1.2569	3.52
	Smoking (yes = 1, no = 0)	0.7045	2.02
	Age (1 yr)	0.0120	1.012
	Systolic blood pressure (1 mm Hg)	0.0152	1.015
	Serum cholesterol (1 mg/dL)	0.0067	1.007
	Body mass index (1 kg/m^2)	0.0237	1.024
2	Gender (male = 1, female = 0)	1.2669	3.55
	Smoking (yes = 1, no = 0)	0.6803	1.97
	Older age* (yes = 1, no = 0)	0.1391	1.15
	Hypertension† (yes = 1, no = 0)	0.5030	1.65
	Hypercholesterolemia‡ (yes = 1, no = 0)	0.4552	1.58
	Obesity§ (yes = 1, no = 0)	0.1876	1.21

*Age ≥ 55 yr.
†Blood pressure ≥ 140 mm Hg systolic or ≥ 90 mm Hg diastolic or antihypertensive therapy.
‡Total serum cholesterol ≥ 240 mg/dL or lipid-lowering treatment.
§Body mass index ≥ 27.8 kg/m^2 in males and ≥ 27.3 kg/m^2 in females.

model (Tables 7-18 and 7-19). Here, the outcome of interest is also incident CHD, but in contrast with the logistic regression analysis (which assumes that all participants had complete follow-up and the cumulative incidence odds were obtained), the regression coefficients in Table 7-21 take into account the *time of occurrence* of each event, as well as the time of censoring for the participants who were not observed for the entire follow-up (see Chapter 2, Section 2.2). Thus, also in contrast with the logistic regression, where the regression coefficients antilogs were interpreted as odds ratios, exponentiation of the regression (beta) coefficients in Table 7-21 results in hazards ratios (analogous to relative risks).

There is a remarkable similarity between the estimates obtained from logistic regression in Tables 7-18 and 7-19 (cumulative incidence odds ratio; time to event and censoring not considered) and the Cox estimates in Table 7-21 (hazard ratio; time to event and censoring taken into account). This similarity is probably due to the following facts: (1) CHD is relatively rare, and thus the odds ratio estimated from logistic regression approximates the hazard ratio (akin to a relative risk) estimated by Cox's regression; (2) losses to follow-up and time to events are likely to be non-differential between the exposure groups, and thus, the biases resulting from time-related factors tend to cancel out, which represents a phenomenon comparable to "compensating bias," described in Section 4.2.

It should be underscored that, unlike the output obtained from logistic regression, there is no intercept in the Cox model. Cox's important contribution was to devise a method for estimating the regression parameters in the proportional hazards model without the need to specify the value or the shape of the baseline hazard (h_0), which is the equivalent of the intercept.[25] Methods have been devised that permit the estimation of the underlying survival function based on the results of a multivariate Cox regression analysis; details on this and other applications of the Cox model can be found in the growing literature and textbooks on survival analysis.[26,27]

The Cox model is also called the *proportional hazards model*. This term emphasizes the "proportionality assumption" (i.e., the assumption that the exposure of interest multiplies the baseline hazards [the hazards in those unexposed] by a constant factor, e^b [see Equation 7.8], at any given point during follow-up). As illustrated in Figure 7-8, this implies that regardless of the value of the baseline hazard at any given point in time, those exposed have a hazard equal to the baseline hazard multiplied by e^b. The need for this assumption is implicit in the fact that *one* hazard ratio is estimated for the entire follow-up. If the hazards are not proportional over time (i.e., if the hazard ratio changes during the follow-up), the model needs to account for this by stratifying according to follow-up time. This situation could be properly described as a case of "time × exposure" interaction (i.e., effect modification [see Chapter 6]) in which time modifies the relationship between exposure and outcome. For a more detailed description of methods to assess the proportionality assumption when applying the Cox model as well as approaches to account for time × exposure interactions, the reader is referred to a more specialized text (e.g., Collett[26] or Parmar and Machin[27]).

7.4.5 Poisson Regression

The Poisson regression model is another method for multiple-regression analysis of cohort data with a dichotomous outcome and one or more categorically defined predictors. It is mostly used in situations in which the outcomes of interest are rates (and rate ratios); it is especially suitable for studying rare diseases in large populations. The model specifies that the magnitude of the rate is an exponential function of a linear combination of covariates and unknown parameters:

$$\text{Rate} = e^{(b_0 + b_1 x_1 + b_2 x_2 + \ldots + b_k x_k)}$$

This equation can be rewritten as the log of the rate being the dependent variable of a linear function:

$$\log(\text{rate}) = b_0 + b_1 x_1 + b_2 x_2 + \ldots + b_k x_k \qquad (\text{Eq. 7.9})$$

Equation 7.9 is also called a *log-linear model*, reflecting the fact that it is simply a log transformation of an outcome variable (a rate in this case) related to a linear equation of predictors. If the "rate" is decomposed into its two components (number of events in the numerator and person-time in the denominator), Equation 7.9 can be rewritten in the following ways:

$$\log(\text{events/person-time}) = b_0 + b_1 x_1 + b_2 x_2 + \ldots + b_k x_k$$
$$\log(\text{events}) - \log(\text{person-time}) = b_0 + b_1 x_1 + b_2 x_2 + \ldots + b_k x_k$$
$$\log(\text{events}) = [\log(\text{person-time})] + b_0 + b_1 x_1 + b_2 x_2 + \ldots + b_k x_k$$
$$\log(\text{events}) = b_0^* + b_1 x_1 + b_2 x_2 + \ldots + b_k x_k$$

In this equation, the log (person-time) is incorporated ("offset" in statistical terms) into the intercept (now noted as b_0^*) of the multiple linear predictor, and the outcome variable is now a count, the number of events (log transformed). For this type of outcome variable (a count) and for reasonably rare events (as it is the case in most epidemiologic studies), it is assumed that the most appropriate basis for the statistical procedure of estimation of the parameters in the previous model is the Poisson distribution. (Several statistical textbooks provide additional details regarding the statistical properties and uses of the Poisson distribution; see, for example Armitage et al.[11])

Again, the interpretation of the Poisson regression coefficients is analogous to those in logistic regression and Cox models, except that where in the latter models the odds ratio and the hazard ratio were, respectively, obtained, in the Poisson regression the *rate ratio* is estimated. For example, when comparing exposed (e.g., $x_1 = 1$) and unexposed ($x_1 = 0$) groups, Equation 7.9 will reduce to the following:

For the exposed: $\log(\text{rate}_{exp}) = b_0 + b_1 \times 1 + b_2 x_2 + \ldots + b_k x_k$

For the unexposed: $\log(\text{rate}_{unexp}) = b_0 + b_1 \times 0 + b_2 x_2 + \ldots + b_k x_k$

Subtracting these equations:

$$\log(\text{rate}_{exp}) - \log(\text{rate}_{unexp}) = b_1$$

And thus,

$$\log\left(\frac{\text{rate}_{exp}}{\text{rate}_{unexp}}\right) = \log(\text{rate ratio}) = b_1$$

Consequently, the antilog of the regression coefficient estimate (e^{b_1}) corresponds to the rate ratio comparing exposed and unexposed, adjusted for all the other variables included in the model ($x_2, \ldots x_k$).

As pointed out previously, all independent (x) variables in the Poisson regression model need to be categorical, as the method is set to use the total amount of person-time and the total number of events per category or cell (representing each unique combination of the predictors). For example, the application of the Poisson regression method to the analysis of CHD incidence in the ARIC study and including the same variables as in model 2 of the Cox regression example (Table 7-21) results in the data shown in Table 7-22. The exponentiation of the Poisson regression coefficients provides estimates of the adjusted rate ratios comparing exposed (i.e., those with the characteristic coded as 1) and unexposed individuals.

To carry out the Poisson regression analyses in Table 7-22, each unique combination of the six independent variables had to be identified (total $2^6 = 64$ cells), the total person-time contributed to by all individuals in each cell had to be added up, and the total number of events among these individuals had to be identified. The cell-specific data look as shown in Table 7-23, in which 8 of the 64 cells are shown, each with its corresponding total person-years (PY; LogPY is the logarithm of that value) and number of CHD events. The calculation of the regression coefficients shown in Table 7-22 was based on these data.

7.4.6 A Note on Models for the Multivariate Analyses of Data from Matched Case-Control Studies and Case-Control Studies Within a Defined Cohort

In *matched case-control studies* (see Section 1.4.5), the multivariate analysis technique most frequently used is *conditional logistic regression*. This model is analogous to the logistic regression model presented previously (Section 7.4.3), except that the

TABLE 7-22 Results from a Poisson regression analysis of binary predictors of coronary heart disease (CHD) incidence in the Washington County cohort of the Atherosclerosis Risk in Communities (ARIC) study, ages 45–64 years at baseline, 1987–1994.

Variable	Poisson regression coefficient	Rate ratio
Intercept	−6.3473	—
Gender (male = 1, female = 0)	1.1852	3.27
Smoking (yes = 1, no = 0)	0.6384	1.89
Older age* (yes = 1, no = 0)	0.2947	1.34
Hypertension† (yes = 1, no = 0)	0.5137	1.67
Hypercholesterolemia‡ (yes = 1, no = 0)	0.6795	1.97
Obesity§ (yes = 1, no = 0)	0.2656	1.30

*Age ≥ 55 yr.
†Blood pressure ≥ 140 mm Hg systolic or ≥ 90 mm Hg diastolic or antihypertensive therapy.
‡Total serum cholesterol ≥ 240 mg/dL or lipid-lowering treatment.
§Body mass index ≥ 27.8 kg/m² in males and ≥ 27.3 kg/m² in females.

TABLE 7-23 Data used for calculating the results shown in Table 7-21.

Cell	Male	Smok	Old age	Hyperten	Hypercho	Obese	PY	CHD	LogPY
1	0	0	0	0	0	0	1740.85	1	7.46213
2	0	0	0	0	0	1	1181.40	2	7.07446
3	0	0	0	0	1	0	539.97	0	6.29152
4	0	0	0	0	1	1	521.93	1	6.25754
.../...									
61	1	1	1	1	0	0	24.48	1	3.19804
62	1	1	1	1	0	1	37.41	0	3.62208
63	1	1	1	1	1	0	171.41	1	5.14405
64	1	1	1	1	1	1	85.37	5	4.44701

parameters (the intercept and regression coefficients) are estimated taking into account ("conditioned on") the pairing or matching of cases and controls with respect to the variables that determined the matching. The interpretation of the coefficients in conditional logistic regression is the same as in ordinary logistic regression, except that these coefficients are to be considered "adjusted" not only for the variables included in the model but also for the matching variables. Details on the statistical properties and applications of the conditional logistic regression model can be found elsewhere (e.g., Hosmer and Lemeshow,[21] Breslow and Day[28]). This model is particularly useful for the analyses of studies in which cases and controls are *individually matched sets* (case-control pairs or triplets, etc.—when more than one control is matched to each case). An example is given by the cross-sectional examination of variables associated with carotid atherosclerosis in the ARIC study.[29] For this analysis, cases (n = 386) were defined as individuals with elevated carotid artery intimal-medial thickness (IMT) based on B-mode ultrasound imaging measurements (see preceding examples in this chapter). Controls in this study were selected among individuals with low IMT and were individually matched to each case on sex, race, age group (45–54 or 55–64 years), study center, and date of examination. Selected results from this study are presented in Table 7-24. Each of the odds ratios in this table was obtained by exponentiating the regression coefficient estimate (e^b) obtained from a logistic regression model conditioned on the matching variables. Although the estimates in Table 7-24 are adjusted for age (and for other matching variables), residual confounding could result from the use of broad age-matching categories. This is the reason why the study investigators also adjusted for age as a continuous variable (see Section 1.4.5, Figure 1-24, and Section 7.6).

In studies in which cases and controls are frequency matched (see Section 1.4.5), a more efficient strategy is simply to use ordinary logistic regression and include the matching variables in the model. An example of a frequency-matched study, cited in Chapter 1, is the examination of the relationship between CMV antibodies and atherosclerosis.[30] Table 7-25 shows the association between CMV antibody levels in serum samples collected in 1974 and the presence of carotid atherosclerosis in the ARIC study's first two examinations (1987–1992).[30] These odds ratios were obtained from the estimated coefficients in logistic regression models that contained the matching variables (*matched odds ratio*) and additional variables adjusted for (*adjusted odds ratio*).

Nested case-control studies, in which the controls are selected among the members of the "risk set," that is, among the cohort members at risk at the time when the case occurs (see Chapter 1, Section 1.4.2), can be considered and analyzed as "matched case-control studies" in which cases and controls are matched by length of follow-up (Figure 1-20). Thus, as in other matched case-control studies, the multivariate analysis technique most frequently indicated is the conditional logistic regression, in which the conditional variable is length of follow-up. This type of conditional logistic regression model is analogous to the Cox proportional hazards regression model.[31] In addition to its inherent logistical advantages (see Chapter 1, Section 1.4.2), the nested case-control

TABLE 7-24 Adjusted odds ratios* for carotid atherosclerosis in relation to selected cardiovascular risk factors in 386 matched pairs† from the Atherosclerosis Risk in Communities (ARIC) study cohort examined between 1987 and 1989.

Variable and reference category	Age-adjusted odds ratio (95% confidence interval)	Multivariate-adjusted‡ odds ratio (95% confidence interval)
Current smoker vs ex- and never-smoker	3.3 (2.3–4.7)	3.9 (2.6–5.9)
Ever smoker vs never-smoker	2.8 (2.0–4.0)	3.1 (2.1–4.6)
Hypertensive vs normotensive	2.7 (1.9–3.8)	2.9 (1.9–4.3)
LDL cholesterol ≥ 160 vs < 100 mg/dL	2.6 (1.6–4.4)	2.0 (1.1–3.7)
100–159 vs < 100 mg/dL	1.6 (1.0–2.6)	1.4 (0.8–2.4)

*Obtained by conditional logistic regression.
†Matched on sex, race, age group (45–54 or 55–64 yr), study center, and date of examination.
‡Adjusted for age (as a continuous variable) and all the other variables listed in the table, in addition to matching variables.
Source: Data from G Heiss et al., Carotid Atherosclerosis Measured by B-Mode Ultrasound in Populations: Associations with Cardiovascular Risk Factors in the ARIC Study. *American Journal of Epidemiology*, Vol 134, pp. 250–256, © 1991.

TABLE 7-25 Intimal-medial thickness case-control status in the Atherosclerosis Risk in Communities (ARIC) study (1987–1992) in relation to high or moderate versus low positive/negative values for cytomegalovirus (CMV) antibodies in serum samples collected in 1974.

CMV antibody levels*	Cases	Controls	Matched OR[†] (95% confidence interval)	Adjusted OR[‡] (95% confidence interval)
Low	31	51	1.0[§]	1.0[§]
Moderate	104	94	1.9 (1.1–3.2)	1.5 (0.8–2.9)
High	15	5	5.2 (1.7–16.0)	5.3 (1.5–18.0)

*Low: positive/negative ratio < 4; moderate: positive/negative ratio 4 to 19; high: positive/negative ratio ≥ 20.
[†]Odds ratios obtained by multiple-logistic regression analysis including the frequency-matching variables age (10-year categories) and gender.
[‡]Odds ratios obtained by multiple-logistic regression analysis including the frequency-matching variables age (10-year categories and gender) plus continuous age, cigarette smoking (current/former vs never), years of education (> 12 vs ≤ 12), hypercholesterolemia, hypertension, diabetes, and overweight.
[§]Reference category.
Source: Data from FJ Nieto et al., Cohort Study of Cytomegalovirus Infection as a Risk Factor for Carotid Intimal-Medial Thickening, a Measure of Subclinical Atherosclerosis, *Circulation*. Vol 94, pp. 922–927, © 1996.

study has become a popular study design as a result of the wide availability in recent years of statistical packages that can carry out this type of conditional analysis.

In the alternative design for case-control studies within a well-defined cohort, the so-called *case-cohort study*, cases occurring in the cohort during follow-up are compared with a random sample of the baseline cohort (*subcohort*) (see Chapter 1, Section 1.4.2). The analytical approach to these data must consider the design's peculiar sampling scheme, namely, that a fraction of the cases may have been included in the subcohort. Fortunately, as described elsewhere,[32,33] the Cox model can be adapted to this situation by allowing for staggered entries (for the cases outside the subcohort).

As an example of this approach, Table 7-26 shows results from a study described at the end of Section 1.4.2. This is a case-cohort study conducted within the ARIC cohort looking at the association between serum antibodies against *Chlamydia pneumoniae*

TABLE 7-26 Estimated crude and adjusted hazard ratios of incident coronary heart disease (and 95% confidence intervals) by level of *C. pneumoniae* antibody titers at baseline, 1987–1991:* A case-cohort study within the Atherosclerosis Risk in Communities cohort study.

	C. pneumoniae IgG antibody titers		
	Negative	1:8–1:32	≥1:64
Adjusted for demographics[†]	1.0	1.2 (0.7–2.1)	1.6 (1.0–2.5)
Adjusted for demographics[†] and risk factors[‡]	1.0	1.1 (0.6–2.3)	1.2 (0.7–2.1)

*Estimated using weighted proportional hazards regression models with staggered entries for cases outside the subcohort and Barlow's robust variance estimates.[32]
[†]Age (continuous), gender, race, and center.
[‡]Smoking, hypercholesterolemia, hypertension, diabetes, and educational level.
Source: Data from FJ Nieto et al., *Chlamydia Pneumoniae* Infection and Incident Coronary Heart Disease: The Atherosclerosis Risk in Communities (ARIC) Study. *American Journal of Epidemiology*. Vol 150, pp. 149–156, © 1999.

and incident CHD over a follow-up of 3 to 5 years.[34] The 246 incident CHD cases were compared with a stratified random sample of 550 participants from the original cohort using a Cox regression analysis, which takes into consideration time-to-event and allows for staggered entries to handle the case-cohort sampling design. As in the previous examples, each of the hazard ratios shown in the table was obtained by exponentiating the corresponding regression coefficient from the Cox regression model. The results shown in Table 7-26 suggest that the apparent increased hazard of CHD in those with high levels of *C. pneumoniae* antibodies at baseline can be largely explained by positive confounding effects by other risk factors.

7.4.7 Modeling Nonlinear Relationships with Linear Regression Models

Epidemiologic studies often use continuous variables to measure physiologic parameters or other characteristics, such as those in the examples discussed in previous sections. Two different definitions of such variables were used to illustrate the application of a number of adjustment models: continuous (e.g., systolic blood pressure levels; Tables 7-16, 7-18, and 7-21, model 1) or dichotomous (e.g., hypertension; Tables 7-19, 7-21, model 2, and 7–22). In this section, the possible limitations of these models and some alternative approaches are briefly discussed.

To illustrate the problems related to the selection of the modeling approach, Figure 7-9A shows a hypothetical observed (assumed to be true) "J-shape" relationship between a given continuous predictor (x) and an outcome variable (y); y here could be any of the dependent variables in the models summarized in Table 7-15—for example, a continuous variable such as the carotid intimal-medial thickness when using linear regression or the log (odds) of carotid atherosclerosis (defined as a binary variable) when using logistic regression. This type of relationship has been found, for example, in epidemiologic studies of body weight and mortality,[35,36] in which a higher risk of mortality has been observed in low-weight individuals (possibly because of underlying chronic morbidity), the lowest risk in individuals of "normal" weight, and a steady increase in mortality in overweight and obese individuals. (Other examples of such J- or U-type relationships are those between serum cholesterol and mortality[37] and between alcohol intake and coronary heart disease.[38])

Figure 7-9B illustrates the problems of using a linear regression model to explain the observed relationship between x and y. In Figure 7-9B, an estimate of the regression coefficient, b, would represent the average linear increase of y (e.g., mortality) per unit increase in the continuous variable x (e.g., body weight) (i.e., the slope of the straight line in Figure 7-9B). Obviously, the estimation of an overall linear regression coefficient, corresponding to the straight line shown in Figure 7-9B, ignores the fact that there is actually a *decrease* in y in the lower x range, a slow increase in y in the mid x range, and a pronounced increase in y in the upper x range. Because the latter is more pronounced than the former, the average value of b will come out positive; however, as readily inferred from Figure 7-9B, this estimate misrepresents the true relationship of x to y, to the extent that it falsely "reverses" the observed negative association for lower values of x and underestimates the strong positive association seen for higher x values.

For the model represented in Figure 7-9C, x is defined as a dichotomous variable, with the categories 0 and 1 represented in the abscissa of the graph. By so modeling x, the model assumes that there is a "threshold" phenomenon: that is, that the relationship between x and y is flat for the lower range of x values and that there is a sudden increase in y at a certain x threshold (which is the cutoff point used to define x as a categorical

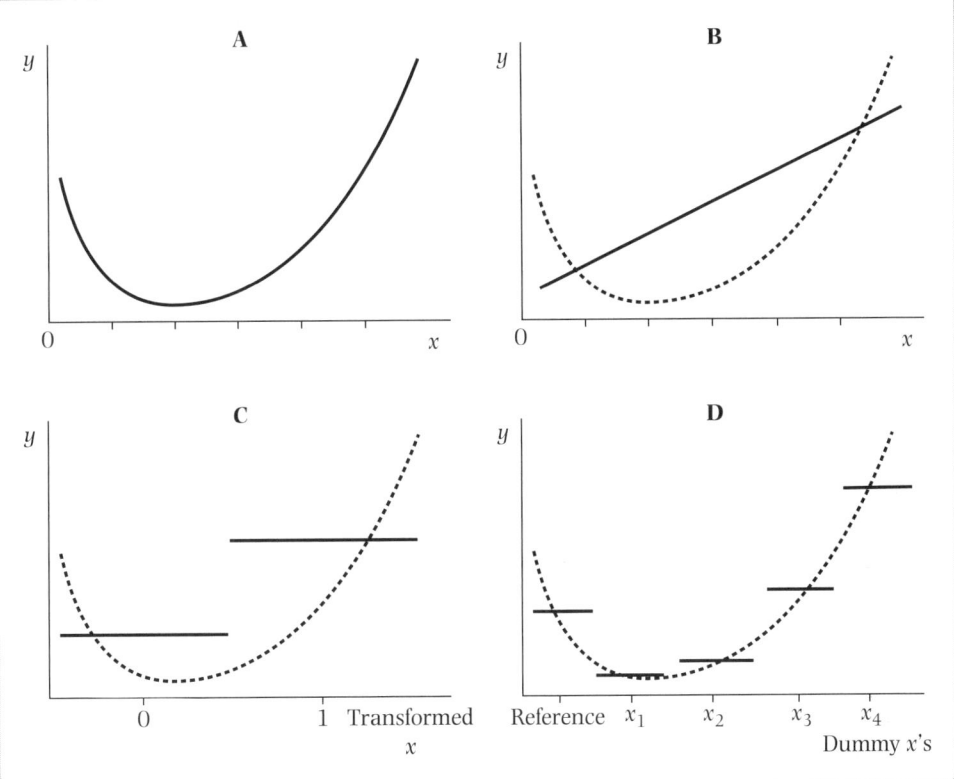

FIGURE 7-9 Hypothetical example of an observed (true) J-shape relationship between x and an outcome variable y (A); B through D illustrate the observed relationship (broken line) with alternative models superimposed: continuous x (B), dichotomous x (C), and dummy variables for x quintiles (D).

variable), after which there is no further increase in y as x increases. The estimated regression coefficient in this case represents the difference in the average y value between the higher and the lower x range categories (see Figure 7-6)—that is, the vertical distance (in y units) between the two horizontal bars depicted in Figure 7-9C. As for the model shown in Figure 7-9B, this one also neglects an important feature of the relationship between x and y, namely that y decreases as x increases for low values of x, whereas the opposite is true for higher values.

Use of Indicator ("Dummy") Variables

To take into account these patterns, more elaborate and complex models are necessary. One option, often used in epidemiology, consists of breaking down the continuous independent variable x into multiple categories (based, e.g., on quartiles or quintiles) and then using one *dummy* variable as an indicator for each category while allowing the "slope" (the change in y) to vary from category to category. Examples of the use of dummy variables for modeling multilevel categories of an independent variable that is not linearly related to the outcome follow. Consider the model illustrated in Figure 7-9D. In this panel, the range of x values has been divided in fifths—that is, in five groups defined by the quintiles, each containing 20% of the individuals ordered according to the value of x from lowest to highest. A set of dummy or indicator variables (categories)

TABLE 7-27 Definitions of dummy variables for the model in Figure 7-9D.

Fifth of x	Dummy variables			
	x_1	x_2	x_3	x_4
1 (reference)	0	0	0	0
2	1	0	0	0
3	0	1	0	0
4	0	0	1	0
5	0	0	0	1

can be then defined, as many as the number of categories for the independent variable minus 1 (4 in this example). One of the categories is chosen as the "reference," and each of the remaining categories is assigned a value of 1 for one of the dummy variables and 0 for the others (Table 7-27). For the category arbitrarily chosen as reference (the lowest fifth in this case), all four dummy variables have 0 values. Each of the dummies represents the remaining fifths. Thus, the model corresponding to Figure 7-9D can be written as follows:

$$y = b_0 + b_1 x_1 + b_2 x_2 + b_3 x_3 + b_4 x_4 \qquad \text{(Eq. 7.10)}$$

These four dummy variables correspond to different categories of a single variable, x. In fact, because of the complete lack of overlap between these "variables" (no one individual can have a value of 1 for more than one such "variable," simply because no individual can belong to more than one of these mutually exclusive fifths), the model in Equation 7.10 can be reduced to the following equations for each of the fifths:

- For the individuals in the bottom fifth, all dummies have a value of 0, and thus $y = b_0$
- For individuals in the second fifth, where only x_1 is equal to 1, $y = b_0 + b_1 x_1$
- For individuals in the third fifth, $y = b_0 + b_2 x_2$
- For individuals in the fourth fifth, $y = b_0 + b_3 x_3$
- For individuals in the top fifth, $y = b_0 + b_4 x_4$

Thus, the regression coefficients have the following interpretation:

- b_0 = the average value of y among individuals in the reference category (bottom fifth).
- b_1 = the average difference in the value of y between individuals in the second fifth and those in the bottom fifth.
- b_2 = the average difference in the value of y between individuals in the third fifth and those in the bottom fifth.
- b_3 = the average difference in the value of y between individuals in the fourth fifth and those in the bottom fifth.
- b_4 = the average difference in the value of y between individuals in the top fifth and those in the bottom fifth.

The difference between each fifth and a different fifth other than the reference is easily obtained by subtraction of the regression coefficients. For example, the difference between the top fifth and the second fifth can be calculated as $b_4 - b_1$.

In Figure 7-9D, b_0 represents the y value corresponding to the horizontal bar for the "reference" category, and each of the other b's represents the vertical distance (in y units) between the horizontal bars for each of the fifths and the reference fifth. In the hypothetical example shown in Figure 7-9D, the values of b_1 and b_2 will be negative (because the average y values in subjects in the second and third fifth are lower than the average y value in the bottom fifth), whereas the values of b_3 and of b_4 will be positive. The choice of the reference category is purely arbitrary and largely inconsequential. For example, because the second fifth is the category with the lowest y value and thus might be considered the "normal" range for x, it could have been chosen as the reference category in the preceding example. If this had been the case, b_0 would have represented the average value of the individuals in this new reference category, and the remaining b's (all positive in this situation) would have been the average differences between each of the other fifths and the second fifth. If, in addition, the model in Equation 7.10 had included other variables, each of the estimates for the difference between each category and the reference category would have been adjusted for these other variables.

A real-life example of breaking down continuous independent variables into several categories when using the multiple-logistic regression model is presented in Table 7-28, which shows results pertaining to the examination of the cross-sectional associations between sociodemographic characteristics and the prevalence of depressive symptoms among Mexican Americans participating in the US Hispanic Health and Nutrition Examination Survey.[39] In Table 7-28, logistic regression coefficients and corresponding odds ratios (and the attached p values—see Wald statistic, Appendix A, Section A.9) are presented side by side. All variables were entered in the model as categorical variables, including variables that could have been entered as continuous (e.g., age, annual household income). With the exception of sex and employment status, all variables in Table 7-28 have more than two categories. For each of these variables, one of the categories is used as the reference (i.e., it has no regression coefficient), with the value of its odds ratio being, by definition, 1.0. All other categories have been modeled as dummy variables. For each of these categories, a logistic regression coefficient is estimated; exponentiation of this coefficient results in an estimate of the odds ratio that compares this category with the reference category. For example, for age, the younger age group (20–24 years) was chosen as reference. The coefficient for "25 to 34 years" is 0.1866, corresponding to an odds ratio of $e^{0.1866}$, or 1.2; for the next age group ("35–44 years"), the coefficient is negative (-0.1112), thus indicating that the log odds in this category is lower than that in the reference, which translates into an odds ratio below 1.0 (OR = $e^{-0.1112}$ = 0.89), and so forth. For years of education and income, the highest categories were chosen as reference; if the authors had chosen the lowest instead, the results would have been the reciprocals of those shown in the table. Very importantly, as discussed previously in this section, by breaking down the continuous variables into dummy variables (categories), it is possible to model adequately the nonlinear relationships observed in these data by using a linear model. For example, the use of five dummy variables (plus a reference category) for age in Table 7-28 suggests the presence of an inverse "J-shape" pattern, as the odds ratio is higher for the category 25 to 34 years than for the reference category (20–24 years), but consistently and increasingly lower for the older age categories.

The use of dummy variables is sometimes mandatory, as when modeling *nonordinal* polychotomous categorical variables such as "marital status" and "place of birth/acculturation" in Table 7-28. For example, one potentially important finding of this analysis is that compared with US-born/Anglo-oriented, the prevalence of depressive state seems

TABLE 7-28 Logistic regression analysis of the association between various sociodemographic characteristics and prevalence of depressive state, Hispanic Health and Nutrition Examination Survey, Mexican Americans aged 20–74 years, 1982–1984.

Characteristic	Logistic regression coefficient	Odds ratio	p Value
Intercept	−3.1187		
Sex (female vs male)	0.8263	2.28	0.0001
Age (years)			
20–24	—	1.00	
25–34	0.1866	1.20	0.11
35–44	−0.1112	0.89	0.60
45–54	−0.1264	0.88	0.52
55–64	−0.1581	0.85	0.32
65–74	−0.3555	0.70	0.19
Marital status			
Married	—	1.00	
Disrupted marriage	0.2999	1.35	0.18
Never married	0.7599	2.14	0.004
Years of education			
0–6	0.8408	2.32	0.002
7–11	0.4470	1.56	0.014
12	0.2443	1.28	0.21
≥ 13	—	1.00	
Annual household income (US$)			
0–4,999	0.7055	2.02	0.019
5,000–9,999	0.7395	2.09	0.009
10,000–19,999	0.4192	1.52	0.08
≥ 20,000	—	1.00	
Employment			
Unemployed vs employed	0.2668	1.31	0.20
Place of birth/acculturation			
US-born/Anglo oriented	—	1.00	
US-born/bicultural	−0.3667	0.69	0.004
Foreign-born/bicultural	−0.6356	0.53	0.026
Foreign-born/Mexican oriented	−0.8729	0.42	0.0003

Source: Data from EK Moscicki et al., Depressive Symptoms Among Mexican-Americans: The Hispanic Health and Nutrition Examination Survey. *American Journal of Epidemiology.* Vol 130, pp. 348–360, © 1989.

to be significantly lower among the foreign born, particularly those who are Mexican oriented. Again, it is important to bear in mind that the estimate for each variable is adjusted for all other variables shown in Table 7-28. Variables not included in the model, however, could still confound these associations (see Section 7.6); furthermore, causal inferences based on the data shown in Table 7-28 may be affected by their cross-sectional nature and its related biases (see Chapter 4, Section 4.4.2).

With respect to continuous or ordinal categorical variables, dummy variables can serve as an intermediary or exploratory step to evaluate whether a straight linear model is appropriate or whether several categories have to be redefined or regrouped. For example, after seeing the results shown in Table 7-28, one could simplify the definition for the variable "income" by grouping the two categories of less than US $10,000 into one, in view of their seemingly homogeneous odds of depression. Furthermore, because of the appearance of an approximately linear increase in the odds of depression according to decreasing levels of education, the authors could have further simplified the model by replacing the three dummy variables for education with a single ordinal variable (coded 1 to 4, or 0 to 3); in this example, the value of the coefficient in the latter case would be interpreted as the decrease in the log odds per unit increase in the level of education. In other words, the antilog of this coefficient would be the estimate of the odds ratio comparing any one pair of adjacent ordinal categories of education (i.e., comparing those with ≥ 13 years versus those with 12 years; or those with 12 years versus those with 7–11 years; or those with 7–11 years versus those with 0–6 years).

The latter approach, frequently used in the analysis of epidemiologic data (as when redefining the levels of certain serum parameters, nutrients, etc., according to quartiles, quintiles, etc.) is essentially equivalent to using a continuous variable, except that the possible values of x are now restricted to the integer values from 1 to 4 or 1 to 5 and so on. The advantages of this approach as compared with a more complex model including a number of dummy variables are that (1) the resulting model is more parsimonious and simpler to explain (see Section 7.7) and (2) the statistical testing of the corresponding regression coefficient (see next section and Appendix A, Section A.9) is the multivariate adjusted analogue of the test for dose response described in Appendix B. It is important to bear in mind, however, the risks of using these ordinal definitions of the independent variables without consideration of the possible presence of patterns such as those schematically represented in Figure 7-9A.

Alternative Modeling Techniques for Nonlinear Associations

The use of more complex mathematical functions constitutes another approach to modeling associations for which a simple linear function (e.g., a straight line) does not seem to represent a proper fit. Examples of these alternative models include the use of quadratic terms (which can model simple curve relationships) or more complex polynomial or other types of functions to model U- or J-shape relationships (e.g., Figure 7-9A). Although a discussion of these models is outside the purview of this book (see, e.g., Armitage et al.[11]), two examples are displayed in Figures 7-10 and 7-11.

Figure 7-10 is based on a study that examined the relationship between BMI and percent body fat in several populations of African descent.[40] Figure 7-10A shows the scatter diagram for the combined male and female subjects from the Nigeria subset in that study, whereas Figures 7-10B and 7-10C show the estimated regression lines separately for males and females. After evaluating different modeling options, the

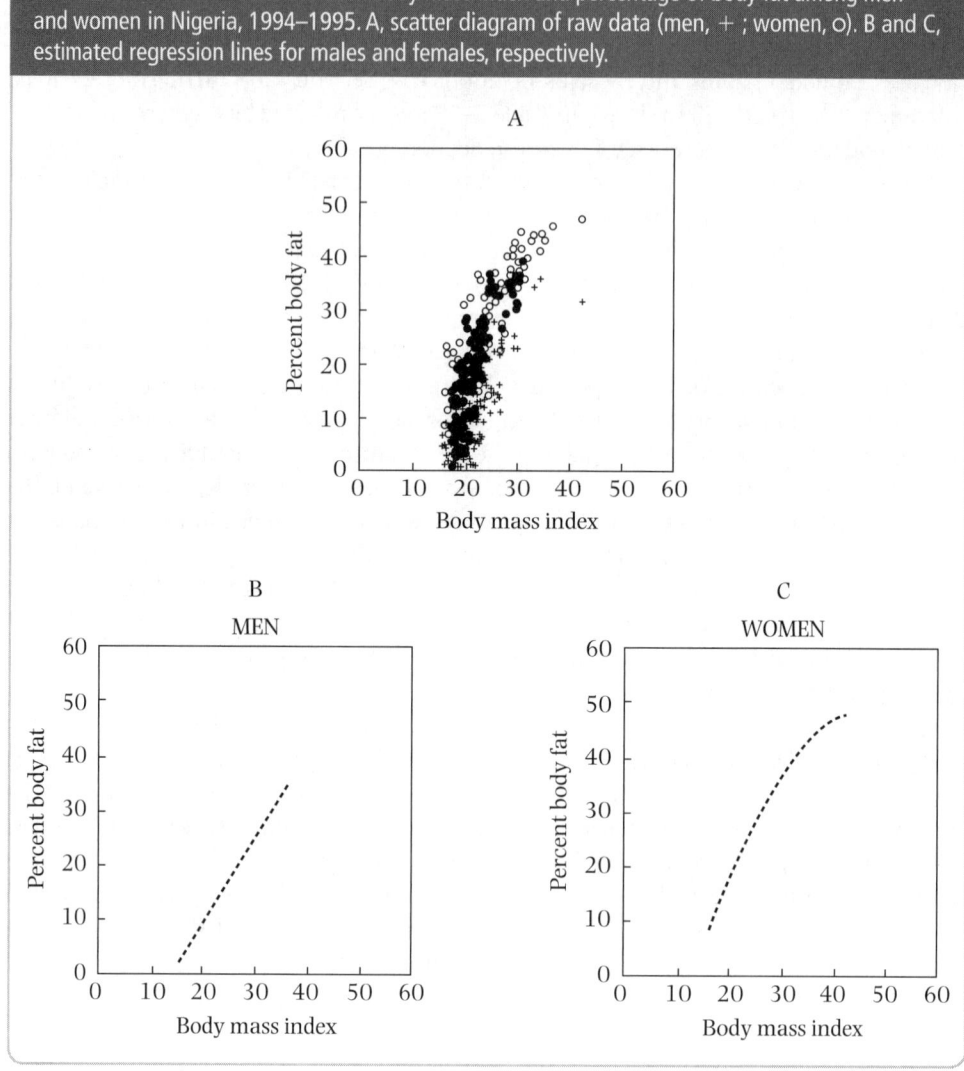

FIGURE 7-10 Relations between body mass index and percentage of body fat among men and women in Nigeria, 1994–1995. A, scatter diagram of raw data (men, +; women, o). B and C, estimated regression lines for males and females, respectively.

Source: Reprinted with permission from A Luke et al., Relation Between Body Mass Index and Body Fat in Black Population Samples from Nigeria, Jamaica, and the United States. *American Journal of Epidemiology*, Vol 145, pp. 620–628, © 1997.

authors concluded that the relationship between BMI and body fat was well described by a simple linear model in men.

$$\% \text{ body fat} = -21.37 + 1.51(\text{BMI})$$

whereas a curvilinear model (quadratic term) was needed for women:

$$\% \text{ body fat} = -44.24 + 4.01(\text{BMI}) - 0.043(\text{BMI})^2$$

Figure 7-11 is from a simulation study of the spread of two sexually transmitted diseases (gonorrhea and *Chlamydia trachomatis*) based on different assumptions regarding transmission patterns.[41] Specifically, Figure 7-11 shows the prevalence of these diseases according to the effective contact rate (a function of the mean and variance of the number of sexual partners); shown in the figure are the estimated (observed) prevalence

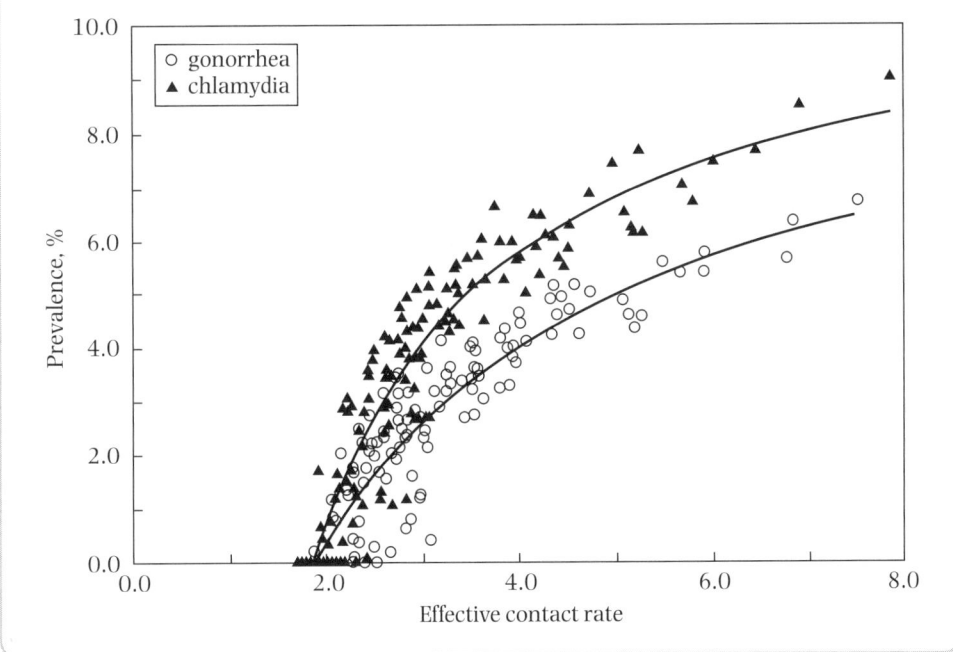

FIGURE 7-11 Simulation models for the spread of gonorrhea and *Chlamydia trachomatis*: the prevalence rates of gonorrhea and chlamydia (as percentages of the model population) as a function of the effective contact rates. Each data point represents one simulation run. The solid lines represent hyperbolic functions of the form $y = [b_0(x - b_1)]/[b_2 + (x - b_1)]$, which were fitted to the data points with a nonlinear curve-fitting program. In this equation, y is prevalence and x is the effective contact rate; the resulting parameter value estimates were for gonorrhea, $b_0 = 10.08$, $b_1 = 1.89$, $b_2 = 3.18$, and for chlamydia, $b_0 = 11.12$, $b_1 = 1.85$, $b_2 = 2.0$.

Source: Reprinted with permission from M Kretzschmar, YTHP van Duynhoven, and AJ Severijnen, Modeling Prevention Strategies for Gonorrhea and Chlamydia Using Stochastic Network Simulations. *American Journal of Epidemiology*, Vol 144, pp. 306–317. © 1996.

in each of the simulations (the dots) and the estimated statistical models that best fit the observed data for either disease. As previously discussed, these complex hyperbolic functions are useful for prediction. On the other hand, none of the parameters from these models (e.g., $b_1 = 1.89$) has a clear interpretation in terms of summarizing the association between the variables of interest (e.g., effective contact rate and prevalence of gonorrhea). The trade-off between simplicity and interpretability on the one hand and proper fit on the other is at the core of the art and science of statistical modeling, as briefly discussed in the summary section of this chapter (Section 7.7).

7.4.8 Statistical Testing and Confidence Intervals of Regression Estimates

The values of the regression parameters in linear regression, whether simple (Section 7.4.1) or multiple (Section 7.4.2) linear regression, are estimated using the *ordinary least-squares* method. This method of estimation is fairly simple and, in the case of simple linear regression, can be carried out with a simple pocket calculator; for multivariate linear regression, however, matrix algebra is required. On the other hand, the simple least-squares method cannot be applied to the other three regression methods described in the previous sections. Logistic regression, Cox regression, and Poisson regression methods require an iterative estimation process based on the *maximum likelihood method* (MLE), a task that is greatly facilitated by using modern computers and statistical software. (For a general introduction to the principles of likelihood and MLE, see Clayton and Hills.[42])

As with any other statistical estimate, the regression parameters obtained using ordinary-least squares or MLE for the regression methods presented in the previous sections are subject to uncertainty because of sampling variability. Thus, in addition to the regression coefficient, the estimation algorithm provides the standard error associated with that parameter estimate (see, e.g., Table 7-17). With the point estimate of the regression coefficient and its standard error (in any of the regression methods described in the preceding sections), hypothesis testing can be performed to assess whether the regression coefficient in question is statistically significant: that is, whether the null hypothesis (H_o: $b = 0$) can be rejected at a certain significance (alpha error) level. This test, called the Wald statistic, is briefly described with some examples in Appendix A, Section A.9. Similarly, a confidence interval for the value of a regression coefficient can be estimated using the point estimate and the standard error of that regression coefficient (see Appendix A). As shown in the examples in the appendix, for multiplicative models (e.g., logistic, Cox, Poisson), the exponentiation of the lower and upper confidence interval for the regression coefficients provides the corresponding confidence limits for the multiplicative measures of association (e.g., odds ratio, hazards ratio, rate ratio).

In addition to the Wald statistic and confidence limits to evaluate the statistical relevance of each regression parameter estimated, other statistical parameters or tests are useful for the comparison of different models; these include the value of the R^2 in the context of linear regression, which gives an estimate of the proportion of the variance of the dependent variable explained by the independent variables, and the *likelihood ratio test*, a significance test comparing models based on MLE-based regression methods. In addition, a number of numerical and graphical techniques can be used to evaluate the statistical assumptions and fit of the data to a particular model or set of independent variables. For more details on these methods, the reader is referred to more advanced textbooks, such as Armitage et al.,[11] Kleinbaum et al.,[13] or Clayton and Hills.[42]

7.5 ALTERNATIVE APPROACHES FOR THE CONTROL OF CONFOUNDING

The preceding sections cover the traditional approaches to control for confounding in epidemiologic studies (either in the design phase of the study—such as matching, or during the analysis—such as stratification and regression). In addition to these traditional methods, new approaches have been proposed in recent years. These include the use of *instrumental variables*—of which the *Mendelian randomization* method is a special case, and the *propensity score* method. In this section, the rationale, methodology, and application examples of these methods as well as their potential caveats are discussed.

7.5.1 Instrumental Variable Method

The instrumental variable method originated in the fields of econometrics and social sciences, and has recently been applied in health services and epidemiologic research. The approach uses directed acyclic graphs techniques (see Section 5.3) to identify the existence of a variable (the so-called *instrument*) that is causally related to the exposure of interest *and* is not related to the outcome *other than through the exposure*. Under such circumstances, by studying the relation between the instrument and the outcome—or more specifically, by regressing the exposure on the instrument and then regressing the outcome on the predicted value of the exposure (as a function of the instrument—see below), one can make causal inferences with regard to the relation between the exposure and the outcome that are not affected by the presence of unmeasured confounding.[43–46]

As illustrated in Figure 7-12, an instrumental variable must meet the following conditions:

1. it is causally associated with the exposure;
2. it affects the outcome *only* through the exposure; and
3. it is not associated with any confounders (known or unknown) of the association between the exposure and the outcome.

An example of the application of the instrumental variable approach has been provided by Glymour et al.[47] These authors were interested in examining the association between childhood schooling (number of years in school) and memory in older age. They used individual-level data on education, mental status, and other covariates from participants in the Health and Retirement Study. The authors were concerned about potential confounding, e.g., by intelligence quotient (IQ) or socioeconomic status that could be related to both childhood education and cognitive function in older age (including memory)—see Figure 7-13A. In order to control for these and other unknown confounders, the authors used an instrumental variable approach. They used compulsory state schooling laws at the time of the study participants' birth as the instrument (Figure 7-13B) based on the following rationale: since there are states that require more years of schooling (by regulating mandatory enrollment age and minimum drop out age), if a relation between the existence of these compulsory schooling regulations during childhood and memory in older age is observed, this finding will strengthen the inference of a causal relationship between schooling and cognitive function later in life. The key assumption for this inference to be valid (condition number 3 above) is

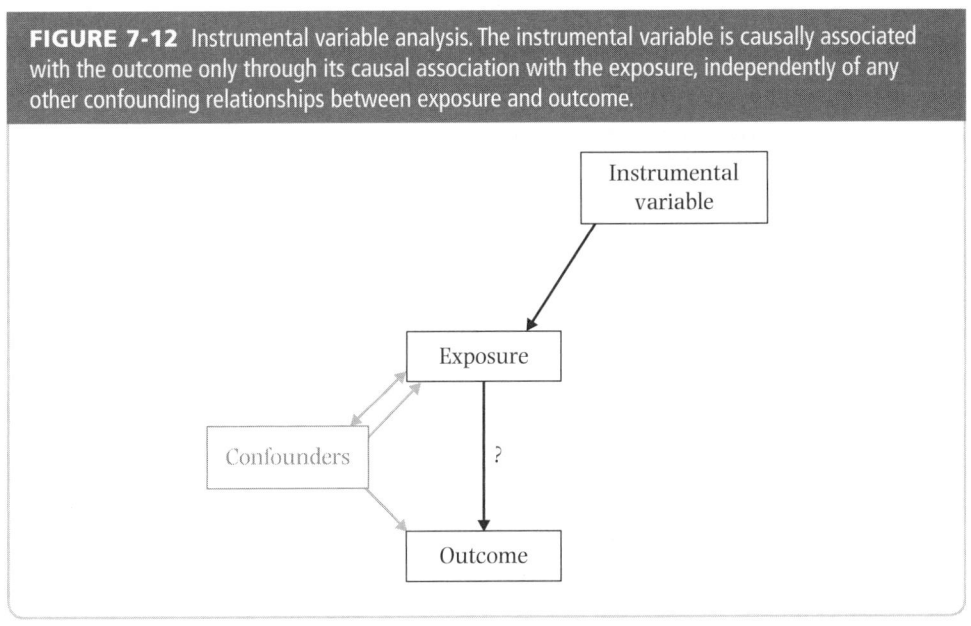

FIGURE 7-12 Instrumental variable analysis. The instrumental variable is causally associated with the outcome only through its causal association with the exposure, independently of any other confounding relationships between exposure and outcome.

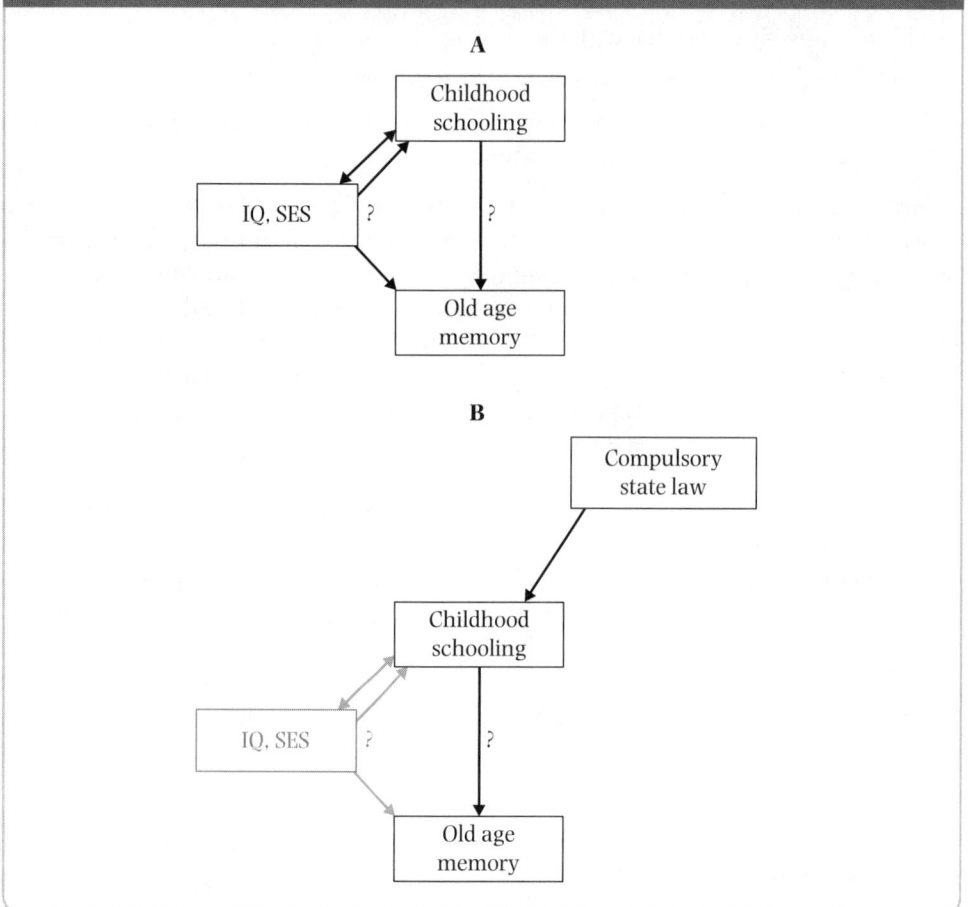

FIGURE 7-13 Example of the application of instrumental variable analysis. When studying the relation between childhood schooling and memory in old age, other factors such as intelligence quotient (IQ) and socioeconomic status (SES) can act as confounders (A). By studying the relation between previous existence of compulsory minimum schooling state laws (the instrument) and epidemiologic data on memory of older people (B), an inference can be made with regard to the relation between schooling and cognitive function in older age independently of measured or unmeasured confounders.

Source: Based on MM Glymour, I Kawachi, CS Jencks, LF Berkman, Does Childhood Schooling Affect Old Age Memory or Mental Status? Using State Schooling Laws as Natural Experiments, *Journal of Epidemiology and Community Health.* 2008;62:532–537.

that state regulations are not related to the individual-level confounding factors that affect the traditional observational study assessing the relation between individual schooling and the old age memory (i.e., IQ, SES and other unmeasured confounders in this example).

The implementation of the instrumental variable approach is not as straightforward as Figure 7-13B would imply, however. The naïve analysis would simply replace the exposure (schooling) with the instrumental variable (state laws) in the regression on the outcome (old age memory). However, while the existence of an association in this analysis would be suggestive, its results will not provide a correct inference with regard to the magnitude of the association of interest (childhood schooling—old age memory). The reason is that childhood schooling depends on many other variables aside from state laws; simply ignoring these other determinants of schooling will tend to dilute the association.

As described in detail elsewhere,[45,47,48] the correct analysis involves a two-step approach as follows: (1) a regression of the instrument on the exposure to obtain "predicted values" of the exposure (years of schooling in this example) as a function of the instrumental variable (see Section 7.4.1); and (2) a regression of the predicted years of schooling (exposure) on the outcome (old age memory). The regression coefficient estimated for predicted years of schooling in the second step thus represents an unbiased estimate of the association between schooling and memory in old age.

In another example, Leigh and Schembri[48] used cigarette price as an instrument to try to estimate the *causal* association between smoking and general health. Whereas the relation between smoking and health can be subject to confounding (e.g., by other unhealthy behaviors), one can assume that the price of cigarettes in the locality where an individual lives is not directly associated with his or her health. The authors of this study conducted a cross-sectional analysis of data from more than 34,000 adult participants in a national survey to study how number cigarettes smoked per day, as predicted by the average cigarette price for the state in which the subject resided, correlated with functional status measured using the SF-12 instrument. The main findings of this study where that higher average cigarette price in each state was associated with lower cigarette consumption and that predicted cigarettes per day (based on cigarette price—the instrument) was strongly and negatively associated with physical functioning; moreover, the latter association was stronger than that for observed cigarette consumption, implying that the true effect of smoking on health may be larger than conventional methods have estimated.[48] The assumption is that, by using a modified estimate of the exposure (predicted by the instrument) that is less prone to confounding, this approach offers a more accurate estimate of the true causal relation between smoking and physical functioning than a standard outcome-exposure regression analysis.

When the instrument is an ecological variable such as in the preceding examples (e.g., compulsory schooling law; price of cigarettes) the instrumental variable approach can be thought of as emulating a "natural experiment."[5] In general, the usefulness of this approach relies on the degree to which it mimics an experimental randomization approach. As illustrated in Figure 7-14, the randomization model is essentially an analogue of the instrumental variable model (Figure 7-12); the variable "treatment assignment" (as determined by randomization) meets the three conditions that define an instrument as described above: (1) it determines who receives what treatment (who is exposed); (2) it affects the outcome through its effect on what treatment is actually received; and (3) it is unrelated to confounders of the treatment-outcome association. A randomized trial, using an *intention-to-treat* approach to study the relation between randomization (treatment allocation) and an outcome, provides an unbiased estimate of the causal effect of treatment on the outcome.[5] Thus, in the preceding examples, compulsory schooling laws or cigarette pricing are considered analogues to randomized treatment assignment to the extent that they can be assumed to be independent of confounding factors that could affect the associations of interest (schooling and cognitive function in older age; smoking and physical functioning) and have an effect on the outcome only through their effects on the exposures of interest.

Conversely, the randomization analogy offers a framework to understand the possible limitations of the instrumental variable approach. Inasmuch as the instrument fails to mimic a randomized treatment assignment, it will be unwarranted to use the

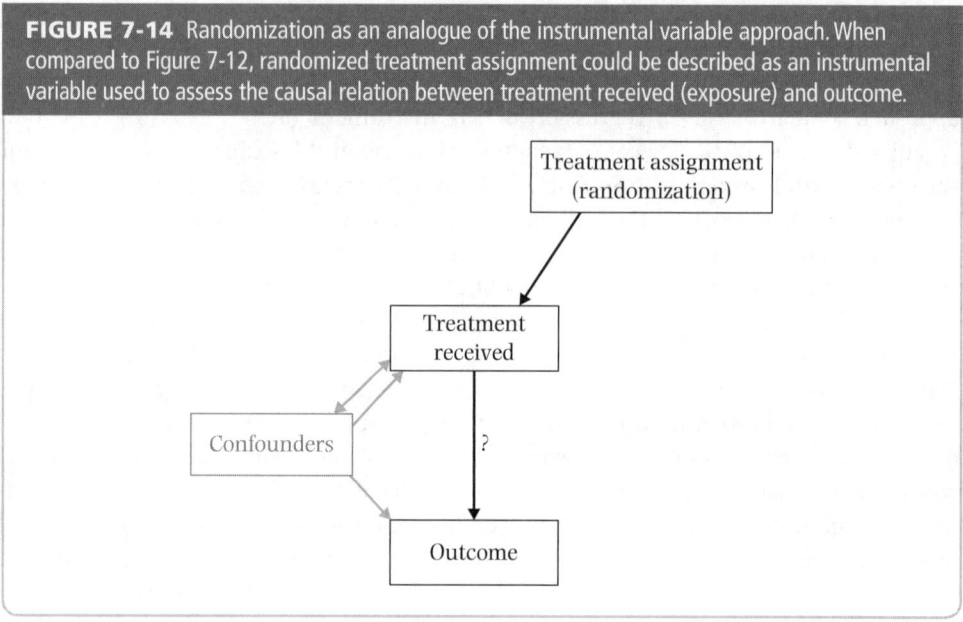

FIGURE 7-14 Randomization as an analogue of the instrumental variable approach. When compared to Figure 7-12, randomized treatment assignment could be described as an instrumental variable used to assess the causal relation between treatment received (exposure) and outcome.

instrumental variable strategy to make valid causal inferences. This could be the case in any one of these two circumstances:

1. When the instrument is only weakly associated with the exposure. This would be the case, for example, if cigarette pricing was only weakly associated with cigarette consumption—e.g., because of people's mobility, the pricing on the current state of residence might not truly reflect long-term smoking habits;[48] or if the level of schooling varies according to other variables other than compulsory schooling law (Figure 7-15A). If this is the case, studying the association between the instrument and the outcome may lead to an incorrect conclusion regarding the true causal nature of the exposure-outcome association, as it will be affected by confounding (or even bias, e.g., dilution bias, ecological bias). Note that this is analogous to the shortcomings of an intention-to-treat analysis of a clinical trial when randomization does not effectively separate the treatment groups—e.g., because of poor compliance or because of crossover, leading to biased estimates of the effects of treatment.
2. When the relationship between the instrument and the outcome is affected by confounding (e.g., when condition no. 3 above is not fulfilled). For example, it is conceivable that states that have more stringent schooling regulations might also have different average SES and a different political environment (e.g., health care and public health programs), which, in turn, would affect health throughout the life-course, including cognitive function in older age (Figure 7-15B).[47] If that were the case, the instrumental variable approach illustrated in Figure 7-13B, would not lead to the correct inferences regarding the association between childhood schooling and old age memory (see Chapter 5).

Because of these potential biases, instrumental variable approaches should be used and interpreted cautiously.[49] In addition to these potential interpretation caveats, another important practical limitation of the instrumental variable method is that it is only applicable when a suitable instrument is available. Like the randomized

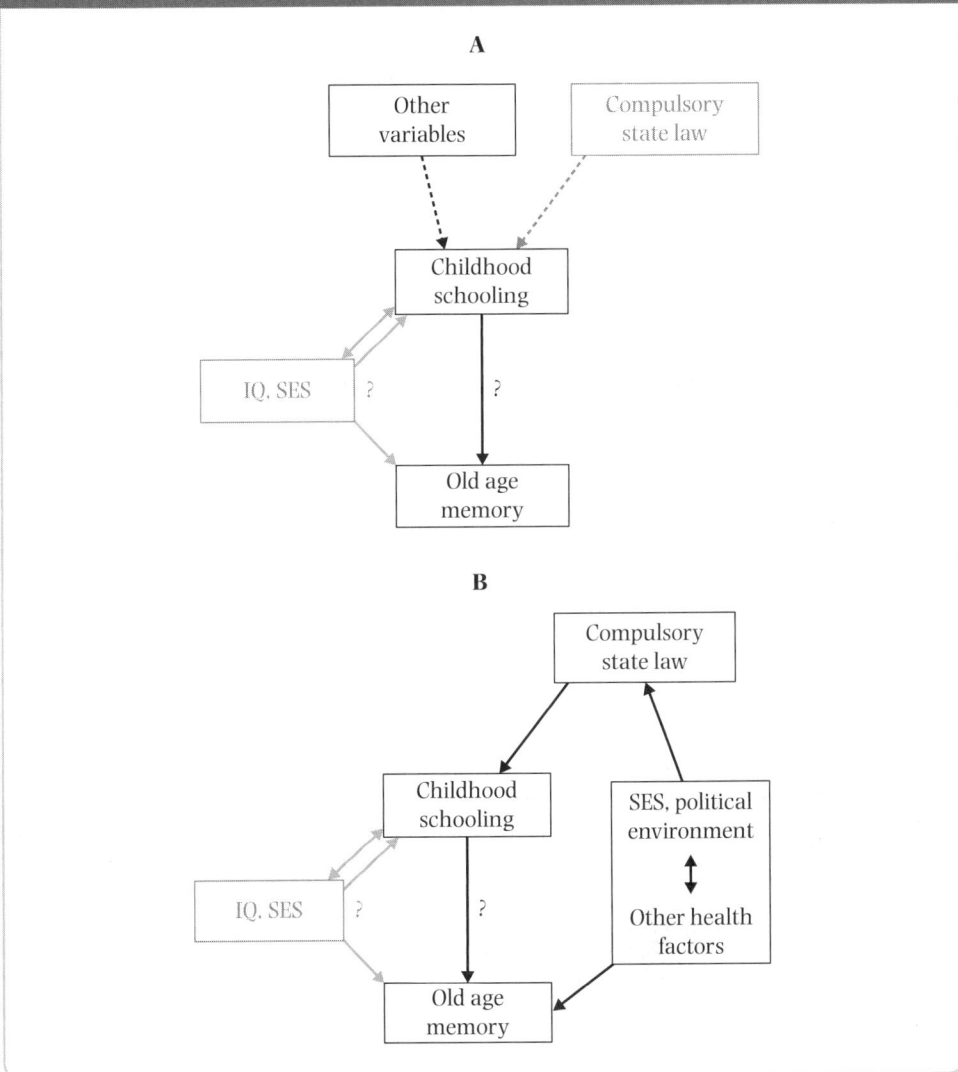

FIGURE 7-15 Limitations of the instrumental variable approach. (A): when the instrument (e.g., compulsory state law) is only weakly associated with the exposure (childhood schooling); (B): when the instrument is associated with other variables that are in turn related to the outcome (old age memory).

trial approach—which is often not feasible or applicable to address many epidemiologic questions—there are instances when there is no identifiable or measurable instrumental variable that could be used in the analysis.

Mendelian Randomization

Mendelian randomization is a special application of the instrumental variable approach when the instrument is a genetic polymorphism known to affect the presence or the level of the exposure of interest (the phenotype).[50] Because chromosomes and genes are randomly segregated during gamete formation and recombined at conception, the association between the suspected genetic polymorphism and the disease will be free of confounding (e.g., by other genetic, behavioral, or environmental characteristics) and thus reflect the true causal exposure–disease association.

One example is the study of the association between plasma homocysteine levels and cardiovascular disease. Observational studies have suggested that high levels of homocysteine (an aminoacid that is a by-product of methionine's metabolism) are associated with both subclinical and clinical atherosclerosis.[51,52] However, because high homocysteine levels might be the result of low folate and vitamin B_{12} dietary intake,[54,55] this association might be affected by confounding (e.g., poor diet resulting from unhealthy lifestyle, low socioeconomic status or other factors). Homocysteine metabolism and its blood levels are also affected by a functional polymorphism of the gene encoding the enzyme methylene tetrahydrofolate reductase (MTHFR).[50] A substitution of cytosine (C) for thyamine (T) at the 677T allele results in a decreased activity of this enzyme; individuals who are homozygous for this polymorphism (MTHFR 677T TT) tend to have higher plasma homocysteine levels. The MTHFR 677T TT genetic variant thus mimics the effect of low folate but is theoretically not subject to the potential confounding from factors affecting dietary intake of vitamins. If an association between the MTHFR 677T TT genotype and cardiovascular disease is observed, this will support the notion that homocysteine is causally related to cardiovascular disease (Figure 7-16) in view of the association between this genotype and homocysteine levels. Note that this situation is analogous to the instrumental variable approach described above (Figure 7-12) and that the MTHFR 677T TT trait meets all required conditions that characterize an instrument: (1) it is associated with a higher level of the exposure (homocysteine level); (2) it affects the outcome (cardiovascular disease) only through its association with the exposure; and (3) it is not affected by confounders of the exposure-outcome association (diet, other lifestyle factors).

Casas et al. used the Mendelian randomization approach represented in Figure 7-16 to test the hypothesis that homocysteine is causally related to stroke.[55] A meta-analysis

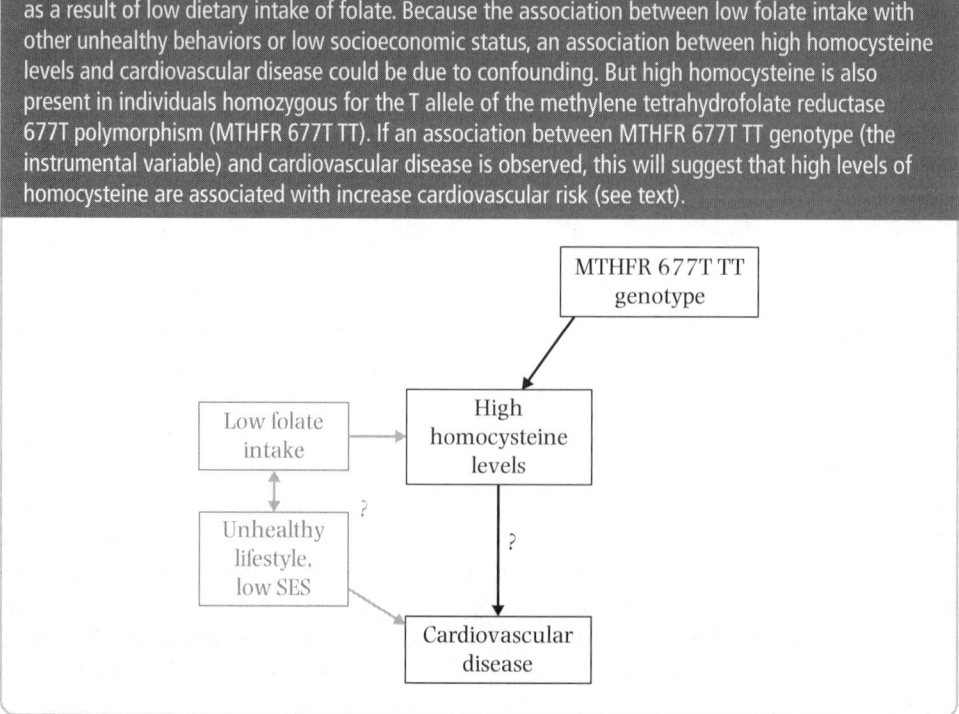

FIGURE 7-16 Example of Mendelian randomization. High levels of plasma homocysteine occur as a result of low dietary intake of folate. Because the association between low folate intake with other unhealthy behaviors or low socioeconomic status, an association between high homocysteine levels and cardiovascular disease could be due to confounding. But high homocysteine is also present in individuals homozygous for the T allele of the methylene tetrahydrofolate reductase 677T polymorphism (MTHFR 677T TT). If an association between MTHFR 677T TT genotype (the instrumental variable) and cardiovascular disease is observed, this will suggest that high levels of homocysteine are associated with increase cardiovascular risk (see text).

of 111 observational studies (see Section 10.4) found that the pooled mean difference in homocysteine concentration between MTHFR C677T TT and CC homozygous individuals was 1.93 micromol/L. The pooled odds ratio of stroke was 1.26 (95% confidence limits 1.14–1.40) for TT versus CC homozygotes—which was very similar to the pooled odds ratio estimate corresponding to a 1.93 micromol/L difference in homocysteine concentration from these same studies (pooled OR = 1.20). The similarity in the strength of the association of the instrument with the outcome, and that of the exposure with the outcome, can be regarded as evidence supporting causality. Taken overall, these results are consistent with a causal relation between homocysteine concentration and risk of stroke.

In another example, Elliott et al. used Mendelian randomization to investigate whether C-reactive protein (CRP, a maker of inflammation) is causally associated with coronary heart disease (CHD).[56] The authors identified single-nucleotide polymorphisms (SNPs) that were associated with increased CRP but that were not related to risk of CHD in a meta-analysis of observational studies. These findings argue against a causal association between CRP and CHD and imply that the widely observed association between high CRP levels and cardiovascular outcomes might be explained by confounding or reverse causation (e.g., rather than a causal factor, high CRP may be a consequence of atherosclerosis—the underlying pathological process in CHD).

It is important to note that Mendelian randomization is not limited to the study of biochemical markers such as homocysteine and CRP levels. It could be applied to any other characteristics (including other physical, mental, or behavioral) for which a genetic polymorphism can be causally linked. For example, this approach was used to assess the hypothesis that alcohol intake is causally related to risk of esophageal cancer.[57] This association has been well established in numerous observational studies and it has been attributed to the carcinogenic effects of acetaldehyde, the principal alcohol metabolite. The ability to metabolize acetaldehyde is encoded by the ALDH2 gene; a single point mutation in ALDH2 results in the ALDH2*2 allele, which produces an inactive protein that is unable to metabolize acetaldehyde. Individuals who are ALDH2*2*2 homozygotes have unpleasant symptoms after consumption of alcohol (including nausea, headaches, drowsiness) that prevent them from heavy drinking; heterozygotes have a limited ability to metabolize acetaldehyde but don't have such an adverse physical reaction following alcohol intake. Lewis and Davey Smith[57] found that, relative to ALDH2*1*1 homozygotes, the risk of esophageal cancer was reduced among *2*2 homozygotes (odds ratio = 0.36) and increased among *1*2 heterozygotes (OR = 3.19). These results not only provide strong evidence in support of the notion that the relation between alcohol intake and esophageal cancer is causal in nature; but they also validate the hypothesis that acetaldehyde plays a carcinogenic role.

Like instrumental variable analysis in general, Mendelian randomization is not free of limitations.[58] The method can't be used unless a genetic trait that is strongly associated with the exposure of interest needs has been identified. Furthermore, the analysis might be confounded by *linkage disequilibrium*, i.e., if the genetic polymorphism under study is associated (linked) with other genetic variants that increase or decrease the risk of the outcome. This phenomenon is known as "population stratification" in the field of genetic epidemiology and would constitute a violation of the third condition for an instrumental variable discussed above. Other possible limitations of Mendelian randomization might occur as a result of phenomena such as pleiotropy and developmental compensation ("canalization"), as discussed in more specialized literature.[58]

7.5.2 Propensity Scores

A propensity score is the predicted probability ("propensity") of exposure in a particular individual based on a set of relevant characteristics.[59] As originally proposed by Rosenbaum and Rubin,[60] the propensity scores can be used to control for confounding in observational cohort studies using one of several different approaches briefly described below. The idea is to try to mimic randomization by making the exposed and the unexposed groups as comparable as possible with respect to relevant confounding variables. Historically, these methods have been particularly popular in cohort studies assessing the effectiveness of drugs or other therapies when random allocation was not done; but they can be equally applied to any other type of exposure (see examples below). These methods have the intuitive appeal of trying to emulate randomization and under certain circumstances provide a more efficient control of confounding, which makes them particularly useful for the study of rare outcomes.

The application of this method involves two steps. In the first step, the exposure variable (e.g., treated or not treated) is modeled as the dependent variable in a multiple regression (typically a logistic regression) including as predictors covariates that are considered as possible confounders of the exposure-outcome association. As described in Section 7.4.3, the intercept and the regression coefficients from this multiple regression can then be used to calculate the predictive probability of exposure as a function of this multivariate set of possible confounding variables. These predicted probabilities of exposure ("propensity scores") can then be applied either to generate a new dataset of matched exposed and unexposed based on propensity score. Because these two groups are *similar* with respect to an overall set of (known) covariates, this approach (described below) could be thought of as analogous to a *simulated randomization*. An alternative approach, also briefly described below, is to use the propensity score as an overall covariate score in a multivariate regression model.

Propensity Score Matching

For this method, a new dataset is created that includes exposed and unexposed individuals matched with respect to the propensity score. This dataset is typically smaller than the original dataset as it only includes exposed and unexposed individuals whose scores matched (i.e., individuals in the extreme ranges of the propensity score in either group for whom a match was not found are excluded.)

An example of this approach is a study of the association between in-hospital smoking cessation counseling and 3-year mortality among 2,342 survivors of a myocardial infarction at 103 acute care hospitals in Ontario, Canada.[61] Of these, 1,588 patients received smoking cessation counseling (treated) before discharge and 754 did not (untreated). This intervention was not randomized and the two groups were quite different with regard to several characteristics that could strongly influence prognosis (Table 7-29, "Overall" columns). The smoking cessation counseling propensity scores were calculated using a set of 33 relevant characteristics (including demographic variables, risk factors, comorbidities, other treatments, etc.). To be considered a match, treated and untreated subjects had to be within 0.2 standard deviation units of the logit of the propensity score. Six hundred and forty-six treated and untreated propensity score-matched pairs were identified. As shown on the right-hand side columns, these matched treated and untreated individuals were very similar with respect to the characteristics shown in Table 7-29, albeit not exactly identical for most of them, as the matching was done on the overall propensity score. (Note that this is the same situation with

TABLE 7-29 Example of propensity score matching: characteristics of myocardial infarction survivors who were given smoking cessation counseling and those who were not, overall and after propensity score matching.

	Overall			Propensity score matched*	
	Smoking cessation counseling (n = 1,588)	No counseling (n = 754)	p value	Smoking cessation counseling (n = 646)	No counseling (n = 646)
Age (mean years)	56.2	60.5	<0.001	58.7	59.1
Female (%)	25.0	29.2	0.032	27.1	27.6
Diabetes (%)	16.4	23.7	<0.001	21.7	20.1
Hyperlipidemia (%)	33.9	31.6	0.254	33.1	33.4
Hypertension (%)	34.1	39.1	0.017	38.2	38.2
Family history CHD (%)	47.5	33.6	<0.001	36.4	33.7
Comorbid					
Stroke/TIA (%)	4.2	8.2	<0.001	7.1	6.0
Cancer (%)	1.3	2.9	0.005	2.0	2.3
Depression (%)	8.2	10.1	0.145	9.8	9.8
CHF (%)	1.5	3.2	0.008	2.2	2.0
White cell count (in 1000)	10.8	11	0.17	10.7	10.9
Prescriptions					
Statin	40.1	25.6	<0.001	28.6	29.3
Beta-blocker	75.1	61.0	<0.001	66.1	65.6
Aspirin	84.4	72.1	<0.001	75.5	73.7

*Matching according to a total of 33 variables, including the variables shown in the table and the following variables: acute pulmonary edema, systolic blood pressure, diastolic blood pressure, heart rate, respiratory rate, angina, dementia, previous myocardial infarction, asthma, peptic ulcer disease, peripheral vascular disease, previous coronary revascularization, hemoglobin, glucose, sodium, potassium, creatinine, angiotensin converting enzyme inhibitor, Plavix.

CHD: coronary hearth disease; CHF: congestive heart failure.

Source: Data from PC Austin, A Tutorial and Case Study in Propensity Score Analysis: An Application to Estimating the Effect of In-Hospital Smoking Cessation Counseling on Mortality. *Multivariate Behavioral Research.* Vol 46, pp. 119–151, © 2011.

randomization: the randomized groups tend to be similar, but not necessarily identical with respect to most characteristics.) In this analysis, the 3-year probability of death in the propensity matched treated and untreated groups were 0.14 and 0.16, respectively (relative risk = 0.88; 95% confidence limits, 0.69–1.13).

In another example, propensity score matching was used to explore whether female gender were at higher risk of mortality following coronary bypass surgery.[62] In this historical cohort study, the in-hospital mortality of 9848 males and 3267 females who underwent bypass surgery at a Texas hospital between 1995 and 2009 was compared. Because of the potential for confounding according to differential severity and co-morbidity profiles between males and females, propensity scores *for being female* were calculated based on a logistic regression model including 20 potentially relevant clinical covariates. Based on these propensity scores, 1800 males were matched to the same number of females. The odds ratio of in-hospital mortality comparing females to males was 1.84 (95% confidence limits, 1.22–2.78). In comparison, a regular logistic regression analysis that included gender and the other 20 variables that were used in the propensity score calculation as covariates, the odds ratio associated with female gender was 1.67 (95% confidence limits, 1.35–2.05).

Covariate Adjustment Using the Propensity Score

For this approach, a multiple regression analysis (e.g., linear, logistic, or Cox regression) is conducted using the propensity score as a covariate—other covariates can also been added if necessary.

For example, in the same smoking cessation counseling study described above,[61] a logistic regression analysis with smoking cessation counseling as the main independent variable and the propensity score added to the model as a covariate, resulted in an estimated adjusted odds ratio of 3-year mortality associated with treatment of 0.79 (95% confidence limits, 0.60–1.05). A logistic regression analysis including treatment and all the 33 covariates that were used in the propensity score calculation resulted in an odds ratio of 0.77 (95% confidence limits, 0.56–1.05) comparing treated to untreated patients.

Propensity score covariate adjustment was also the approach used in a study of the risk of diabetes mellitus associated with statin use.[63] A total of 153,840 participants in the Women's Health Initiative without diabetes at baseline (7% of whom were taking statins) were followed for a total of 1,004,466 person-years. Statin propensity score was estimated based on a logistic regression that included age, body mass index, self-report of hypertension, self-report of cardiovascular disease, family history of diabetes, and smoking. In unadjusted analysis using Cox proportional hazards regression (Section 7.4.4), statin use was associated with a relative hazard of incident diabetes mellitus of 1.71 (95% confidence limits, 1.61–1.83); after adjustment using the propensity score, the estimated relative hazard was attenuated but remained statistically significant (1.38, 95% confidence limits, 1.29–1.47). In adjusted analyses introducing all the same covariates used to construct the propensity score as separate terms in the Cox regression (instead of the propensity score as such), the corresponding hazard ratio was 1.48 (95% confidence limits, 1.38–1.59).

The approaches described in the preceding paragraphs are two of the possible ways propensity scores can be used to control for confounding. Other alternative approaches also based on the propensity scores (not described here) are *stratification on the propensity score* and *weighting by the inverse of the propensity score*.[62,64]

Partly because of their intuitive appeal in their ability to handle a large number of covariates, propensity score-based methods are becoming increasingly popular and widely used.[59] Compared to traditional regression methods for control of confounding that include all known relevant covariates, the propensity score methods have the disadvantage of losing useful information about predictors of outcomes[59]—i.e., not explicitly examining the association between single covariates and the outcome. In any event, as shown in the above examples and elsewhere,[59,61,64,65] the results of analyses using these methods tend to be very similar to those using conventional multiple regression methods. Finally, propensity scores-based methods are fundamentally limited to the control of known confounders on which information is available and, thus, like all the other methods described in this chapter, subject to potential residual confounding by unknown or misspecified confounding variables (see next section).

7.6 INCOMPLETE ADJUSTMENT: RESIDUAL CONFOUNDING

The issue of residual confounding, which occurs when adjustment does not completely remove the confounding effect due to a given variable or set of variables, has been introduced in Chapter 5, Section 5.5.4. The sources for incomplete adjustment and/or residual confounding are diverse, and some of the most important ones are discussed here.

1. *Improper definition of the categories of the confounding variable.* This occurs, for example, when attempting to adjust for a continuous variable using categories that are too broad. For example, Table 7-30 shows the results of different alternatives for age adjustment when exploring the cross-sectional relationship between menopausal status and prevalent coronary heart disease (CHD) using unpublished data from the ARIC study. The decrease in odds ratio when adjusting for age as a continuous variable indicates that the "age-adjusted" estimates using categorical definitions of age did not completely remove its confounding effect. The inference that the best alternative for the age adjustment in Table 7-30 is the model using age as a continuous variable obviously requires assuming that CHD prevalence increases linearly with age throughout the entire age range of study participants. This is an approximately correct assumption in this particular example, given the relatively narrow age range of the study population (middle-aged women). This may not be the case, however, in other situations. For example, if the age range of individuals in the study covered the entire life span, a linear model would not be reasonable, as the rate at which the increase in CHD risk varies by age is different between younger and older individuals. In this situation, a model similar to model 3 in Table 7-30 (defining age categorically) might have been the most appropriate. Another example of potential residual confounding relates to the adjustment for smoking using categorical definitions such as "current," "former," or "never." The variability in cumulative dose *within* the first two categories (i.e., in average number of cigarettes per day, pack-years, and time since quitting) may be large, thus resulting in important residual confounding when evaluating relationships between variables confounded by smoking.

2. *The variable used for adjustment is an imperfect surrogate of the condition or characteristic the investigator wishes to adjust for.* When using a given variable in an epidemiologic

TABLE 7-30 Cross-sectional relationship between natural menopause and prevalent coronary heart disease (CHD), Atherosclerosis Risk in Communities (ARIC) Study, ages 45–64, 1987–1989.

Model		OR	95% Confidence interval
1	Crude	4.54	2.67–7.85
2	Adjusted for age using two categories: 45–54 and 55–64 years (Mantel-Haenszel)	3.35	1.60–6.01
3	Adjusted for age using four categories: 45–49, 50–54, 55–59, and 60–64 years (Mantel-Haenszel)	3.04	1.37–6.11
4	Adjusted for age as a continuous variable (logistic regression)	2.47	1.31–4.63

study, it is important to consider the issue of its construct validity (i.e., the extent to which it represents the exposure or the outcome it purports to represent).[66] A typical example leading to residual confounding is the use of education to adjust for social class when evaluating ethnic differences (e.g., black–white differences) in a given outcome, as residual differences in access to goods and income level may exist between ethnic/racial groups, even *within* each educational-level category.[67]

3. *Other important confounders are not included in the model.* If some of the confounding variables are left out of the model, the adjusted estimates will obviously still be confounded. The results in the first row of Table 7-26, for example, are adjusted for demographic variables; if these had been the only results provided (either because of missing data on the additional possible confounders considered in the second model or because these data, although available, had been deemed unimportant by the investigators), their interpretation would have been that a high level of *C. pneumoniae* antibodies was associated with a 60% increase in the "adjusted" hazard ratio of CHD. Even the second model, which implies that the association is either weak or nonexistent, may be subject to residual confounding, because of the failure to include additional (unmeasured or unknown) confounders. Another example is the study showing an association between frequent sexual activity and lower mortality[68] that was discussed in Chapter 5, Section 5.5.4. As mentioned in that section, the lower mortality of study participants with a higher frequency of sexual intercourse persisted when a number of putative confounding variables were adjusted for using multiple logistic regression. In their discussion, the authors of that study speculated that unknown confounders might account for the results. Although they did not discuss which specific variables might account for residual confounding, at least two possibilities can be suggested. First, social class, an important determinant of both disease and mortality, has been taken into consideration in only a very crude manner by a dichotomous occupational variable ("manual" and "nonmanual" occupations); thus, substantial residual confounding may have remained. In addition, the only prevalent disease adjusted for was CHD; other diseases affecting both sexual activity and mortality (e.g., diabetes, perhaps psychiatric conditions) apparently were not considered and could result in residual confounding of the reported results.

4. *Misclassification of confounding variables.* Another source of residual confounding is misclassification of confounders, which results in imperfect adjustment.[69] Thus, for example, if there is no causal association between exposure and outcome, but the confounded association is reflected by a risk ratio or odds ratio greater than 1.0, adjustment for misclassified confounders may not result in an adjusted risk ratio or odds ratio of 1.0. An example of this phenomenon, based on hypothetical data, is presented in Table 7-31. The left hand side of this table shows the same data from Table 7-1; in this example, although the crude odds ratio suggested that males were at a 71% higher risk of malaria than females, this association all but vanished in occupation-stratified analyses; the occupation-adjusted OR_{MH} was 1.01 (see Sections 7.2 and 7.3.3). When misclassification of the confounder occurs (right-hand side of the table), the resulting "adjusted" OR_{MH} (1.30) is affected by residual confounding and fails to remove the confounding effect of occupation completely. The example in Table 7-31 is one of the simplest cases of misclassification: non-differential and only in one direction. More complex patterns of misclassification (e.g., bidirectional and/or differential) may lead

to unpredictable consequences with respect to the magnitude of bias in the "adjusted" estimates.

Methods to assess the impact of residual confounding resulting from confounder misclassification have been described.[70] These methods allow the estimation of how much confounding is likely to remain based on the change in estimates after adjusting for the imperfect confounding measure.

7.7 OVER-ADJUSTMENT

As mentioned in Chapter 5 (Section 5.5.3), adjustment for a given variable implies an adjustment, at least partially, for other variables related to it. Thus, when adjusting for educational level, adjustment for income is to a certain extent also carried out. As mentioned previously, depending on the specific characteristics of the study population, adjustment for residence will result in adjustment for related variables, such as

TABLE 7-31 Hypothetical data showing residual confounding resulting from nondifferential misclassification of a confounder (occupational status).

All cases and controls

	Cases	Controls	Total	
Males	88	68	156	OR = 1.71
Females	62	82	144	
Total	150	150	300	

Correctly classified occupational status*   **Misclassified occupational status†**

Mostly outdoor occupations

	Cases	Controls	Total		Cases	Controls	Total	
Males	53	15	68	OR = 1.06	35†	10	45	OR = 1.00
Females	10	3	13		7	2	9	
Total	63	18	81		42	12	54	

Mostly indoor occupations

	Cases	Controls	Total		Cases	Controls	Total	
Males	35	53	88	OR = 1.00	53†	58	111	OR = 1.33
Females	52	79	131		55	80	135	
Total	87	132	219		108	138	246	

"Correct" $OR_{MH} = 1.01$ "Misclassified" $OR_{MH} = 1.30$

*See Table 7-1.
†Nondifferential misclassification: one-third of all individuals with mostly outdoor occupation (regardless of case-control or gender status) are misclassified to mostly indoor occupation. (All the misclassified numbers are rounded to the nearest integer.) For example, of the 53 male cases in outdoor occupations, 18 ($\approx 53 \times 0.333$) are misclassified to mostly indoor, which leaves 35 subjects in that cell; in turn, as many as 53 male cases (35 correctly classified + 18 misclassified) are now included in the corresponding indoor occupation stratum.

socioeconomic status or ethnic background. *Over-adjustment* (or *overmatching*, for a variable adjusted for by matching) is said to occur when adjustment is inadvertently carried out for a variable that is either in the causal pathway between the exposure and the outcome (thus being an "intermediate" cause) or so strongly related to either the exposure or the outcome that their true relationship is distorted.[71] Over-adjustment can, therefore, obscure a true effect or create an apparent effect when none exists.[72]

An example is given by the adjustment for hypertension when examining the association between overweight and hemorrhagic stroke. As hypertension is likely to be an important mechanism explaining this association, adjustment for it may lead to obscuring the obesity–stroke relationship. As discussed in Chapter 5 (Section 5.2.3), it would nevertheless be appropriate to adjust for an intermediate cause or a mechanistic link when assessing the presence of residual effects due to alternative mechanisms.

Over-adjustment may also occur when adjusting for a variable closely related to the exposure of interest. An example that epitomizes gross over-adjustment is the adjustment for residence when studying the relationship of air pollution to respiratory disease. Other examples include situations when different variables representing overlapping constructs are simultaneously adjusted, as when including education, income, occupation, and aggregate (ecologic) measures of income or other socioeconomic indicators in the same regression model. Because all of these variables are markers of "social class," their collinearity would render the corresponding regression coefficients hard to interpret, or even meaningless.

The issue of over-adjustment underscores the need to consider the biologic underpinnings of a postulated relationship, as well as to carry out a thorough assessment of the relationships between the postulated confounding variable on the one hand and the exposure and outcome variables on the other (see Chapter 5, Section 5.3).

7.8 CONCLUSION

> *Our aim is to discover and ascertain the nature and substance of the soul, and, in the next place, all the accidents belonging to it.*
>
> Aristotle (quoted in Durrant[73(p.15)])

Statistical models are conceptual and mathematical summaries that are meant to express the presence of a certain pattern or association between the elements of a system (e.g., suspected risk factors and disease outcome). The epidemiologist uses statistical models "to concisely summarize broad patterns in data and to interpret the degree of evidence in a data set relevant to a particular hypothesis."[74 (p.1064)] When trying to identify patterns of associations between exposures and outcomes in epidemiology, the goal of the modeling process is usually to find the most *parsimonious* statistical model (i.e., the simplest model that satisfactorily describes the data). One simple way to understand this idea is to conceive the statistical model as a *sketch* or a *caricature* of the association under investigation. Thus, statistical modeling could be seen as a process analogous to that of a cartoonist trying to find the few lines that capture the essence of the character being portrayed, as illustrated in Figure 7-17. The four panels in this figure can be conceived as four "models" of former US president William J. Clinton. The model in Figure 7-17A is the simplest but fails to represent effectively the person that it is trying to portray (most people would not recognize President Clinton if shown only this picture). Some, but not all people, would recognize Clinton if shown Figure 7-17B, and probably almost everyone would recognize him in the sketch in Figure 7-17C. Thus, when looking for a succinct, parsimonious model to describe the essence of Clinton's portrait, those shown in Figures 7-17B or 7-17C would be the best choices. The "model" in Figure 7-17D fits "the data" better, but at the expense of making each of the elements in the sketch less useful in portraying the *essence* of the character.

This process is similar when using statistical modeling in epidemiologic analysis. As discussed by Zeger,[74] statistical models should be considered as "tools for science" rather than "laws of nature": "Statistical models for data are *never true*. The question of whether a model is true is irrelevant. A more appropriate question is whether we obtain the correct scientific conclusion if we pretend that that process under study behaves according to a particular statistical model."[74(p.1064)]

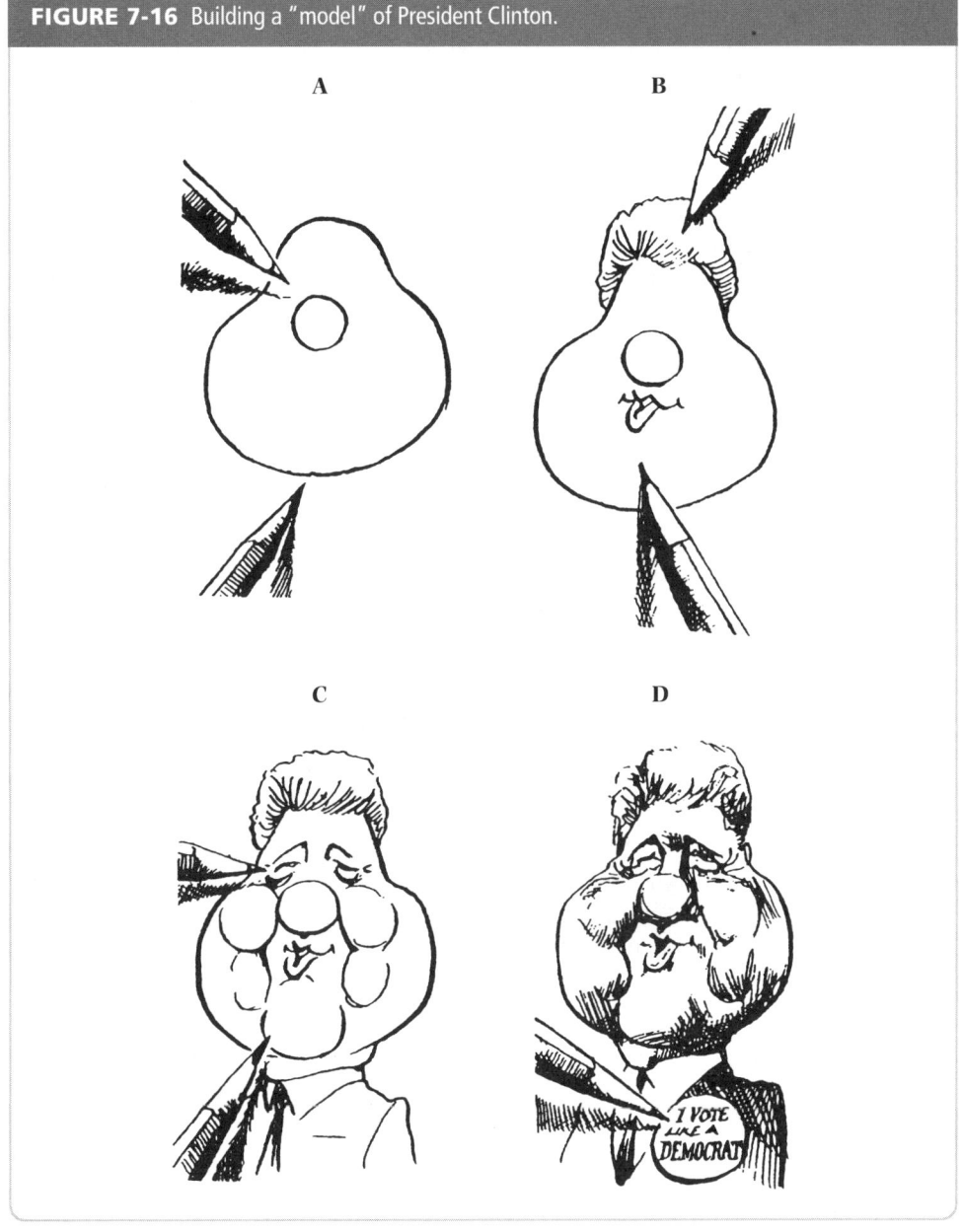

FIGURE 7-16 Building a "model" of President Clinton.

Source: Copyright © Kevin "KAL" Kallaugher, 1986, Baltimore Sun, Cartoonists and Writers Syndicate.

Thus, the key question is whether the model fits the data reasonably well in order to help the investigator to derive appropriate inferences. This means that whether the estimated value of the parameter (e.g., $b_1 = 0.0025$ mm in Table 7-16, model 1) is a *perfect* estimate of the "true" relationship between systolic blood pressure (SBP) and carotid intimal-medial thickness (IMT) or whether the true relationship between these two variables is *exactly* linear (e.g., Figure 7-4) is not that important. Often, the relevant questions are whether there is a more or less linear increment and what the approximate average increment is on y per unit of x after controlling for certain covariates. It should be again emphasized, however, that, as in the example in Figure 7-9, a model should never be adopted just because it is simple if it does not describe the association of interest properly (e.g., Figures 7-9B or 7-9C).

The attractiveness of simple linear models is precisely their simplicity and the interpretability of the parameters, such as the straight line that expresses the expected increase in carotid IMT for a given increase in SBP (Figure 7-4). Assuming that the model is appropriate (i.e., that the association is linear), it is possible to calculate the parameters (intercept and linear regression coefficient of the line—the model) that would best fit the data (Equation 7.2). Thus, the assumption is that the line in Figure 7-4 reflects the true *essence* of the relationship between SBP and IMT and that the scatter around the line (the observed data) is just *noise* (i.e., within-individual variability or random error).

The same logic applies to situations that incorporate the mutual relations among different correlates of both "exposure" (e.g., SBP) and "outcome" (e.g., IMT), such as models 2 to 4 in Table 7-16. These *multivariate* or multiple-regression models, while still assuming that the relationship between these variables is linear, define a multidimensional space where the mutual correlations between the independent and dependent variables can be accounted for. Thus, each estimate from these multiple-regression models (each regression coefficient) is said to be *adjusted* for all of the other variables in the model, although it is important to always consider the potential limitations of this kind of inference, as discussed in Sections 7.6 and 7.7. This discussion applies to all generalized linear models that were presented in preceding sections in this chapter (see Table 7-15), which differ only with regard to the type of dependent variable and, consequently, the interpretation of the corresponding regression coefficient.

It may, of course, be found that the data do not fit one of these simple "linear" models. For example, if the type of scatter in Figures 7-9, 7-10, or 7-11 is observed, it would probably be necessary to use some of the more complex modeling approaches that were discussed in Section 7.4.7 (dummy variables, quadratic terms, etc.). Furthermore, if it is suspected that two or more of the covariates in the model interact (i.e., if one *modifies the effect* of the other), stratification or inclusion of interaction terms will be needed to account for such interactions.

Again, the investigator has to take a stand in the trade-off between fit and simplicity (interpretability) of the model. Ignoring the possibility that a linear association may not be a good way to describe the association of interest may lead to seriously misleading conclusions. The need to examine the data carefully cannot be sufficiently emphasized. The use of dummy variables to examine patterns of associations across the range of values of continuous variables was discussed briefly in Section 7.4.7. More advanced statistical textbooks cover in great detail other statistical tools to assess the goodness of fit of the models described previously here (see, for example, Draper and Smith[14] for linear models, Hosmer and Lemeshow[21] for logistic models, and Collett[26] for Cox regression). If a straight line is not an appropriate model, more complex models need to be adopted, such as those seen in Figures 7-10 and 7–11, a process that could be seen as analogous to going from B to C or D in Figure 7-9.

The preceding discussion pertains to the use of statistical models in identifying and describing associations between exposures and outcomes in epidemiology; however, statistical models can also be used for *prediction*, as discussed with examples in the logistic regression section in this chapter (Section 7.4.3). In this case, obtaining a model as parsimonious as possible is no longer the primary goal. In fact, to obtain an accurate prediction of the *expected* value of a dependent variable, the more complex the model, the better. Because the interpretation of the parameters in themselves is not the goal, complex models (e.g., Figures 7-10 and 7-11) are perfectly suitable for prediction. Again, using the analogy of the cartoonist (Figure 7-17), if the goal was to identify the subject accurately (e.g., if the cartoonist was working for the police in creating—predicting—a suspect's portrait), the most complex "model" of the type shown in Figure 7-9D would be a more appropriate choice—an actual photograph would be even better.

7.8.1 Selecting the Right Statistical Model

So far, this discussion has focused mainly on modeling issues with respect to the *shape* of the relationship between a certain independent variable and a dependent variable. Obviously, however, this is not the only issue in statistical modeling. Other fundamental decisions in any multivariate or multiple-regression analysis are (1) the choice of the

TABLE 7-32 Commonly used analytic techniques available to the epidemiologist for the assessment of relationships between exposures and outcomes.

Type of study	Type of dependent variable (outcome)	Multivariate technique	Adjusted measure of association
Any	Continuous biological parameter	ANOVA Linear regression	Difference in means Linear regression coefficient
Cross-sectional	Diseased/nondiseased	Direct adjustment Indirect adjustment Mantel-Haenszel Logistic regression	Prevalence rate ratio Standardized prevalence ratio Odds ratio Odds ratio
Case-control	Diseased/nondiseased	Mantel-Haenszel Logistic regression	Odds ratio Odds ratio
Cohort	Cumulative incidence (by the end of follow-up)	Direct adjustment Indirect adjustment Mantel-Haenszel Logistic regression	Relative risk Standardized incidence ratio Odds ratio Odds ratio
	Cumulative incidence (Time-to-event data)	Cox model	Hazard ratio
	Incidence rate (per person-time)	Mantel-Haenszel Poisson regression	Rate ratio Rate ratio
Nested Case-control Case-cohort	Time-dependent disease status (Time-to-event data)	Conditional logistic regression Cox model with staggered entries	Hazard ratio

specific regression/stratification-based technique and (2) the choice of the variables to be included in the multivariate equation or stratification scheme.

The choice of the adjustment technique (stratification or regression based) is often a matter of convenience and personal preference. The choice of a particular adjustment technique over all others described in the preceding sections of this chapter (and others not covered here) is often based on the type of study design, the type of variables (dependent and independent) under investigation, and the type of measure of association that one wishes to obtain. Table 7-32 summarizes how the adjustment techniques described in this chapter relate to the main study designs, variable types, and measures of association.

Analysis of variance methods (not discussed here) and linear regression models are indicated when the outcome variable is continuous. When the outcome is a binary variable (as is often the case in epidemiology), the adjustment techniques based on the popular multiplicative models described previously (e.g., Mantel-Haenszel summary odds ratio or rate ratio, logistic regression, Cox regression, Poisson regression) tend to provide similar results. This is illustrated by the similarity of results obtained in Tables 7-16, 7-18, 7-19, 7-21, and 7-22. A similar example can be found in Kahn and Sempos,[16] where different stratification-based and multiple-regression-based adjustment methods were used to obtain the adjusted estimates of the associations of three risk factors (hypertension, age, and male sex) with coronary heart disease in a subset of participants from the Framingham Heart Study. All methods resulted in comparable estimates leading to similar conclusions. As discussed by Greenland,[75] many of these methods often used in epidemiology (e.g., Mantel-Haenszel, logistic, Poisson, Cox) are based on similar assumptions (i.e., multiplicative relationships between risk factors and disease) and have similar epidemiologic meanings. Thus, it is not surprising that, with the exception of unusually extreme circumstances (e.g., gross violations of the basic assumptions of the model, extreme outliers), these methods will often produce similar results.

The issue of *which independent variables (confounders) ought to be included* in the model is at the core of the discussion on the topic of confounding in general (Chapter 5) and of residual confounding in particular (Section 7.6). A detailed discussion of the statistical techniques which could be helpful in choosing a particular set of variables for a model is outside of the scope of this textbook. A useful overview was provided by Greenland.[75]

Finally, an important recommendation when choosing a particular statistical model is to conduct a *sensitivity analysis* (i.e., to check whether similar results are obtained when different models or assumptions are used for the analysis).[75,76]

Because of the increased ease and availability of computers and computer software, the last few years have seen a flourishing of the options for and frequency of use of multivariate analysis in the biomedical literature. These highly sophisticated mathematical models, however, rarely eliminate the need to examine carefully the raw data by means of scatter diagrams, simple $n \times k$ tables, and stratified analyses.

REFERENCES

1. Miettinen OS, Cook EF. Confounding: Essence and detection. *Am J Epidemiol.* 1981;114:593–603.
2. Greenland S. Absence of confounding does not correspond to collapsibility of the rate ratio or rate difference. *Epidemiology.* 1996;7:498–501.
3. Reif JS, Dunn K, Ogilvie GK, Harris CK. Passive smoking and canine lung cancer risk. *Am J Epidemiol.* 1992;135:234–239.
4. Shapiro S, Slone D, Rosenberg L, et al. Oral-contraceptive use in relation to myocardial infarction. *Lancet.* 1979;1:743–747.
5. Gordis L. *Epidemiology*, 4th ed. Philadelphia, PA: Elsevier Saunders; 2008.
6. Armstrong BG. Comparing standardized mortality ratios. *Ann Epidemiol.* 1995;5:60–64.
7. Mantel N, Haenszel W. Statistical aspects of the analysis of data from retrospective studies of disease. *J Natl Cancer Inst.* 1959;22:719–748.
8. Pandey DK, Shekelle R, Selwyn BJ, et al. Dietary vitamin C and beta-carotene and risk of death in middle-aged men: The Western Electric Study. *Am J Epidemiol.* 1995;142:1269–1278.
9. Sorlie PD, Adam E, Melnick SL, et al. Cytomegalovirus/herpesvirus and carotid atherosclerosis: The ARIC Study. *J Med Virol.* 1994;42:33–37.
10. Kannel WB, McGee D, Gordon T. A general cardiovascular risk profile: The Framingham Study. *Am J Cardiol.* 1976;38:46–51.
11. Armitage P, Berry, G, Matthews JNS. *Statistical Methods in Medical Research*, 4th ed. Oxford, UK: Blackwell Publishing; 2002.
12. Nieto FJ, Diez-Roux A, Szklo M, et al. Short- and long-term prediction of clinical and subclinical atherosclerosis by traditional risk factors. *J Clin Epidemiol.* 1999;52:559–567.
13. Kleinbaum DG, Kupper LL, Nizam A, Muller KE. *Applied Regression Analysis and Other Multivariable Methods*, 4th ed.. Belmont, CA: Thomson, Brooks/Cole; 2008.
14. Draper N, Smith H. *Applied regression analysis*, 3rd ed. New York, NY: John Wiley; 1998.
15. Keys A. *Seven Countries: A Multivariate Analysis of Death and Coronary Heart Disease.* Cambridge, MA: Harvard University Press; 1980.
16. Kahn HA, Sempos CT, *Statistical Methods in Epidemiology.* 2nd ed. New York, NY: Oxford University Press; 1989.
17. Nieto FJ, Szklo M, Folsom AR, et al. Leukocyte count correlates in middle-aged adults: The Atherosclerosis Risk in Communities (ARIC) Study. *Am J Epidemiol.* 1992;136:525–537.
18. Feldstein M. A binary multiple regression method for analyzing factors affecting perinatal mortality and other outcomes of pregnancy. *J Roy Stat Soc [A].* 1966;129:61–73.
19. The Atherosclerosis Risk in Communities (ARIC) Study: Design and objectives: The ARIC investigators. *Am J Epidemiol.* 1989;129:687–702.
20. Chambless LE, Heiss G, Folsom AR, et al. Association of coronary heart disease incidence with carotid arterial wall thickness and major risk factors: The Atherosclerosis Risk in Communities (ARIC) Study, 1987–1993. *Am J Epidemiol.* 1997;146:483–494.
21. Hosmer D, Lemeshow S. *Applied Logistic Regression* 2nd ed. New York, NY: John Wiley; 2000.
22. Schlesselman J. *Case Control Studies: Design, Conduct, Analysis.* New York, NY: Oxford University Press; 1982.
23. Gibas A, Blewett DR, Schoenfeld DA, Dienstag JL. Prevalence and incidence of viral hepatitis in health workers in the prehepatitis B vaccination era. *Am J Epidemiol.* 1992;136:603–610.

24. Spiegelman D, Hertzmark E. Easy SAS calculations for risk or prevalence ratios and differences. *Am J Epidemiol.* 2005;162:199–200.
25. Cox D. Regression models and life table (with discussion). *J Roy Stat Soc [B].* 1972;34:187–220.
26. Collett D. *Modelling Survival Data in Medical Research*. London, UK: Chapman & Hall; 1994.
27. Parmar M, Machin D. *Survival Analysis: A Practical Approach*. Chichester, UK: John Wiley; 1995.
28. Breslow NE, Day NE. Statistical methods in cancer research: Volume I: The analysis of case-control studies. *IARC Sci Publ.* 1980.
29. Heiss G, Sharrett AR, Barnes R, et al. Carotid atherosclerosis measured by B-mode ultrasound in populations: associations with cardiovascular risk factors in the ARIC study. *Am J Epidemiol.* 1991;134: 250–256.
30. Nieto FJ, Adam E, Sorlie P, et al. Cohort study of cytomegalovirus infection as a risk factor for carotid intimal-medial thickening, a measure of subclinical atherosclerosis. *Circulation.* 1996;94:922–927.
31. Pearce N. Incidence density matching with a simple SAS computer program. *Int J Epidemiol.* 1989; 18:981–984.
32. Barlow WE. Robust variance estimation for the case-cohort design. *Biometrics.* 1994;50:1064–1072.
33. Thomas D. New techniques for the analysis of cohort studies. *Epidemiol Rev.* 1998;20:122–134.
34. Nieto FJ, Folsom AR, Sorlie PD, et al. Chlamydia pneumoniae infection and incident coronary heart disease: The Atherosclerosis Risk in Communities Study. *Am J Epidemiol.* 1999;150:149–156.
35. Waaler HT. Height, weight and mortality: The Norwegian experience. *Acta Med Scand Suppl.* 1984; 679:1–56.
36. Allison DB, Faith MS, Heo M, Kotler DP. Hypothesis concerning the U-shaped relation between body mass index and mortality. *Am J Epidemiol.* 1997;146:339–349.
37. Fagot-Campagna A, Hanson RL, Narayan KM, et al. Serum cholesterol and mortality rates in a Native American population with low cholesterol concentrations: A U-shaped association. *Circulation.* 1997; 96:1408–1415.
38. Thun MJ, Peto R, Lopez AD, et al. Alcohol consumption and mortality among middle-aged and elderly U.S. adults. *N Engl J Med.* 1997;337:1705–1714.
39. Moscicki EK, Locke BZ, Rae DS, Boyd JH. Depressive symptoms among Mexican Americans: The Hispanic Health and Nutrition Examination Survey. *Am J Epidemiol.* 1989;130:348–360.
40. Luke A, Durazo-Arvizu R, Rotimi C, et al. Relation between body mass index and body fat in black population samples from Nigeria, Jamaica, and the United States. *Am J Epidemiol.* 1997;145:620–628.
41. Kretzschmar M, van Duynhoven YT, Severijnen AJ. Modeling prevention strategies for gonorrhea and Chlamydia using stochastic network simulations. *Am J Epidemiol.* 1996;144:306–317.
42. Clayton D, Hills, M. *Statistical Models in Epidemiology*. Oxford, UK: Oxford University Press; 1993.
43. Zohoori N, Savitz DA. Econometric approaches to epidemiologic data: relating endogeneity and unobserved heterogeneity to confounding. *Ann Epidemiol* 1997;7:251–257.
44. Greenland S. An introduction to instrumental variables for epidemiologists. *Int J Epidemiol.* 2000;29:722–729.

45. Martens EP, Pestman WR, de Boer A, et al. Instrumental variables, applications and limitations. *Epidemiology*. 2006;17:260–267.
46. Porta M, *Dictionary of Epidemiology*, 5th edition. NY: Oxford University Press; 2008.
47. Glymour MM, Kawachi I, Jencks CS, Berkman LF. Does childhood schooling affect old age memory or mental status? Using state schooling laws as natural experiments. *J Epidemiol Community Health*. 2008;62:532–537.
48. Leigh JP, Schembri M. Instrumental variable technique: cigarette price provided better estimates of effects of smoking on SF-12. *J Clin Epidemiol*. 2004;284–293.
49. Hernán MA, Robins JM. Instruments for causal inference, an epidemiologist's dream. *Epidemiology*. 2006;17:360–372.
50. Davey Smith G, Ebrahim S. 'Mendelian randomization': Can genetic epidemiology contribute to understanding environmental determinants of disease? *Int J Epidemiol*. 2003;32:1–22.
51. Malinow MR, Nieto FJ, Szklo M, et al. Carotid artery intimal-medial thickening and plasma homocyst(e)ine in asymptomatic adults. The Atherosclerosis Risk in Communities Study. *Circulation*. 1993;87:1107–1113.
52. Ford ES, Smith SJ, Stroup DF, et al. Homocyst(e)ine and cardiovascular disease: A systematic review of the evidence with special emphasis on case-control studies and nested case-control studies. *Int J Epidemiol*. 2002;31:59–70.
53. Shimakawa T, Nieto FJ, Malinow MR, et al. Vitamin intake: a possible determinant of plasma homocyst(e)ine among middle-aged adults. *Ann Epidemiol*. 1997;7:285–293.
54. Homocysteine Lowering Trialists' Collaboration. lowering blood homocysteine with folic acid based supplements: Meta-analysis of randomized controlled trials. *BMJ*. 1998;316:894–898.
55. Casas JP, Bautista LE, Smeeth L, et al. Homocysteine and stroke: evidence on a causal link from Mendelian randomisation. *Lancet*. 2005;365:224–232.
56. Elliott P, Chambers JC, Zhang W, et al. Genetic loci associated with C-reactive protein levels and risk of coronary heart disease. *JAMA*. 2009;302:37–48.
57. Lewis SJ, Davey Smith G. Alcohol, ALDH2, and esophageal cancer: A meta-analysis which illustrates the potential and limitations of a Mendelian randomization approach. *Cancer Epidemiol Biomarkers Prev*. 2005;14:1967–1971.
58. Lewis SJ. Mendelian randomization as applied to coronary heart disease, including recent advances incorporating new technology. *Circ Cardiovasc Genet*. 2010;3:109–117.
59. Stürmer T, Joshi M, Glynn RJ, et al. A review of the application of propensity score methods yielded increasing use, advantages in specific settings, but not substantially different estimates compared with conventional multivariable methods. *J Clin Epidemiol* 2006;59:437–447.
60. Rosenbaum PR, Rubin DB. The central role of the propensity score in observational studies for causal effect. *Biometrika*. 1983;70:41–55.
61. Austin PC. A tutorial and case study in propensity score analysis: an application to estimating the effect of in-hospital smoking cessation counseling on mortality. *Multivariate Behav Res*. 2011;46:119–151.
62. Alam M, Lee VV, Elayda MA, et al. Association of gender with morbidity and mortality after isolated coronary artery bypass grafting. A propensity score matched analysis. *Int J Cardiol*. 2012; In press.
63. Culver AL, Ockene IS, Balasubramanian R, et al. Statin use and risk of diabetes mellitus in postmenopausal women in the Women's Health Inititative. *Arch Intern Med*. 2012;172:144–152.

64. Williamson E, Morley R, Lucas A, Carpenter J. Propensity scores: from naïve enthusiasm to intuitive understanding. *Stat Methods Med Res*. 2011; Jan 24:1–21.

65. Shah BR, Laupacis A, Hux JE, Austin PC. Propensity score methods gave similar results to traditional regression modeling in observational studies: a systematic review. *J Clin Epidemiol*. 2005;58:550–559.

66. Krieger N, Williams DR, Moss NE. Measuring social class in US public health research: Concepts, methodologies, and guidelines. *Annu Rev Public Health*. 1997;18:341–378.

67. Kaufman JS, Cooper RS, McGee DL. Socioeconomic status and health in blacks and whites: The problem of residual confounding and the resiliency of race. *Epidemiology*. 1997;8:621–628.

68. Davey Smith G, Frankel S, Yarnell J. Sex and death: Are they related? Findings from the Caerphilly Cohort Study. *Br Med J*. 1997;315:1641–1644.

69. Greenland S. The effect of misclassification in the presence of covariates. *Am J Epidemiol*. 1980;112: 564–569.

70. Savitz DA, Baron AE. Estimating and correcting for confounder misclassification. *Am J Epidemiol*. 1989;129:1062–1071.

71. Last J. *A Dictionary of Epidemiology*, 4th ed. New York, NY: Oxford University Press; 2000.

72. Breslow N. Design and analysis of case-control studies. *Ann Rev Public Health*. 1982;3:29–54.

73. Durrant M. *Aristotle's De Anima in Focus*. London, UK: Routledge; 1993.

74. Zeger SL. Statistical reasoning in epidemiology. *Am J Epidemiol*. 1991;134:1062–1066.

75. Greenland S. Modeling and variable selection in epidemiologic analysis. *Am J Public Health*. 1989; 79:340–349.

76. Robins JM, Greenland S. The role of model selection in causal inference from nonexperimental data. *Am J Epidemiol*. 1986;123:392–402.

EXERCISES

1. The association between activities of daily living and the prevalence of low back pain was studied cross-sectionally in a sample of middle aged and older adult residents in a suburban area. One of the activities of interest was "gardening." Current prevalent low back pain was defined based on the reporting of at least one episode of low back pain during the last month. The following table shows the distribution of individuals according to the prevalence of low back pain ("outcome") and whether they frequently engaged in gardening activities ("exposure"). Because the authors of the study were concerned with the possible confounding effect of age, the data were stratified by age as follows:

	Frequent gardening	Low back pain	
		Yes	No
Age < 65 years	Yes	70	299
	No	20	198
Age ≥ 65 years	Yes	55	15
	No	40	25

   a. Use the data presented in this stratified table to assess whether age meets each of the criteria to be a confounder, and justify your answers.

   1st criteria: *Age is related to the "exposure."*

   2nd criteria: *Age is related to the "outcome."*

   3rd criteria: (Describe) _____

   b. Use the data shown in the previous table to calculate the *crude odds ratio* of low back pain (i.e., not considering age), comparing those who do frequent gardening with those who do not.

   c. Based on the data shown in the previous table, use the Mantel-Haenszel method to calculate the *age-adjusted* odds ratio of low back pain comparing those who do frequent gardening with those who do not.

   d. Was it appropriate to carry out this adjustment?

   e. Which of the following statements best describe the preceding data?

   ☐ Age is a negative confounder of the association between gardening and low back pain.

   ☐ Age is a positive confounder of the association between gardening and low back pain.

   ☐ Age is an effect modifier of the association between gardening and low back pain.

   ☐ Age is both a confounder and an effect modifier of the association between gardening and low back pain.

   Justify your answer.

2. Fukushima et al. conducted a case-control study of the relationship of peak (as opposed to average) alcohol drinking and risk of Parkinson's disease. The 124 cases were patients within 6 years of the onset of the disease and were recruited from 11 collaborating Japanese hospitals. Controls were inpatients and outpatients without neurodegenerative diseases, and numbered 327. The odds ratios expressing the relationship of peak alcohol drinking to Parkinson's disease are shown in the table:

Odds ratios for Parkinson's disease in relation to alcohol drinking during peak period

Frequency of alcohol drinking during peak period	No. (%) Cases (N = 124)	No. (%) Controls (N = 327)	Crude OR* (95% CI)	Adjusted† OR
Nondrinker	115 (53.7)	181 (55.4)	1.00	1.00
< 6 days/week	63 (29.4)	77 (23.6)	1.29 (0.86, 1.93)	1.29 (0.78, 2.13)
≥ 6 days/week	36 (16.8)	69 (21.1)	0.82 (0.51, 1.30)	0.96 (0.50, 1.81)
P for trend			0.70	0.96

*Odds ratio
†Adjusted for sex, age, region of residence, pack-years of smoking, years of education, body mass index, alcohol flushing status, and medication history for hypertension, hypercholesterolemia, and diabetes.
(Modified from W Fukushima, Y Miyake, K Tanaka, et al. *BMC Neurology.* 2010;10:111–119)

a. Examining only the point estimates of OR, what can be inferred when comparing the crude with the adjusted ORs?

b. Examining the point estimates for both the crude and the adjusted ORs, was it appropriate to do a linear trend test?

3. The table shows the relationship of smoking to coronary heart disease incidence rates in the Atherosclerosis Risk in Communities (ARIC) Study.[‡]

Age, field center- and race-adjusted average coronary heart disease incidence rates/1000 person-years, ARIC

Smoking	Rate	
	Women	Men
Current	5.3	11.5
Never	1.3	4.7

[‡]Modified from: LE Chambless, G Heiss, AR Folsom, et al. Association of coronary heart disease incidence with carotid arterial wall thickness and major risk factors. *Am J Epidemiol.* 1997;146:483–494.

a. Using the direct method and a standard population of 5000 current smokers and 2000 never smokers, calculate the smoking-adjusted rates/1000 person-years, the smoking-adjusted rate ratio and absolute difference in rates. For these calculations, assume that women represent the "unexposed" category.

	Standard population	Expected number of cases	
Smoking		Women	Men
Current	5000		
Never	2000		
Total	7000		
Smoking adjusted rate			
Rate ratio		1.0	
Absolute difference in rates		0	

b. Using the data in the first table, calculate the smoking stratum specific rate ratios and absolute differences between men and women.

c. Assuming that men are the "exposed" category and women the "unexposed" category, and further assuming that these relative and absolute differences are valid (i.e, free of additional confounding and bias), how do you interpret the first table's findings?

d. Now repeat all these calculations using a standard population formed by 10,000 never smokers and 500 current smokers.

	Standard population	Expected number of cases	
Smoking		Women	Men
Current	500		
Never	10,000		
Total	10,500		
Smoking adjusted rate			
Rate ratio		1.0	
Absolute difference in rates		0	

e. How do you explain the differences/similarities between this table and the previous table?

f. From the comparison between the results in this table and the previous table, what can be inferred about the use of standard populations?

4. The questions that follow are based on the data below.

   a. Using the data below, calculate "age-standardized" incidence rate ratios in populations A and B. For this calculations, an external study population should be used as the source of the "standard rates." Note that the age-specific incidence rates are exactly the same in these two study populations.

					Expected numbers of incident cases	
Age	Population A	Population B	Incidence rates/1000 in A and B	"Standard" rates/1000	Population A	Population B
45–54	2000	400	10.0	5.0		
55–64	800	600	15.0	7.0		
65–74	400	2500	25.0	20.0		
Total population	3200	3500		12/1000		
Total number of cases						
Standardized incidence ratio						

   b. What is the interpretation of the standardized incidence (or mortality) ratio?

   c. Why, in spite of having the same age-specific incidence rates, there was such a fairly large difference in the standardized incidence ratio between populations A and B?

5. Gallagher et al. conducted a clinical trial of 458 children to assess the effectiveness of a sun protective cream ("sunscreen") with regard to the development of new nevi during a 3-year follow-up.[§] Parents of children assigned to the intervention group were told to apply sunscreen (SPF) 30 when sun exposure was expected to last 30 minutes or longer. Parents of control children were not given any advice pertaining to use of sunscreen. The table shows data based on Gallagher et al.'s study.

	Sunscreen group		Control group		[Control – sunscreen] mean difference
Sunburn score	No. (%)	Mean no. of new nevi	No. (%)	Mean no. of new nevi	
Low	50 (22.5)	20	180 (76.0)	50	30
High	172 (77.5)	60	56 (24.0)	40	30
Total	222 (100.0)	51	136 (100.0)	59.5	8.5

[§]Gallagher RP, Jason K, Rivers JK, et al. Broad-spectrum sunscreen use and the development of new nevi in white children: a randomized controlled trial. *JAMA* 2000;283:2955–2960.

a. By mere inspection of the table would you conclude that sunburn score is a confounding variable? Why?

☐ Yes

☐ No

b. Using the data in this table, and as standard weights ("standard population") the sum of the sunscreen and control groups shown in the table, calculate the sunburn score-adjusted difference in mean number of new nevi between the sunscreen and the control groups.

c. If another set of standard weights had been used, would the same sunburn score-adjusted difference be observed? Why?

☐ Yes

☐ No

The authors also examined the development of new nevi according to the percent of the childrens' faces covered by freckles. The results are shown in the table.

Number of new nevi in the sunscreen and control group			
	No. of new nevi		
Freckles %	Sunscreen	Control	Difference
10	24	24	0
20	20	28	−8
30	20	30	−10
40	16	30	−14

d. What important information would be lost if only freckle-adjusted mean differences in the development of new nevi had been reported by the authors?

6. In the hypothetical results of an individually matched case-control study shown in the table, the authors selected three controls per case. Calculate the odds ratio using the Mantel-Haenszel method to adjust for matching variables.

Exposed?	Case	Cont	Total	No. of matched sets	Num	Den
Yes	1	0	4	40		
No	0	3				
Yes	1	1	4	60		
No	0	2				
Yes	1	2	4	12		
No	0	1				
Yes	1	3	4	10		
No	0	0				
Yes	0	0	4	30		
No	1	3				
Yes	0	1	4	5		
No	1	2				
Yes	0	2	4	7		
No	1	1				
Yes	0	3	4	20		
No	1	0				

Numerator =

Denominator =

OR_{MH} =

7. In a study of the determinants of serum glucose levels in a population of women, four variables were found to be significantly associated in multiple logistic regression analyses with impaired glucose tolerance (serum glucose ≥7.8 mmol/L). The following results were obtained when four variables were simultaneously included in the model with impaired glucose tolerance as the dependent variable:

Variable	Logistic regression coefficient	Standard error
Body mass index (kg/m^2)	0.077	0.032
Waist/hip ratio (ratio increase of 1.0)	3.625	1.670
Diabetogenic drugs: yes = 1; no = 0	0.599	0.302
Regular exercise: no = 1; yes = 0	1.664	0.740

a. State in words the meaning (interpretation) of the logistic regression coefficients for waist/hip ratio (3.625) and regular exercise (1.664).

b. Based on the information in the table, calculate the odds ratios and their corresponding 95% confidence limits for each of the variables, as indicated in the following table:

Variable	Odds ratio	95% CL
Body mass index (kg/m²)	....	....
Waist/hip ratio	....	....
Diabetogenic drugs: yes = 1; no = 0	....	....
Regular exercise: no = 1; yes = 0	....	....

c. State in words the meaning of the odds ratio for waist-to-hip ratio and for regular exercise.

d. Based on the data previously described, the investigators concluded, "In our study, waist/hip ratio was more strongly associated with impaired glucose tolerance than with body mass index." Do you agree with this conclusion? Why?

e. Calculate the odds ratio and the 95% confidence limits for an increase in 0.01 in the waist/hip ratio. (It is suggested that you use the answer to this question to reconsider your answer to the previous question.)

8. Plasma fibrinogen concentration has been shown to be a predictor of incident clinical atherosclerotic disease. In a study looking at correlates of plasma fibrinogen levels in a group of middle-age adults, multiple linear regression methods were used to explore what other risk factors may be associated with plasma fibrinogen levels. The following table shows some of the results from this study. In the analyses under "Model 1," only demographic variables (age, sex, and race) were included. In model 2, cigarette smoking was added. In model 3, body mass index was added.

Multiple linear regression analyses of predictors of plasma fibrinogen levels (in mg/dL)				
Characteristic	Label	Model 1	Model 2	Model 3
		Estimated regression coefficient		
Age (1 year)	b1	0.019	0.020	0.018
Sex (women = 1, men = 0)	b2	29.1	28.4	29.0
Race (blacks = 1, whites = 0)	b3	15.8	15.9	6.8
Cigarettes per day** 1–19	b4	—	11.3	12.2
≥20	b5	—	18.5	17.3
Body mass index (1 kg/m²)	b6	—	—	4.7

**Reference category: nonsmokers.

a. State in words the interpretation of b_1 (the coefficient for age) and b_4 (the coefficient for 1–20 cigarettes/day) in model 3.

b. Which of the corresponding statements best corresponds to these results?

- ☐ Body mass index but not cigarette smoking is an effect modifier of the association between race and plasma fibrinogen levels.
- ☐ Both body mass index and smoking are positive confounders of the association between race and plasma fibrinogen levels.
- ☐ Body mass index but not cigarette smoking is a positive confounder of the association between race and plasma fibrinogen levels.
- ☐ Body mass index but not cigarette smoking is a negative confounder of the association between race and plasma fibrinogen levels.
- ☐ There is evidence of an interaction between body mass index and cigarette smoking in relationship to plasma fibrinogen levels.

CHAPTER 8

Quality Assurance and Control

8.1 INTRODUCTION

As with other types of empirical research, the *validity* of the inferences made from results of epidemiologic research depends on the accuracy of its methods and procedures. In epidemiologic jargon, the term *validity* (or *accuracy*) refers to absence of bias. The most common biases and some approaches to prevent their occurrence so as to maximize the validity of the study's results and inferences were discussed in Chapter 4. This chapter extends the discussion of issues related to the accuracy of data collection and data processing that should be considered when designing and conducting epidemiologic studies. In addition to validity or lack of bias, this chapter also addresses issues related to assessing and ensuring *reliability* (precision, reproducibility) of the data collected.

The terms *quality assurance* and *quality control* are sometimes used interchangeably or, even more often, lumped together under a common term, *quality control*. However, for systematization purposes in this chapter, the activities to ensure quality of the data before data collection are regarded as quality assurance, and the efforts to monitor and maintain the quality of the data during the conduct of the study are regarded as quality control.

Quality assurance and quality control activities are key components of epidemiologic research and are best understood in the context of the key features of an epidemiologic study design. The important features of a study design, aptly described in Kahn and Sempos's textbook,[1] provide the background for further elaboration in the context of this chapter (Table 8-1). Most components of a study can be said to relate to quality assurance or quality control in one way or another in the broad context of validity and reliability of epidemiologic research. This chapter, however, focuses on the activities more traditionally regarded as belonging to the realms of quality assurance or control (i.e., items 7 and 8 in Table 8-1). For an additional systematic review on this topic, see Whitney et al.[2]

To illustrate some of the issues covered in the discussion that follows, Appendix D includes a verbatim transcription of the quality assurance and control manual for two procedures carried out in a multicenter cohort study of atherosclerosis, the Atherosclerosis Risk in Communities (ARIC) study:[3] blood pressure and venipuncture.

8.2 QUALITY ASSURANCE

Quality assurance activities before data collection relate to standardizing procedures and thus preventing or at least minimizing systematic or random errors in collecting and analyzing data. Traditionally, these activities have comprised detailed protocol preparation, development of data collection instruments and procedures and their manuals of operation, and training and certification of staff. (The development of manuals specifying quality control activities can also be regarded as a quality assurance activity.)

TABLE 8-1 Key features of the design of an epidemiologic study.

Activity (quality assurance, QA, or quality control, QC)	Comments
1. Formulation of study's main hypothesis/hypotheses (QA)	The hypothesis should specify the independent (e.g., risk factor) and the dependent (e.g., disease outcome) variables. If the investigators plan to analyze interaction, the study's hypothesis should specify the potential effect modifier(s).
2. A priori specification of potential confounding variables (QA)	A review of the pertinent literature may assist the investigators in identifying the main confounding variables, and thus help in choosing the most appropriate study design (e.g., matched vs unmatched case-control) and in selecting the data that need to be collected.
3. Definition of the characteristics of the study population for external validity (generalizability) purposes (QA)	The ability to generalize results to other populations is conditional on several circumstances, including differences in the distribution of effect modifiers and the characteristics of the study population. A detailed characterization of the study participants allows data "consumers" to decide whether findings are applicable to their target population.
4. Definition of the design strategy (e.g., cohort, case-control, case-cohort) and of the groups to be compared, and specification of selection procedures for internal validity (comparability) purposes (QA)	Selection of groups to be compared relates to prevention of selection bias and the level of confounding to be expected. The strategy for the search of confounders in addition to those suggested by previous studies should be specified.
5. Definition of the design strategy and samples for studies of reliability and validity (QA/QC)	The approach for selection of samples for studies of repeat measurements (reliability) of comparison with "gold standards" (validity) should be specified.
6. Specification of the study power necessary to detect the hypothesized association(s) at a given level of significance (QA)	The estimation of sample size is an important guidepost to decide whether the study has sufficient power at a given alpha error level, and it should take into account the potential interaction(s), if specified in the study hypothesis.
7. Standardization of procedures (QA)	This includes preparation of written manuals that contain a detailed description of the procedures for selection of the study population and data collection, as well as training and certification of staff.
8. Activities during data collection, including analysis of quality control data and remedial actions (QC)	These include ongoing monitoring of data collection procedures, as well as conducting studies on samples to assess validity and reliability of measurements, which may result in retraining and recertification of study staff.

(continues)

TABLE 8-1 Key features of the design of an epidemiologic study *(continued)*.

Activity (quality assurance, QA, or quality control, QC)	Comments
9. Data analysis	Data analysis should be done according to a preestablished plan. Efforts should be made to establish analytic strategies in advance (e.g., the choice of "cutoff" points when using continuous or ordinal data to create discrete categories). Analysis should proceed from the more parsimonious strategies (description of data, stratification, calculation of unadjusted measures of association, simple adjustment approaches) to the more complex models (e.g., Cox, logistic regression). Investigators should also specify analytic strategies to evaluate validity and reliability of procedures.
10. Reporting of data	Findings should be reported as soon as possible after data collection activities are finished so as to preserve the timeliness of the study. To avoid publication bias, data should be reported regardless of the direction of findings (see Chapter 10, Section 10.5). The study instruments and quality control data should be available to the scientific community on request.

Source: Data from HA Kahn and CT Sempos, *Statistical Methods in Epidemiology*, © 1989.

The design of quality assurance activities should be followed by pretesting and pilot-studying these activities. Results of pretests and pilot studies, in turn, assist in modifying and/or making adjustments to these procedures so as to make them more efficient, valid, and reliable.

8.2.1 Study Protocol and Manuals of Operation

The *study protocol* consists of a description of the general components of the investigation, including those shown in Table 8-1. It provides a global picture of the strategies leading to the development of more detailed manuals of operation. The protocol describes the general design and procedures used in the study (including those related to sampling and recruiting study participants) and assists the staff in understanding the context in which their specific activities are carried out.

Manuals of operation should contain detailed descriptions of exactly how the procedures specific to each data collection activity are to be carried out so as to maximize the likelihood that tasks will be performed as uniformly as possible. For example, the description of the procedures for blood pressure measurements should include the calibration of the sphygmomanometer, the position of the participant, the amount of resting time before and between measurements, the size of the cuff, and the position of the cuff on the arm. With regard to interviews, the manual of operations should contain instructions as to exactly how each question should be asked during the course of the interview ("question-by-question" instructions or, to use epidemiologic jargon, "q by q's"). Standardization of procedures is particularly critical in multicenter studies in which several technicians carry out the same exams or administer the same questionnaires to study participants recruited and examined at different clinics or locations. Detailed manuals of operation are important to achieve the highest possible level of uniformity and standardization of data collection procedures in the entire study population.

In large studies involving different measurements, the manuals of operation may be activity-specific: that is, separate manuals of operation may be prepared for different data-related activities, such as interviews, collection and processing of blood samples, and pulmonary function testing. Manuals of operation must also be developed for reading and classifying data, as when coding electrocardiographic findings using the Minnesota Code[4] or assigning a disease to different diagnostic categories, such as "definite," "probable," or "absent" myocardial infarction.[5] A manual may also have to be developed specifying how "derived" variables are created for the purposes of the study, that is, analytical variables based on combinations of "raw" variables obtained during data collection. An example is the definition of *hypertension* (present or absent) based on measured blood pressure levels *or* a participant's report of physician-diagnosed hypertension *or* use of antihypertensive medications.

8.2.2 Data Collection Instruments

Development (or choice) of data collection instruments and their corresponding operation manuals is a key step in the study design and should be carried out according to well-established rules, as in the case of designing a questionnaire.[6,7]

Whenever possible, it is advisable to choose data collection instruments and procedures that have been used effectively in previous studies to measure both suspected risk factors and disease outcomes. Examples include the questionnaire to identify angina pectoris developed by Rose[8] (the so-called "Rose questionnaire"), the American Thoracic Society questionnaire to assess respiratory symptoms,[9] the blood pressure measurement procedures followed by the National Health Examination Surveys,[10] and the food frequency questionnaires designed by Block et al.[11] or Willett et al.[12] to assess dietary habits. Validity and reliability of such previously tested instruments and procedures are sometimes known,[12] allowing to some extent the assessment of, and even correction for, possible bias and misclassification (discussed later). (Note, however, that reliability and validity values are often dependent on the specific study population for which they have been estimated, and thus may not be generalizable to populations distinct from the study population [e.g., populations with different educational levels].)

In addition, the use of established instruments and procedures permits comparing findings of the study with those of previous studies, thus facilitating the preparation of systematic reviews.[13]

On occasion, a well-established instrument is modified to suit a study's purposes. For example, modification of a questionnaire may be done either to include or exclude variables or to reduce interview time. The extent to which the modified version maintains the reliability and validity of the original instrument can be assessed by comparing results using the two instruments in the same sample. Such assessment, however, may be affected by the lack of independence between the two instruments when they are applied to the same individuals (i.e., responses to the questionnaire administered last may be influenced by the study participants' recall of the responses to the first questionnaire). Sometimes, a questionnaire designed in English has to be translated to another language (e.g., Chinese, Spanish) for application to a minority subgroup.[14] When that is the case, reverse translation to English is helpful to establish the accuracy of the translation.[15,16] When instruments effectively used in the past are not available, making it necessary to create special instruments to suit the purposes of the study, pilot studies of the validity and reliability of the instruments and related measurement procedures should be carried out, preferably before data collection activities begin (Section 8.2.4).

8.2.3 Training of Staff

Training of each staff person should aim at making him or her thoroughly familiar with the procedures under his or her responsibility. These procedures include not only data collection and processing procedures but also setting up appointments for interviews or visits to study clinics, preparing materials for the interviewers and other data collectors, calibrating instruments, and assigning interviewers to study participants. Training should also involve laboratory technicians and those in charge of reading and classifying data obtained from exams such as electrocardiograms and imaging studies. In multicenter studies, training of technicians from all field centers is usually done at a central location. Training culminates with the certification of the staff member to perform the specific procedure. Particularly in studies with a relatively long duration (such as concurrent prospective studies; see Gordis[17]), periodic recertification is carried out, with retraining of any staff member whose performance in conducting recertification tasks is deemed to be inadequate. Because retraining and recertification are done when data collection activities are already ongoing, however, they are usually classified as quality control rather than quality assurance activities.

Careful training of all study personnel involved in data collection is required for standardization of data collection and classification procedures and should emphasize adherence to the procedures specified in the manuals of operation (discussed previously). A thorough training of data collectors is key to prevent misclassification, which may occur if data collection procedures are not used in a standardized manner. Use of standardized procedures is particularly important to ensure that, if misclassification occurs, it will be nondifferential (Chapter 4, Section 4.3.3).

8.2.4 Pretesting and Pilot Studies

Verification of the feasibility and efficiency of the study procedures is carried out through pretests and pilot studies. Often, the terms *pretesting* and *pilot testing* are used interchangeably; however, a useful distinction is that the pretest involves assessing specific procedures on a "grab" or convenience sample (e.g., on staff persons themselves or their friends or relatives) in order to detect major flaws, whereas the pilot study is a formal "rehearsal" of study procedures that attempts to reproduce the entire flow of operations in a sample as similar as possible to study participants. Results of pretesting and pilot studies are used to assess participant recruitment and data collection procedures and, if necessary, to correct these procedures before fieldwork begins. For example, after pretesting and carrying out a pilot study of a questionnaire, the following elements can be assessed: flow of questions (including skip patterns), presence of sensitive questions, appropriateness of categorization of variables, clarity of wording to the respondent and the interviewer, and clarity of the "question-by-question" instructions to the interviewer.

Pilot studies also allow evaluating alternative strategies for participant recruitment and data collection. For example, a pilot study can be carried out to assess whether telephone interviews are a good alternative to the more expensive and time-consuming in-person interviews.

A summary of some of the key quality assurance steps is shown in Exhibit 8-1.

8.3 QUALITY CONTROL

Quality control activities begin after data collection and processing start. Monitoring of quality control data is the basis for possible remedial actions aimed at minimizing bias and reliability problems. Quality control strategies include observation of procedures performed by staff members, which allows the identification of obvious protocol deviations, and special studies of validity and reliability usually carried out in samples of study subjects at specified intervals throughout data collection and processing (see Appendix D). What follows is a summary of the most common quality control strategies and indices. The in-depth statistical discussion of reliability and validity indices is beyond the scope of this textbook; instead, the focus of the following sections is on their applicability, interpretation, and limitations.

8.3.1 Observation Monitoring and Monitoring of Trends

To identify problems in the implementation of study procedures by interviewers, technicians, and data processors, supervisors can monitor the quality of these procedures by "over-the-shoulder" observation of staff. For example, observation monitoring of the quality of blood pressure measurements is often done by "double stethoscoping" (i.e., using a stethoscope that allows two observers to measure blood pressure levels simultaneously). Observation monitoring of interviews to assess interviewers' adherence to protocol and accuracy of recorded responses can be done by taping all interviews and reviewing a random sample of them.

Another monitoring technique routinely performed in epidemiologic studies, particularly in multicenter studies in which participants are recruited and data collected over prolonged periods, is the statistical assessment of trends over time in the performance of each observer (interviewer and clinic or laboratory technician).[2] In the ARIC study, for example, the Coordinating Center routinely (quarterly) performs calculation of statistics on blood pressure and other variables measured by each technician for all study participants. After adjustment for age, sex, and other relevant characteristics, the temporal

---

EXHIBIT 8-1 Steps in quality assurance.

1. Specify study hypothesis.

2. Specify general design to test study hypothesis → Develop an overall study protocol.

3. Choose or prepare specific instruments, and develop procedures for data collection and processing → Develop operation manuals.

4. Train staff → Certify staff.

5. Using certified staff, pretest and pilot-study data collection and processing, instruments and procedures; pilot-study alternative strategies for data collection (eg, telephone vs mail interviews).

6. If necessary, modify 2 and 3, and retrain staff on the basis of results of 5.

trends in these statistics are analyzed for each technician (see Appendix D). If drifts are detected which cannot be explained by changes in the demographic composition of the participant pools, the corresponding clinic coordinator is notified, and a review of the protocol adherence for the affected technician is conducted.

Each type of measurement may require a special quality monitoring approach. For blood pressure and anthropometric measurements, for example, the routine assessment of digit preference is carried out in a straightforward manner. For studies using specialized reading centers for the reading and scoring of measurements performed at different field centers (e.g., ultrasound, magnetic resonance imaging, X-rays), monitoring data quality over time is more complicated because both field center data collection and centralized reading/scoring procedures can be sources of errors and variability.[2] Monitoring of laboratory data quality may require using external or internal standards (pools), as discussed later in this chapter.

8.3.2 Validity Studies

In epidemiologic studies, particularly those conducted on large numbers of individuals, a compromise between accuracy on the one hand, and costs and participants' burden on the other, is often necessary. Highly accurate diagnostic procedures are often too invasive and/or expensive for use in large samples of healthy individuals; accurate information on complex lifestyle characteristics or habits usually requires the use of lengthy (and therefore time-consuming) questionnaires. Thus, epidemiologists must frequently settle for less invasive or less time-consuming instruments or procedures that, although cheaper and more acceptable to study participants, may result in errors in the assessment of the variables of interest. Validity studies in subsamples of participants who undergo both the study-wide procedure and a more accurate procedure serving as a "gold standard" allow assessing the impact of these errors on the study estimates.

Some of the approaches applicable to the evaluation of validity in the context of epidemiologic studies are described next. In Section 8.4, the most commonly used indices of validity are described.

Standardized Pools for Laboratory Measurements

When using blood or other biological specimens, a possible approach for conducting a validity study is to take advantage of a well-established external quality control program conducted in a masked fashion. This approach consists of using the same biological (e.g., serum) pool to compare measurements obtained from applying study procedures with those resulting from the application of the "gold standard" procedures. The reference values serving as the "gold standard" may be measured in a pool *external* to the study—such as a pool provided by the Centers for Disease Control and Prevention [CDC] serum cholesterol standardization program.[18] Alternatively, an *internal* pool can be created by combining specimens obtained from study participants and tested by a "standard" laboratory outside the study. Usually, each sample unit in the pool is formed by biologic specimens contributed to by several participants so as to use as small an amount of specimen of each study individual as possible (see Figure 8-1). Ideally, deviations, if any, of the study measurements from the "true" (standard) results should be random during data collection and measurement activities; importantly, these deviations should not vary by presence and level of key variables, such as the main exposure and outcome of interest and participant accrual or follow-up time, lest differential misclassification occur (Chapter 4, Section 4.3.3). An example of the use of an "internal" pool is a validity study based on a mass serum cholesterol screening program involving 1880 Washington County, Maryland, residents. Screening measurements were done on blood obtained by the fingerstick method in a nonfasting state. In a subset of 49 screenees who also participated in a major cardiovascular study, serum cholesterol could also be assayed in a nationally recognized standard laboratory (Comstock, personal communication, 1991). The standard measurements were done in fasting state under carefully controlled conditions. The validity (i.e., sensitivity and specificity; see Section 8.4.1) of the screening measurements resulting in a classification according to presence of hypercholesterolemia (yes or no) could thus be evaluated by using the standard laboratory values as the "gold standard."

An example of a study that participated in the CDC serum cholesterol standardization program is the study by Burke et al.[19] of time trends in mean cholesterol levels in participants in the Minnesota Heart Survey (MHS). In this study, values obtained from applying MHS procedures were compared with those obtained from applying "gold standard" (CDC) procedures. MHS values were found to be lower than CDC values, and the difference was found to be greater at the beginning than at the end of the study. This phenomenon of

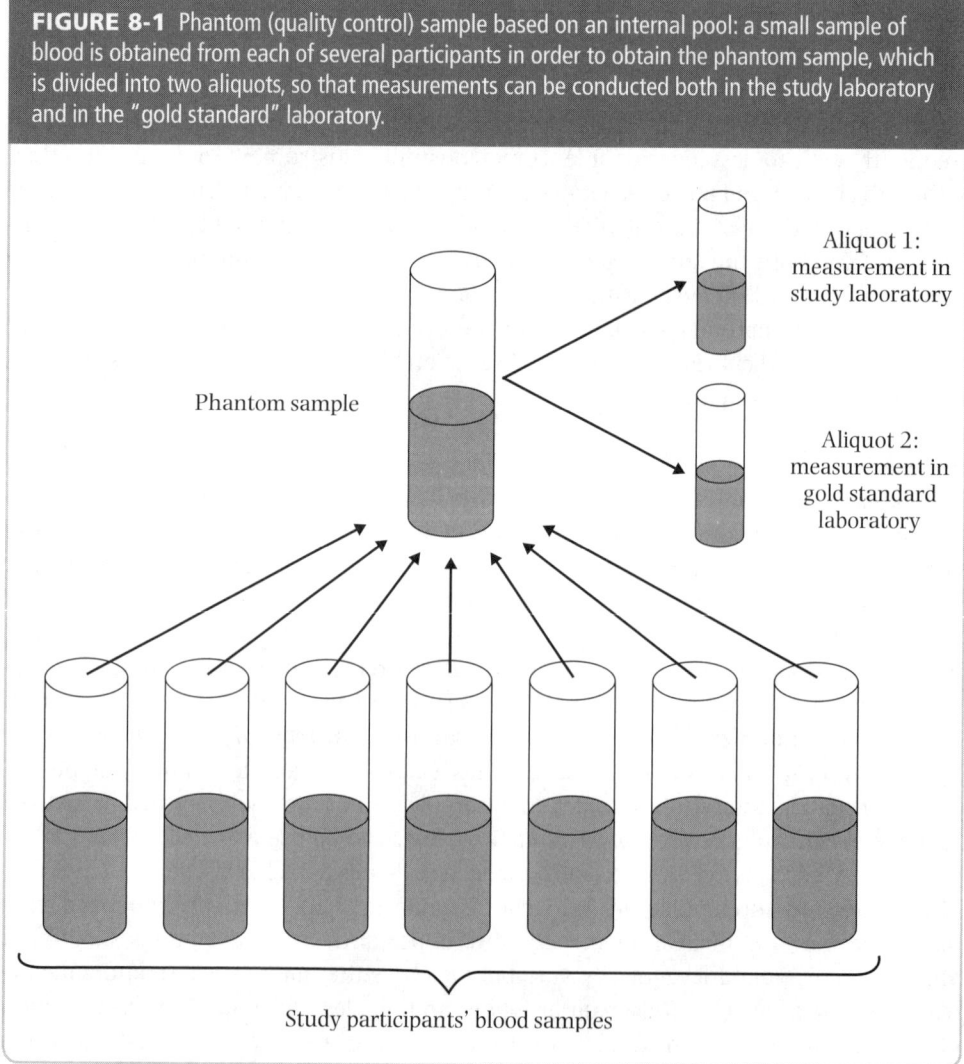

FIGURE 8-1 Phantom (quality control) sample based on an internal pool: a small sample of blood is obtained from each of several participants in order to obtain the phantom sample, which is divided into two aliquots, so that measurements can be conducted both in the study laboratory and in the "gold standard" laboratory.

differential bias over time, generically referred to as a temporal "drift," is schematically shown in Figure 8-2. After the magnitude of the "drift" is estimated using the standard, statistical techniques can be used to estimate "corrected" values. Thus, with correction for the temporal drift, the temporal decrease in serum cholesterol over time in the MHS was estimated to be even larger than that observed without the correction.[19]

Other Approaches to Examine Validity

The approach of comparing study-wide data with "gold standard" results in samples of study participants is not limited to laboratory measurements; it applies to questionnaire data as well. For example, in a case-control study assessing the relationship of hormone replacement therapy to breast cancer, information given by study participants was verified by contacting the physicians who had written these prescriptions.[20] Another example is given by a study that assessed the validity of Willett's food frequency questionnaire in a sample of 173 women selected from among the over 90,000 participants in the Nurses' Health Study.[12] All study participants responded to the 61-item food frequency questionnaire, which is relatively simple and easy to administer and that measures the approximate average frequency of intake of selected food items. In addition, the women in the sample kept a 1-week diet diary, which was then used as the "gold standard" to assess the validity of the food frequency questionnaire applied to the entire cohort. (This sample was also given the same food frequency questionnaire twice over a 1-year period to assess its reliability; see Section 8.3.3.)

In some studies, "validation" is sought only for "positive" responses given by study participants. Assessing samples of both "positive" and "negative" answers is important, however, because it allows estimation of both sensitivity and specificity of the study's data collection strategy (see Section 8.4.1)—as, for example, when confirming interview data given by both participants who report and those who do not report oral contraceptive pill use. In addition, information should be collected separately for the groups being compared (e.g., cases and controls or exposed and unexposed) to assess whether misclassification, if present, is non-differential or differential (see Chapter 4, Section 4.3.3).

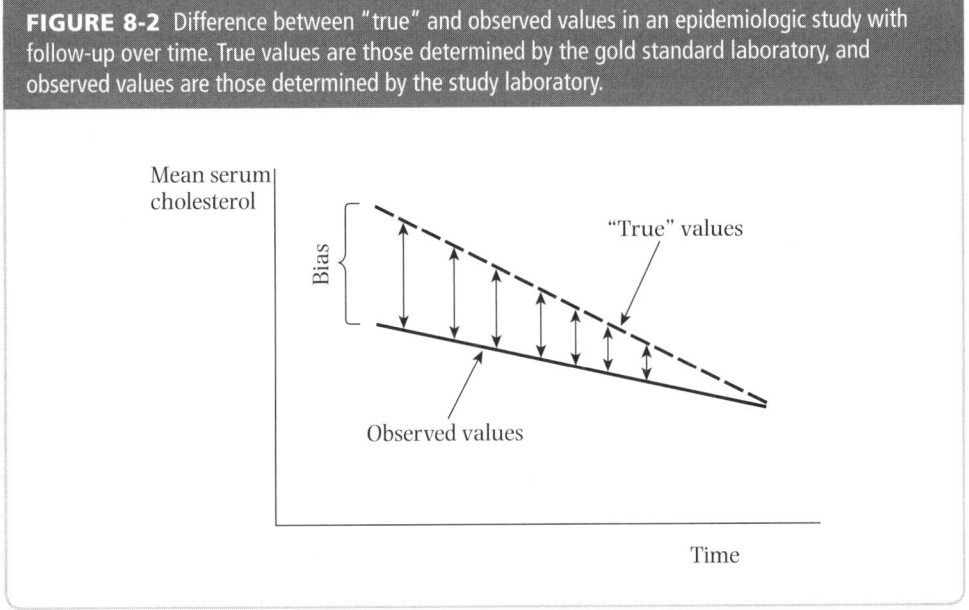

FIGURE 8-2 Difference between "true" and observed values in an epidemiologic study with follow-up over time. True values are those determined by the gold standard laboratory, and observed values are those determined by the study laboratory.

Availability of Validity Data from Previous Studies

On occasion, data on validity of a given procedure are available from previous studies. For example, data have been published on self-reported hypertension ever diagnosed by a health professional in approximately 8400 participants of the National Health and Nutrition Examination Survey III (NHANES III), a nationwide inquiry conducted in the United States between 1988 and 1991.[21] Availability of "gold standard" data comprising the actual blood pressure levels measured in these participants makes it possible to estimate the sensitivity and specificity of the participants' self-reports both for the total sample and according to sociodemographic characteristics (see Section 8.4.1).

Similarly, a study of the validity of self-reported anthropometric variables was conducted in participants of the Lipid Research Clinics (LRC) Family Study, whose weights and heights were both self-reported and measured.[22] As in the previous example, the authors of this study examined the validity of self-reported weight and height information according to the participant's age and gender and identified important differences (see Section 8.4.1).

Studies that rely on self-reported information, such as that on hypertension or weight/height, may use the estimates of validity of previous studies to evaluate the possible misclassification resulting from the use of such information in their own study population. In this case, it is necessary to judge whether the estimates of validity obtained in these previous studies (e.g., NHANES III or the LRC Family Study) are relevant and applicable to the study population in question, as briefly discussed in the following paragraphs.

Importance and Limitations of Validity Studies

As extensively illustrated in Chapter 4, the presence and strength of associations observed in epidemiologic studies are a function of the validity (and reliability) of key study variables, which in turn determines the presence and degree of misclassification (see Chapter 4, Section 4.3.3). Thus, an important element in the causal inferential process is the knowledge of the validity of exposure, outcome, main confounding variables, and effect modifiers. That many variables, even those considered as fairly "objective," have a relatively poor validity has been clearly shown (Table 8-2).[23] Consider, for example, a case-control study in which information on smoking is obtained from next of kin, rather than directly from cases and controls. In this study, assume that the prevalence of smoking in controls is 10%. Assume, in addition, that the "true" odds ratio associated with smoking (2.25) can be obtained by using data from direct personal interviews with the cases and controls themselves. Using the sensitivity and specificity figures for smoking shown in Table 8-2 (bottom row), if misclassification were nondifferential, the study's observed (biased) relative odds would be almost 30% closer to the null hypothesis (i.e., 1.63) than would the true value. (For the calculation of biased estimates based on sensitivity and specificity figures, see Chapter 4, Section 4.3.3.) A weaker association might have been missed altogether with these same levels of sensitivity and specificity–even though the sensitivity (94%) and specificity (88%) levels are reasonably high! As also mentioned in Chapter 4, Section 4.3.3, knowledge of the sensitivity and specificity levels of misclassified variables (as shown in Table 8-2) allows the correction of a biased estimate. When sensitivity and specificity values of a certain procedure are not known, sensitivity analysis* can be carried out whereby certain values

---

*Note that "sensitivity analysis" in this context is distinct from examination of sensitivity in validity studies (Chapter 10, Section 10.3).

are assumed, and their impact on the measure of association is evaluated (see Chapter 10, Section 10.3). It should be emphasized that assessment of validity levels is crucial to the continuous efforts to develop ever more accurate data collection procedures without sacrificing their efficiency.

Notwithstanding the importance of carrying out validity studies, it should be emphasized that these studies, especially (but not exclusively) those dealing with questionnaire data, may have important limitations. Thus, their results should be interpreted with caution. First, the "gold standard" itself may not be entirely valid. In validation studies of dietary information, for example, diary data, often used as gold standard, may have its own limitations with regard to measuring food intake.[24] Similarly, the use of information from medical charts, which are not primarily collected for research purposes, to "validate" data collected by interview may be problematic; as these records are not tightly standardized, they often lack relevant information. As a consequence, even important data from medical records regarding the patients' medical history may have limited accuracy. For information on habits or behaviors (e.g., past history of smoking) that are not routinely collected and recorded in medical records, self-reports from participants may well be more accurate.

Another problem related to validity studies is that although these studies are usually attempted on a random sample of participants, the study sample frequently constitutes a selected group of especially willing individuals. Because the "gold standard" procedure tends to be more invasive and burdensome—which, in addition to its cost, may be precisely why it has not been used as the primary means of study-wide data collection in the first place—often validity studies primarily include compliant volunteers. As a

TABLE 8-2 Examples of reported sensitivities and specificities of tests used in epidemiologic studies.

Test	Validation approach*	Sensitivity (%)	Specificity (%)
	Cohort		
Glucose tolerance by University Group Diabetes Project Criteria	World Health Organization criteria	91	94
Pap smear	Biopsy	86	91
Peptic ulcer by questionnaire	Radiologic diagnosis	50	98
Protoporphyrin assay-microhematocrit	Blood lead concentration	95	73
Rose questionnaire	Clinical interview	44	93
	Case-control		
Circumcision status by questionnaire	Physician's examination	83	44
Smoking status by next of kin	Personal questionnaire	94	88

*For bibliographic sources of original validation studies, see Copeland et al. (source).
Source: Data from KT Copeland et al., Bias Due to Misclassification in the Estimation of Relative Risk. *American Journal of Epidemiology*, Vol 105, pp. 488–495, © 1977.

result, validity levels estimated in these participants may not be representative of the true validity levels in the entire study population, particularly for questionnaire data. For example, in the validation study of Willett's dietary questionnaire described previously, 224 female nurses randomly selected among the Boston participants were invited to participate (participants from other locations were excluded for logistical reasons); of these, 51 declined, dropped out, or had missing information on key items for the validation study. Thus, the 173 women on whom the validity and reproducibility were eventually assessed (77% of those originally invited from the Boston subset) may be unrepresentative of all study participants.

An additional concern is that the usually small sample size and resulting statistical imprecision of validity studies limit the applicability of their findings. This is especially problematic if the derived estimates of sensitivity and specificity are used to "correct" the study's observed estimate of the measure of association. A correction based on validation estimates that are markedly affected by random error may do more harm than good: in other words, the "corrected" estimate may be even less "correct" than the original one. A related problem is that, although it is usually assumed that the estimates obtained in a validation study apply equally to the whole study population, this may not be the case if sensitivity and specificity of the procedure varied according to certain characteristics of the study population (e.g., the accuracy of self-reports of weight may be affected by the participants' true weight). Yet, the sample size for a validation study that allowed for stratification for all possible relevant variables would likely be too large and, thus, not practical vis-à-vis the resources available to most studies. Similarly, caution should be used when extrapolating the results of a validation study from one population to another, particularly if the data collection instrument is a questionnaire. For example, the validity of Willett's food frequency questionnaire, even if estimated accurately and precisely in a cohort of nurses, may not be generalizable to other study populations with different sociodemographic characteristics and health-related attitudes and awareness. Particularly problematic is the application to different cultures of validity figures for interview instruments obtained from a given study population. Often, culture-specific instruments need to be developed: an example is the food frequency questionnaire developed by Martin-Moreno et al.[25] for use in the Spanish population.

8.3.3 Reliability Studies

In contrast with validity studies, reliability studies assess the extent to which results agree when obtained by different observers, study instruments or procedures, or by the same observer, study instrument, or procedure at different points in time. To assess reliability, it is important to consider all sources of variability in an epidemiological study. Ideally, the only source of variability in a study should be that *between study participants*. Unfortunately, other sources of variability also influence any given measurement in most real-life situations; these include

- *Variability due to imprecision of the observer or the method*, which can be classified in two types:
  1. *Within-observer (or intra-observer) or within-method variability*, such as the variability of a laboratory determination conducted twice on the same sample by the same technician using the same technique. Within-observer variability also pertains to the variability of a response to a question by the same study participants when the same interview is conducted at different points in time by the same interviewer (assuming that the response is not time dependent).

2. *Between-observer (or inter-observer) or between-method variability*, such as the variability of a laboratory determination conducted on the same sample by two (or more) different technicians using the same assay or the variability of a laboratory determination done on the same individuals by the same technician using different assays.

- *Variability within study participants*, such as variability in habits and behaviors (e.g., day-to-day dietary intake variability) or physiologic variability in hormone or blood pressure levels. For example, Figure 8-3 shows systolic blood pressure values of two individuals over time. In this hypothetical example, one of the individuals is hypertensive, and the other is not (i.e., their average blood pressure levels are respectively equal or above, and below the cutoff level for the definition of systolic hypertension, 140 mm Hg). Because of the physiologic within-individual blood pressure variability, however, participant A's blood pressure occasionally dips below the hypertension cutoff level. If the measurement turns out to be at one of those moments (and if the participant does not have a hypertensive diastolic level and is not being medicated for hypertension), that participant will be erroneously classified as "normotensive." In this example, the within-individual variability masks the between-individual variability, that is, the difference in "true" average values which distinguish participants A and B as hypertensive and normotensive, respectively. Unlike observer or method variability, within-individual variability is real; however, it has consequences similar to those resulting from variability due to measurement errors in that it introduces "noise" in detecting differences between study participants, the usual goal in epidemiologic research. Like errors due to the measurement method (originating from the observer, the participant, the instrument, or the procedure), intra-individual variability masks the true between-individual variability and by doing so also produces misclassification. Whereas quality assurance procedures attempt to prevent or minimize within- and between-observer or method variability, physiologic within-individual variability is not amenable to prevention. Its influence, however, can be minimized by standardizing the timing of data collection for measures with known temporal fluctuations, such as physiologic measures that have circadian rhythms (e.g., levels of salivary cortisol or blood pressure), or by standardizing measurement conditions for variables affected by stress or activity (e.g., blood pressure should be measured after a resting time in a quiet environment). If possible, it is highly advisable to collect data at several points in time and use the average of all values. This would tend to prevent the nondifferential misclassification also known as *regression dilution bias* resulting from random variation over time in the values of a suspected risk factor or confounder (see Section 8.5). Statistical correction for this type of bias is also possible under certain conditions.[26]

All of these sources of variability, if present, tend to decrease the reliability of the measured value of a given variable; for any given measurement, they will add to the variability of the "true value" for the individual in question when compared with the rest of the individuals in the study population.

Reliability studies during data collection and processing activities usually consist of obtaining random repeat measurements, often referred to as "phantom" measurements. Figure 8-4 schematically illustrates an approach to reliability studies in the case of a biologic specimen.[27] Reliability studies may include repeated measures in the same individual to assess within-individual variability. Measurements of within-laboratory

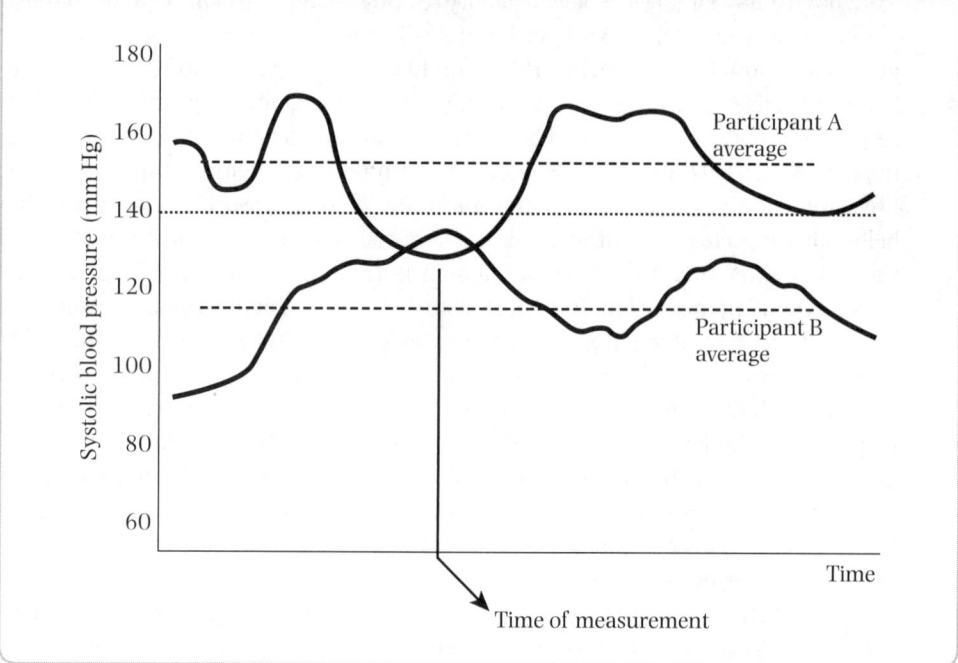

FIGURE 8-3 Hypothetical systolic blood pressure values of two individuals over time. Participant A is "hypertensive" (average or usual systolic blood pressure, 154 mm Hg – higher than standard cutoff, 140 mm Hg); participant B is "normotensive" (average systolic blood pressure, 115 mm Hg). If they are measured at the time indicated by the arrow, misclassification will result due to within-individual variability: participant A will be misclassified as "normotensive" (systolic blood pressure < 140 mm Hg); moreover, participant B's blood pressure will be considered higher than participant A's blood pressure.

(or technician) reliability can be done by splitting a phantom sample into two aliquots, which are then measured by the same laboratory (or technician) on separate occasions (Figure 8-4, aliquots 1.1 and 1.2). An additional split aliquot (aliquot 1.3) can be sent to another laboratory (or technician) to assess between-laboratory reliability. It is important that all of these repeat determinations in phantom samples be conducted in a masked fashion. Typically, phantoms are interspaced in the general pool of samples that are sent to a given laboratory or technician so that masking can be achieved.

As for laboratory determinations, reliability studies of other types of measurements (e.g., radiological imaging, height) can be conducted by repeat exams or repeat readings. Within-individual variability for many of these exams is limited or null (e.g., the short-term variability of a radiological image of a tumor or of height). Sources of variability that should be assessed include the exam procedures (e.g., the participant's positioning in the machine) and the reading (or interpretation of the image)—see examples in Section 8.4.2 that illustrate the assessment of reliability of readers of polysomnographic studies to determine the presence of sleep-related breathing disorders.

Assessing the reliability of each type of measurement has its own singularities and challenges. Anthropometric determinations, such as adult height for example, have little (if any) within-individual variability (at least in the short term); assessment of between-observer variability is fairly straightforward. On the other hand, assessment of within-observer reliability of such measurements may be challenging because it is difficult to "mask" the reader, as he or she may recognize the study participant as

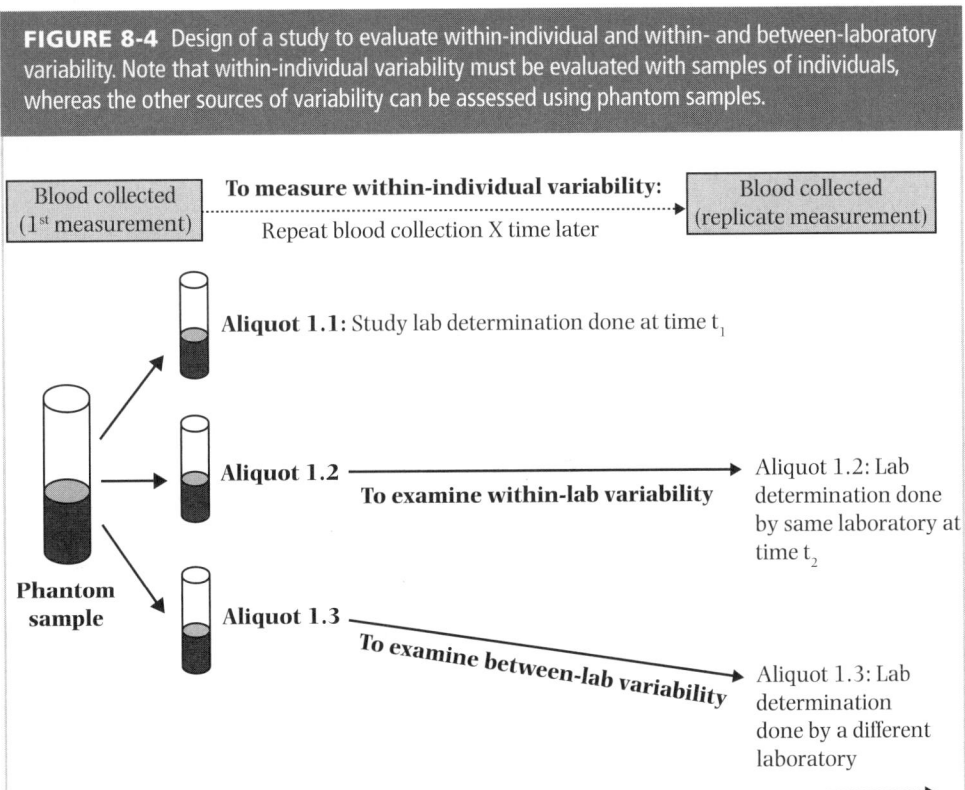

FIGURE 8-4 Design of a study to evaluate within-individual and within- and between-laboratory variability. Note that within-individual variability must be evaluated with samples of individuals, whereas the other sources of variability can be assessed using phantom samples.

Source: Based on LE Chambless et al., Short-Term Intraindividual Variability in Lipoprotein Measurements: The Atherosclerosis Risk in Communities (ARIC) Study. *American Journal of Epidemiology*, Vol 136, pp. 1069–1081, © 1992.

a "repeat" measurement (and thus remember the previous reading and/or make an effort to be more "precise" than usual). Similarly, studying the reliability of answers to questionnaires is difficult, as the participant's recall of his or her previous answers will influence the responses to the repeat questionnaire (whether it is administered by the same or by a different interviewer).

As with validity studies, if the sample is of sufficient size, it is important to assess whether reliability estimates obtained for a sample of study participants differ according to relevant characteristics, which may result in differential levels of misclassification. For example, the reliability of Willett's food frequency questionnaire was compared across subgroups of participants in the Nurses' Health Study, defined according to age, smoking and alcohol intake status, and tertiles of relative body weight.[28] In this study, no important differences in reproducibility of nutrient intake estimates among these different categories were observed, suggesting that the measurement errors resulting from the imperfect reliability of nutrient intake information were probably nondifferential (see Chapter 4, Section 4.3.3).

Finally, as with results of validity studies, it is important to be cautious when generalizing results from a reliability study of a given instrument to another study population: like validity, reliability may be a function of the characteristics of the study population. Even though it is appropriate to use published reliability and validity estimates in the planning stages of the study, it is recommended that, whenever possible, reliability and validity of key instruments, particularly questionnaires, be assessed in study participants. In addition, it is important to evaluate within-individual variability, as it may also differ according to certain population characteristics, thus further affecting the generalizability of reliability results. For example, the daily variability in levels of serum gonadal hormones (e.g., estrogens) is much larger in premenopausal than in postmenopausal women; thus, regardless of the measurement assays, reliability of levels of gonadal hormones for younger women is not applicable to older women.

8.4 INDICES OF VALIDITY AND RELIABILITY

In this section, some of the most frequently used indices of validity and reliability are briefly described, along with examples from published studies. Some of these indices, such as sensitivity and specificity, relate to the assessment of validity, whereas others, such as kappa or intraclass correlation, are usually applied in the evaluation of reliability (Table 8-3); however, some of these indices are used interchangeably to evaluate validity and reliability. For example, indices that are typically used as reliability indices, such as percent agreement or intraclass correlation coefficient (ICC), are sometimes used to report validity results. In real life, a true "gold standard" may not be available, thus sometimes making it difficult to distinguish between validity and reliability measures. When a "gold standard" is not clearly identified, "validity" results are often referred to as *inter-method reliability estimates*.

8.4.1 Indices of Validity/Reliability for Categorical Data

Sensitivity and Specificity

Sensitivity and specificity are the two traditional indices of validity when the definitions of exposure and outcome variables are categorical. The study exposure or outcome categorization is contrasted with that of a more accurate method (the "gold standard," which is assumed to represent the "true" value and thus to be free of error). Sensitivity and specificity are measures also frequently used in the context of the evaluation of diagnostic and screening tools; in that context, basic epidemiology textbooks usually describe them in relationship to the assessment of disease status (the "outcome"). As quality control measures in an analytic epidemiologic study, however, these indices apply to the evaluation of both exposure and outcome variables.

The definitions of the terms *sensitivity* and *specificity* were presented in Chapter 4, Exhibit 4-1. The calculation of sensitivity and specificity for a binary variable is again schematically shown in Table 8-4. (Appendix A, Section A.10 shows the method for the calculation of the confidence interval for estimates of sensitivity and specificity.)

An example is shown in Table 8-5, based on a study done in Washington County, Maryland, and previously discussed in Section 8.3.2, in which fingerstick tests were compared with standard laboratory ("gold standard") measurements of serum cholesterol. For Table 8-5, abnormal values are defined as those corresponding to 200 mg/dL or higher. Sensitivity and specificity for these data were found to be $18/19 = 0.95$ and $11/30 = 0.37$, respectively. Although the screening test's ability to identify truly hyper-cholesterolemic individuals was quite acceptable, its ability to identify "normals" was poor (63% of normal—which represent the complement of specificity—were false positives).

In the study of the validity of self-reported weight and height information among participants in the LRC Family Study mentioned previously,[22] participants were classified

TABLE 8-3 Summary of indices or graphic approaches most frequently used for the assessment of validity and reliability.

		Mostly used to assess . . .	
Type of variable	Index or technique	Validity	Reliability
Categorical	Sensitivity/specificity	+ +	
	Youden's J statistic	+ +	+
	Percent agreement	+	+ +
	Percent positive agreement	+	+ +
	Kappa statistic	+	+ +
Continuous	Scatter plot (correlation graph)	+	+ +
	Linear correlation coefficient (Pearson)	+	+
	Ordinal correlation coefficient (Spearman)	+	+
	Intraclass correlation coefficient	+	+ +
	Mean within-pair difference	+	+ +
	Coefficient of variation		+ +
	Bland-Altman plot	+ +	+ +

Note: + +, the index is indicated and used to measure the magnitude of validity or reliability; +, although the index is used to measure the magnitude of either validity or reliability, its indication is somewhat questionable.

in four categories according to their body mass index (BMI), measured as kg/m^2: "underweight" (BMI < 20 kg/m^2), "normal" (BMI = 20–24.9 kg/m^2), "overweight" (BMI = 25–29.9 kg/m^2), and "obese" (BMI ≥ 30 kg/m^2). BMI was calculated on the basis of either self-reported or measured weight and height. The cross-tabulation between self-reported and measured BMI categories is presented in Table 8-6. Based on these data and using measured BMI as the "gold standard," the validity of binary definitions of self-reported overweight and obesity can be estimated by constructing the two-by-two tables shown in Table 8-7. The validity estimates differ according to the cutoff adopted. For example, for definition A, *overweight* was defined as BMI ≥ 25 kg/m^2, resulting in a sensitivity of 3234/3741 =([2086 +280 + 59 + 809] ÷ [2086 + 280 + 59 + 809 + 505 + 2])= 0.86 and a specificity of 3580/3714 = 0.96. For definition B (right-hand side of Table 8-7), "obesity" was defined as BMI ≥ 30 kg/m^2, with sensitivity and specificity estimates of 0.74 and 0.99, respectively. In this example, sensitivity is lower than specificity: that is, there is a lower proportion of "false positives" than of "false negatives," probably as a consequence of the stigma associated with obesity in our society, resulting in a higher proportion of individuals underestimating than of those overestimating their weight.

Other issues related to sensitivity and specificity that should be underscored include the following. First, the dependence of sensitivity and specificity estimates on the cutoff level used shows that there is a certain arbitrariness in assessing and reporting the validity of binary definitions of continuous exposure and outcome variables. This problem should not be confused, however, with the dependence of "predictive values" on the prevalence of the condition.* Unlike positive and negative predictive values,

TABLE 8-4 Schematic representation of the calculation of sensitivity and specificity for a binary variable.

Study's result	Gold standard's result		Total
	Positive	Negative	
Positive	a	b	a + b
Negative	c	d	c + d
Total	a + c	b + d	N

Sensitivity = a/(a + c)
Specificity = d/(b + d)

TABLE 8-5 Comparison of screening values of serum cholesterol under field conditions and values done in a standard laboratory.

Screening values	Standard laboratory values		
	Abnormal*	Normal	Total
Abnormal*	18	19	37
Normal	1	11	12
Total	19	30	49

Sensitivity = 5 18/19 = 5 0.95
Specificity = 5 11/30 = 5 0.37

*Abnormal: serum cholesterol ≥ 200 mg/dL for screening and standard laboratory, respectively.
Source: Unpublished data from GW Comstock, 1991.

sensitivity and specificity are conditioned on the table's bottom totals (the "true" numbers of positives and negatives) and thus are theoretically independent of the prevalence of the condition. However, the common belief that sensitivity and specificity are inherent (fixed) properties of the test (or diagnostic criteria or procedure) itself, regardless of the characteristics of the study population, may be an oversimplification. This is particularly true for conditions based on a continuous scale that

---

*Positive and negative predictive values are measures used in the context of the evaluation of screening and diagnostic procedures, in addition to sensitivity and specificity. *Positive predictive value* (PPV) is the proportion of true positives among individuals who test positive (e.g., in Table 8-7, definition A, 3234/[3234 + 134] = 0.96). *Negative predictive value* (NPV) is the proportion of true negatives out of the total who test negative (e.g., in Table 8-7, definition A, 507/[507 + 3580] = 0.12). An important feature of these indices is that, in addition to their dependence on the sensitivity/specificity of the test in question, they are a function of the prevalence of the condition. For example, in Table 8-7, the prevalence of overweight (definition A) is 50.2% (3741/7455); if the prevalence had been 10% instead, even at the same self-reported weight and height sensitivity and specificity levels as those from the LRC Family Study, the PPV would have been only 0.71. (This can be shown as follows: using the notation from Table 8-4, and assuming the same total N = 7455, the expected value of cell *a* would be 641.1 (7455 × 0.10 × 0.86) and that of cell *b* would be 268.4 [7455 × (1 − 0.10) × (1 − 0.96)]; thus PPV = 641.1/(641.1 + 268.4) = 0.70.)

These indices have limited relevance in the context of evaluating the influence of validity on estimates of measures of association and are thus not discussed here. A detailed discussion of their interpretation and use, as well as a discussion of the likelihood ratio and other validity issues more relevant to screening and clinical decision making, can be found in basic clinical epidemiology textbooks.[29,30]

TABLE 8-6 Cross-tabulation of self-reported and measured four body mass index (BMI) categories: 7455 adult participants of the Lipid Research Clinics Family Study, 1975–1978.

BMI based on self-reports	Measured BMI category				
	Underweight	Normal	Overweight	Obese	Total
Underweight	462	178	0	0	640
Normal	72	2868	505	2	3447
Overweight	0	134	2086	280	2500
Obese	0	0	59	809	868
Total	534	3180	2650	1091	7455

Note: Underweight, BMI < 20 kg/m^2; Normal, BMI = 20 − 24.9 kg/m^2; Overweight, BMI = 25–29.9 kg/m^2; Obese, BMI ≥ 30 kg/m^2.
Source: Data from FJ Nieto-Garcia, TL Bush, and PM Keyl, Body Mass Definitions of Obesity: Sensitivity and Specificity Using Self-Reported Weight and Height. *Epidemiology*, Vol 1, pp. 146–152, © 1990.

TABLE 8-7 Cross-tabulation of self-reported and measured binary body mass index (BMI) categories: 7455 adult participants of the Lipid Research Clinics Family Study, 1975–1978 (see Table 8-6).

Definition A: overweight*			Definition B: obese†		
	Measured BMI category			Measured BMI category	
BMI based on self-report	Overweight	Nonoverweight	BMI based on self-report	Obese	Nonobese
Overweight	3234	134	Obese	809	59
Nonoverweight	507	3580	Nonobese	282	6305
Total	3741	3714	Total	1091	6364

*Overweight: BMI ≥ 25 kg/m^2 (that is, for the purposes of this example, "overweight" also includes "obese")
†Obese: BMI ≥ 30 kg/m^2.
Source: Data from FJ Nieto-Garcia, TL Bush, and PM Keyl, Body Mass Definitions of Obesity: Sensitivity and Specificity Using Self-Reported Weight and Height. *Epidemiology*, Vol 1, pp. 146–152, © 1990.

is more or less arbitrarily changed into a binary one (e.g., obesity, hypertension).[31,32] For a continuous trait, the probability of misclassifying a true positive as a negative (i.e., 1 − sensitivity, or cell c in Table 8-4) tends to be higher for individuals whose true values are near the chosen cutoff value, such as hypertensives with systolic blood pressure values close to the traditional cutoff point to define "high" values (e.g., 140 mm Hg). Thus, even for the same test (or diagnostic procedure) and the same cutoff point, the degree of misclassification will be larger if the distribution of values (i.e., the "spectrum of severity" of the condition) is closer to that of the truly negative, as illustrated in Figure 8-5.

Thus, the sensitivity and specificity of a given definition of a condition (i.e., based on a cutoff in a continuous distribution) depend on the distribution of the severity of the condition. The validity of a test can also vary from population to population when the test is not a direct marker of the condition. For example, the specificity of positive occult blood in the stool *for the diagnosis of colon cancer* varies according to the prevalence of other conditions that also cause gastrointestinal bleeding, such as peptic ulcer or parasitic disorders. Similarly, the ability of the purified protein derivative (PPD) test to diagnose human tuberculosis accurately is a function of the prevalence of atypical mycobacterial infections in the study population.

As discussed previously, another limitation of sensitivity and specificity estimates obtained in validation studies, especially when the information is obtained by questionnaire, is that these measures can vary according to the characteristics of the individuals in question. As a result, their external validity (generalizability) is limited. Examples are shown in Table 8-8. In Nieto-García's et al. study,[22] the validity of the definition of *obesity* (BMI ≥ 30 kg/m^2) based on self-reported weight and height information varied substantially according to age and gender. Sensitivity estimates using "measured" BMI as the gold standard (74% overall) ranged from more than 80% in young adults of either sex to less than 40% in older males.

Table 8-8 also shows the marked differences in the sensitivity of self-reported hypertension depending on ethnicity and health care utilization (indicated by a doctor's visit in the previous year) in the NHANES III survey. On the basis of these data, the authors concluded that "use of self-reported hypertension as a proxy for hypertension prevalence . . . is appropriate among non-Hispanic whites and non-Hispanic black women and persons who had a medical contact in the past 12 months. However, self-reported hypertension is not appropriate . . . among Mexican-Americans and individuals without access to regular medical care."[21(p.684)] These examples illustrate the influence of key sociodemographic variables on estimates of validity and serve as an empirical demonstration of the problems related to the extrapolation of validity estimates to populations with characteristics different from those in which validity was assessed. In addition, the large variability of validity estimates according to demographic variables, such as those shown in Table 8-8, suggests that if these variables represent the exposures of interest (or are correlated with them), differential misclassification may arise (see Chapter 4, Section 4.3.3).

Finally, it is important to emphasize that, as discussed previously in Section 8.3.2, the validity of some information items that are widely used in clinical settings or epidemiologic studies cannot be taken for granted. Table 8-2 shows some examples of results from validation studies of diverse clinical or medical history data, as summarized in a review by Copeland et al.[23] Some of the tests included in Table 8-2 suffer from poor sensitivity but have acceptable specificity, such as self-reported peptic ulcer and Rose's questionnaire for angina pectoris. These miss 50% or more of the cases identified by X-rays or clinical interviews, respectively, while correctly identifying almost all non-cases. On the other hand, other tests suffer from the opposite problem, such as the self-report of circumcision status, which tends to identify more than 80% of truly positive cases (according to a physician's examination), while at the same time labeling a large proportion of true negatives as (false) positives (1 − specificity = 56%). The poor specificity of self-reported circumcision status underscores the fact that even items of information expected to be highly valid because of their "objective" nature are subject to error. Further illustration is given by findings from a study by Fikree et al.[33] on the validity of husbands' report of their wives' pregnancy outcomes. In this study, carried out on a sample of 857 couples selected from a working population in Burlington, Vermont, the wives' reports were used as the standard against which the husbands' reports were evaluated. The sensitivity of men's report of low birth weight pregnancies was 74%. That of spontaneous abortions was 71.2%, and that of induced abortions was 35.1%. The validity was poorer among

FIGURE 8-5 Two hypothetical situations leading to different estimates of sensitivity depending on the spectrum of severity of a given condition (e.g., systolic blood pressure in the abscissa) even though the same test and cutoff (e.g., systolic blood pressure ≥ 140 mm Hg for the definition of hypertension) is used in both situations.

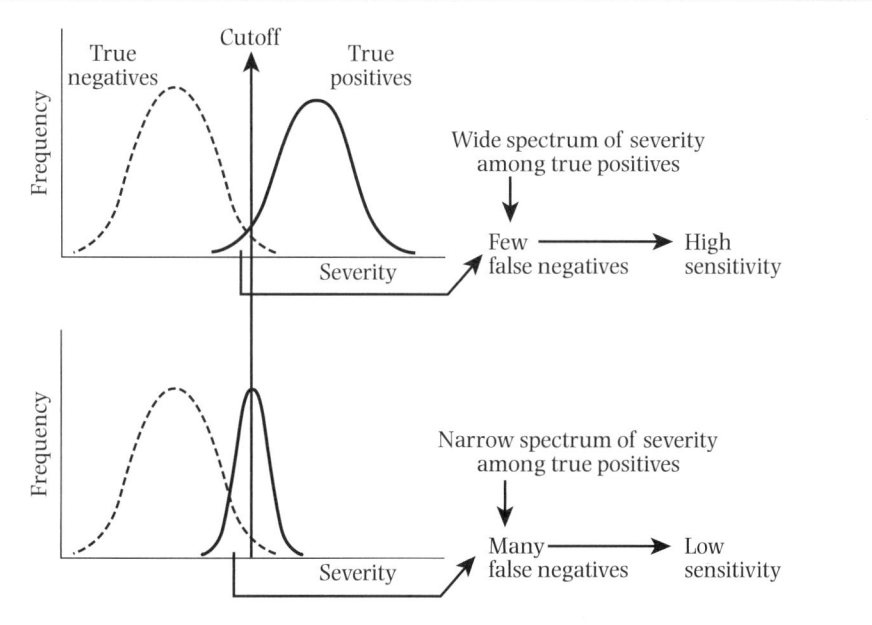

the younger and lower-educated individuals. The authors of this study concluded that it "would be prudent to avoid the use of husbands as proxy informants of their wives' reproductive histories."[33(p.237)]

Youden's J Statistic

Described by Youden[34] in 1950, the J statistic is a summary index of validity that combines sensitivity and specificity. It is calculated as

$$J = \text{Sensitivity} + \text{Specificity} - 1.0$$

For example, for the data shown in Table 8-5

$$J = (18/19) + (11/30) - 1.0 = 0.947 + 0.367 - 1.0 = 0.314 \text{ (or 31.4\%)}$$

The value 1.0 is subtracted from the sum of sensitivity and specificity so that the maximum value of the index becomes 1 when there is perfect agreement. Although theoretically the value of J can be negative, down to -1 (i.e., in the presence of perfect disagreement, when the test always disagrees with the "gold standard"), a more realistic minimum for the range of J in real life is $J = 0$, obtained when the test performs no better than chance alone (i.e., sensitivity and specificity = 0.5). This index gives equal weight to sensitivity and specificity, thus assuming that both are equally important components of validity. For example, for the data shown in Table 8-7, the values of J for the self-reported information are 0.82 and 0.73 for "overweight" and "obese," respectively. (The latter is almost identical to the estimated sensitivity of obesity based on self-report [0.74] because of the virtually perfect specificity [0.99]; in this case, a value that is essentially canceled out by subtracting 1.0 in the calculation.)

TABLE 8-8 Examples of results from subgroup analyses of sensitivity of information obtained by self-reports in two epidemiologic studies.

			Males	Females
Study	Category		Sensitivity (%)	
Nieto-García et al. "Obesity" based on self-reported weight and height*	Age (yr)	20–29	81	82
		30–39	73	85
		40–49	69	82
		50–59	65	81
		60–69	46	75
		70–79	38	68
Vargas et al. "Hypertension" based on self-report[†]	White			
	Doctor visit last year	Yes	71	73
		No	43	57
	Black			
	Doctor visit last year	Yes	80	74
		No	36	73
	Mexican American			
	Doctor visit last year	Yes	61	65
		No	21	65

*Based on data from the Lipid Research Clinics Family Study (see text); true "obesity" defined as measured body mass index $\geq$ 30 kg/m^2.
Source: FJ Nieto-Garcia, et al., Body Mass Definitions of Obesity: Sensitivity and Specificity Using Self-Reported Weight and Height. *Epidemiology*, Vol 1, pp. 146–152, 1990.
[†]Based on data from NHANES III (see text); true "hypertension" defined as measured systolic blood pressure $\geq$ 140 mm Hg, diastolic blood pressure $\geq$ 90 mm Hg, or use of antihypertensive medication.
Source: CM Vargas, et al., Validity of Self-Reported Hypertension in the National Health and Nutrition Survey III, 1988-91. *Preventive Medicine*, Vol 26, pp. 678–685, © 1997.

The formulas for the calculation of the confidence interval for a J statistic estimate are provided in Appendix A, Section A.11.

Because the J statistic assigns equal weight to sensitivity and specificity, alternative indices need to be used when these validity components are deemed not to be equally important in a given situation.

Percent Agreement

Percent agreement between two sets of observations is obtained by dividing the number of paired observations in the agreement cells by the total number of paired observations (Figure 8-6). As an example of calculation of percent agreement, Table 8-9 shows results of repeat readings of B-mode ultrasound images of the left carotid bifurcation, conducted to examine reliability of atherosclerotic plaque identification in the ARIC study.[35] When using a binary definition of the variable (plaque or normal), as in the example shown in Table 8-9, the percent agreement can be calculated simply as

$$\text{Percent agreement} = \frac{140 + 725}{986} \times 100 = 87.7\%$$

Not only is the percent agreement the simplest method of summarizing agreement for categorical variables, but it has the added advantage that it can be calculated for any number of categories, not just two, as in the preceding example. Thus, in the carotid ultrasound reading reliability study,[35] readers who detected a carotid plaque were also asked to assess the presence of acoustic shadowing (an attenuation of echoes behind the plaque often reflecting the presence of plaque calcification—i.e., an advanced atherosclerotic plaque). The results of the reproducibility readings of the left carotid bifurcation in this study when the finer definition of the plaque is used are shown in Table 8-10; the percent agreement in this case can be calculated as

$$\text{Percent agreement} = \frac{17 + 104 + 725}{986} \times 100 = 85.8\%$$

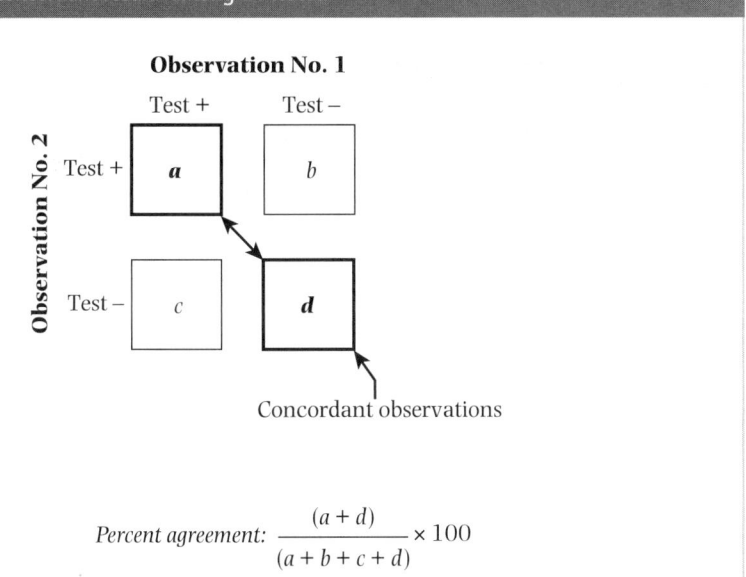

FIGURE 8-6 Percent agreement for paired binary test results (positive vs negative) (e.g., those obtained by two different observers or methods or by the same observer at two different points in time): proportion of concordant results among all tested.

TABLE 8-9 Agreement between the first and the second readings to identify atherosclerosis plaque in the left carotid bifurcation by B-mode ultrasound examination in the Atherosclerosis Risk in Communities (ARIC) Study.

		First reading		
		Plaque	Normal	Total
	Plaque	140	52	192
Second reading	Normal	69	725	794
	Total	209	777	986

Source: Data from R Li et al., Reproducibility of Extracranial Carotid Atherosclerosis Lesions Assessed by B-Mode Ultrasound: The Atherosclerosis Risk in Communities. *Ultrasound in Medicine & Biology*, Vol 22, pp. 791–799, © 1996.

Results from another reliability evaluation, based on data from a study of the relationship between p53 protein overexpression and breast cancer risk factor profile, are shown in Table 8-11.[36] As part of the quality control procedures in this study, 49 breast tumor sections were stained twice, and the resulting cross-tabulation of the results after the first and second staining shows the percent agreement to be $[(14 + 7 + 21)/49] \times 100 = 85.7\%$.

Although the percent agreement is the epitome of reliability indices for categorical variables, it can also be used to assess validity: that is, it can be used to examine the agreement between the test results and a presumed "gold standard"; when this is done, the calculation is obviously carried out without conditioning on the latter (as is the case with sensitivity/specificity calculations). For example, in Table 8-5, percent agreement is merely the percentage of the observations falling in the agreement cells over the total, or $[(18 + 11)/49] \times 100 = 59.2\%$. Likewise, in the validity study results shown in Table 8-6, the percent agreement between the weight categories based on self-report and measured weight and height is $[(462 + 2868 + 2086 + 809)/7455] \times 100 = 83.5\%$.

TABLE 8-10 Agreement between the first and the second readings to identify atherosclerosis plaque with or without acoustic shadowing in the left carotid bifurcation by B-mode ultrasound examination in the Atherosclerosis Risk in Communities (ARIC) Study.

		First reading			
		P + S*	Plaque only	Normal	Total
Second reading	P + S*	17	14	6	37
	Plaque only	5	104	46	155
	Normal	5	64	725	794
	Total	27	182	777	986

*Plaque plus (acoustic) shadowing.
Source: Data from R Li et al., Reproducibility of Extracranial Carotid Atherosclerosis Lesions Assessed by B-Mode Ultrasound: The Atherosclerosis Risk in Communities Study. Ultrasound in Medicine & Biology, Vol 22, pp. 791–799, © 1996.

TABLE 8-11 Reproducibility of the staining procedure for p53 overexpression in 49 breast cancer sections: Netherlands OC Study.

		First staining			
		p53+	p53±	p53−	Total
Second staining	p53+	14	1		15
	p53±		7	2	9
	p53−		4	21	25
	Total	14	12	23	49

Note: p53+, p53 overexpression; p53±, weak overexpression; p53−, no p53 overexpression.
Source: Data from K van der Kooy et al., p53 Protein Overexpression in Relation to Risk Factors for Breast Cancer. American Journal of Epidemiology, Vol 144, pp. 924–933, © 1996.

A limitation of the percent agreement approach is that its values tend to be high whenever the proportion of negative–negative results is high (resulting from a low prevalence of positivity in the study population), particularly when the specificity is high. For example, in Table 8-7, the percent agreement is higher for definition B (95.4%) than for definition A (91.4%), even though sensitivity was 12 points lower in B than in A (74% and 86%, respectively); this can be explained partly by the fact that the prevalence of the condition is lower in B than in A, thus inflating the negative–negative cell, and partly by the fact that the specificity is higher in B than in A (it is close to 100% for the former). As further illustration, Table 8-12 shows the hypothetical situation of a population in which the prevalence of obesity was 20 times lower than that observed in the LRC population but the sensitivity and specificity levels were *the same* as those observed in Table 8-7, definition B (except for rounding). In this situation, the percent agreement will increase from 95.4% to about 99%; that is, it will be almost perfect solely as a result of the decreased prevalence. In an analogous fashion, the percent agreement also tends to be high when the prevalence of the condition is very high (resulting in a high proportion of positive–positive observations), particularly when the sensitivity is high.

As for sensitivity and specificity, standard errors and confidence limits for percent agreement are calculated following standard procedures for an observed proportion (see Appendix A, Section A.10).

Percent Positive Agreement

In part to overcome the limitations of the percent agreement as a reliability index when the prevalence of the condition is either very low or very high, at least two measures of *positive agreement* (PPA) have been proposed:[37]

TABLE 8-12 Hypothetical results based on the example shown in Table 8-7 (Definition B), assuming the same validity figures but a prevalence of obesity approximately 20 times lower than that found in the Lipid Research Clinics population.

BMI based on self-report	Measured BMI category		Total
	Obese	Nonobese	
Obese	41	69	110
Nonobese	14	7331	7345
Total	55	7400	7455

$$\text{Percent agreement} = \frac{(41 + 7331)}{7455} \times 100 = 98.9\%$$

$$\text{PPA*} = \frac{2 \times 41}{(55 + 110)} \times 100 = 49.7\%$$

$$\text{Chamberlain's PPA*} = \frac{41}{(41 + 69 + 14)} \times 100 = 33.1\%$$

*Percent positive agreement.

1. *Percent positive agreement:* the number of occurrences for which both observers report a positive result, out of the average number of positives by either observer. Using the notation in Table 8-4, this is formulated as follows:

$$\text{PPA} = \frac{a}{\left(\frac{(a+c)+(a+b)}{2}\right)} \times 100 = \frac{2a}{[(a+c)+(a+b)]} \times 100$$

$$= \frac{2a}{(2a+b+c)} \times 100$$

(An intuitive understanding of the PPA formula is that "$2a$" represents positives identified by both observers, whereas "b" and "c" are the positives identified by only one observer.)

2. *Chamberlain's percent positive agreement:* the number of occurrences for which both observers report positive results out of the total number of observations for which at least one observer does so.[38]

$$\text{Chamberlain's PPA} = \frac{a}{(a+b+c)} \times 100$$

The calculation of these two indices is illustrated in the example shown in Table 8-12. Notice that the two indices are closely related algebraically:

$$\text{Chamberlain's PPA} = \frac{\text{PPA}}{(2-\text{PPA})}$$

Kappa Statistic

The preceding measures of agreement have an important limitation. They do not take into account the agreement that may occur by chance alone: that is, they do not take into consideration the fact that even if both readings were completely unrelated (e.g., both observers scoring at random), they would occasionally agree just by chance. A measure that corrects for this chance agreement is the kappa statistic (κ) defined as the fraction of the *observed* agreement not due to chance in relation to the *maximum* non-chance agreement when using a categorical classification of a variable.[39–41] This definition is readily grasped by consideration of the formula for the calculation of (κ):

$$\kappa = \frac{P_o - P_e}{1.0 - P_e}$$

where P_o is the proportion of *observed* agreement and P_e is the chance agreement, that is, the proportion of agreement *expected* to occur by chance alone. Their difference (the numerator of kappa) is thus the non-chance observed agreement, whereas $1.0 - P_e$ (the denominator) is the maximum non-chance agreement.

The kappa statistic is calculated from the cells shown in the diagonal of a cross-tabulation table, representing complete concordance between the two sets of observations. The chance agreement is the agreement that would be expected if both observers rated the responses at random. The total chance agreement is the sum of the chance agreement for each cell on the diagonal. The number expected in each cell by chance alone is the product of the corresponding marginal totals divided by the grand total. (This is the same method as that used for calculating the expected values under the null hypothesis for a chi-square test in a contingency table.) For example, the chance agreement for the "plaque–plaque" cell in Table 8-9 is $(209 \times 192)/986$, or 40.7, and that for the "normal–normal" cell is $(777 \times 794)/986$, or 625.7.* The total expected chance agreement is thus $(40.7 + 625.7)/986 = 0.676$. A shortcut for the calculation of the proportion chance agreement for each cell is to divide the products of the marginals by the square of the total: that is, to combine both steps—calculation of the expected number and that of the expected *proportion*—into one. For example, for the data in Table 8-9, the expected proportion for the "plaque–plaque" cell is $[209 \times 192]/986^2$, and that for the "normal–normal" cell is $[777 \times 794]/986^2$. The total chance agreement is therefore $[209 \times 192 + 777 \times 794]/986^2 = 0.676$.) Because, as shown previously, the observed agreement for this table was 0.877,

$$\kappa = \frac{0.877 - 0.676}{1.0 - 0.676} = 0.62$$

Formulas for the standard error and confidence interval of kappa are given in Appendix A, Section A.12.

Possible values of kappa range from -1 to 1, although values below 0 are not realistic in practice (the observed agreement would be worse than by chance alone). For the interpretation of a given value of kappa, different classifications have been proposed[40,42–44] (Figure 8-7). Of these, probably the most widely used is that proposed by Landis and Koch.[42] It is important to realize, however, that these classifications are arbitrary[45]; for any given value of kappa, the degree of misclassification/bias that would result from using the corresponding instrument/reader will depend on other circumstances, such as the prevalence of the condition and the distribution of the marginals (discussed later).

Like the percent agreement, the kappa can be estimated from 3×3, 4×4, or $k \times k$ tables. For example, the value of kappa for the repeat readings of the ultrasound examinations of the left carotid bifurcation in the ARIC study shown in Table 8-10 can be calculated as follows:

Observed agreement (see above) = 0.858

$$\text{Chance agreement} = \frac{[(27 \times 37) + (182 \times 155) + (777 \times 794)]}{(986)^2} = 0.665$$

$$\kappa = \frac{(0.858 - 0.665)}{(1 - 0.665)} = 0.576$$

Also like percent agreement, kappa is primarily used for the assessment of reliability—that is, when there is no clear-cut standard and it is appropriate to give equal weight to both sets of readings. It is also occasionally used for the assessment of validity, however, to compare the test results with those from a "gold standard." As previously discussed, the

---

*To understand better the probability that both readings would coincide by chance, it can be calculated for the "plaque–plaque" cell as follows (a similar calculation can be done for the "normal–normal" cell): the proportions of plaque identified by the first and second readings in Table 8-9 are $209/986 = 0.212$ and $192/986 = 0.195$. Thus, if both readings were entirely independent (i.e., coinciding only by chance), the joint probability that both would identify plaque is $0.212 \times 0.195 = 0.041$, which translates into an expected chance agreement of $0.041 \times 986 = 40.7$ for plaque–plaque readings.

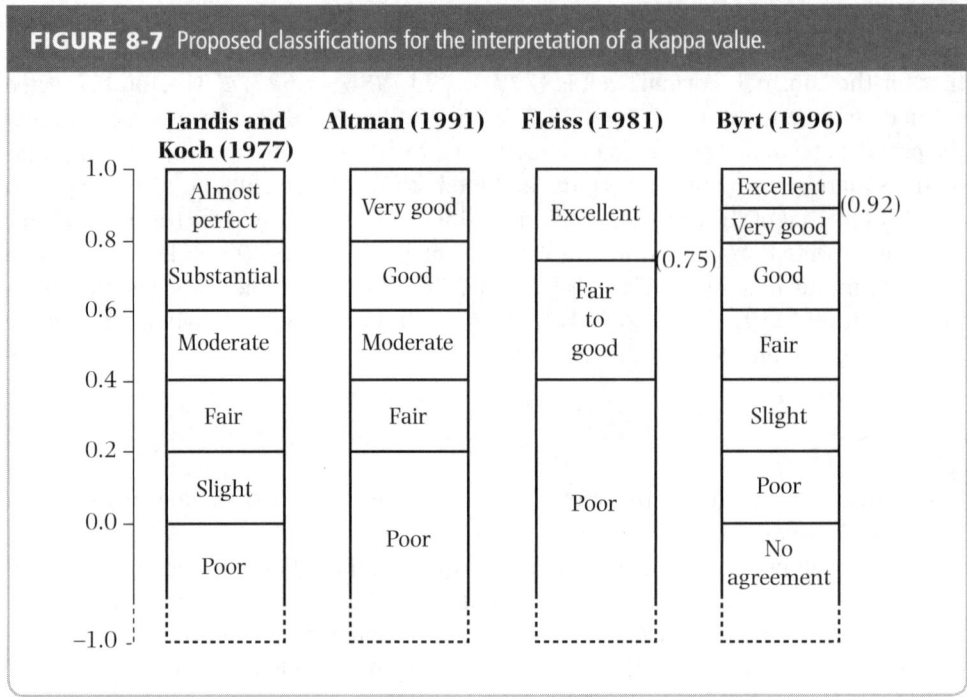

FIGURE 8-7 Proposed classifications for the interpretation of a kappa value.

observed agreement between BMI categories based on self-report and the "gold standard" (measured BMI) in Table 8-6 is 0.835. The expected chance agreement would be

$$\frac{[(534 \times 640) + (3180 \times 3447) + (2650 \times 2500) + (1091 \times 868)]}{7455^2} = 0.340$$

Thus,

$$\kappa = \frac{(0.835 - 0.340)}{(1 - 0.340)} = 0.75$$

Kappa is also frequently used in situations in which, although a "gold standard" exists, it is subject to non-negligible error, and thus, the investigator is reluctant to take it at face value (as assumed when sensitivity and specificity of the "test" are calculated). (As mentioned previously, in this situation, it may be preferable to refer to the comparison between the "gold standard" and the test as an evaluation of "inter-method reliability" rather than of validity.) An example is a study using serum cotinine levels as the "gold standard" to assess the "validity" of self-reported current smoking among pregnant women;[46] because in this example the "gold standard" is also subject to errors stemming from both laboratory and within-individual variability, kappa was calculated and shown to be 0.83. In addition, to assess indirectly which method (self-report or serum cotinine) had better predictive validity (and reliability), the authors compared the magnitude of their correlation with an outcome known to be strongly related to maternal smoking: infant birthweight. The correlation between serum cotinine and birthweight ($r = 0.246$) was only slightly higher than that observed between smoking self-report and birthweight ($r = 0.200$), suggesting that, in this study population, serum cotinine and self-report are similarly adequate as markers of current smoking exposure. (The limitations of inferences based on the value of the correlation coefficient are discussed in Section 8.4.2.)

TABLE 8-13 Agreement between reported disability and observed performance in a sample of 626 individuals aged 72 years and older in Barcelona, Spain.

Reported "need of help" to walk

		Performance: 4-meter walk				
	Unable	Able	Sensitivity*	Specificity*	% Agreement	Kappa
Yes	15	12	0.58	0.98	96	0.55
No	11	571				

Reported "difficulty" in walking

		Performance: 4-meter walk				
	Slow†	Quick†	Sensitivity	Specificity	% Agreement	Kappa
Yes	85	75	0.60	0.83	78	0.41
No	56	367				

Reported "difficulty" in standing up from a chair

		Performance: 5 consecutive rises from a chair				
	Unable	Able	Sensitivity	Specificity	% Agreement	Kappa
Yes	71	41	0.63	0.92	86	0.55
No	42	455	(0.54–0.72)‡	(0.89–0.94)‡	(83–89)‡	(0.47–0.63)‡

*Sensitivity and specificity were calculated considering the physical performance test as the "gold standard."
†"Slow" and "quick" were identified according to whether the subject walked 4 meters in more or less than 7.5 seconds, respectively.
‡Confidence interval for these estimates are presented and their calculation illustrated in Appendix A, Sections A.10 and A.12.
Source: Data from M Ferrer et al., Comparison of Performance-Based and Self-Related Functional Capacity in Spanish Elderly. *American Journal of Epidemiology,* Vol 149, pp. 228–235. © 1999

Another example of the application of kappa to evaluate inter-method reliability is a study comparing performance-based and self-rated functional capacity in an older population of Barcelona, Spain.[47] Selected results from this study are shown in Table 8-13. The authors reported measures of both validity (sensitivity and specificity) and reliability (percent agreement and kappa), thus leaving to the reader the judgment as to whether performance evaluation at one point in time was an appropriate gold standard.

Extensions of the kappa statistic to evaluate the agreement between multiple ratings (or multiple repeat measurements) are available.[40] An example of this application of kappa can be found in a study assessing the reliability of diagnostic classification of emergency visits and its implications for studies of air pollution.[48] The agreement (kappa) between the diagnosis obtained from the hospital database and that made by six external raters (full-time emergency physicians) according to diagnostic category and day's pollution level was efficiently displayed by the authors (as shown in Figure 8-8).

Weighted Kappa

When study results can be expressed by more than two categories, certain types of disagreement may be more serious than others; in this situation, consideration should be given to the use of the weighted kappa. An example of its application is the comparison

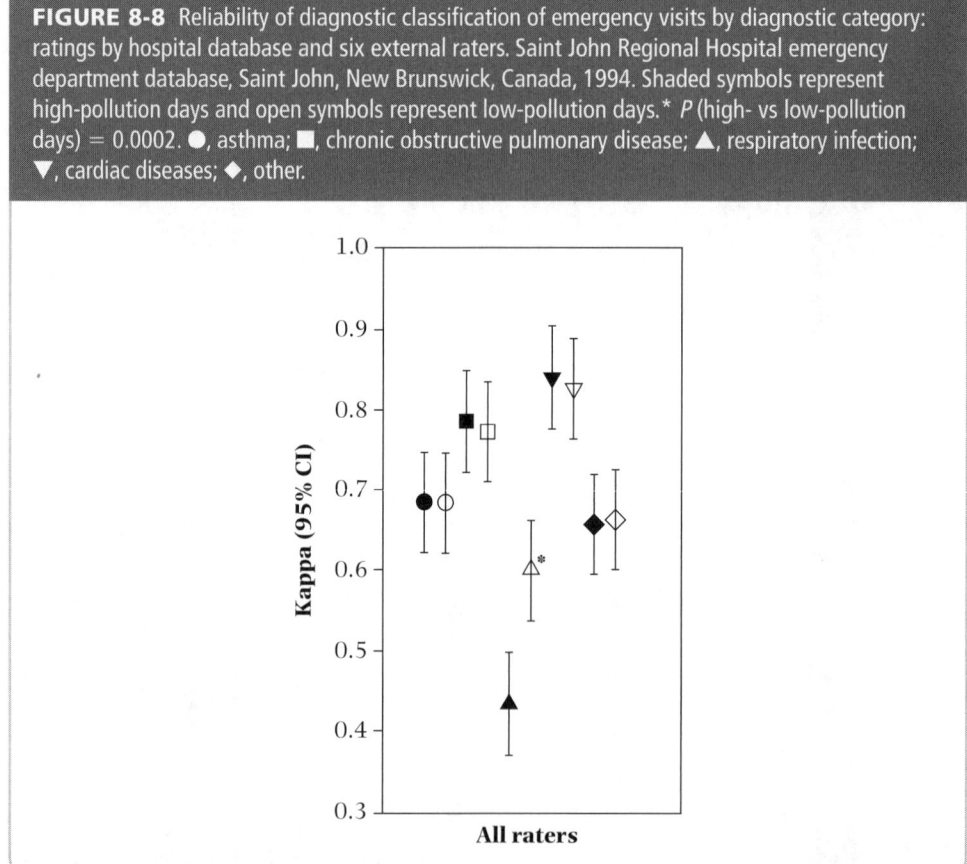

FIGURE 8-8 Reliability of diagnostic classification of emergency visits by diagnostic category: ratings by hospital database and six external raters. Saint John Regional Hospital emergency department database, Saint John, New Brunswick, Canada, 1994. Shaded symbols represent high-pollution days and open symbols represent low-pollution days.* *P* (high- vs low-pollution days) = 0.0002. ●, asthma; ■, chronic obstructive pulmonary disease; ▲, respiratory infection; ▼, cardiac diseases; ◆, other.

Source: Reprinted with permission from DM Stieb et al., Assessing Diagnostic Classification in an Emergency Department: Implications for Daily Time Series Studies of Air Pollution. *American Journal of Epidemiology*, Vol 148, pp. 666–670, © 1998

between self-reported and measured BMI, previously discussed (see Table 8-6). When the kappa statistic for these data was calculated above ($\kappa = 0.75$), it was assumed that only total agreement (the diagonal in Table 8-6) was worth considering: that is, any type of disagreement, regardless of its magnitude, was regarded as such. An alternative approach when calculating the value for kappa is to assign different weights to different levels of disagreement and thus to assume that cells that are adjacent to the diagonal represent some sort of "partial" agreement. For example, Table 8-14 shows the same data as in Table 8-6 but also indicates that full weight (1.0) was assigned to the diagonal cells representing perfect agreement, a weight of 0.75 to disagreement between adjacent categories, a weight of 0.5 for disagreement corresponding to a "distance" of two categories, and a weight of 0 for disagreement of three categories. The calculation of the *observed agreement* in Table 8-14 is analogous to the calculation of a weighted mean in that it consists of merely multiplying the number in each cell by the corresponding weight, summing up all products, and dividing the sum by the grand total. Starting in the first row with the cell denoting "Underweight" for both assays, and proceeding from left to right in each row, the observed agreement (P_{ow}, in which the letters *o* and *w* denote "observed" and "weighted," respectively) is

$$P_{ow} = (462 \times 1 + 178 \times 0.75 + 0 + 0 + 72 \times 0.75 + 2868 \times 1$$
$$+ 505 \times 0.75 + 2 \times 0.5 + 0 + 134 \times 0.75 + 2086 \times 1 + 280$$
$$\times 0.75 + 0 + 0 + 59 \times 0.75 + 809 \times 1)/7455 = 0.959$$

The calculation of P_{ow} can be simplified by rearranging this equation, grouping the cells with equal weights (and omitting those with zeros):

$$P_{ow} = [(462 + 2868 + 2086 + 809) \times 1 + (178 + 72 + 505$$
$$+ 134 + 280 + 59) \times 0.75 + (2) \times 0.5]/7455 = 0.959$$

The calculation of the *chance agreement* (P_{ew}, in which the letter *e* denotes "expected" by chance alone) in this example is done as follows: (1) multiply the marginal totals corresponding to cells showing a weight of 1.0; then sum these products, and multiply this sum by the weight of 1.0; (2) do the same for the cells with weights of 0.75 and for the cells with weights of 0.5 (i.e., including those with observed value of 0); and (3) sum all of these, and divide the sum by the square of the grand total, as follows:

$$P_{ew} = [(534 \times 640 + 3180 \times 3447 + \ldots) \times 1 + (534 \times 3447 + \ldots) \times 0.75$$
$$+ (2650 \times 640 + 1091 \times 3447 + 534 \times 2500 + 3180 \times 868)$$
$$\times 868) \times 0.5]/7455^2 = 0.776$$

After the *weighted* observed and chance agreement values are obtained, the formula for the weighted kappa (κ_w) is identical to that for the unweighted kappa:

$$\kappa_w = \frac{P_{ow} - P_{ew}}{1.0 - P_{ew}}$$

Using this formula to calculate a weighted kappa for Table 8-14 yields

$$\kappa_w = \frac{0.959 - 0.776}{1.0 - 0.776} = 0.82$$

In this example, the weight of 0.5 assigned to a disagreement of two categories was used only as a hypothetical example for the calculation of weighted kappa; in real life, one would be unlikely to assign any weight at all to disagreements between such extreme categories as "obese" versus "normal" or "overweight" versus "underweight." In general, the weights assigned to cells, although somewhat arbitrary, should be chosen on the basis of the investigators' perception of how serious the disagreement is *in the context of how the data will be used*. For example, in a clinical setting where a confirmatory breast cancer diagnosis from biopsy specimens may be followed by mastectomy, nothing short of perfect agreement may be acceptable. (In practice, in this situation, disagreement between two observers is usually adjudicated by an additional observer or observers.) As a different example, the inclusion of either "definite" or "probable" myocardial infarction cases in the numerator of incidence rates for analyzing associations with risk factors in a cohort study (see, e.g., White et al.[5]) may well be acceptable, thus justifying the use of a weighting score similar to that shown in Table 8-15 for the calculation of kappa between two raters. In this example, the weighting scheme is set up recognizing that the disagreement between "probable" or "definite" on the one hand, and "absent" on the other, is deemed to be more serious than that between "definite" and "probable." In the hypothetical example shown in Table 8-15, perfect agreement in myocardial infarction diagnoses between two observers was assigned a weight of 1.0 (as in the calculation of the unweighted kappa); the "definite" versus "probable"

TABLE 8-14 Calculation of weighted kappa: cross-tabulation of self-reported and measured four body mass index (BMI) categories among 7455 adult participants of the Lipid Research Clinics Family Study, 1975–1978 (See Table 8-6).

BMI based on self-reports	Measured BMI category				
	Underweight	Normal	Overweight	Obese	Total
Underweight	462 (1.0)*	178 (0.75)	0 (0.5)	0 (0)	640
Normal	72 (0.75)	2868 (1.0)	505 (0.75)	2 (0.5)	3447
Overweight	0 (0.5)	134 (0.75)	2086 (1.0)	280 (0.75)	2500
Obese	0 (0)	0 (0.5)	59 (0.75)	809 (1.0)	868
Total	534	3180	2650	1091	7455

*Observed number (weight for the calculation of kappa).

TABLE 8-15 Agreement weights for calculation of kappa: a hypothetical example of classification of myocardial infarction by certainty of diagnosis.

Observer no. 2	Observer no. 1		
	Definite	Probable	Absent
Definite	1.0	0.75	0
Probable	0.75	1.0	0
Absent	0	0	1.0

disagreement was arbitrarily assigned an "agreement" weight of 0.75, which recognized its lesser seriousness vis-à-vis the weight of 0 assigned to the disagreement between the "absent" and the other categories. If an additional and even "softer" diagnostic category, "possible," was also used, the disagreement between, for example, "definite" and "possible" might be given a smaller weight (e.g., 0.5) than that assigned to the "definite-probable" cells. A similar approach could be used for the data shown in Table 8-10, in which the disagreement between the readings "plaque + shadowing" and "plaque" might not be considered as severe as that between either of the two and "normal."

In any event, the value of weighted kappa will obviously depend on the weighting scheme that is chosen. This arbitrariness has been criticized and is one of the weaknesses of weighted kappa,[49] particularly when continuous variables are grouped into multiple ordinal categories (e.g., the BMI categories in Table 8-6). In the latter case, it will be best to use certain weighting schemes for kappa* that are equivalent to the intraclass correlation coefficient described in Section 8.4.2.

Dependence of Kappa on Prevalence

An important limitation of kappa when comparing the reliability of a diagnostic procedure (or exposure) in different populations is its dependence on the prevalence of true "positivity" in each population. Following is an example that illustrates how differences in prevalence affect the values of kappa.

Consider a given condition Y, which is to be screened independently by two observers (A and B) in two different populations I and II, each with a size of 1000 individuals. Prevalence rates in these populations are 5% and 30%, respectively, such as can be found in younger and older target populations with regard to hypertension. Thus, the numbers of true positives are 50 for population I and 300 for population II. The sensitivity and specificity of each observer (assumed not to vary with the prevalence of Y) are, for observer A, 80% and 90%, respectively, and for observer B, 90% and 96%, respectively.

These sensitivity levels can be applied to the true positives in populations I and II to obtain the results shown in Table 8-16. For example, for population I, as seen in the row total, the sensitivity of observer A being 0.80, 40 of the 50 true positive subjects are correctly classified by him or her, whereas 10 are mistakenly classified as (false) negatives. For observer B, who has a sensitivity of 0.90, these numbers are, respectively, 45 and 5. The concordance cell—that is, the number of persons who are classified as "positive" by both observers A and B—is merely the joint sensitivity applied to the total group of positive cases: for example, for population I, $(0.80 \times 0.90) \times 50 = 0.72 \times 50 = 36$. With three of these numbers—that is, those classified as "positive" by A, those classified as "positive" by B, and those jointly classified as "positive"—it is possible to calculate the other cells in Table 8-16.

---

*It has been shown by Fleiss[40] that for ordinal multilevel variables, when the weights, w_{ij} ($i = 1, \ldots, k; j = 1, \ldots, k$), are defined as

$$w_{ij} = 1 - \frac{(i-j)^2}{(k-1)^2}$$

where k is the number of categories in the contingency table for the readers indexed by i and j, the value of the weighted kappa is identical to that of the intraclass correlation coefficient (see Section 8.4.2).

TABLE 8-16 Results of measurements conducted by observers A and B* in true positives in populations with different prevalence rates of the condition measured, each with a population size of 1000.

	Population I (prevalence = 5%)			Population II (prevalence = 30%)		
	Observer A			Observer A		
Observer B	Pos	Neg	Total	Pos	Neg	Total
Positive	36‡	9	45§	216‡	54	270§
Negative	4	1	5	24	6	30
Total	40**	10	50†	240**	60	300†

*Observer A has an 80% sensitivity and 90% specificity; observer B has a 90% sensitivity and a 96% specificity.
†Number of true positives, obtained by multiplying the prevalence times the total population size: for example, for population I, 0.05 × 1000.
‡Obtained by applying the joint sensitivity of observers A and B to the total number of true positives: for example, for population I, (0.80 × 0.90) × 50.
§Obtained by applying the sensitivity level of observer B to the total number of true positives in populations I and II: for example, for population I, 0.90 × 50.
**Obtained by applying the sensitivity level of observer A to the total number of true positives in populations I and II: for example, for population I, 0.80 × 50.

In Table 8-17, similar calculations are done for the true negatives, using the specificity values for observers A and B. Again, the number of true negatives so classified by both observers is obtained by applying the joint probability of both observers detecting a true negative (0.90 for A times 0.96 for B) to the total number of true negatives in each population: for example, in population I (0.90 × 0.96) × 950 = 821. (Some rounding is used.)

The total results shown in Table 8-18 are obtained by summing the data from Tables 8-16 and 8-17. Kappa calculations for populations I and II, using the data shown in Table 8-18, yield the following values:

Population I

$$\kappa = \frac{0.862 - 0.804}{1.0 - 0.804} = 0.296$$

Population II

$$\kappa = \frac{0.830 - 0.577}{1.0 - 0.577} = 0.598$$

Thus, for the same sensitivity and specificity of the observers, the kappa value is greater (about twice in this example) in the population in which the prevalence of positivity is higher (population II) than in that in which it is lower (population I). A formula that expresses the value of kappa as a function of prevalence and the sensitivity/specificity of both observers has been developed,[41] demonstrating that, for fixed sensitivity and specificity levels, kappa tends toward 0 as the prevalence approaches either 0 or 1.

An additional problem is that, paradoxically, high values of kappa can be obtained when the marginals of the contingency table are unbalanced;[50,51] thus, kappa tends to be higher when the observed positivity prevalence is different between observers A and B than when both observers report similar prevalence. Kappa therefore unduly rewards a differential assessment of positivity between observers.

TABLE 8-17 Results of measurements conducted by observers A and B* in true negatives in populations with different prevalence rates of the condition measured, each with a population size of 1000.

	Population I (prevalence = 5%)			Population II (prevalence = 30%)		
	Observer A			Observer A		
Observer B	Pos	Neg	Total	Pos	Neg	Total
Pos	4	34	38	3	25	28
Neg	91	**821‡**	**912§**	67	**605‡**	**672§**
Total	95	**855****	950†	70	**630****	700†

*Observer A has an 80% sensitivity and 90% specificity; observer B has a 90% sensitivity and a 96% specificity.
†Number of true negatives, obtained by subtracting the number of true positives (Table 8-16) from the total population size: for example, for population I, 1000 − 50.
‡Obtained by applying the joint specificity of observers A and B to the total number of true negatives: for example, for population I, (0.90 × 0.96) × 950. (Results are rounded.)
§Obtained by applying the specificity level of observer B to the total number of true negatives in populations I and II: for example, for population I, 0.96 × 950.
**Obtained by applying the specificity level of observer A to the total number of true negatives in populations I and II: for example, for population I, 0.90 × 950.

TABLE 8-18 Results of measurements by observers A and B for total populations I and II obtained by combining results from Tables 8-16 and 8-17.

	Population I (prevalence = 5%)			Population II (prevalence = 30%)		
	Observer A			Observer A		
Observer B	Pos	Neg	Total	Pos	Neg	Total
Pos	40	43	83	219	79	298
Neg	95	822	917	91	611	702
Total	135	865	1000	310	690	1000

The previous discussion suggests that comparisons of kappa values among populations or across different manifestations of a condition (e.g., symptoms) may be unwarranted; it follows that using a specific kappa value obtained in a given target population to predict the value for another population is warranted only if prevalence rates of the condition(s) of interest are similar in both populations *and* if different raters (or repeat readings) provide reasonably similar prevalence estimates of positivity. For example, in the ARIC carotid ultrasound reliability study,[35] the authors assessed the reliability of plaque identification (with or without shadowing) not only in the left carotid bifurcation (see Table 8-10) but also in the common and the internal carotid sites. The weighted kappa results for the three arterial segments are shown in Table 8-19. Both readings resulted in reasonably similar prevalence percentages of plaque for each carotid artery site. For each reading, however, there are important differences in plaque prevalence across sites. Thus, in comparing these kappa values across arterial segments, the authors aptly noted that "the

TABLE 8-19 Weighted kappa and prevalence of plaque (with or without shadowing) in two readings of B-mode ultrasound exams in three carotid artery segments, Atherosclerosis Risk in Communities (ARIC) Study.

Carotid segment	First reading prevalence of plaque %	Second reading prevalence of plaque %	Weighted kappa
Common carotid	5.0	6.0	0.47
Carotid bifurcation*	21.2	19.5	0.60
Internal carotid	7.7	7.3	0.69

*See data in Table 8-10. Note that this weighted kappa value is slightly greater than the unweighted value of 0.576 (see text).
Source: Data from R Li et al., Reproducibility of Extracranial Carotid Atherosclerosis Lesions Assessed by B-Mode Ultrasound: The Atherosclerosis Risk in Communities Study. *Ultrasound in Medicine & Biology*, Vol 22, pp. 791–799, © 1996.

low weighted kappa coefficient . . . in the common carotid artery may be partially due to the low prevalence of lesions in this segment."[35(pp.796,797)] (On the other hand, although the prevalence is almost as low in the internal carotid as in the common carotid, the highest kappa is found in the former, probably as a function of the fact that the actual images in the internal carotid were of better quality than those in the other sites.)

Notwithstanding these limitations, kappa does provide a useful estimate of the degree of agreement between two observers or tests over and above the agreement that is expected to occur purely by chance, which explains its popularity. Furthermore, under certain conditions and partly because of its dependence on prevalence, kappa may be useful as an index to predict the degree to which non-differential misclassification attenuates the odds ratio:[41] that is, it can be used to assess the validity of the value of the measure of association based on data obtained with a given instrument or test.

In summary, although clearly a useful measure of reliability for categorical variables, kappa should be used and interpreted with caution. Most experts agree in recommending its use in conjunction with other measures of agreement, such as the percent agreement indices described previously here. When using it, however, it is important to take into consideration its variability as a function of the prevalence of the condition and of the degree of similarity between observers with regard to the prevalence of positivity.[35,37,45,51]

8.4.2 Indices of Validity/Reliability for Continuous Data

This section describes some of the available methods to evaluate the validity and/or the reliability of a given continuous measurement. The indices most frequently used for these purposes are listed in Table 8-3 and are briefly described later. As indicated in Table 8-3, some of these indices can be used for the assessment of validity (e.g., when measurements in serum samples done in a certain laboratory are compared with measurements in the same samples obtained at a reference laboratory; see Section 8.3.2), whereas others are more often used in reliability studies (e.g., for assessment of within-observer, between-observer, or within-individual repeated measurements of a continuous parameter; see Section 8.3.3).

The data shown in Table 8-20 are used to illustrate the reliability measures discussed in this section. Shown in this table are partial data obtained during a reliability study of polysomnography (PSG) scoring in the Sleep Heart Health Study (SHHS) project,

TABLE 8-20 Data from a reliability study of sleep-breathing disorders variables obtained from home polysomnography recordings.

Study no.	Apnea-hypopnea index*			Arousal index†		
	Scorer A		Scorer B	Scorer A		Scorer B
	First reading	Second reading		First reading	Repeat reading	
1	1.25	0.99	1.38	7.08	7.65	8.56
2	1.61	1.57	2.05	18.60	23.72	19.91
3	5.64	5.60	5.50	20.39	39.18	25.17
4	0.00	0.32	0.00	16.39	26.77	22.68
5	12.51	11.84	11.03	27.95	22.64	17.21
6	22.13	21.64	21.34	29.57	34.20	27.15
7	2.68	1.77	2.39	13.50	14.31	18.66
8	2.19	2.18	2.04	24.50	21.35	20.58
9	8.52	8.67	8.64	14.63	13.42	15.61
10	0.33	0.16	0.16	11.15	13.12	13.10
11	0.00		0.00	19.52		19.05
12	2.70		2.46	18.91		18.59
13	3.03		2.11	17.98		10.78
14	3.49		3.30	15.78		12.64
15	1.12		0.98	0.00		7.04
16	4.94		4.09	8.15		10.75
17	9.52		8.47	20.36		20.61
18	27.90		25.47	36.62		34.90
19	5.58		5.21	18.31		20.84
20	6.59		6.94	17.56		24.28
21	1.08		1.32	8.14		22.94
22	5.46		5.16	17.30		19.38
23	0.00		0.00	16.39		22.68
24	2.32		1.64	29.29		65.09
25	1.93		1.38	18.80		18.75
26	17.68		18.74	10.92		20.97
27	2.54		1.70	12.53		13.38
28	6.50		6.34	24.94		43.92
29	2.09		2.35	18.66		18.02
30	11.09		9.25	12.50		23.25

⌊ Within scorer ⌋   ⌊ Within scorer ⌋
⌊_____ Between scorer _____⌋   ⌊_____ Between scorer _____⌋

Note: Partial data obtained as part of a formal reliability study in the Sleep Heart Health Study (SF Quan, et al., The Sleep Heart Health Study: Design, Rationale and Methods. *Sleep*, Vol 20, pp. 1077–1085, 1997; CW Whitney, et al., Reliability of Scoring Disturbance Indices and Sleep Staging. *Sleep*, Vol 21, pp. 749–757, 1998). These data, kindly provided by the SHHS investigators, are presented for didactic purposes. Derived validity/reliability indices are not to be interpreted as an accurate and complete representation of the reliability of the scoring procedures in the SHHS, for which readers are referred to the original report (see Whitney, et al., above).
*Apnea-hypopnea index: average number of apnea and hypopnea episodes per hour of sleep (apnea, cessation of airflow for ≥ 10 seconds; hypopnea, decrease in airflow or thoracoabdominal excursion of $\geq 30\%$ for ≥ 10 seconds, accompanied by a $\geq 4\%$ decrease in oxygen saturation).
†Arousal index: average number of sleep arousals per hour of sleep.

a population-based study of the cardiovascular consequences of sleep-disordered breathing (e.g., sleep apnea).[52] In the SHHS, the PSG recordings obtained from 6440 participants in six field centers were sent to a central reading center for scoring (sleep staging and calculation of indices of sleep-disordered breathing). The design and results of the reliability study conducted in the SHHS have been described in detail[53] and have included both the within- and between-scorer reliability of sleep-disordered breathing variables and sleep staging. For the purposes of this example, Table 8-20 shows only data on two measures of sleep-disordered breathing (apnea-hypopnea index [AHI] and arousal index [AI]) for 30 PSG studies that were read by two of the scorers (scorers A and B) to assess between-scorer reliability, as well as 10 studies that were read twice by one of the scorers (scorer A) as part of the within-scorer reliability study.

The validity/reliability measures described in the following paragraphs are one of two types. The first type consists of indices based on assessing the *linear correlation* between the two sets of values being compared (correlation plot, correlation coefficients). The second type consists of measures based on the *pair-wise comparison* of the numerical values of the two measures being compared (mean difference, coefficient of variation, and Bland-Altman plot).

Correlation Graph (Scatter Diagram)

The simplest way to compare two sets of readings is merely to plot the values for each method and carefully examine the patterns observed in the scatter plot. For example, Figures 8-9A and 8-9B show the correlation between the AHI and AI values obtained by scorers A and B. Figures 8-9C and 8-9D correspond to the within-scorer reliability: that is, these charts show the AHI and AI values resulting from the 10 repeat readings done by scorer A. They show that AHI readings (Figures 8-9A and 8-9C) are strongly correlated (as expressed by their being almost perfectly superimposed to the 45° lines, which corresponds to a perfect agreement). For AI, although there appears to be a correlation, a significant scatter is seen around the ideal 45° lines. (The diagonals or identity lines in Figure 8-9 [going through the origin with a 45° slope] are equivalent to regression lines [see Chapter 7, Section 7.4.1] with intercept = 0 and regression coefficient = 1.0 unit.)

Although simple correlation graphs are useful to get a sense of the degree of agreement between two measures, they are not as sensitive as alternative graphic techniques (see Bland-Altman plot later in this chapter) for the detection of certain patterns in the data.

Linear Correlation Coefficient, Rank Correlation, Linear Regression

Pearson's product-moment correlation coefficient (usually denoted by r) is a measure of the degree to which a set of paired observations in a scatter diagram approaches the situation in which every point falls exactly on a straight line.[43,54] The possible range of values of r is from -1 (when there is a perfect negative correlation between the two observers) to $+1$ (when there is a perfect positive correlation). The closer the r values are to 0, the weaker the correlation (either negative or positive) between the two sets of values. For example, the r values for the scatter diagrams in Figure 8-9 are:

AHI:	Between scorer (A), $n = 30$:	$r = 0.995$
	Within scorer (C), $n = 10$:	$r = 0.999$
AI:	Between scorer (B), $n = 30$:	$r = 0.655$
	Within scorer (D), $n = 10$:	$r = 0.710$

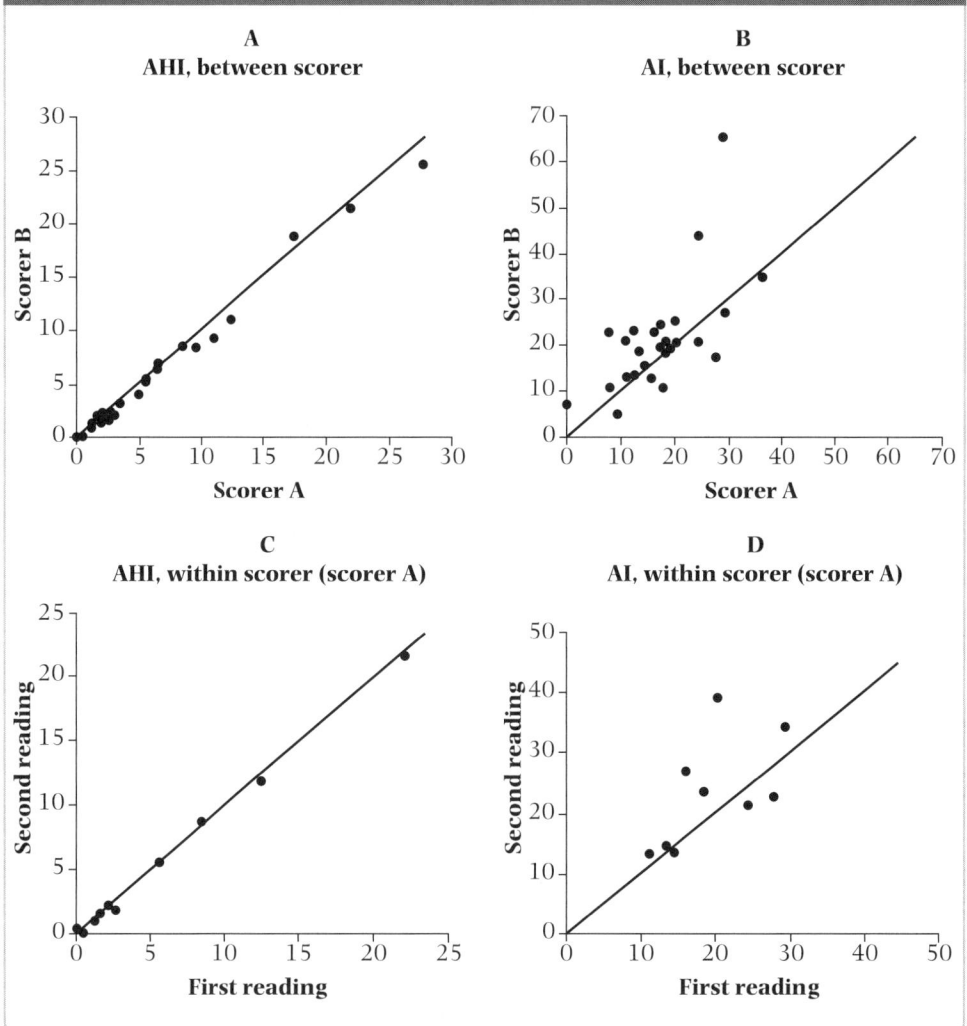

FIGURE 8-9 Scatter diagrams for between- and within-scorer reliability for data shown in Table 8-20. A: between-scorer AHI values (scorers A and B); B: between-scorer AI values (scorers A and B); C: within-scorer AHI values for repeat readings by scorer A; D: within-scorer AI values for repeat readings by scorer A. The straight diagonal lines in these plots represent the identity lines, that is, where the points would be if agreement was perfect. AHI and AI are expressed as the average number of episodes per hour of sleep.

Calculation of the Pearson correlation coefficient is fairly straightforward and can be done using most available statistical packages and even most pocket calculators carrying scientific functions.

Although Pearson's r is probably one of the most frequently used measures of agreement for continuous variables in the biomedical literature (in both validity and reliability studies), it is also one of the least appropriate.[55–58] Its main limitations can be summarized as follows.

First, Pearson's r is an index of linear association, but it is not necessarily a good measure of agreement. It is insensitive to systematic differences (bias) between two

FIGURE 8-10 Correlation coefficients are equally high when both observers read the same value (A) and when there is a systematic difference between observers but readings vary simultaneously (B and C).

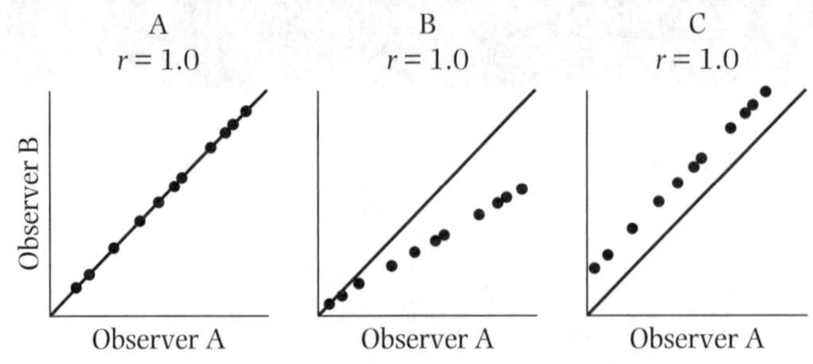

observers or readings, as illustrated in Figure 8-10. The values of the correlation coefficients ($r = 1.0$) in this figure indicate perfect linear correlation between the two observers in all three panels. However, perfect agreement of values occurs only in Figure 8-10A, in which all the observations fall in the identity line (i.e., for each pair of observations, observer B value = observer A value). In Figure 8-10B, the points fall in a perfect straight line, but the slope of the line is different from 1.0: that is, compared with observer A, observer B tends to read the higher values at lower levels. The situation illustrated in Figure 8-10C also shows lack of agreement due to systematic readings by observer B at higher levels across the entire range of values (which results in a regression line with an intercept different from zero).

The latter situation (Figure 8-10C) is particularly likely in the presence of systematic differences among readers, drifts over time in the readers' ability to apply the study criteria, wearing out of reagents used in certain laboratory techniques, and so forth. In these situations, the exclusive use of Pearson's r may produce a misleading assessment of agreement. A real-life example relates to the LRC data (see Tables 8-6 and 8-7), in which the Pearson correlation coefficient between "self-reported" and "measured" BMI was found to be 0.96. Other studies have shown similarly strong correlations between these approaches of measuring BMI and body weight, leading some authors to conclude that self-reported weights are remarkably accurate and may obviate the need for costly and time consuming anthropometric measurements in epidemiological investigations.[59,60] This conclusion may be misleading, however, because even though the correlation is high, there is a systematic tendency of individuals to underestimate their weights (usually paralleled by an overestimation of their heights). As a result, in Table 8-6, there is a larger number of individuals above (and to the right) of the perfect agreement diagonal than below it. It follows that if the BMI based on self-reports is used to define categorical adiposity variables, this systematic error will result in less than perfect agreement (and thus misclassification). For the data shown in Table 8-6, kappa was 0.75—notwithstanding, as mentioned previously, the almost perfect correlation between self-reports and measured weight and height (Pearson $r = 0.96$).

Second, the value of r is very sensitive to the range of values. The influence of the range of values on the Pearson's r is illustrated in Figures 8-11A and 8-11B. In this hypothetical example, both readers are assumed to be similarly reliable. Nonetheless, because sample values have a broader distribution in Figure 8-11B than in Figure 8-11A,

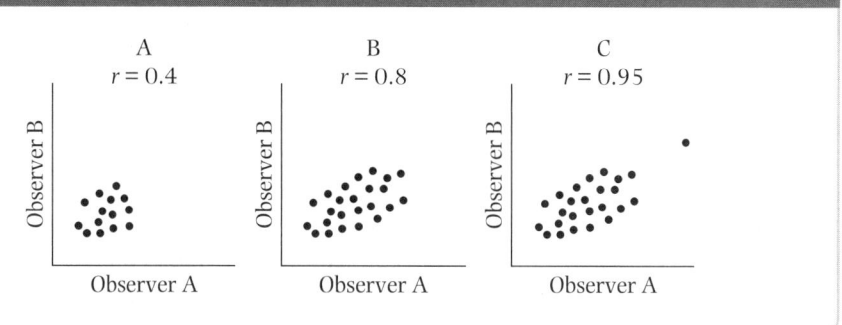

Figure 8-11 Pearson's correlation coefficient is very sensitive to the range of values and to the presence of outliers (extreme values). Hypothetical examples.

the correlation coefficients will be higher for the former. This can also be illustrated using real data from Figure 8-9B. As mentioned previously, Pearson's r for the total set of 30 repeat readings of AI by scorers A and B was 0.655. If, however, this set is split into two subsets, one including the studies in which scorer B read values of AI < 15 per hour ($n = 8$) and another in which scorer B read values of AI ≥ 15 per hour ($n = 22$), the correlation coefficients are estimated at 0.59 and 0.51, respectively: that is, *both r's are smaller* than the r based on the entire set of 30 observations, which does not make a lot of intuitive sense.

As a corollary of its dependence on the range of values, Pearson's correlation coefficient is unduly sensitive to extreme values (outliers). Thus, for example, Figure 8-11C is a repetition of Figure 8-11B, but with one additional observation with an extreme value; this outlier has an enormous influence in defining the regression line and the value of the correlation coefficient, which increases from 0.8 in Figure 8-11B to 0.95 in Figure 8-11C.

Despite its undesirable properties, Pearson's correlation coefficient is often used as the main, if not the sole, measure of reliability reported in biomedical or epidemiologic studies. This may have to do with tradition, pattern recognition, and imitation ("everybody uses it").[56] Some argue that r is an appropriate measure for reliability studies when the objective is to see whether two different sets of readings would classify (order) subjects in the same manner; thus, if Pearson's r is high, it would be justified to use the distribution of study values to classify subjects. If that is the case, however, the *Spearman correlation coefficient* (also called "ordinal" or "rank correlation coefficient" and denoted by r_s) is more appropriate. This coefficient takes the value of $+1$ when the paired ranks are exactly in the same order, a value of -1 when the ranks are exactly in an inverse order, and a value of 0 when there is no correlation between the ordering of the two sets of paired values. For example, the r_s values for the scatter diagrams in Figure 8-9 are 0.984 (AHI, between), 0.58 (AI, between), 0.976 (AHI, within), and 0.757 (AI, within). Although more congruous with the goal of assessing consistency of the ranking and less influenced by outlying values, the Spearman correlation coefficient does not address the other limitation of Pearson's r previously discussed, namely its insensitivity to lack of agreement due to systematic differences in values between the readers.

Finally, because of its relatively frequent occurrence in the biomedical literature, it is worth discussing the use of statistical significance testing to evaluate a correlation coefficient (Pearson's or Spearman's) in the context of validity/reliability studies. The calculation of a *p* value for a correlation coefficient (i.e., evaluating the null hypothesis H_0: *r* = 0.0) is not useful in this context for both theoretical and practical reasons: (1) the null hypothesis—that there is *no relationship* between two tests (or two observers) supposedly measuring the *same* variable or construct is illogical and demonstrating that it can be rejected is not very informative; (2) even when the reliability is fairly poor (e.g., $r \leq 0.3$ or 0.4), the corresponding *p* value may well be "significant" if the sample size is reasonably large. Thus, a highly significant *p* value may be mistakenly interpreted as evidence of "high reliability" when in fact its only interpretation is that it is relatively safe to reject a (meaningless, anyway) null hypothesis. Testing the hypothesis of quasi-perfect correlation (e.g., H_0: *r* = 0.95) has been proposed as an alternative and more useful approach.[57] Another logical alternative is to calculate confidence limits for the value of the correlation coefficient rather than its associated *p* value.

The preceding discussion suggests that the correlation coefficient should be used judiciously. More specifically, its interpretation is greatly enhanced by a consideration of possible systematic differences between measurements. The use of a scatter diagram of the data is helpful in detecting these systematic differences, the presence of outlying values, and differences between variables with regard to the range of their values. Other indices of reliability that avoid some of the pitfalls inherent to Pearson's *r* are discussed next.

An alternative to Pearson's *r* is *linear regression*, which provides a measure of the regression function's intercept and slope (see Chapter 7, Section 7.4.1), thus allowing the assessment of situations such as those illustrated in Figure 8-10B and Figure 8-10C, in which the intercept is not zero or in which there is a systematic difference between readers. Linear regression, however, is not problem free when used to analyze reliability data: for example (and importantly), it neglects the fact that measurement errors may occur for both dependent and independent variables.[55] (In ordinal linear regression, the so-called independent variable, *x*, is assumed to be error free, and only errors [statistical variability] in the "dependent" variable are considered; see Chapter 7, Section 7.4.1.) Linear regression is more useful for "calibration" purposes than to assess reliability: that is, it is more useful to predict outcomes or to obtain "corrected" values once a systematic difference is identified and quantified.

Intraclass Correlation Coefficient

The intraclass correlation coefficient (ICC) or reliability coefficient (R) is an estimate of the fraction of the total measurement variability caused by variation among individuals.[40,58] Ideally, an epidemiologic study should use highly standardized procedures and data collection methods known to be valid and reliable. Under these optimal circumstances, most of the variability can be attributed to differences among study participants (between-individual variability) (see Section 8.3.3).

The general formula for the ICC is thus

$$\text{ICC} = \frac{V_b}{V_T} = \frac{V_b}{V_b + V_e}$$

in which V_b = variance between individuals, V_T = total variance, which includes both V_b and V_e, and V_e = unwanted variance ("error"). V_e will include different components depending on the design of the study (see Figure 8-4). For example, in a within-laboratory reliability study, it will include the variance due to laboratory/method error. In a within-individual reliability study (i.e., repeat readings or determinations by the same reader or technique obtained in the same individual), it will be the estimated variance within individuals. It can also be combinations of these, as, for example, in a study assessing both the laboratory and within-individual variability of hemostasis and inflammation plasma parameters.[61]

The ICC is akin to the kappa statistic for continuous variables and has the same range of possible values (from -1.0 or more realistically from 0 to $+1.0$, in case of perfect agreement). It has the advantage over the Pearson's or Spearman's correlation coefficient in that it is a true measure of agreement, combining information on both the correlation and the systematic differences between readings.[58] As in the case of Pearson's correlation coefficient, however, ICC is affected by the range of values in the study population. In the previous formula, when V_b is small, ICC also will be small. This is particularly important in studies within populations in which the exposure values are either very high or very low. For example, a high intake of animal fat in some populations may result in uniformly high serum cholesterol levels. A low reliability coefficient resulting from a small variability of the exposure levels may negatively influence the power of an epidemiologic study and thus make it difficult to assess an association. Obviously, the ICC will also be low when there is substantial intra-individual variability of the factor of interest, as in the case of gonadal hormone levels in premenopausal women.

ICC can be calculated from an analysis of variance (ANOVA) table, although a more simple formula based on the standard deviations of the two sets of observations, and the sum and the standard deviation of the paired differences, has been provided[58] (see Appendix E). Based on this formula, for example, the ICC for the between-reader reliability study data shown in Table 8-20 can be estimated as 0.99 for AHI and 0.58 for AI. Like kappa, the ICC can also be extended to calculate the reliability between more than two observers or readings. For example, in the actual (full) reliability study of sleep scoring in the SHHS,[53] the reported ICC between the three scorers was 0.99 for AHI and 0.54 for AI.

As an additional example, Table 8-21 shows the ICC for three lipid measurements in a sample of the ARIC study cohort baseline examination.[27] The high ICC obtained for total cholesterol and total high-density lipoprotein (HDL) cholesterol in this study suggests that the proportion of the variance due to within-individual variability or laboratory error for these analytes is small; on the other hand, the ICC for an HDL cholesterol fraction (HDL_2) was found to be much lower.

An additional reliability measure, which is closely related to the intraclass correlation coefficient, the Cronbach alpha, is widely used by researchers in the social sciences.[62,63]

TABLE 8-21 Intraclass correlation coefficients (ICCs) and coefficients of variation (CVs) for selected analytes in the Atherosclerosis Risk in Communities (ARIC) Study.*

Analyte	ICC	CV (%)
Total cholesterol	0.94	5.1
HDL cholesterol	0.94	6.8
HDL_2	0.77	24.8

*Includes both within-individual and laboratory variability.
Source: Data from LE Chambless et al., Short-Term Intraindividual Variability in Lipoprotein Measurements: The Atherosclerosis Risk in Communities (ARIC) Study. *American Journal of Epidemiology*, Vol 136, pp. 1069–1081, © 1992

Mean Difference and Paired t-Test

The average of the differences between the two values of the pairs of observations is a measure of the degree of *systematic* differences between the two sets of readings. A paired *t*-test statistic can be calculated simply by dividing the mean value of all paired differences denoted by $\bar{x}$ by its standard error (i.e., the standard deviation [s] over the square root of the sample size):

$$t\text{-test} = \frac{\bar{x}_{(1-2)}}{s_{(1-2)}/\sqrt{n}}$$

This index is typically used when assessing *validity*, as it provides a direct estimate of the degree of *bias* for one of the sets of measurements when it is justified to use the other set as a gold standard. On the other hand, it can also be used in the context of paired *reliability* studies, as when assessing systematic differences between readers of a test. For example, for the between-reader reliability study in Table 8-20, scorers A's and B's mean differences were 0.367 (standard deviation [SD] = 0.703) for AHI and −3.327 (SD = 8.661) for AI. Although their magnitude is rather small, particularly for AHI, both differences were found to be statistically significant at conventional levels ($p < 0.05$), thus suggesting the existence of a systematic between-scorer variability. In Whitney et al.'s report,[53] this index was used to assess within-scorer reliability.

Caution should be exercised when using the mean difference as a measure of validity or reliability without a careful examination of the data (e.g., looking at a scatter diagram or a Bland-Altman plot; see later in this Chapter), as its value can be heavily dependent on extreme values.

Coefficient of Variability

Another index of reliability often used in epidemiologic studies is the coefficient of variability (CV), which is the standard deviation expressed as a percentage of the mean value of two sets of paired observations. In an analysis of reliability data, it is calculated for each pair of observations and then averaged over all pairs of original and replicate measures. Its estimation is very straightforward. The variance of each pair of measurements is

$$V_i = \sum_{j=1}^{2}(x_{ij} - \bar{x}_i)^2$$

in which i is a given pair of repeat measurements (indexed by j) on the same sample or individual, x_{i1} and x_{i2} are the values of these two measurements, and $\bar{x}_i$ is their mean.

The standard deviation (SD) for each pair of observations is the square root of V_i; thus, for each pair of measurements, the coefficient of variability (expressed as a percentage) is

$$CV_i = \frac{SD_i}{\bar{x}_i} \times 100$$

For example, for the last pair (pair 30) of between-scorer readings of AHI in Table 8-20 (11.09 and 9.25, mean 10.17), these calculations are as follows:

$$V_{30} = (11.09 - 10.17)^2 + (9.25 - 10.17)^2 = 1.693$$

with the resulting coefficient of variability for that pair

$$CV_{30} = \frac{\sqrt{1.693}}{10.17} \times 100 = 12.8\%$$

This calculation would have to be repeated for all pairs of measurements, and the overall coefficient of variability would be the average of all pair-wise coefficients of variability. The lower the coefficient of variability, the less variation there is between the replicate measurements. Obviously, if there were no differences whatsoever between paired values (perfect agreement), the value of the coefficient of variability would be zero. The overall between-scorer coefficients of variability for all 30 paired observations shown in Table 8-20 are 10.1% for AHI and 22.8% for AI. In addition to the intraclass correlation coefficients discussed previously, Table 8-21 shows the coefficients of variability for serum total cholesterol, HDL cholesterol, and HDL_2 in the ARIC cohort reliability study.[27] Consistently with the intraclass correlation coefficients, the coefficients of variability are fairly low for total cholesterol and total HDL cholesterol but high for the HDL cholesterol fraction, HDL_2, indicating substantial imprecision in the measurement of the latter fraction.

Bland-Altman Plot

This is a very useful graphical technique that is a good complement to the ordinary scatter diagram (discussed previously) for the examination of patterns of disagreement between repeated measurements (or between a given measurement and the "gold standard"). It consists of a scatter plot where the difference between the paired measurements (A − B in the ordinate) is plotted against their mean value [(A + B)/2, in the abscissa]. From this plot, it is much easier than in a regular scatter diagram to assess the magnitude of disagreement (including systematic differences), spot outliers, and to see whether there is any trend.[55,56] For example, Figures 8-12A and 8-12B show the Bland-Altman plots for the between-scorer measurements of AHI and AI data from Table 8-20. Compared with the corresponding scatter diagrams (Figures 8-9A and 8-9B), these pictures reveal more clearly some interesting features of the data, as follows:

- There is a slight systematic difference between the two measurements, as represented by the departure from zero of the horizontal line corresponding to the mean difference.

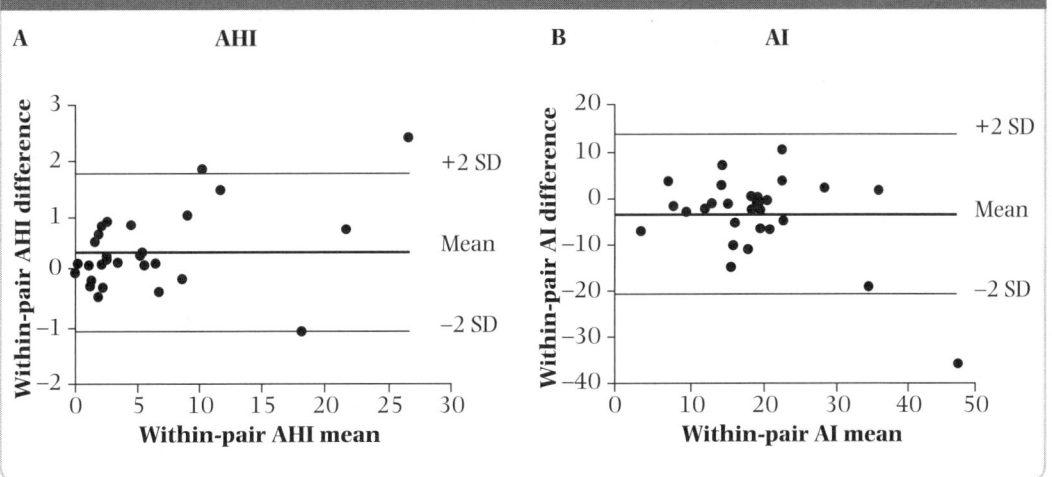

FIGURE 8-12 Bland-Altman plots for AHI and AI for the between-scorer reliability study data from Table 8-20. The horizontal lines represent the mean within-pair difference (0.367 and −3.327, for AHI and AI, respectively) and the mean ±2 standard deviations (1 SD = 0.703 for AHI and 8.661 for AI). AHI and AI are expressed as the average number of episodes per hour of sleep. (Note that the scales in the ordinates of AHI and AI are different.)

- Outliers may be present: in Figure 8-12, there is one measurement with mean AHI greater than 25 and one with mean AI greater than 40 that are clearly outside the range of mean difference ± 2 SD.
- The graphs provide a clearer idea of the magnitude of disagreement in comparison with the actual measurement. In Figure 8-12A, for example, all but one (or perhaps two or three) AHI mean differences are within the (mean ± 2 SD) range, which spans approximately three AHI units; the latter is a relatively low value in the range of AHI values in the abscissa. In contrast, the (mean difference ± SD) range for AI (Figure 8-12B), whereas containing also all but one observation, spans almost 35 AI units, which is practically the entire range of AI values observed in these individuals.
- The AHI plot in Figure 8-12A suggests that disagreement between the scorers increases as the actual value of AHI increases. This pattern is not as evident for AI, however (Figure 8-12B).

If this graphic approach is used when one of the measurements can be considered a gold standard, one may want to represent the latter in the abscissa instead of the mean of both measurements. In this case, the vertical departure from zero will represent the magnitude of bias of the test value with respect to the gold standard.

An alternative to the Bland-Altman approach that allows the evaluation of agreement between more than two sets of observations and is based on an extension of the Kaplan-Meier method has been suggested by Luiz et al. and is described in detail elsewhere.[64]

8.5 REGRESSION TO THE MEAN

The phenomenon known as *regression to the mean* permeates many of the problems and analytical approaches described in the previous sections and deserves a brief discussion here. This is a well-known phenomenon, aptly discussed by Oldham in 1962,[65] which expresses the tendency for high values of continuous variables (e.g., blood pressure) measured at any given point in time to decrease and, for low values to increase, when repeated measurements are done. This tendency may result from either intra-individual variability (as illustrated in Figure 8-3) or random measurement errors. As an example, when measurements of blood pressure levels in a group of individuals are repeated, many values converge (*regress*) toward the mean. A corollary of this is that caution is needed when analyzing data on repeated measurements over time and when analyzing correlation of these data with baseline values.[66] In addition, regression to the mean underscores the desirability of using the average of repeated measurements rather than single measurements for physiologic parameters that fluctuate (as is the case of blood pressure, among many other examples). This is particularly important in studies in which a cutoff point is used as a study inclusion criterion, such as the cutoff to define hypertension in clinical trials of hypertension management. Many individuals eligible on the basis of one measurement would not be eligible if the mean of repeated measurements of blood pressure were used instead. When regression to the mean occurs, the initial follow-up phase of a clinical trial aimed at examining the effectiveness of an antihypertensive medication may show a decrease in blood pressure levels in both the active intervention and the placebo groups (Figure 8-13). An example is given by the Hypertension Detection and Follow-up Program, in which a decline in systolic blood pressure was seen in both the intervention and the control groups and in all four sex-ethnic groups (white men and women and African American men and women).[67]

8.6 FINAL CONSIDERATIONS

It should be emphasized that validity and reliability are two entirely different issues. For example, poor validity may be consistent with an excellent reliability, i.e., every time the procedure is repeated, the same or very similar, albeit always inaccurate results are found.

In addition, assessment of the same summary measures, such as the kappa statistic, may not be sufficient to implement a specific corrective action. Consider, for example, a situation in which agreement between experienced readers in the interpretation of mammographic images results in a high kappa value (e.g., $\kappa = 0.9$), denoting that the agreement is "almost perfect" according to Landis and Koch's classification (Figure 8-7).[42] However, the reviewers disagree with regard to ten observations. For quality control, it may be useful to ask why two experienced readers, using the same protocols, arrived at different results from ten study participants. Can the results be explained by these participants' characteristics, e.g., obesity interfering with the quality of the mammographic images? Were the discrepant results due to one or both of the readers' state of mind when they were interpreting the results? And so on. This example underscores the contrast between reporting a summary measure (kappa) and the practical aspects of conducting research, and suggests that, in addition to examining the actual reasons for the discrepant findings, strategies that allow a more complete examination of data, such as Bland-Altman plot, should be favored over more concise summary measures, such as Kappa.

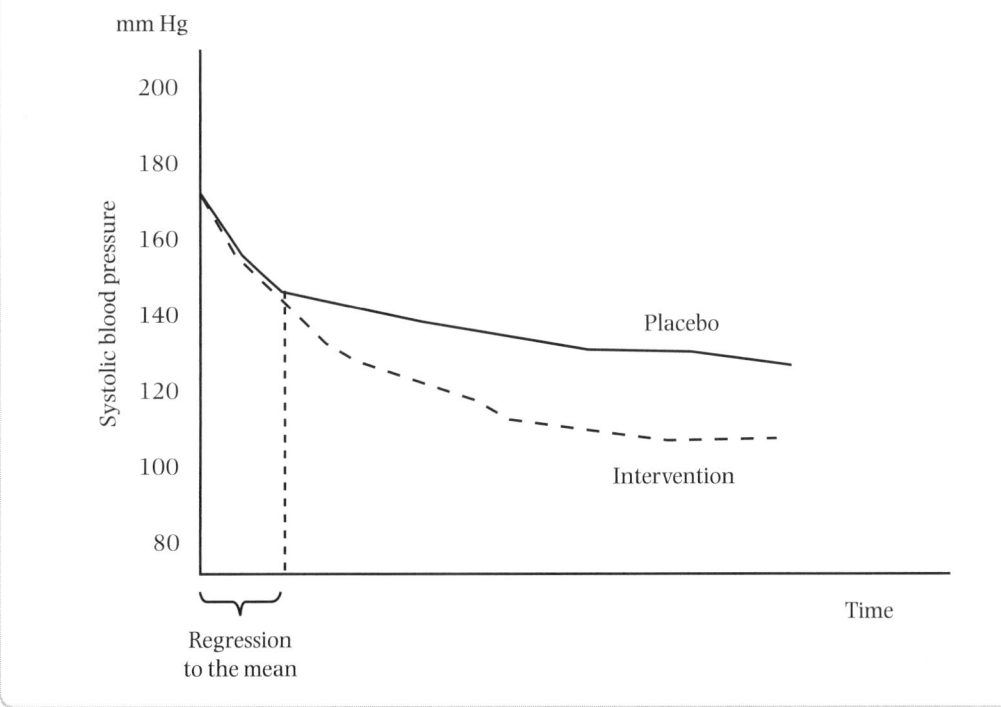

FIGURE 8-13 Schematic representation of regression to the mean in a randomized clinical trial. In a clinical trial of an anti-hypertensive drug, individuals are selected on the basis of a blood pressure value above a certain cut-off point defining hypertension (e.g., systolic blood pressure ≥160 mm Hg, denoting severe hypertension). Some individuals are, thus, chosen when their blood pressure levels are above their average values. As a result, in the initial phases of follow-up, blood pressure will decline in both intervention and placebo groups regardless of the effectiveness of the drug.

REFERENCES

1. Kahn HA, Sempos CT. *Statistical Methods in Epidemiology*. New York, NY: Oxford University Press; 1989.
2. Whitney CW, Lind BK, Wahl PW. Quality assurance and quality control in longitudinal studies. *Epidemiol Rev*. 1998;20:71–80.
3. The Atherosclerosis Risk in Communities (ARIC) Study: Design and objectives: The ARIC investigators. *Am J Epidemiol*. 1989;129:687–702.
4. Prineas R, Crow RS, Blackburn H. *The Minnesota Code Manual of Electrocardiographic Findings*. Littleton, MA: John Wright PSG; 1982.
5. White AD, Folsom AR, Chambless LE, et al. Community surveillance of coronary heart disease in the Atherosclerosis Risk in Communities (ARIC) Study: Methods and initial two years' experience. *J Clin Epidemiol*. 1996;49:223–233.
6. Sudman S, Bradburn NM. *Asking Questions*. San Francisco, CA: Jossey-Bass Publishers; 1982.
7. Converse J, Presser S. *Survey Questions: Handcrafting the Standardized Questionnaire*. Newbury Park, CA: Sage Publications; 1986.
8. Rose GA. Chest pain questionnaire. *Milbank Mem Fund Q*. 1965;43:32–39.
9. Comstock GW, Tockman MS, Helsing KJ, Hennesy KM. Standardized respiratory questionnaires: Comparison of the old with the new. *Am Rev Respir Dis*. 1979;119:45–53.
10. Burt VL, Cutler JA, Higgins M, et al. Trends in the prevalence, awareness, treatment, and control of hypertension in the adult US population: Data from the health examination surveys, 1960 to 1991. *Hypertension*. 1995;26:60–69.
11. Block G, Hartman AM, Dresser CM, et al. A data-based approach to diet questionnaire design and testing. *Am J Epidemiol*. 1986;124:453–469.
12. Willett WC, Sampson L, Stampfer MJ, et al. Reproducibility and validity of a semiquantitative food frequency questionnaire. *Am J Epidemiol*. 1985;122:51–65.
13. Dickersin K, Berlin JA. Meta-analysis: State-of-the-science. *Epidemiol Rev*. 1992;14:154–176.
14. Bild D, Bluemke DA, Burke GL, et al. Multi-ethnic Study of Atherosclerosis: objectives and design. *Am J Epidemiol*. 2002;156:871–881.
15. Ramirez-Anaya M, Macias ME, Velazquez-Gonzalez E. Validation of a Mexican Spanish version of the Children's Dermatology Life Quality Index. *Pediatr Dermatol*. 2010;27:143–147.
16. Laliberté S, Lamoureux J, Sullivan MJ, et al. French translation of the Multidimensional Pain Inventory: L'inventaire multidimensionnel de la douler. *Pain Res Manag*. 2008;13:497–505.
17. Gordis L. *Epidemiology*, 4th ed. Philadelphia, PA: Elsevier Saunders; 2008.
18. Lippel K, Ahmed S, Albers JJ, et al. External quality-control survey of cholesterol analyses performed by 12 lipid research clinics. *Clin Chem*. 1978;24:1477–1484.
19. Burke GL, Sprafka JM, Folsom AR, et al. Trends in serum cholesterol levels from 1980 to 1987: The Minnesota Heart Survey. *N Engl J Med*. 1991;324:941–946.
20. Brinton LA, Hoover RN, Szklo M, Fraumeni JF Jr. Menopausal estrogen use and risk of breast cancer. *Cancer*. 1981;47:2517–2522.
21. Vargas CM, Burt VL, Gillum RF, Pamuk ER. Validity of self-reported hypertension in the National Health and Nutrition Examination Survey III, 1988–1991. *Prev Med*. 1997;26(5 Pt 1):678–685.
22. Nieto-García FJ, Bush TL, Keyl PM. Body mass definitions of obesity: Sensitivity and specificity using self-reported weight and height. *Epidemiology*. 1990;1:146–152.

23. Copeland KT, Checkoway H, McMichael AJ, Holbrook RH. Bias due to misclassification in the estimation of relative risk. *Am J Epidemiol.* 1977;105:488–495.
24. Block G. A review of validations of dietary assessment methods. *Am J Epidemiol.* 1982;115:492–505.
25. Martin-Moreno JM, Boyle P, Gorgojo L, et al. Development and validation of a food frequency questionnaire in Spain. *Int J Epidemiol.* 1993;22:512–519.
26. Frost C, White IR. The effect of measurement error in risk factors that change over time in cohort studies: Do simple methods overcorrect for "regression dilution"? *Int J Epidemiol.* 2005;34:1359–1368.
27. Chambless LE, McMahon RP, Brown SA, et al. Short-term intraindividual variability in lipoprotein measurements: The Atherosclerosis Risk in Communities (ARIC) Study. *Am J Epidemiol.* 1992;136: 1069–1081.
28. Colditz GA, Willett WC, Stampfer MJ, et al. The influence of age, relative weight, smoking, and alcohol intake on the reproducibility of a dietary questionnaire. *Int J Epidemiol.* 1987;16:392–398.
29. Sackett DL. *Clinical Epidemiology: A Basic Science for Clinical Medicine.* Boston, MA: Little, Brown; 1991.
30. Fletcher R, Fletcher, SW, Wagner, EH. *Clinical Epidemiology: The Essentials*, 2nd ed. Baltimore, MD: Williams & Wilkins; 1988.
31. Ransohoff DF, Feinstein AR. Problems of spectrum and bias in evaluating the efficacy of diagnostic tests. *N Engl J Med.* 1978;299:926–930.
32. Brenner H, Gefeller O. Variation of sensitivity, specificity, likelihood ratios and predictive values with disease prevalence. *Stat Med.* 1997;16:981–991.
33. Fikree FF, Gray RH, Shah F. Can men be trusted? A comparison of pregnancy histories reported by husbands and wives. *Am J Epidemiol.* 1993;138:237–242.
34. Youden WJ. Index for rating diagnostic tests. *Cancer.* 1950;3:32–35.
35. Li R, Cai J, Tegeler C, et al. Reproducibility of extracranial carotid atherosclerotic lesions assessed by B-mode ultrasound: The Atherosclerosis Risk in Communities Study. *Ultrasound Med Biol.* 1996;22: 791–799.
36. van der Kooy K, Rookus MA, Peterse HL, van Leeuwen FE. p53 protein overexpression in relation to risk factors for breast cancer. *Am J Epidemiol.* 1996;144:924–933.
37. Cicchetti DV, Feinstein AR. High agreement but low kappa: II: Resolving the paradoxes. *J Clin Epidemiol.* 1990;43:551–558.
38. Chamberlain J, Rogers P, Price JL, et al. Validity of clinical examination and mammography as screening tests for breast cancer. *Lancet.* 1975;2:1026–1030.
39. Cohen J. A coefficient of agreement for nominal scales. *Educ Psychol Meas.* 1960;20:37–46.
40. Fleiss J. *Statistical Methods for Rates and Proportions*, 2nd ed. New York, NY: John Wiley and Sons; 1981.
41. Thompson WD, Walter SD. A reappraisal of the kappa coefficient. *J Clin Epidemiol.* 1988;41:949–958.
42. Landis JR, Koch GG. The measurement of observer agreement for categorical data. *Biometrics.* 1977; 33:159–174.
43. Altman DG. *Practical Statistics for Medical Research.* London, UK: Chapman and Hall; 1991.
44. Byrt T. How good is that agreement? *Epidemiology.* 1996;7:561.
45. Seigel DG, Podgor MJ, Remaley NA. Acceptable values of kappa for comparison of two groups. *Am J Epidemiol.* 1992;135:571–578.
46. Klebanoff MA, Levine RJ, Clemens JD, et al. Serum cotinine concentration and self-reported smoking during pregnancy. *Am J Epidemiol.* 1998;148:259–262.

47. Ferrer M, Lamarca R, Orfila F, Alonso J. Comparison of performance-based and self-rated functional capacity in Spanish elderly. *Am J Epidemiol.* 1999;149:228–235.
48. Stieb DM, Beveridge RC, Rowe BH, et al. Assessing diagnostic classification in an emergency department: Implications for daily time series studies of air pollution. *Am J Epidemiol.* 1998;148:666–670.
49. Maclure M, Willett WC. Misinterpretation and misuse of the kappa statistic. *Am J Epidemiol.* 1987;126:161–169.
50. Feinstein AR, Cicchetti DV. High agreement but low kappa: I: The problems of two paradoxes. *J Clin Epidemiol.* 1990;43:543–549.
51. Byrt T, Bishop J, Carlin JB. Bias, prevalence and kappa. *J Clin Epidemiol.* 1993;46:423–429.
52. Quan SF, Howard BV, Iber C, et al. The Sleep Heart Health Study: Design, rationale, and methods. *Sleep.* 1997;20:1077–1085.
53. Whitney CW, Gottlieb DJ, Redline S, et al. Reliability of scoring respiratory disturbance indices and sleep staging. *Sleep.* 1998;21:749–757.
54. Armitage P, Berry G. *Statistical methods in medical research*, 3rd ed. London, UK: Blackwell; 1994.
55. Altman DG, Bland JM. Measurement in medicine: The analysis of method comparison studies. *The Statistician.* 1983;32:307–317.
56. Bland JM, Altman DG. Statistical methods for assessing agreement between two methods of clinical measurement. *Lancet.* 1986;1:307–310.
57. Hebert JR, Miller DR. The inappropriateness of conventional use of the correlation coefficient in assessing validity and reliability of dietary assessment methods. *Eur J Epidemiol.* 1991;7:339–343.
58. Deyo RA, Diehr P, Patrick DL. Reproducibility and responsiveness of health status measures: Statistics and strategies for evaluation. *Control Clin Trials.* 1991;12(4 suppl):142S–158S.
59. Stunkard AJ, Albaum JM. The accuracy of self-reported weights. *Am J Clin Nutr.* 1981;34:1593–1599.
60. Palta M, Prineas RJ, Berman R, Hannan P. Comparison of self-reported and measured height and weight. *Am J Epidemiol.* 1982;115:223–230.
61. Sakkinen PA, Macy EM, Callas PW, et al. Analytical and biologic variability in measures of hemostasis, fibrinolysis, and inflammation: Assessment and implications for epidemiology. *Am J Epidemiol.* 1999;149:261–267.
62. Cronbach LJ. Coefficient alpha and the internal structure of tests. *Psychometrika.* 1951;16:297–334.
63. Cronbach LJ, Shavelson RJ. My current thoughts on coefficient alpha and successor procedures. *Educational and Psychological Measurement.* 2004;64:391–418.
64. Luiz RR, Costa AJL, Kale PL, et al. Assessment of agreement of a quantitative variable: a new graphical approach. *J Clin Epidemiol.* 2003;56:963–967.
65. Oldham PD. A note on the analysis of repeated measurements of the same subjects. *J Chron Dis.* 1962;15:969–977.
66. Nieto-García FJ, Edwards LA. On the spurious correlation between changes in blood pressure and initial values. *J Clin Epidemiol.* 1990;43:727–728.
67. Five-year findings of the hypertension detection and follow-up program: III: Reduction in stroke incidence among persons with high blood pressure: Hypertension Detection and Follow-up Program Cooperative Group. *JAMA.* 1982;247:633–638.

EXERCISES

1. The relationship between serum cholesterol and coronary heart disease seems to follow a "dose–response" (graded) pattern. A serum cholesterol concentration test based on blood obtained by finger-stick in nonfasting individuals was considered for use in a large cohort study of risk factors for coronary heart disease. Also discussed in Section 8.3.2 of this chapter, a pilot study was conducted comparing results from this test with those obtained by assaying serum cholesterol in a nationally recognized standard laboratory. The standard examinations were done in the fasting state on plasma under carefully controlled conditions. The results are shown in the table. In this table, "positive" values refer to a serum cholesterol concentration of ≥ 200 mg/dL.

Finger-stick values	Standard laboratory values		
	Positive	Negative	Total
Positive	18	19	37
Negative	1	11	12
Total	19	30	49

   a. Calculate the sensitivity, specificity, and predictive values of the finger-stick test by using the standard laboratory values as the gold standard.
   b. On the basis of this pilot study, would you recommend the use of the finger-stick test in the study? State the reasons for your recommendation and the potential impact of using this test on the study's results.
   c. Would you have analyzed the results of this pilot study differently? Why and how?

2. Define quality assurance and quality control, and next to each activity shown in the table check whether it should be regarded as a quality assurance or a quality control activity.

Activity	Quality assurance	Quality control
Preparation of manuals of operation	......	......
Over-the-shoulder observation of interviews during the study's data collection phase	......	......
Determination of interobserver reliability during the study's data collection phase	......	......
Certification of interviewers	......	......
Recertification of interviewers	......	......
Examination of intralaboratory reliability using phantom (repeat) blood samples collected from the study participants	......	......

   (continues)

(continued)

Activity	Quality assurance	Quality control
Assessment of the validity of two data collection instruments to decide which instrument should be used in the study	......	......
Duplicate readings (with adjudication by a third reader) of X-rays for confirmation of an outcome in an ongoing cohort study	......	......
Training of interviewers	......	......
Pretest of a questionnaire	......	......

3. In an ongoing epidemiologic study, the inter-observer reliability of body mass index (BMI, measured in kg/m^2) was examined, based on three categories: "normal" (BMI, <25), "overweight" (25–29.9), and "obese" ($\geq$30). Two independent observers measured weight and height on the same day in 30 volunteers. The results are shown in the following table:

		Observer A			
		Normal	Overweight	Obese	Total
Observer B	Normal	10			10
	Overweight		12	2	14
	Obese		1	5	6
	Total	10	13	7	30

   a. Calculate the unweighted as well as the weighted kappa values. For the latter, use weights of 1.0 for perfect agreement and 0.7 for a one-category difference.
   b. Given these kappa values, which additional action would you pursue?
   c. Under which circumstances would you use the weighted kappa?
4. In a hypothetical study, two technicians used a stethoscope that allows two observers to measure levels of blood pressure simultaneously to determine inter-observer agreement of systolic blood pressure measures. Both technicians were trained using the same protocol and by the same experienced third technician. The results are as follows:

	Levels of systolic blood pressure (mmHg)	
Study participant no.	Technician A	Technician B
1	122	125
2	130	129
3	118	116
4	136	135
5	114	112
6	116	118
7	124	122
8	110	111
9	140	142
10	146	145

a. Calculate the coefficient of variability for this set of blood pressure measurements.

b. What can be concluded from your observation of these values and from the coefficient of variability?

PART FIVE
Issues of Reporting and Application of Epidemiologic Results

CHAPTER 9 Communicating Results of Epidemiologic Studies 369

CHAPTER 10 Epidemiologic Issues in the Interface with Public Health Policy 391

Communicating Results of Epidemiologic Studies

CHAPTER 9

9.1 INTRODUCTION

Oral and written communication of research results is not only frequently full of specialized jargon but is also often characterized by systematic mistakes that might properly be classified as biases. This chapter reviews some basic concepts and approaches that are relevant to the reporting of epidemiologic results and discusses common mistakes made when communicating empirical findings. Although some of these mistakes may be a function of errors made during the design and conduct of the study and are thus difficult, if not impossible, to rectify, many can be prevented during the preparation of the report of study results. This chapter is not meant to be prescriptive but rather it attempts to cover some issues that should be considered when preparing a report of epidemiologic findings.

9.2 WHAT TO REPORT

Notwithstanding the necessary flexibility in style and content of reports of epidemiologic studies, Exhibit 9-1 summarizes some of the key issues that are worth considering when preparing such reports. Obviously, not all of the items listed in Exhibit 9-1 are relevant to all reports of empirical findings. In the following paragraphs, selected issues summarized in Exhibit 9-1 that are often neglected when describing the study rationale, design, and results are briefly discussed.

9.2.1 Study Objectives and/or Hypotheses

The study objectives and hypotheses that guided the conduct of the study need to be explicitly stated, usually at the end of the Introduction section. One common way to structure the Introduction section of the paper is to link previous evidence on the subject (from epidemiologic and other studies, such as animal experiments) with the specific questions that justify the present study.

If the study does not have specific hypotheses—that is, if it is an exploratory study of multiple exposure–outcome relationships (i.e., a "fishing expedition" in the epidemiology jargon)—this too should be clearly stated in the Introduction. In many large epidemiologic studies and surveys, dozens or hundreds of variables can be cross-tabulated in search of possible associations. For example, up to 1000 two-by-two tables showing pooled data can be generated from a survey with information on 100 two-level exposure variables and 10 possible binary outcomes (e.g., the prevalence rates of 10 different diseases). Theoretically, even if none of these exposure variables is truly associated with the outcomes, chance alone will determine that in approximately 50 of the 1000 cross-tabulations a statistical association will be found to be significant at $p \leq 0.05$ level. Selective publication of only these "significant" findings will lead to publication bias (see Chapter 10, Section 10.5).

> **EXHIBIT 9-1** Issues to be considered when preparing epidemiologic reports.
>
> 1. *Introduction*
>   a. Succinctly review rationale for study: • biologic plausibility*
>   • what is new about study
>   b. State hypothesis/hypotheses [specify interaction(s), if part of the hypothesis].
> 2. *Methods*
>   a. Describe study population characteristics (e.g., age, gender), setting (e.g., hospital patients, population-based sample), and time frame of the study.
>   b. Describe inclusion and exclusion criteria.
>   c. Describe data collection procedures; give accuracy/reliability figures for these procedures, if known.
>   d. Specify criterion/criteria for identification of confounding variables.
>   e. Describe statistical methods; explain criterion/criteria for categorization of study variables.
>   f. Give rationale for believing that the assumptions underlying the selected model are reasonable (e.g., for the use of the Cox model, that the hazard ratio is constant over the follow-up time).
> 3. *Results*
>   a. Present descriptive data with minimum modeling (frequency distributions, medians, means, unadjusted differences).
>   b. Present stratified data.
>   c. Present data using more complex models, but use the most parsimonious model warranted by the data (e.g., Mantel-Haenszel-adjusted odds ratio if only one or two categorical variables need to be adjusted for).
>   d. When postulating interactions a priori (or exploring their presence a posteriori), consider assessing both multiplicative and additive interactions.
> 4. *Discussion*
>   a. Review main results of study, and emphasize similarities and dissimilarities with the literature.
>   b. Review strengths and limitations of study. Consider bias and confounding as alternative explanations for the results. Comment on possible misclassification of data in the context of the known or estimated validity and reliability of the data collection instruments and procedures used in the study.
>   c. Suggest specific ways to rectify some of the shortcomings of previous research and the present study, so as to help future investigators to address the same question(s).
>   d. If appropriate and warranted by the data, discuss the implications for public health policy or medical practice of the study results.

*"Biologic" if the disease process investigated is biological or physiological in nature. For epidemiologic studies dealing with psychosocial aspects, for example, the relevant aspects will be based on the psychosocial theoretical model underlying the hypothesis under study.

Source: Based on HA Kahn and CT Sempos, *Statistical Methods in Epidemiology*, 2nd ed. © 1989.

For example, Friedman et al.[1] published a paper reporting for the first time a strong graded relationship between leukocyte count and risk of myocardial infarction. In their discussion of these findings, then unexpected, Friedman et al. aptly opened their Discussion section with the following statement: "Our finding that the leukocyte count is a predictor of myocardial infarction should be viewed in the context of the exploratory study that we have been carrying out. In searching through approximately 750 assorted variables for new predictors of infarction. . . ."[1(p.1278)]

In fact, Friedman et al.'s results were subsequently replicated in a number of other studies. Although the causal nature of the association remains controversial,[2] its biologic plausibility has been strengthened by studies showing a relationship between inflammatory markers and coronary heart disease.[3,4] On the other hand, how many other findings in the medical/epidemiologic literature are just the product of a chance finding in a "fishing expedition," create a short lived uproar in the mass media, and are then never replicated?

This argument also applies to the reporting of interactions. Because an apparent effect modification may occur by chance (see Chapter 6, Section 6.10), the reader needs to consider whether it was a chance event resulting from multiple stratified cross-tabulations between the study variables, rather than an expected finding based on a previously established and plausible hypothesis.

9.2.2 Description of Validity and Reliability of Data Collection Instruments

When describing the data collection procedures, it is important to report the corresponding measures of validity and reliability whenever possible (see Chapter 8). Avoid statements such as "the validity/reliability of [the questionnaire] has been reported elsewhere [Reference]" or "the instrument has been validated previously [Reference]," as such wording is not informative for the reader without time or access to the source article. Moreover, these statements may be interpreted as meaning that the instrument is "valid" and "reliable," when in fact they may relate to a questionnaire with poor to moderate validity/reliability (e.g., Kappa or intraclass correlation coefficients of 0.20–0.40, as seen in validation studies of dietary data, for example). In the case of questionnaires, a special problem is that their validity and reliability may be a function of the characteristics of the study population (e.g., educational level)—that is, validity/reliability figures obtained from a given population may not be applicable to another population (see Chapter 8, Sections 8.3.2 and 8.3.3). Similarly, as discussed in Chapter 8, the validity/reliability of certain instruments or tests may be different between populations as a function of the underlying distribution of the trait. It is, therefore, important not only that results of validity/ reliability studies be reported but also that a summary of the characteristics of the individuals who participated in these studies be provided. Obviously, reports of study findings should also include internal results of quality control sub-studies, if available (see Chapter 8).

9.2.3 Rationale for the Choice of Confounders

Reports of epidemiologic observational studies frequently fail to describe the criteria for selection of confounding variables. For example, was the choice of potentially confounding variables initially based on the literature and subsequently verified in the study data? Were new potential confounders explored in the study that had not been considered in previous studies? And if so, which analytic approaches were used to examine confounding (see Chapter 5, Section 5.4.)?

Sometimes, direct acyclic graphs may help in framing the analysis of confounding in the context of a theoretical causal model and should be presented whenever appropriate (see Chapter 5, Section 5.3). Generally, authors should avoid selecting confounders on the basis of results of significance testing (see Chapter 5, Section 5.5.6).

9.2.4 Criteria for Selection of the Cutoff Points When Establishing Categories for Continuous or Ordinal Variables

Common approaches for categorizing continuous or ordinal variables are the use of either established standards (e.g., abnormal ST–T segment elevations observed in an electrocardiogram tracing to define myocardial ischemia) or study data distributions (e.g., use of percentiles as cutoff points). On occasion, investigators choose cutoff points that have been widely used for clinical purposes or in previous epidemiologic research (e.g., defining hypertension as values of ≥ 140 mm Hg systolic or ≥ 90 mm Hg diastolic blood pressure levels or defining hypercholesterolemia as serum cholesterol levels ≥ 200 mg/dL). When no such cutoff points exist and particularly when investigating novel risk factor-disease associations, the investigator may be interested in using exploratory techniques for optimizing and exploring the consequences of different cutoff choices for categorical[5] or ordinal[6] regression analyses. In any case, the report should explicitly describe the criteria or method used for this purpose; failure to define criteria clearly for selection of categories of the variables of interest may suggest that data were regrouped over and over again until the results were to the investigator's liking (e.g., until they achieved statistical significance).

9.2.5 Unmodeled and Parsimoniously Modeled Versus Fully Modeled Data

To provide adequate background information to put the study findings in proper perspective, unmodeled and parsimoniously modeled results should be presented, including the characteristics of the study population and both univariate and stratified distributions of key study variables and findings. Authors should avoid the temptation of reporting only the results of full statistical modeling. Because unadjusted results undergo minimum modeling and are thus more "representative" of the study population, it could even be argued that if adjusted and unadjusted results are similar only the latter should be presented. Otherwise, it is advantageous to show unadjusted along with adjusted results; this strategy not only allows additional insight into the strength of a possible confounding effect but may also help in elucidating underlying mechanisms. An illustration of the advantage of showing both unadjusted and adjusted measures of association is given by a study of the relationship of social class to carotid atherosclerotic disease.[7] The weakening of the relationship resulting from adjustment for major cardiovascular risk factors (e.g., hypertension, smoking, and hypercholesterolemia) gives a measure of the importance of these factors as mediating factors. Because the relationship may indeed be explained (at least partly) by these risk factors, it is inappropriate to show only the adjusted results.

Another example is that, assuming no measurement errors, the difference in the magnitude of birth weight-adjusted and unadjusted associations of maternal smoking with perinatal mortality reflects the importance of low birth weight as a mechanism explaining the association (Chapter 5, Figures 5-4 and 5-5). Ideally, the role of each individual potential confounder should be assessed so as to pinpoint the exact source of confounding and/or to assess the mechanism linking the risk factor to the outcome. Procedures and rationale for evaluating the influence of a given variable reflecting a mechanism linking the risk factor of interest to the outcome or the degree of positive confounding were discussed in Chapter 5, Sections 5.2.3 and 5.3.

Another issue related to confounding is that, although logistic regression is often used in cross-sectional analysis of prevalence,* prevalence odds ratio may be misinterpreted as a prevalence ratio. For example, authors may describe a prevalence odds ratio of 3.0 as meaning that "the disease is three times more *likely* to be present in the exposed than in the unexposed." Yet, studies of associations based on prevalence rates usually deal with fairly common conditions, such as those encountered in cross-sectional surveys. Under these circumstances, the prevalence odds ratio is a *biased* estimate of the prevalence ratio (See Chapter 3, Section 3.2.1). For example, in a cross-sectional study including individuals aged 65 years or older, hypertension was found to be prevalent in 66% of African American women and 52% of white women.[8] Thus, the prevalence of hypertension was approximately 1.3 times greater in African American women than in white women; the prevalence odds ratio, however, was estimated at 1.8, which may lead to the erroneous inference that the prevalence of hypertension in this study was 80% greater in African American than in white women. Regardless of the accuracy of the interpretation of the odds ratio, prevalence ratios (and relative risks) are usually preferred, as they are easier to grasp by readers who are unfamiliar with epidemiology,

---

*Or in prospective studies when incidence ratios are estimated without consideration of time to event, or in case-based case-control studies.

such as practicing physicians to whom many epidemiologic papers are aimed. As also mentioned in Chapter 7, Section 7.4.3, an alternative to logistic regression for the calculation of adjusted risk and prevalence ratios has been described.[9]

Finally, it should be emphasized that, from the public health viewpoint, reporting the unadjusted results may be of greater interest. Consider, for example, a comparison of Alzheimer's disease rates between two groups of interest, the objective of which is to assist in the planning of health services. Would it be useful to the health planner to conclude that, after age adjustment, there is no difference between the groups? Obviously not, as the adjusted rates would not accurately express the differential disease burden in the two groups.

9.2.6 Assessment of Interaction

All too often, the widespread use of logistic regression, Cox regression, and related models results in an almost exclusive focus on multiplicative interaction. As discussed in Chapter 6 (Section 6.6), however, the evaluation of additive interaction is of importance to public health practitioners[10,11] and should be carried out regardless of the statistical model used to analyze epidemiologic data. It is important to bear in mind that the use of logistic regression or other "multiplicative" models does not preclude the assessment of additive interaction.[12]

9.3 HOW TO REPORT

9.3.1 Avoiding Scientific Arrogance

When reporting results of individual studies, particularly those of observational studies, epidemiologists frequently do not sufficiently recognize that no study can stand alone and that replication is needed to minimize the effects of chance, design, or analytic problems. One individual study supplies at best only one piece of a huge, almost limitless puzzle. Thus, in general, it is advisable to avoid definitive statements, such as "this study unequivocally demonstrates that . . . ," when interpreting the results of a single observational study. In general, caution is called for when interpreting results of observational research.

9.3.2 Avoiding Verbosity

As in all scientific communication, it is important to be as concise as possible when reporting results from epidemiologic studies. In an editorial written a few years ago, Friedman[13] underscored the importance of writing scientific reports in a manner as concise as possible without loss of meaning or clarity. Consider the 73-word paragraph that follows; it comes from a paper submitted to an epidemiology journal:[13]

> Other investigations exploring the association between multiparity and scleroderma have obtained information on multiparity using surrogate measures. The amount of money spent on diapers, without consideration of inflation, has been used as a proxy by several groups of investigators, and all have reported that no significant differences were observed once the data were stratified by age at last full time pregnancy. Similar results were found in the analysis reported here.

A significant reduction of its length (to about 40 words) recommended by Friedman[13] not only preserved the paragraph's meaning but may have improved its clarity:

> Other investigators have used surrogate measures of multiparity, such as the amount of money spent on diapers, without consideration of inflation. As with our study, all

revealed no significant differences once the data were stratified by age at last full time pregnancy.

Friedman has subsequently renewed his call for the avoidance of verbosity[14] and invited the readers to read a paper by Lewis et al.[15] as an exemplar of concise, yet clear writing.

9.3.3 Improving Readability

Another way to make communication of epidemiologic findings more efficient, particularly when it is expected that some of the readers will lack familiarity with the terms used in the article, is to use as simple a language as possible. Several readability formulas are available to determine the educational grade level of the intended readership.[16,17] Consider, for example, applying the SMOG grading formula for tailoring an English-written report to the educational level of the readers[18]—an approach that reminds us of the need to keep the language simple when communicating with the public at large. The formula is easy to apply: (1) Select 30 sentences from the paper's text—10 at the beginning of the text, 10 in the middle, and 10 near the end; (2) count words with three or more syllables; (3) take the square root of this count; and (4) add 3 to this square root to obtain the US-equivalent grade level needed for understanding the report. For example, if there are 100 such words, the educational level needed will be

$$\text{SMOG Index} = \sqrt{100} + 3 = 13$$

that is, at least completion of high school. By applying this formula, Freimuth[16] concluded that patients receiving educational pamphlets about mammography from the Fox Chase Cancer Center would need to have at least 2 years of high school to be able to understand them. Although there is an obvious difference in the educational level of readers of scientific papers and that of the usual target readers of health education pamphlets, the SMOG formula and related formulas may be useful to epidemiologists who need to interface with the lay public (e.g., to communicate with the press or to have their views understood in a court of law).

In view of their culture specificity and assuming that epidemiologic literature is read all over the world, jargon and abbreviations should be avoided or used sparingly only when they achieve a universal acceptance/permanence status, as in the case of the terms DNA, IgG, or HIV. Widely used abbreviations such as CHD (for coronary heart disease) or SES (for socioeconomic status) may be acceptable, provided that they are properly spelled out at their first appearance in the article. Even the widespread use of commonly recognized abbreviations may lead to some confusion, however; for example, in Spanish-speaking countries, the abbreviation *AIDS* for "acquired immunodeficiency syndrome" becomes *SIDA* (*síndrome de inmunodeficiencia adquirida*), which in turn may be interpreted by English-speaking readers as a misspelling of the abbreviation *SIDS*, denoting "sudden infant death syndrome." In any case, authors should always be reminded that the abuse of abbreviations, although shortening the length of the manuscript, tends to decrease its readability, particularly for readers not entirely familiar with the specific research topic. Consider the following paragraph, taken from the (structured) abstract of a paper published in a major medical journal,[19] that the use of abbreviations makes virtually incomprehensible to the average reader:

> Methods and Results: Relative LV myocardial MMP activity was determined in the normal ($n = 8$) and idiopathic DCM ($n = 7$) human LV myocardium by substrate

zymography. Relative LV myocardial abundance of interstitial collagenase (MMP-1), stromelysin (MMP-3), 72 kD gelatinase (MMP-2), 92 kD gelatinase (MMP-9), TIMP-1, and TIMP-2 were measured with quantitative immunoblotting. LV myocardial MMP zymographic activity increased with DCM compared with normal (984 ± 149 versus 413 ± 64 pixels, $P < .05$). With DCM, LV myocardial abundance of MMP-1 decreased to 16 ± 6% ($P < .05$), MMP-3 increased to 563 ± 212% ($P < .05$), MMP-9 increased to 422 ± 64% ($P < .05$), and MMP-2 was unchanged when compared with normal. LV myocardial abundance of TIMP-1 and TIMP-2 increased by > 500% with DCM. A high-molecular-weight immunoreactive band for both TIMP-1 and TIMP-2, suggesting a TIMP/MMP complex, was increased > 600% with DCM.

9.3.4 Deriving Appropriate Inferences

Common inferential mistakes in epidemiologic reports include the implication that a statistical association can be automatically interpreted as causal, the use of statistical significance as the main criterion to judge whether an association is present, and the comparison of the "strength" of associations for different risk factors using the size of the regression coefficients or derived risk estimates.

The Presence of an Association (Even If Statistically Significant) Does Not Necessarily Reflect Causality

The fact that statistical associations are not necessarily causal is extensively discussed in basic epidemiology and statistics textbooks (e.g., Gordis,[20] Armitage and Berry[21]) and Chapters 4, 5, and 10 in this textbook. However, epidemiologists often use the word *effect* as a proxy/or *association* (or otherwise imply causality from statistical associations: e.g., "A decrease in *X* resulted in a decrease in *Y*"), even if it is not warranted, given that most etiologic studies are observational in nature.[22]

Even more troubling because of its frequent occurrence is the often implicit assumption that an adjusted estimate is free of confounding. Caution about inferring that confounding has been eliminated is crucial because even if multivariate models are used as an attempt to adjust for all known confounding variables, the possibility of residual confounding must almost always be explicitly considered (as discussed in detail in Chapter 7, Section 7.6).

Statistical Significance Is Not a Measure of the Strength of an Association

It is a common mistake to describe an association that is not statistically significant as nonexistent. For example, it may be correctly reported in a paper's abstract that a *statistically significant* association has not been found between depressed mood and subsequent breast cancer, as the estimated relative risk was 1.5, with the lower 95% confidence limit barely overlapping the null hypothesis.* Yet it would be erroneous if this finding were subsequently interpreted by other authors as evidence of lack of association. Similarly, on the basis of the hypothetical results shown in Table 9-1, particularly because of the suggestion of a graded association for every outcome examined, it would be a mistake to conclude (based on whether or not the lower confidence limit overlapped the null hypothesis) that smoking was related to mortality due to lung cancer and coronary heart

---

*The 95% confidence interval is a statistic that estimates precision and not a test for the statistical significance of a point estimate; however, when the 95% confidence interval of an association measure, such as the relative risk, does not overlap the null value, it is often used as a proxy for the presence of "statistical significance" ($p < 0.05$).

disease *but not to mortality from stroke*. It is important to remember that statistical significance and the width of the confidence limits are strongly dependent on the sample size; a smaller number of stroke deaths, compared with coronary disease deaths, could explain why the latter but not the former association was found to be statistically significant in a situation such as that shown in the hypothetical example in Table 9-1.

The inference that there is no association when the association is not statistically significant, or when the confidence interval overlaps the null hypothesis value, fails to consider the important fact that the likelihood of the values within the confidence interval is maximum for the point estimate.[23] It is our impression that many authors who publish in the medical (and even in the epidemiologic) literature view the 95% confidence interval as some kind of *flat* (and *closed*) range of possible values of the parameter of interest. In other words, all of these "possible values" included in the range are assumed to be equally likely (Figure 9-1A). Thus, in the previous hypothetical example (estimated relative risk for current smoking and stroke = 2.1; 95% confidence interval: 0.9, 4.9), because the 95% confidence interval includes the null hypothesis (i.e., relative risk = 1.0), this result may be mistakenly interpreted as reflecting "lack of association." This is an erroneous interpretation because the likelihood of any given value of the true parameter being estimated is not uniform across the range of values contained in the confidence interval. It is *maximum at the point estimate* (e.g., relative risk = 2.1 for current smokers in Table 9-1) and declines as the values move away from it (Figure 9-1B). The relative risk value of 0.9 (the lower bound of the confidence interval) is very unlikely (as is the uppermost value—relative risk = 4.9). Moreover, values *outside* of the 95% confidence limits are also plausible (albeit less likely). If the sample size in the study had been larger, the same estimate of the relative risk = 2.1 might have been associated with a 95% confidence interval not including the null hypothesis value (e.g., 1.1, 3.9). The confidence interval merely expresses the statistical uncertainty of the point estimate and should not be mechanically and erroneously interpreted as a range of equally likely possible values.

The Magnitude of the Association Estimates Across Variables May Not Be Directly Comparable

The issue of comparing different variables with regard to the strength of their association with a given outcome has been introduced in Chapter 3, Section 3.5, to which the reader is referred. An extension of that discussion follows.

For an example of a situation in which it is inappropriate to compare the values of a measure of association between variables, consider the results of the logistic regression analysis shown in Chapter 7, Table 7-17: the inference that the association for gender is stronger than that for age, based on the fact that the odds ratio is higher for the

TABLE 9-1 Age-adjusted mortality rate ratios for current and former cigarette smokers versus nonsmokers, according to cause of death, hypothetical example.

	Mortality rate ratio (95% confidence interval)		
Cause of death	**Current smokers**	**Former smokers**	**Nonsmokers**
Lung cancer	8.0 (3.0, 21.3)	2.5 (0.9, 6.9)	1.0
Coronary heart disease	2.3 (1.6, 3.3)	1.5 (1.1, 2.0)	1.0
Stroke	2.1 (0.9, 4.9)	1.4 (0.8, 2.5)	1.0

former (3.70) than for the latter (1.011) variable, is clearly unwarranted in view of the striking difference in the nature of these variables and the width of the units used (in the example shown in that table, male/female versus 1 year of age). Although this example highlights the difficulties when comparing discrete with continuous variables, the comparison between continuous variables, too, is a function of the width of unit used for each variable; thus, in Table 7-17, it would be unwarranted to compare the increase in coronary heart disease odds related to a change in total serum cholesterol of 1 mg/dL (odds ratio = 1.007) with that related to a change of 1 kg/m² in body mass index (odds ratio = 1.024), as these "units" (the "widths" for which the odds ratios in this example are calculated) are rather arbitrary. For example, if instead of 1 mg/dL one were to adopt 10 mg/dL as the unit for serum cholesterol, the corresponding odds ratio (based on Table 7-17 results) would be $e^{(10 \times 0.0074)} = 1.08$—that is, larger than the odds ratio for 1 kg/m² in body mass index.

On occasion, authors attempt to overcome this problem by calculating the so-called *standardized regression coefficients* for continuous variables. These are obtained by using one standard deviation as the unit for each variable (or simply multiplying each regression coefficient by the variable's standard deviation); it is argued that this strategy permits comparing different variables within a study or the same variable across studies.[24] This

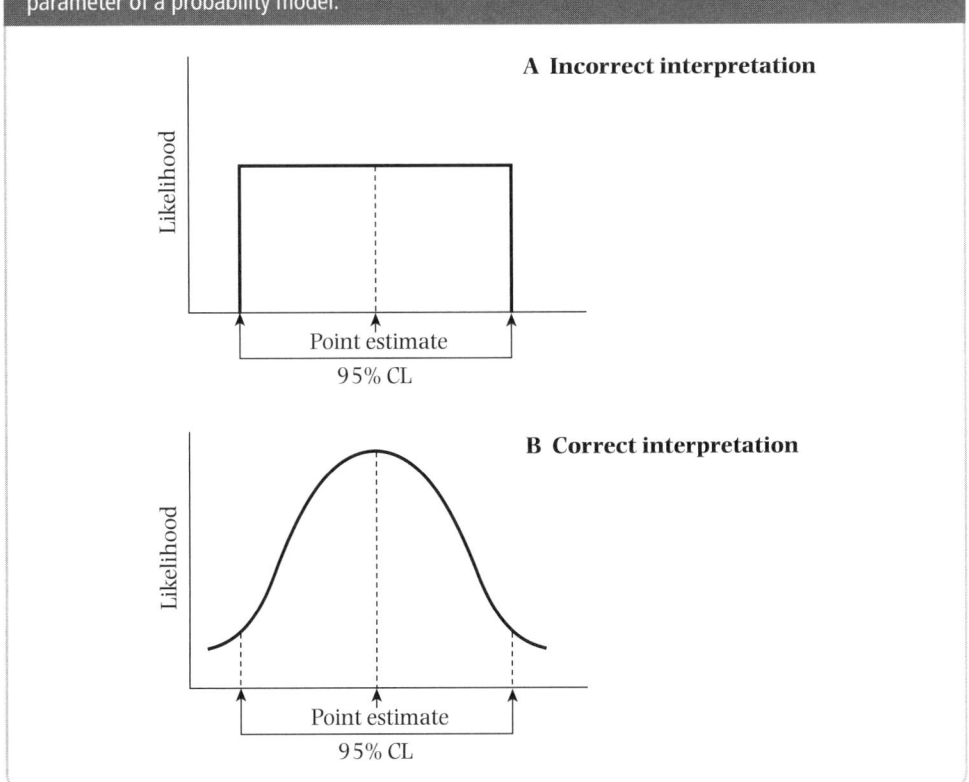

FIGURE 9-1 Incorrect and correct interpretation of the confidence limit (CL): the likelihood of any given value within the range is not uniform (as shown in A); it is maximum at the point estimate of the parameter being measured and declines as values move away from it (B). (Likelihood is a measure of the *support* provided by a body of data for a particular value of the parameter of a probability model.

Note: For more details on this fundamental statistical concept, the reader should refer to more specialized textbooks (e.g., Clayton and Hills: D Clayton & M Hills, *Statistical Models in Epidemiology*, New York, NY: Oxford University Press, 1993).

approach, however, has serious problems,[25] including the following: (1) when different variables in the same study are compared, smaller standard deviation units will result from variables with less variability than from those with more variability, and (2) when the same variable is compared across different studies, the standard deviation is heavily dependent on the characteristics of the study population, the distribution of the variable, and design characteristics of each study; thus the regression coefficients may not be really "standardized" or comparable across studies.

An additional and more fundamental problem is that these comparisons do not take the biologic nature of each factor into consideration.[26] As discussed in Chapter 3, Section 3.5, the unique biological nature of each variable makes it difficult to compare its association strength with that of other variables. Consider, for example, a study in which a 1 mg/dL change in total serum cholesterol is compared with a blood pressure change of 1 mm Hg with regard to coronary disease risk; because the mechanisms by which these variables produce both the underlying disease process (atherosclerosis) and its clinical manifestation (e.g., myocardial infarction) may be quite different, this comparison would be difficult, if not impossible, to justify.

In Chapter 3, Section 3.5, an approach was suggested for comparing different variables that consisted of estimating the exposure intensity necessary for each risk factor of interest to produce an association of the same magnitude as that of well-established risk factors. In addition, Greenland et al.[27] have suggested a method that compares the increase in the level of each factor needed to change the risk of the outcome by a certain fixed amount, such as 50%.

An additional example of the application of a similar type of approach is the study by Sharrett et al.,[28] who used cross-sectional data from the Multiethnic Study of Atherosclerosis to compare the relative importance of smoking (and diabetes) and low-density lipoprotein cholesterol (LDLc) in different phases of the natural history of atherosclerosis. Based on the fact that LDLc is essential to the atherosclerotic process, these authors used LDLc to estimate the "LDL-equivalent" associations* of smoking (and diabetes) with various manifestations of atherosclerosis indicative of its severity. They estimated, for example, that it would take a 238 mg/dL difference in LDLc value to replicate the association of smoking with severe atherosclerotic disease (ankle-brachial index indicative of lower extremity arterial disease). Notwithstanding the study's cross-sectional nature, based on these findings as well as previous literature, the authors suggested that, although LDL is key to the initiation of atherosclerosis—and in this study, LDLc also seemed to have an important role in vulnerability to plaque rupture—smoking is more strongly related to plaque progression to thicker, more fibrous lesions (see also Chapter 10, Section 10.2.4, under "Differences in the Stage of the Natural History of the Underlying Process").

9.3.5 Tables and Figures

There is no standard way of reporting findings in tables and figures, and the need to address different audiences (e.g., peers vs the lay public) and use different vehicles (e.g., scientific journals vs newsletters) calls for flexibility; however, there seem to be some simple rules that, if not always followed, should be systematically considered.

---

*The LDL-equivalent calculation done by the authors is straightforward. For example, if smoking doubled the odds of lower extremity arterial disease (LEAD), the method calculates the amount of LDLc associated with a doubling of the smoking-LEAD odds ratio.

Tables

The following are general guidelines concerning the presentation of tables:

- *Labels and headings.* Tables should be clearly labeled, with self-explanatory titles. Optimally, readers should be able to understand the table even if it is examined in isolation. Regrettably, however, to understand and interpret tables published in the literature, often the entire paper or at least the Methods section must be re-reviewed (e.g., the relevant subgroups are not well defined, or the outcome is not specified or defined in the table). Generous use of footnotes to render the table self-explanatory is recommended.
- *Units.* Categories for discrete variables and units for continuous variables should be specified. For example, an odds ratio next to the variable "age" is meaningless unless it is also stated whether the unit is 1 year of age or some other age grouping. Likewise, an odds ratio next to the variable "race" is not very informative unless the categories being compared are explicitly stated.
- *Comparability with other reports.* Often it is useful to present results in a way that would make them comparable with results of most previous reports. For example, it may be more useful to present age using conventional (e.g., 25–34 and 35–44) than unconventional groupings (e.g., 23–32 and 33–42).
- *Comparing statistics between groups.* Another useful strategy, and one that facilitates grasping the meaning of the results, is to present side by side the statistics that provide the main comparison(s) of interest. For example, when one is presenting cohort study results, the ease of comparing rate/person-years side by side makes the (blank) Table A below more "reader friendly" than Table B.

TABLE A Preferred presentation.

No. of person-years		Rate/person-years	
Exposed	Unexposed	Exposed	Unexposed

TABLE B Less desirable presentation.

Exposed		Unexposed	
No. of person-years	Rate/person-years	No. of person-years	Rate/person-years

The same principle applies to frequency distributions. Data on diabetes according to smoking status[29] can be presented as shown on the right-hand side of Table 9-2 or in a less desirable format on the left.

- *Avoidance of redundancy.* Although there is some controversy regarding the advantages of reporting statistical testing results vis-à-vis precision estimates (i.e., confidence intervals),[30] avoidance of redundancy is not controversial; thus, for example, it is usually undesirable to show in the same table values for chi-square, standard error, and *p* values. Another type of redundancy is the text's repetition of all or most of the table results, often including *p* values or confidence limits. Whereas some repetition of this sort may be useful, the text ought to emphasize mainly the patterns of associations, rather than repeating what is clearly seen in the tables.

TABLE 9-2 Number and percent distributions of individuals with and without diabetes mellitus, according to smoking at baseline.

	Less desirable presentation				Preferred presentation			
	Diabetes		No diabetes		No.		%	
Smoking	No.	%	No.	%	Diabetes	No Diabetes	Diabetes	No Diabetes
Current	90	19.6	2307	18.2	90	2307	19.6	18.2
Former	70	12.7	1136	9.1	70	1136	12.7	9.1
Never	155	27.0	2553	20.4	155	2553	27.0	20.4
Unknown	287	40.7	6566	52.3	287	6566	40.7	52.3

Source: Data from ES Ford and F DeStefano, Risk Factors for Mortality from All Causes and from Coronary Heart Disease among Persons with Diabetes. Findings from the National Health and Nutrition Examination Survey I. *American Journal of Epidemiology,* Vol 133, pp. 1220–1230, © 1991.

- *Shifting denominators.* In most studies, the number of individuals for whom information is missing differs from variable to variable. When this situation occurs, totals should be given for each variable so as to allow the reader to judge whether the magnitude of the loss is such as to cast doubt on the precision and accuracy of the information. A useful strategy is to add a "not stated" or "unknown" category for each variable; alternatively, the apparent inconsistencies in the denominators can be explained in footnotes.
- *Presenting data parsimoniously.* A choice often exists between presenting an "intermediate" statistic or a more easily interpretable one. For example, given the choice of presenting either a beta coefficient from a logistic regression model or the corresponding odds ratio, the latter is usually preferable, particularly when the purpose of the communication is to present an adjusted measure of association rather than a formula needed for prediction. (Even in linear regression, a table heading along the lines of "absolute differences in outcome Y [units] associated with changes in selected variables" with the units for the independent variables specified in the body of the table is more informative than merely "linear regression coefficient.") Another example is the customary reporting of a beta coefficient for an "interaction term," which is difficult to interpret outside of the predictive context of the regression formula (Table 9-3A). It is usually more useful to show stratified results (Table 9-3B).

Some of the principles just discussed are illustrated in the hypothetical example shown in Table 9-4A and Table 9-4B (preferred). In Table 9-4A, beta coefficients rather than hazard ratios (relative risks) are given; no units for the variables are shown, and three somewhat redundant statistics are given (standard error, chi-square, and p values). In Table 9-4B, on the other hand, the units that correspond to the hazard ratios are given, and instead of the three statistics, only 95% confidence intervals are shown.

Figures

The rules that guide presentation of data in tabular form generally also apply to figures. Some of the issues that should be considered specifically when preparing figures for presentation are discussed next.

TABLE 9-3 Colon cancer incidence rates per 1000 per 5 years among 1963 census participants 45 to 64 years of age at baseline, by sex and residence, Washington County, Maryland, 1963–1975.

A

Characteristic	No.	Colon cancer incidence rates/1000	
		Crude	Adjusted
Total	17,968	6.5	6.5
Sex			
Men	8674	5.5	5.2
Women	9294	7.3	5.6
Residence			
Rural	8702	7.6	9.7
Urban	9266	5.4	4.5
Interaction term (sex × residence)			−4.6

B

Sex	No.	Colon cancer incidence rates/1000			
		Crude		Adjusted	
		Rural	Urban	Rural	Urban
Men	8674	5.5	5.6	5.9	5.6
Women	9294	9.7	5.2	10.1	5.2

Source: Unpublished data from GW Comstock.

TABLE 9-4 Multiple risk equation for coronary artery disease: Cox regression model relating baseline risk factors to the incidence of coronary heart disease.

A

Variable	Beta coefficient	Standard error	χ^2	p value
Age	0.149	0.027	29.97	0.0000
Cholesterol	0.013	0.003	15.36	0.0001
Smoking	0.380	0.125	9.28	0.0020
Parental history of coronary heart disease	0.152	0.392	0.15	0.7000

B

Variable	Risk comparison	Hazard ratio	95% confidence interval
Age	10-year difference	4.5	2.6–7.6
Cholesterol	40 mg/dL difference	1.7	1.3–2.2
Smoking	20 cigarettes/day vs nonsmokers	2.1	1.3–3.5
Parental history of coronary heart disease	Present vs absent	1.2	0.5–2.5

- *Use of figure format.* Avoid abusing figures and graphs—that is, displaying data in a graphical format when they could easily be reported in the text. An example of this type of superfluous graphical display is illustrated in Figure 9-2. The information in this figure obviously could be succinctly described in the text. Figure 9-2 exemplifies what Tufte[31] has called a "low data–ink ratio": too much ink for very little data.
- *Titles and labels.* As with tables, figure titles should be as self-explanatory as possible. Ordinates and abscissas should be labeled in their units. When the plot includes several lines, it is useful to organize and place the legends in a manner as closely related as possible to the order and place of the corresponding categories in the actual figure. For example, in Figure 9-3A, the legend for each of the curves is at the bottom of the figure, and the reader has to go back and forth from the graph to the legend to relate each curve to the corresponding group. On the other hand, in Figure 9-3B, the legends are next to the curves, but the order in which the curves appear and the order for the sex/race legends are opposite. By placing the sex/race identification next to the actual curves, Figure 9-3C seems to be the most readily understandable. It should also be emphasized that the greater number of curves in a figure the more difficult it is to decipher it. For example, in Figure 9-3, additional stratification by, for example, two age groups would render it difficult to understand without careful and time-consuming inspection, thus defeating the main purpose of a figure: to allow data to be more readily grasped. In this situation, it would be preferable to present two different figures—one for each age group (or one for each gender or ethnic background, depending on the primary comparison of interest).
- *Ordinate scale.* The scale in the ordinate should be consistent with the measure being plotted. For example, when the main interest is on measures expressing relative differences (e.g., relative risks or odds ratios) plotted with bar charts, a baseline value of 1.0 and a logarithmic scale should be used. An example is shown in Figure 9-4 in which three alternative ways to plot the relative risks corresponding to two different levels associated with a certain variable (relative risk = 0.5 and relative risk = 2.0) are compared. In Figure 9-4A, in which the baseline value is 0 (an "unreal" value in a relative scale), the visual impression conveyed by the bars is that the relative risk on the right-hand side is four times higher than that on the left-hand side, which is senseless in view of the fact that these two relative risks go in opposite directions.

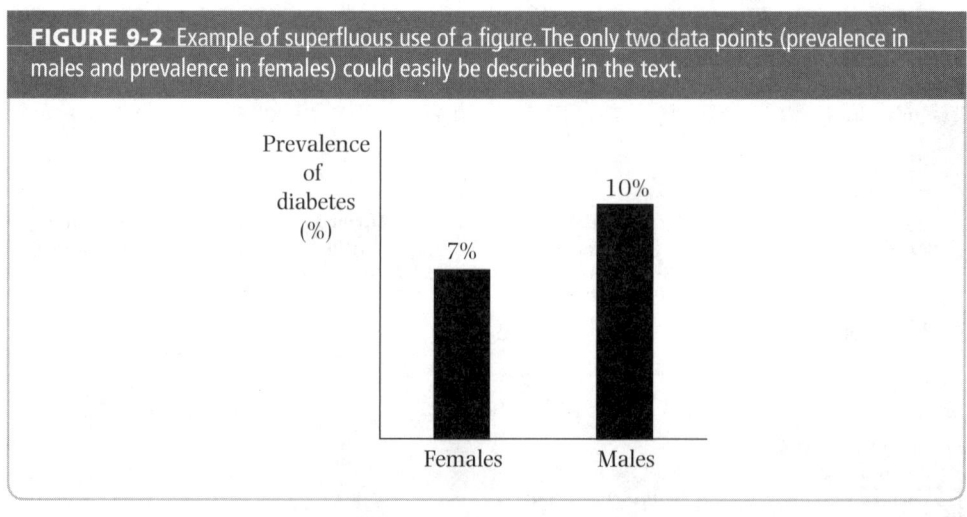

FIGURE 9-2 Example of superfluous use of a figure. The only two data points (prevalence in males and prevalence in females) could easily be described in the text.

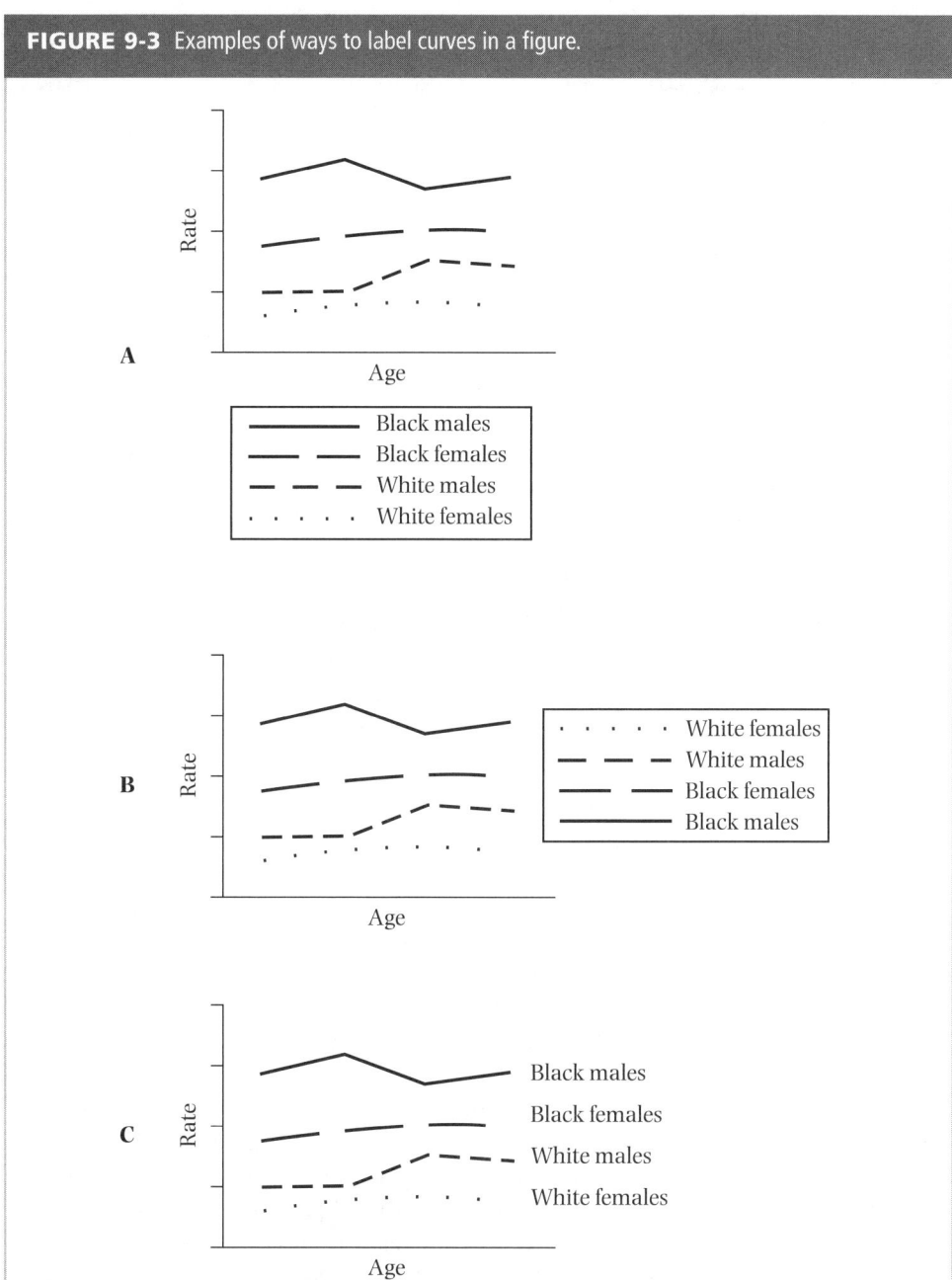

FIGURE 9-3 Examples of ways to label curves in a figure.

The plot in Figure 9-4B, although an improvement over that shown in Figure 9-4A in that its baseline corresponds to the correct null relative risk value (relative risk = 1.0), is still a distorted representation of the magnitude of the relative risks, as it uses an arithmetic scale on the ordinate. The height of the bar corresponding to the relative risk of 2.0 is twice that corresponding to a relative risk of 0.5, when in fact both relative differences are of the same magnitude, albeit in opposite directions. The correct representation is seen in Figure 9-4C, in which a logarithmic scale is used in the ordinate. Even if all relative risks are in the same direction,

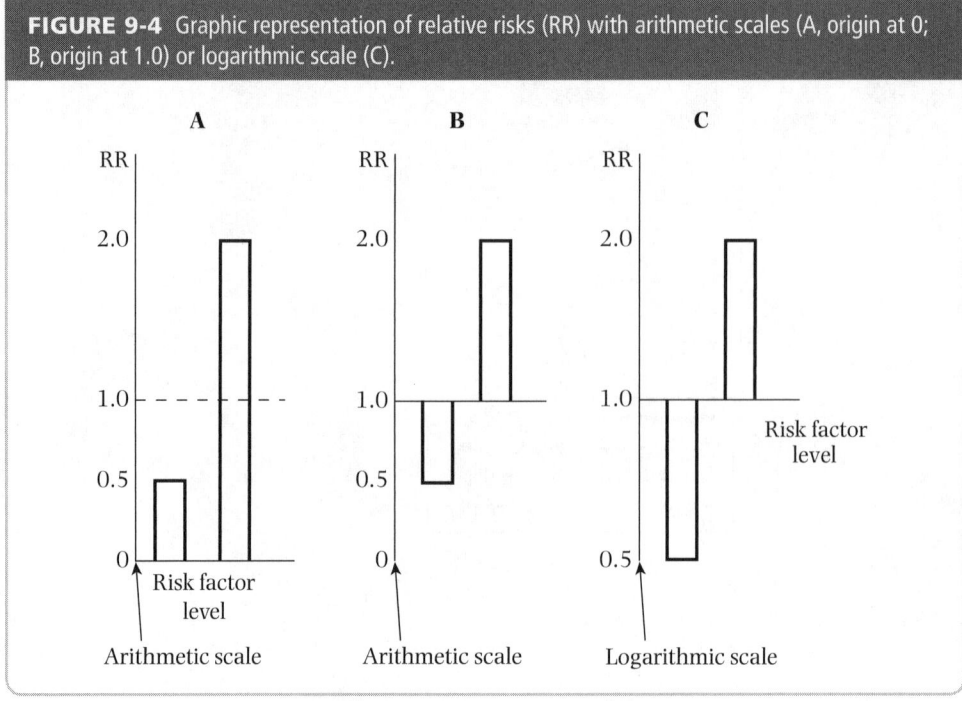

FIGURE 9-4 Graphic representation of relative risks (RR) with arithmetic scales (A, origin at 0; B, origin at 1.0) or logarithmic scale (C).

the use of an arithmetic scale in the ordinate is generally inappropriate when the main focus is the assessment of linear trends in relative differences (ratios). An example is given in Figure 9-5. In Figure 9-5A, in which an arithmetic scale is used, the visual impression is that the relative risk increases more rapidly at the higher levels of the risk factor. When a logarithmic scale is used instead (Figure 9-5B), the correct impression is obtained: the relative risk increase is linear. The curvature in Figure 9-5A is the product of the exponential nature of all relative measures of effect. Although the trained eye may correctly infer that the pattern in Figure 9-5A is linear in an exponential scale, the use of a logarithmic scale on the ordinate, as seen in Figure 9-5B, is less prone to misinterpretation. (An exception to the rule that relative risks or odds ratios are best represented using a log scale in a figure is when the authors wish to emphasize absolute differences, such as in studies of effectiveness—the formula of which is akin to that of percent attributable risk in the exposed. The focus on absolute—rather than relative—excesses justifying the use of an arithmetic scale also applies to the evaluation of additive interactions by means of plotting relative risks or odds ratios, as illustrated in Figure 6-3 of Chapter 6.)

Sometimes, the use of a logarithmic ordinate scale may be pragmatically necessary so as to include all data in the graph, as illustrated in Figure 1-7, Chapter 1. The use of a logarithmic rather than an arithmetic scale in the ordinate allows plotting the wide range of rates included in the analysis of age, cohort, and period effects (from 2–3 per 100,000 in those 40–44 years old from the 1920–1930 birth cohorts to 200–500 per 100,000 in those ≥ 80 years old from the 1905–1910 birth cohorts). It must be emphasized that when a log scale is used, a given difference should be interpreted as a relative difference (ratio) between the rates; in the example shown in Figure 1-7, the fact that the slope of each line tends to be steeper for the older than for the younger age groups in men

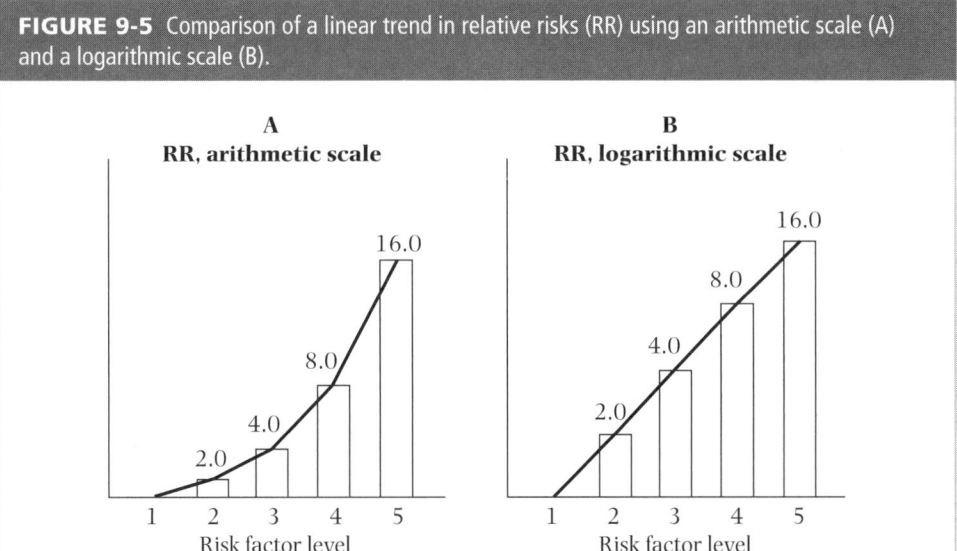

FIGURE 9-5 Comparison of a linear trend in relative risks (RR) using an arithmetic scale (A) and a logarithmic scale (B).

(perhaps with the exception of the 40–44 age group) means that the relative increase (rate ratio, see Chapter 3) from older to recent birth cohorts tends to be larger in older than in younger men (the opposite seems to be true among women).

9.4 CONCLUSION

Epidemiologists must communicate results of empirical research not only to their peers but also to other consumers of epidemiologic data, including practicing physicians, public health personnel, law professionals, and the general public. Scientific journals with a readership traditionally formed by clinical practitioners, such as the *New England Journal of Medicine* and the *Journal of the American Medical Association*, are devoting more and more pages to reports of epidemiologic studies. The use of epidemiologic data by the legal profession is also on the increase. Christoffel and Teret,[32] for example, found that the number of times a word starting with *epidemiol* appeared in federal or state courts increased from close to 0 in 1970 to more than 80 in 1990. It is virtually certain that this increase has been continuing ever since. Thus, epidemiologists should concern themselves not only with the conduct of scientifically valid studies but also with clearly expressing their results to audiences with varying degrees of scientific sophistication. Epidemiologic papers using simple, unambiguous language are likely to be more easily understood by individuals both inside and outside the discipline and are thus more likely to perform their major function: to be used.

REFERENCES

1. Friedman GD, Klatsky AL, Siegelaub AB. The leukocyte count as a predictor of myocardial infarction. *N Engl J Med.* 1974;290:1275–1278.
2. Nieto FJ, Szklo M, Folsom AR, et al. Leukocyte count correlates in middle-aged adults: The Atherosclerosis Risk in Communities (ARIC) Study. *Am J Epidemiol.* 1992;136:525–537.
3. Yeh ET. High-sensitivity C-reactive protein as a risk assessment tool for cardiovascular disease. *Clin Cardiol.* 2005;28:408–412.
4. Koenig W, Rosenson RS. Acute-phase reactants and coronary heart disease. *Semin Vasc Med.* 2002;2:417–428.
5. Wartenberg D, Northridge M. Defining exposure in case-control studies: A new approach. *Am J Epidemiol.* 1991;133:1058–1071.
6. Pastor R, Guallar E. Use of two-segmented logistic regression to estimate change-points in epidemiologic studies. *Am J Epidemiol.* 1998;148:631–642.
7. Diez-Roux AV, Nieto FJ, Tyroler HA, et al. Social inequalities and atherosclerosis: The atherosclerosis risk in communities study. *Am J Epidemiol.* 1995;141:960–972.
8. Svetkey LP, George LK, Burchett BM, et al. Black/white differences in hypertension in the elderly: An epidemiologic analysis in central North Carolina. *Am J Epidemiol.* 1993;137:64–73.
9. Spiegelman D, Hertzmark E. Easy SAS calculations for risk or prevalence ratios and differences. *Am J Epidemiol.* 2005;162:199–200.
10. Saracci R. Interaction and synergism. *Am J Epidemiol.* 1980;112:465–466.
11. Rothman KJ, Greenland S, Walker AM. Concepts of interaction. *Am J Epidemiol.* 1980;112:467–470.
12. Thompson WD. Statistical analysis of case-control studies. *Epidemiol Rev.* 1994;16:33–50.
13. Friedman GD. Be kind to your reader. *Am J Epidemiol.* 1990;132:591–593.
14. Friedman GD. Please read the following paper and write this way! *Am J Epidemiol.* 2005;161:405.
15. Lewis SA, Antoniak M, Venn AJ, et al. Secondhand smoke, dietary fruit intake, road traffic exposures, and the prevalence of asthma: A cross-sectional study in young children. *Am J Epidemiol.* 2005;161:406–411.
16. Freimuth VS. Assessing the readability of health education messages. *Public Health Rep.* 1979;94:568–570.
17. Johnson ME, Mailloux SL, Fisher DG. The readability of HIV/AIDS educational materials targeted to drug users. *Am J Public Health.* 1997;87:112–113.
18. McLaughlin G. SMOG grading: A new readability formula. *J Reading.* 1969;12:639–646.
19. Thomas CV, Coker ML, Zellner JL, et al. Increased matrix metalloproteinase activity and selective upregulation in LV myocardium from patients with end-stage dilated cardiomyopathy. *Circulation.* 1998;97:1708–1715.
20. Gordis L. *Epidemiology*, 4th ed. Philadelphia, PA: Elsevier Saunders; 2008.
21. Armitage P, Berry G. *Statistical Methods in Medical Research*, 3rd ed. London, UK: Blackwell; 1994.
22. Petitti DB. Associations are not effects. *Am J Epidemiol.* 1991;133:101–102.
23. Rothman KJ, Lanes S, Robins J. Casual inference. *Epidemiology.* 1993;4:555–556.
24. Newman TB, Browner WS. In defense of standardized regression coefficients. *Epidemiology.* 1991;2:383–386.
25. Greenland S, Maclure M, Schlesselman JJ, et al. Standardized regression coefficients: A further critique and review of some alternatives. *Epidemiology.* 1991;2:387–392.
26. Criqui MH. On the use of standardized regression coefficients. *Epidemiology.* 1991;2:393.

27. Greenland S, Schlesselman JJ, Criqui MH. The fallacy of employing standardized regression coefficients and correlations as measures of effect. *Am J Epidemiol.* 1986;123:203–208.
28. Sharrett AR, Ding J, Criqui MH, et al. Smoking, diabetes, and blood cholesterol differ in their associations with subclinical atherosclerosis: The Multiethnic Study of Atherosclerosis (MESA). *Atherosclerosis.* 2006;186:441–447.
29. Ford ES, DeStefano F. Risk factors for mortality from all causes and from coronary heart disease among persons with diabetes: Findings from the National Health and Nutrition Examination Survey I Epidemiologic Follow-up Study. *Am J Epidemiol.* 1991;133:1220–1230.
30. Savitz DA, Tolo KA, Poole C. Statistical significance testing in the American Journal of Epidemiology, 1970–1990. *Am J Epidemiol.* 1994;139:1047–1052.
31. Tufte E. *The Visual Display of Quantitative Information.* Cheshire, CT: Graphics Press; 1983.
32. Christoffel T, Teret SP. Epidemiology and the law: courts and confidence intervals. *Am J Public Health.* 1991;81:1661–1666.

EXERCISES

1. The following table shows results of a cohort study examining the relationship between alcohol and liver cancer:

Relationship between alcohol and liver cancer			
Alcohol	Number of subjects	Number who develop liver cancer on follow-up	Relative risk
Yes	560	15	8.4
No	1575	5	1.0

   Identify and describe the flaws in this table.

2. Rewrite the following sentence, which appeared in the Discussion section of a paper, in fewer words:
   "As a result of the confounding effect of smoking, a relationship of alcohol with respiratory cancer was observed. However, upon adjustment for smoking (treating smoking as an ordinal variable in terms of number of cigarettes smoked), the relationship disappeared entirely." (40 words)

3. High nevus density is a risk factor for cutaneous malignant melanoma. In 1993, Gallagher et al. conducted a clinical trial of the effectiveness of high-sun protection factor sunscreen in preventing the development of new nevi in white children in grades 1 and 4 in Vancouver, British Columbia, Canada.* Children assigned to the control group received neither sunscreen nor advice about its use. The results pertaining to a 3-year follow-up (June 1993 through May 1996), stratified by the percentage of the children's face covered by freckles, were presented by the authors in table format, as follows:

	Average number of new nevi on follow-up		Difference in average number of new nevi (sunscreen minus control)	Difference in average number of new nevi as a percentage of the number of new nevi in controls
Freckles %	Sunscreen	Control		
10	24	24	......	......
20	20	28	......	......
30	20	30	......	......
40	16	30	......	......

   a. For each category of percentage of the face covered by freckles, calculate the difference in the average number of new nevi between sunscreen and control children, as a percentage of the average number of new nevi in the control group.

---

*RP Gallagher, K Jason, JK Rivers et al. Broad spectrum sunscreen use and the development of new nevi in white children. *JAMA.* 2000;283:2955–2960.

b. Using the data presented in the table, construct and label a graph to show the number of nevi by group to which children were randomly allocated and by percentage of the face covered with freckles. Assume no losses to follow-up. Also assume that the percentage of face covered by freckles is a continuous variable, and the categories in the table represent the midpoint of the interval. Do not forget the title.

c. Based on the table (and the figure), how would you report (in words) the joint associations of high-sun protection factor sunscreen and freckling (with regard to the number of new nevi) in a scientific meeting (assuming no random variability and no bias)?

4. a. For each category of leisure activity status and separately for those with and those without chronic bronchitis in the table, plot the total mortality odds ratios and 95% confidence intervals found in the Whitehall study,[†] which was the basis for one of the exercises in Chapter 6:

Leisure activity status	Multiply adjusted rate ratio (95% confidence interval)
	No chronic bronchitis
Inactive	1.21 (1.1, 1.3)
Moderate	1.06 (1.0, 1.2)
Active (reference)	1.0
	Chronic bronchitis
Inactive	0.70 (0.3, 1.4)
Moderate	0.73 (0.3, 1.6)
Active (reference)	1.0

b. Assuming no bias and no confounding, what would you conclude about the possible association between moderate leisure activity status and mortality?

5. The table shows results for selected variables in a case-control study conducted by Cox and Sneyd.[‡] Variables were simultaneously and reciprocally adjusted for year of age, sex, ethnicity, and family history of colorectal cancer using logistic regression. When asked to describe the findings in this table, a hypothetical reader described them as follows: "No associations were found for history of ulcerative colitis or Crohn's disease (Odds Ratio, OR = 1.29; 95% confidence interval, CI: 0.56, 3.00, age (OR = 0.99, CI: 0.98, 1.01), sex (OR = 0.81, CI: 0.64, 1.02) and smoking (past smoking OR = 1.06, CI: 0.82, 1.36; current smoking OR = 0.69, CI: 0.46, 1.03). Family history of colorectal cancer was significantly related to colorectal cancer (OR = 1.46, CI: 1.08, 1.96)."

[†] GD Batty, MJ Shipley, MG Marmot, et al. Leisure time physical activity and disease-specific mortality among men with chronic bronchitis: Evidence from the Whitehall study. *Am J Pub Health*. 2003;93:817–821.
[‡] B Cox, MJ Sneyd School milk and risk of colorectal cancer: A national case-control study. *Am J Epidemiol*. 2011;173:394–403.

CHAPTER 9 | Communicating Results of Epidemiologic Studies

Odds ratios for selected variables[§]		
Characteristic	**Odds ratio**	**95% confidence interval**
Age (individual years)	0.99	0.98, 1.01
Sex		
Male	1.00	
Female	0.81	0.64, 1.02
Family history of colorectal cancer		
No	1.00	
Yes	1.46	1.08, 1.96
Smoking		
Never	1.00	
Past	1.06	0.82, 1.36
Current	0.69	0.46, 1.03
History of ulcerative colitis or Crohn's disease		
No	1.00	
Yes	1.29	0.56, 3.00

a. Can you identify some problems with this description that render it less than ideal?

[§]Based on: B Cox, MJ Sneyd. School milk and risk of colorectal cancer: A national case-control study. *Am J Epidemiol.* 2011;173:394–403.

Epidemiologic Issues in the Interface with Public Health Policy

CHAPTER 10

10.1 INTRODUCTION

Epidemiology has played a major role in shaping public health policy and prevention, with examples spanning from Snow's classic 19th century cholera studies leading to the closing of the Broad Street water pump[1] to the United States Preventive Services Task Force recommendations for the primary prevention of cardiovascular diseases by promotion of physical activity and a healthful diet.[2] The translation of study findings into the practice of public health, however, is not an easy task. Policy makers typically grade the quality of the evidence to decide whether it is strong enough to support implementing a program or service (Exhibit 10-1). Randomized clinical trials are considered as providing the best level of evidence,[3,4] but their application to study questions relevant to health policy is frequently limited by ethical or feasibility concerns. Moreover, even decisions based on results from such trials are often difficult, as underscored by the inconsistent results from large clinical trials on the effectiveness of mammography as a screening tool for breast cancer.[5,6]

The problems associated with experimental evidence are compounded when nonexperimental study designs are used, as in these studies confounding and bias are more

EXHIBIT 10-1 Levels of evidence

Grade	Level of evidence	Description of level
A	1a	Systematic review (with homogeneity) of randomized clinical trials
	1b	Individual RCT (with narrow confidence interval)
	1c	"Natural experiments," i.e., interventions with dramatic effects (e.g., streptomycin for tuberculosis meningitis; insulin for diabetes)
	2a	Systematic review (with homogeneity) of cohort studies
	2b	Individual cohort study or randomized clinical trial of lesser quality (e.g., with < 80% follow-up)
B	2c	Outcomes research (based on existing records)
	3a	Systematic review (with homogeneity) of case-control studies
	3b	Individual case-control study
C	4a	Temporal (before-after) series with controls, and cohort and case-control studies of lesser quality
	4b	Temporal (before-after) series without controls
D	5	Expert opinion without explicit critical appraisal, or not based on logical deduction

Source: Based on: The Canadian Task Force on the Periodic Health Examination. *Canadian Guide to Clinical Preventive Health Care*. Canada: Health Canada; 1994; U.S. Preventive Services Task Force. *Guide to Clinical Preventive Services*. U.S. Department of Health and Human Services, Office of Disease Prevention and Health Promotion; 2003; M Bigby M Szklo Evidence-Based Dermatology. In: IM Freedberg, AZ Eisen, K Wolff et al. (eds). *Fitzpatrick's Dermatology in General Medicine*, 6th ed. New York, NY: McGraw-Hill Medical Publishing Division; 2003, pp. 2302.

likely to occur. Other challenges to the inferential process leading to policy recommendations are common to both experimental and nonexperimental studies, such as lack of consistency across studies, particularly in the presence of weak associations or modest effectiveness.

In this chapter, some epidemiologic issues related to the use of exposure–outcome association data in the development of policy recommendations are discussed. Descriptions of Rothman's causality model[7] and of Hill's guidelines to infer causality[8] in the context of their application to the decision-making process are also part of this chapter. Other relevant topics, such as weak associations and homogeneity among studies, are discussed along with the causality guidelines. It should be emphasized that this chapter does not elaborate on many issues that are of interest to health policy students and experts, such as the influence of politics on policy, or the role of public health or other agencies. Instead, it tries to emphasize the relevance to prevention of topics that are largely of specific concern to those involved in epidemiologic teaching and research. Although many of the examples discussed in this chapter refer to primary prevention, several concepts discussed here are also applicable to secondary prevention and clinical practice.

10.2 CAUSALITY: APPLICATION TO PUBLIC HEALTH AND HEALTH POLICY

Inferring whether an association is causal is key to the use of epidemiologic findings in primary prevention and other interventions that aim at modifying the probability of the outcomes of interest. An in-depth discussion of the different models of causal inference is beyond the scope of this book and can be found elsewhere.[9] For practical purposes, the inductive process of prediction—which consists of generalizing results obtained in one or more studies to different target or reference populations—remains the premier approach that public health professionals and policy makers use.

Criteria to define causality were pioneered by Koch as an effort to identify biologic agents responsible for infectious diseases.[10,11] Koch's postulates required that the organism had to be recovered from each case of disease, that the organism had to be cultured *in vitro* from each case, that reinoculation of the purified organism had to cause disease in another host, and that the organism had to be reisolated from the latter. The validity of Koch's paradigm, as expressed by his postulates, has been shown for several infectious diseases. In contradistinction to Koch's paradigm focusing on single causal agents, however, almost a century later, MacMahon, Pugh, and Ipsen[12] proposed the concept of "web of causation" as a way to emphasize the importance of multiple causes of disease. As stated persuasively by Gordis,[13] risk factors in isolation are rarely either sufficient or necessary to cause disease. Even when necessary causes are present, they are usually not sufficient to produce disease—a fact that is particularly true for conditions, such as tuberculosis and stomach cancer, that in certain populations are rare manifestations of common exposures (*Mycobacterium tuberculosis* and *Helicobacter pylori*, respectively).

The web of causality for stomach cancer sharply underscores the interconnections between multiple risk factors. Although *H. pylori* infection appears to be a necessary causal agent for noncardia gastric cancer,[14] its high prevalence and the relative rarity of this neoplasm strongly suggest involvement of other factors, which may include, for example, smoking and exposure of gastric mucosa to N-nitroso compounds. A possible chain of causality may start with low socioeconomic status and household crowding resulting in exposure to *H. pylori*. A subsequent event may be the ingestion of nitrate-rich foods, such as cured meats; these, in turn, are reduced to nitrites by bacteria found in human saliva and in the stomach, the growth of which is facilitated by a change in acidity brought about by smoking and excessive salt intake. Nitrites then react with secondary amines found in several ingested foods (such as pork-based products) to form N-nitroso carcinogenic compounds. A potent inhibitor of this reaction is vitamin C; thus, its deficiency may yet be another factor that contributes to the formation of these carcinogens and, thus, to the web of causation in non-cardia gastric cancer.[15]

10.2.1 Rothman's Causality Model

The pathogenesis of stomach cancer underscores the importance of assessing a constellation of risk factors, or *component causes*, acting jointly to form what Rothman has named a *sufficient cause*, defined as "a set of minimal conditions and events that inevitably produce disease."[7(p.8)] These conditions or events can act either simultaneously or sequentially, such as for example in the case of initiators and promoters of cancer.

On the basis of Rothman's model, several *sufficient causes* can be postulated for stomach cancer, which are represented in "pie" graphs of *component causes* (Figure 10-1). Each of the complete circles in Figure 10-1 represents a sufficient cause composed of a constellation of component causes. Because the sum of the known component causes of stomach cancer used in these hypothetical examples may not be sufficient to complete a sufficient cause constellation, a variable X_z—which represents one or more

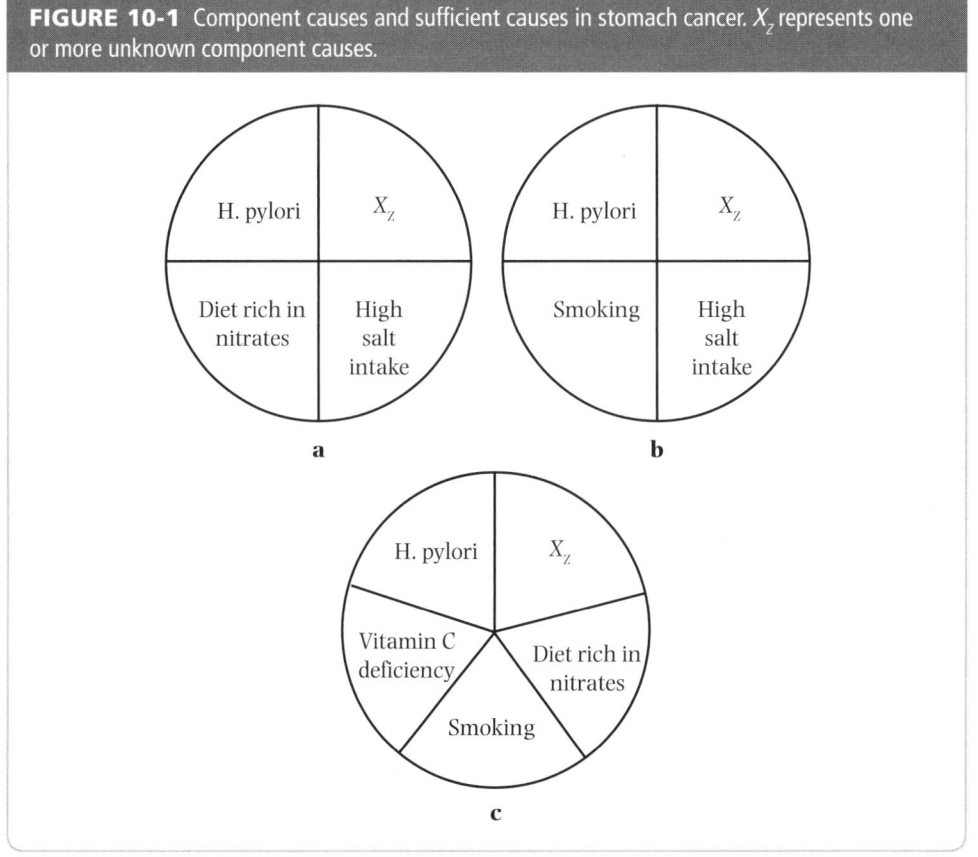

FIGURE 10-1 Component causes and sufficient causes in stomach cancer. X_z represents one or more unknown component causes.

unknown factors acting as component causes—has been added to each complete circle in the figure, as follows.

1. *Sufficient Cause 1*, formed by the component causes, *H. pylori* (a *necessary* component cause), diet rich in nitrates, high salt intake, and X_z (Figure 10-1a).
2. *Sufficient Cause 2*, formed by *H. pylori*, smoking, high salt intake, and X_z (Figure 10-1b).
3. *Sufficient Cause 3*, formed by *H. pylori*, vitamin C deficiency, smoking, diet rich in nitrates, and X_z (Figure 10-1c).

H. pylori, assumed to be a necessary cause, appears as a component cause in all sufficient cause constellations.

When considering Rothman's sufficient causes in the context of preventive activities, the following two issues should be pointed out:

1. Elimination of even a single component cause in a given sufficient cause constellation is useful for preventive purposes, as it will by definition remove the "set of minimal events and conditions," which form that sufficient cause. Consider, for instance, Figure 10-1b: if salt intake were not high, stomach cancer may not occur even if the necessary cause (*H. pylori*) and the other component causes (smoking and X_z) were present. This notion is supported by the fact that, as pointed out previously, although the prevalence of *H. pylori* is very common in certain populations (expressed as a percent), the incidence of stomach cancer in these same populations is fairly rare (expressed as per 100,000).[16]
2. As aptly stated by MacMahon, Pugh, and Ipsen[12(p.18)] several decades ago, "to effect preventive measures, it is not necessary to understand causal mechanisms in their entirety." This important concept is exemplified by Snow's recommendations pertaining to London's water supply many years before Pasteur's discoveries and by Casal and Goldberger's discovery of the nutritional deficiency nature of pellagra well before the actual vitamin involved was discovered.[17,18] Other examples of instances in which identification of an epidemiologic chain amenable to prevention interventions preceded the discovery of the actual causal factor have been discussed by Wynder.[17]

10.2.2 Proximate, Intermediate, and Distal (Upstream) Causes, and Prevention

Several researchers[19,20] have criticized epidemiology's modern tendency toward reductionism, with a primary focus on proximate component causes, particularly those related to biologic markers of risk. These reductionistic approaches tend to be in tune with clinically oriented, "high-risk" strategies for prevention. In contrast, the study of more upstream causes may provide clues for the development of prevention strategies at the level of the total target population. As argued by Rose,[21,22] the population-wide approach based on distal causes—for example, those related to social determinants of disease—might be the most effective prevention strategy for the total population. An example is stroke prevention by either hypertension prevention or treatment. A model representing the chain of causality for stroke is proposed in Figure 10-2. In addition to the distal and proximal sufficient causes, this model also recognizes that there may be an intermediate sufficient cause. In addition, it considers the time sequence of distal,

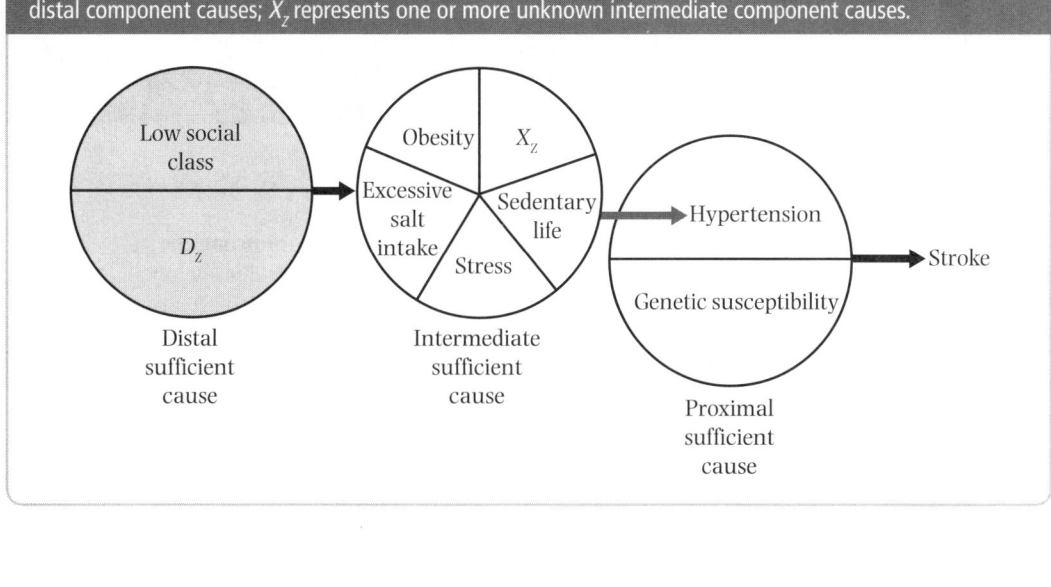

FIGURE 10-2 Component causes and sufficient causes in stroke. D_z represents one or more unknown distal component causes; X_z represents one or more unknown intermediate component causes.

intermediate, and proximal causes. In this example, the component causes, low social class and D_z, are conceptualized as a distal sufficient cause, which in turn results in the intermediate sufficient cause formed by obesity, excessive salt intake, stress, sedentary life, and X_z. This intermediate sufficient cause is responsible for a proximal component cause, hypertension, which along with genetic susceptibility, is part of the proximal sufficient cause of stroke. As previously, the subscript Z represents component causes needed to complete each sufficient cause constellation above and beyond known component causes.

Using this example, the focus of a typical "high-risk" preventive strategy could, for example, be one of the most proximate causes—severe hypertension—that would be identified and treated. Although the relative risk of stroke associated with severe hypertension is high, the prevalence of this type of hypertension is much lower than that of prehypertension plus moderate hypertension, which, notwithstanding its weaker association with stroke, is related to a much higher attributable risk in the population (Figure 10-3). Exhibit 10-2 shows that, although the relative risk of stroke associated with stage 2 hypertension is very high (4.0), its attributable risk is less than that associated with prehypertension, notwithstanding the latter's much lower relative risk (1.5); this is because the prevalence of prehypertension (50%) is much higher than that of stage-2 hypertension (approximately 5%).[23]

The use of a population-wide strategy, consisting of primary prevention by intervention on the distal or intermediate component causes represented in Figure 10-2 could shift the entire blood pressure distribution curve to the left. Examples of this strategy include an improvement in the socioeconomic status of the target population, regulating salt content in processed foods, or promoting the development of urban environments and public transportation options that encourage residents' physical activity. As a result, the prevalence of both prehypertension, moderate and severe hypertension in the total population would decrease (Figure 10-4), resulting in a decrease in stroke incidence of a much greater magnitude than that achieved by the "high-risk" approach. It has been estimated, for example, that a 33% decrease in average salt intake in the population at large would result in a 22% reduction in the incidence of stroke; in comparison, even

FIGURE 10-3 The "high risk" approach focuses on individuals with severe hypertension. Although the relative risk for stroke is high in individuals with severe hypertension (compared to those with normal blood pressure), the prevalence of severe hypertension in the total population is low, and thus the associated population attributable risk is low. Most cases of stroke originate among those with moderate hypertension, the prevalence of which is high.

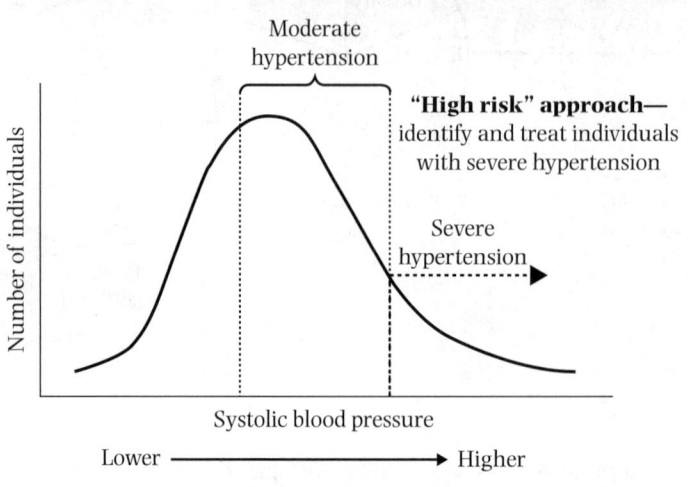

EXHIBIT 10-2 Relative risks and attributable risks for severe (stage 2) hypertension and prehypertension.

$$AR_{POP} = \frac{\text{Prevalence}_{RF}(RR - 1.0)}{\text{Prevalence}_{RF}(RR - 1.0) + 1.0}$$

Stage 2 hypertension (SBP = 160 + or DBP = 100+ mmHg)* and stroke

- Relative risk ~4.0

- Prevalence ~ 5%

$$AR_{POP} = \frac{0.05(4.0 - 1.0)}{0.05(4.0 - 1.0) + 1.0} \times 100 = 13\%$$

Prehypertension (SBP 120–139 or DBP 80–98 mmHg)* and stroke

- Relative risk ~ 1.5

- Prevalence ~ 50%

$$AR_{POP} = \frac{0.50(1.5 - 1.0)}{0.50(1.5 - 1.0) + 1.0} \times 100 = 20\%$$

*Based on: AV Chobanian, GL Bakris, and HR Black, The Seventh Report of the Joint National Committee on Prevention, Detection, Evaluation and Treatment of High Blood Pressure: The JNC 7 Report. *Journal of the American Medical Association*, 2003;289:2560–2572.

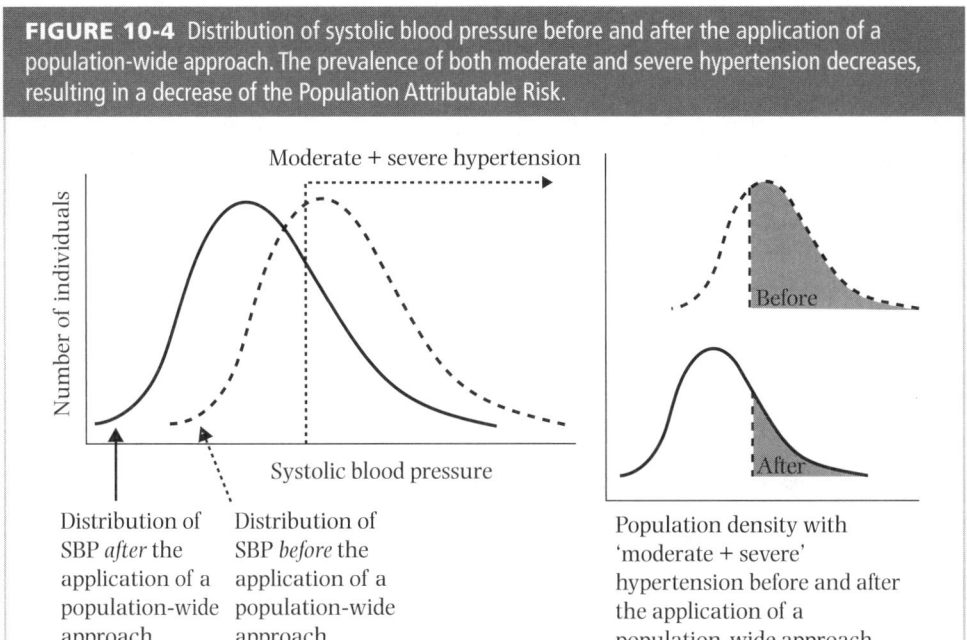

FIGURE 10-4 Distribution of systolic blood pressure before and after the application of a population-wide approach. The prevalence of both moderate and severe hypertension decreases, resulting in a decrease of the Population Attributable Risk.

if all hypertensive patients were identified and successfully treated, this would reduce stroke incidence by only 15%.[24] Similar decreases in all other modifiable hypertension component causes would obviously be expected to have even a greater impact on stroke (and coronary heart disease [CHD]) incidence than salt reduction alone. Thus, when distal or even intermediate component causes are known, primary prevention based on these causes is generally more effective than intervention on proximal causes.

Because screening aims at identifying individuals who already have the disease, it can be regarded as the embodiment of the "high-risk" approach. Taking this approach even further is selective screening, based on two or more steps.[25] In a two-step screening, the first step is the identification of "high-risk" individuals—for example, those with a given trait T—and the second, the application of the screening test. In the example illustrated in Table 10-1, 100,000 women aged 50–64 years undergo selective screening for incident breast cancer based first on identification of those with a family history (comprising 53% of this population) who, in a second phase, are referred to a mammographic exam. Based on published data, the sensitivity and specificity for the discrimination of incident breast cancer are assumed to be, respectively, 0.54 and 0.53 for family history,[26] and 0.93 and 0.99 for mammography.[27] At the end of this two-step screening approach, the overall ("program") sensitivity is estimated to be 0.50. If mammography had been applied to the total population (and not just to those with a positive family history), approximately 11 true cases would have been missed (obtained by multiplying the total number of true cases by the complement of the sensitivity). With the two-step approach exemplified in the table, 64 additional cases are missed (i.e., 69 + 6 − 11), thus, underscoring the loss of sensitivity resulting from this "high–high-risk" strategy. This example highlights the notion that the main reason for using a high-risk strategy is related to cost-effectiveness, rather than to effectiveness alone.

TABLE 10-1 Program validity of a "high-risk" approach in incident breast cancer screening in a population of 100,000 women aged 50–64 years. "High-risk" is defined by presence of a family history of breast cancer with sensitivity = 0.54 and specificity = 0.53.* Those with a family history undergo mammography, with sensitivity = 0.93 and specificity = 0.99.† Yearly incidence of breast cancer is assumed to be about 150/100,000.

Step 1. Identification of individuals with a positive family history

Family history	Disease present	Disease absent	Total
Present	81	52,920	53,001
Absent	69	46,930	46,999
Total	150	99,850	100,000
	Sensitivity = 0.54	Specificity = 0.53	

Step 2. Mammography in those with a positive family history

Test	Disease present	Disease absent	Total
Positive	75	529	604
Negative	6	52,391	52,397
Total	81	52,920	53,001
	Sensitivity = 0.93	Specificity = 0.99	

Program's sensitivity = 75 ÷ 150 = 0.50
(also calculated as the product of the two sensitivity values, or 0.54 × 0.93 = 0.50)

Program's specificity = [46,930 + 52,391] ÷ 99,850 = 0.995
(also calculated as the complement of the product of the complements of the specificities: 1 − [1 − 0.53] × [1 − 0.99] = 0.995)

*LC Hartmann, TA Sellers, MH Frost, et al., Benign Breast Disease and the Risk of Breast Cancer. *New England Journal of Medicine*, 2005;353:229–237.
†AI Mushlin, RW Kouides, and DE Shapiro, Estimating the Accuracy of Mammography: A Meta-Analysis. *American Journal of Preventive Medicine*, 1998;14:143–153.

10.2.3 Social Determinants

Epidemiology as a formal discipline started in 19th century Great Britain with a heavy emphasis on the importance of the unequal distribution of morbidity and mortality by social class. The recent renewed interest in the study of social determinants of health and disease—which had previously peaked in the 1960s and 1970s[28,29]—has focused on a multilevel causality framework, whereby the exclusive emphasis on proximate causes (e.g., smoking in relation to coronary thrombosis, hypertension as a cause of stroke) has been changed to reflect the interdependence between proximate and more distal or upstream (ecological) variables (e.g., high serum cholesterol levels resulting from difficult access to healthy foods, which, in turn, is at least partly determined by social class) (see Chapter 1, Section 1.3). The model subscribed to by social epidemiologists favors neither a reductionistic ("proximate cause-oriented") nor a purely ecological, socially determined approach (based on upstream causes), but rather a consideration of both types of component causes in the search for sufficient causes.[20]

A growing methodologic interest in the interface between individual-level (usually proximate) and group-level (usually distal or intermediate) variables has led to the development of analytical strategies that take into consideration both types of variables. Excellent summaries of these strategies can be found in the literature.[30,31]

10.2.4 Hill's Guidelines

The so-called Hill's criteria, which have been referred to more aptly by Gordis as "guidelines,"[13] were originally published as part of the first Surgeon General Report on Smoking and Health[32] and comprise a series of aspects of a statistical association that, when present, may strengthen the inference that the statistical association is also causal;[8] however, with the exception of "temporality" (discussed later), failure to satisfy any or even most of these guidelines does not necessarily constitute evidence that the association is not causal.[13,33]

Notwithstanding the renewed interest in models of causality over the last few years (see, for example, Greenland and Brumback[34]), Hill's guidelines remain as the cornerstone of causal inference for the practical epidemiologist and health policy expert. The overarching implicit questions that these guidelines seek to address are whether confounding and bias are reasonable alternative explanations for an observed statistical association and, if not, whether a cause–effect relationship can be inferred. What follows is an attempt to expand the discussion on Hill's guidelines and its related issues of meta-analysis and publication bias, with a particular emphasis on consistency of associations across studies. Another issue related to the process of causal inference, sensitivity analysis, is also briefly discussed.

1. *Experimental evidence*: Because randomized trials in humans usually offer the best protection against confounding and bias, they are widely regarded as the "gold standard" for determining causal associations; thus, they are thought to provide the highest level of evidence for developing recommendations pertaining to preventive and clinical interventions (Exhibit 10-1).[3,4] In epidemiologic or public health research, however, random allocation is often either not feasible (e.g., when studying social class as a determinant) or ethically acceptable (e.g., when studying the consequences of a potentially harmful environmental exposure); as a result, these trials are typically limited to assessing interventions that are expected to have a beneficial effect. Internal validity of a randomized trial is optimal when single interventions (e.g., a drug or a vaccine) are studied; from this viewpoint, it may be considered as the epitome of reductionism in epidemiology. In addition to the problems related to open trials of effectiveness, such as poor compliance and "cross-overs," when interventions pertain to only part of the component causes of sufficient cause constellations, results of randomized trials can be erroneously generalized. A possible example is the Finnish trial of smokers, which could not confirm experimentally the results of observational studies suggesting that a diet rich in beta-carotene and alpha-tocopherol reduced lung cancer incidence.[35] Although this trial's results may have accurately expressed these nutrients' lack of efficacy, they may have alternatively reflected the fact that, without considering their complex relationships (including possible interactions) with other dietary components, intake of beta-carotene or alpha-tocopherol may not be not enough to influence a sufficient cause of lung cancer. In other words, the trial likely provided the response to the question asked by its authors (i.e., that using these nutrients as simple pills is not effective in preventing cancer in smokers); however, this response should not necessarily lead to the inference that

alpha-tocopherol and/or beta-carotene are not protective if consumed in their natural states as part of a healthy diet.

2. *Temporality*: The presence of the right temporal sequence, "possible cause → possible effect," per se does not constitute proof that the first event caused the second. Thus, for example, the fact that a given viral infection occurring in early life (e.g., measles) precedes a chronic disease (e.g., degenerative arthritis) cannot be said to constitute strong evidence of the former causing the latter. On the other hand, of all of the guidelines by which to judge whether the relationship is causal, the demonstration that the exposure preceded the outcome under investigation is the only one that, if not met, eliminates the possibility of a causal connection. Yet, it is often difficult to establish temporality in epidemiologic studies, particularly when assessing diseases with long subclinical phases and insidious onsets, such as chronic renal disease or chronic lymphocytic leukemia. A special type of temporal bias, discussed in Chapter 4, Section 4.4.2, is "reverse causality," which occurs when the presumed outcome (disease) is responsible for the occurrence of the exposure of interest. Thus, for example, a chronic disease may go undiagnosed for years with a single symptom (e.g., a moderate loss of appetite) that may result in the hypothesized exposure (e.g., an exposure related to a change in diet). Although case-control studies are more amenable to this bias, it may also occur in cohort studies when ascertainment of the disease onset is difficult and the diagnosis is based on symptomatic disease, which may occur long after the subclinical onset of the disease.

3. *Strength of the association*: The rationale for using strength of the association as a guideline to infer causality is that it is more difficult to explain away a stronger than a weaker association on the basis of confounding or bias. Thus, the relationship of lung cancer to active smoking, expressed by a high relative risk, is more likely to be causal than that of CHD to environmental tobacco smoking (passive smoking), for which the relative risk is estimated at between 1.1 and 1.5.[36] As for Hill's guidelines in general (with the exception of temporality), however, observation of a weak association (e.g., those characterized by relative risks below 2.0) does not negate the possibility of causality. For public health purposes, careful consideration of whether a weak association is causal is justified by the possibility that it may result in a high population attributable risk if the exposure prevalence is high (see Chapter 3, Section 3.2.2). As an example, a relative risk of CHD related to environmental tobacco smoke of 1.2–1.3 and an exposure prevalence of 26%[37] would result in a population attributable risk of about 13%, which given the very large absolute number of new coronary events is far from negligible.[38]

The importance of considering the scale (relative versus absolute excess) when assessing the impact of potentially causal—albeit weak—associations is particularly manifest when assessing interactions. With the widespread use of ratio-based models, assessment of interaction has become virtually synonymous with assessment of multiplicative interaction. Yet, as shown in Chapter 6, Section 6.6, evaluation of additive interactions is crucial for public health purposes and can be readily done in the context of ratio-based models.[39,40]

4. *Dose-response (graded pattern)*: The observation of a straightforward monotonic relationship between exposure dose and risk of an outcome is regarded as strong evidence that a cause–effect relationship exists (Figure 10-5A). There are numerous examples of this type of pattern in the epidemiologic literature (e.g., smoking and lung cancer, blood pressure and stroke). In a meta-analysis of the relationship between birth weight and leukemia (discussed later), the authors used the observation of consistent linear dose-response associations across studies as further evidence that the association was likely causal (Figure 10-6).[41] Causal relationships, however, may also be characterized by other types of patterns reflecting the biologic mechanisms underpinning these relationships. Thus, for example, the association between alcohol intake and cardiovascular mortality seems to follow a J-shaped relationship (Figure 10-5B) probably because at low intake levels alcohol may be protective against atherosclerotic disease through an increase in serum high-density lipoprotein concentration, platelet activation inhibition (and thus coagulation inhibition), and antioxidant activity; however, at higher levels its harmful effects on blood pressure may predominate.[42] Another type of pattern is that in which the excess risk only appears above a certain exposure level (i.e., a certain threshold) (Figure 10-5C). As an example, in early analyses of the Framingham study data, relative weight seemed to be related to an increased incidence of atherothrombotic brain infarction in men aged 50–59 years only at high levels (Figure 10-7).[43] An exposure-outcome association pattern may, in addition, be dose-independent, for example, that seen in allergic disorders to certain environmental exposures, such as medications, pollen, and others.

Although confounding or bias are regarded as having less explanatory value when there is a linear dose-response pattern of the type shown in Figure 10-5A, it must be emphasized that this may not be the case if there is a correlation between the level of the exposure of interest and the level of a confounder (or the level of information bias). An example is the relationship of excessive alcohol intake to lung cancer, which may show a graded pattern because of

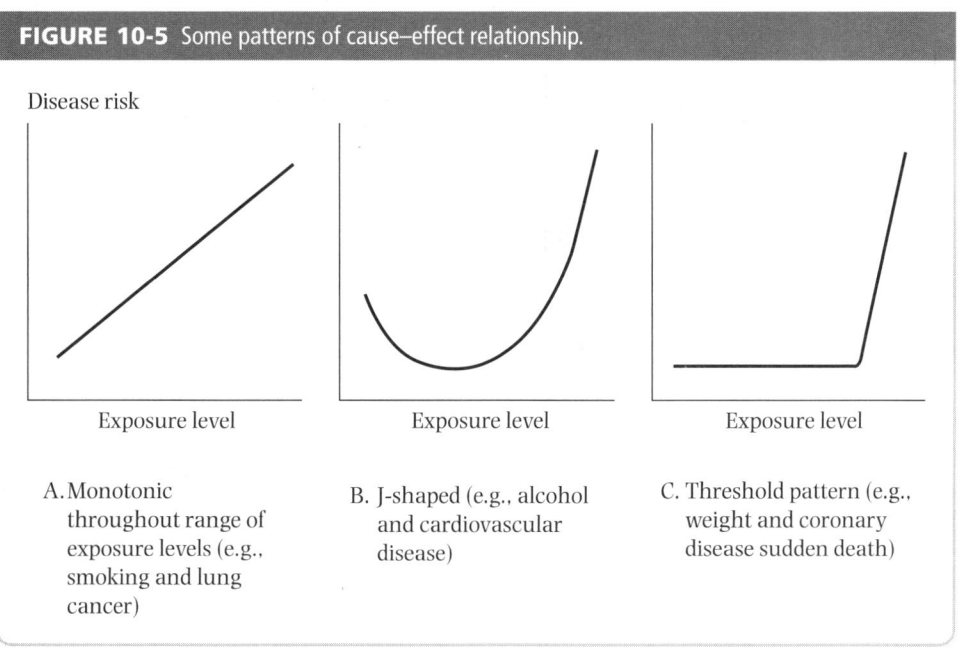

FIGURE 10-5 Some patterns of cause–effect relationship.

A. Monotonic throughout range of exposure levels (e.g., smoking and lung cancer)

B. J-shaped (e.g., alcohol and cardiovascular disease)

C. Threshold pattern (e.g., weight and coronary disease sudden death)

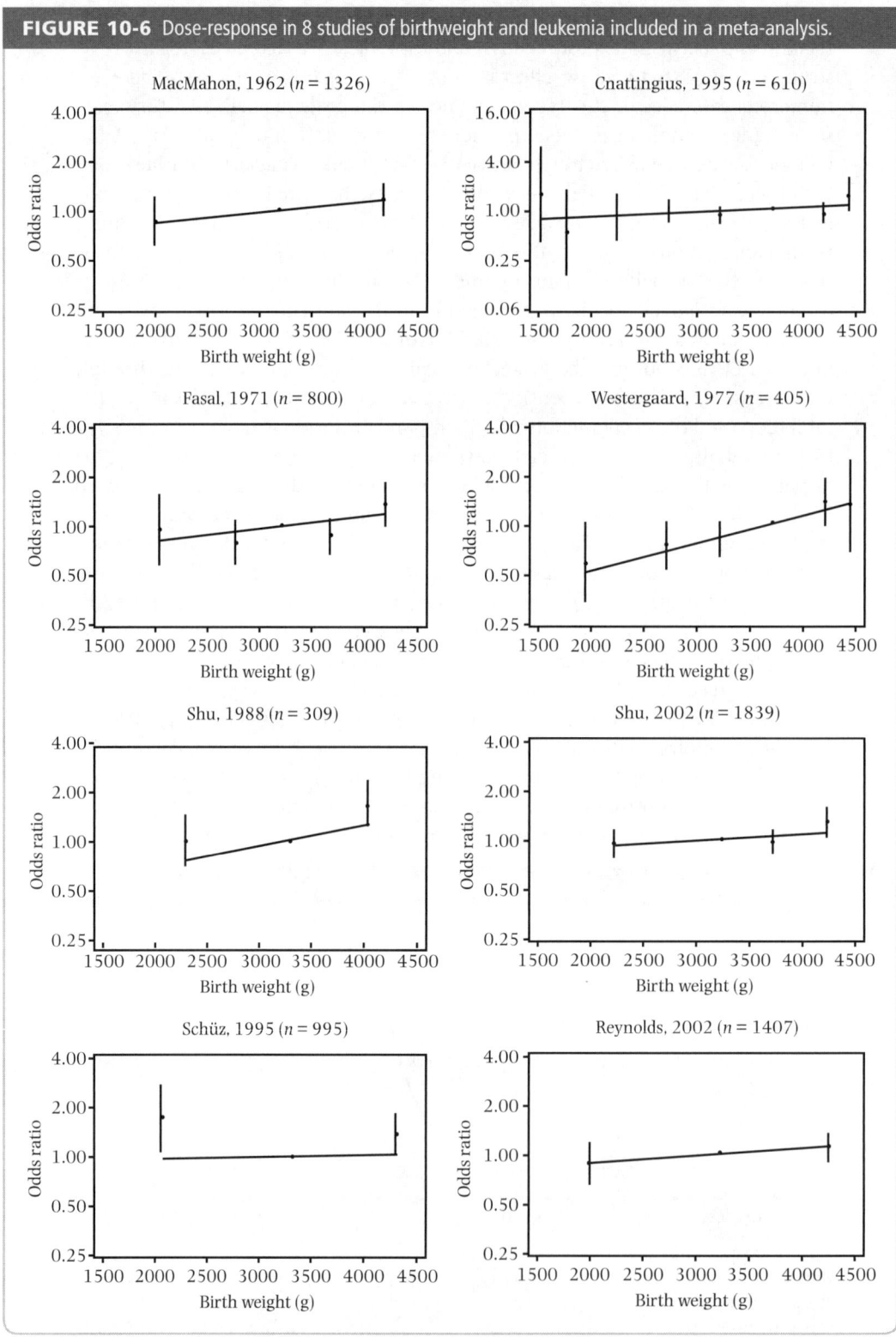

FIGURE 10-6 Dose-response in 8 studies of birthweight and leukemia included in a meta-analysis.

Source: Data from LL Hjalgrim, T Westergaard, and K Rostgaard, Birth Weight as a Risk Factor for Childhood Leukemia: A Meta-Analysis of 18 Studies. *American Journal of Epidemiology*, Vol 158, pp. 724–735, © 2003.

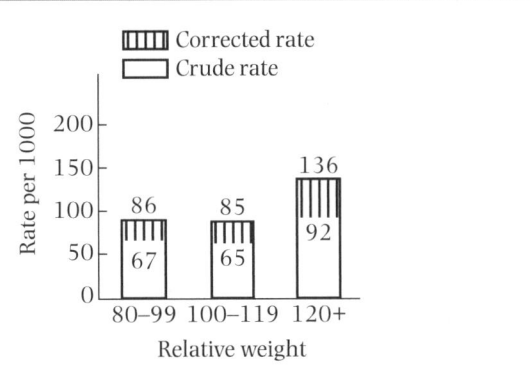

FIGURE 10-7 Risk of atherothrombotic brain infarction in relation to relative weight,* men aged 50–59 years. The Framingham Study.

*Relative weight was determined by comparing the weight of the individual to the median for the age and sex group applicable.
Source: Courtesy of the Harvard University Press. TR Dawber. *The Framingham Study. The Epidemiology of Atherosclerotic Disease*. Cambridge, MA, Harvard University Press, 1980.

the graded relationship between alcohol (the putative risk factor of interest) and the confounder (smoking). In addition, as previously discussed (Chapter 4, Section 4.3.3), both nondifferential misclassification when there are more than two exposure categories and differential misclassification may produce a spuriously graded relationship between exposure and outcome.

5. *Biologic plausibility*: For an association to be causal, it has to be plausible (i.e., consistent with the laws of biology). Biologic plausibility may well be one of the most problematic guidelines supporting causality, however, as it is based on a priori evidence that may not stand the test of time. Thus, for example, vis-à-vis the state-of-the-art scientific knowledge of his time, Snow's hypothesis that cholera was produced by a live organism lacked biologic plausibility altogether. Weed and Hursting[44] go as far as to suggest the dispensability of the biologic plausibility criterion and cite Schlesselman's contention that it "may occasionally impede acceptance of new facts."[45(p.201)]

   Notwithstanding these limitations, biologic plausibility is a useful guideline when it is consistent with the epidemiologic patterns of the exposure–outcome associations. Consider, for example, the J-shaped relationship of alcohol to cardiovascular mortality mentioned previously. Its biologic plausibility is based on the known dose-dependent relationships of alcohol to serum high-density lipoprotein, coagulation factors, and blood pressure, as well as on the knowledge of the roles of these factors in the causal pathways resulting in atherosclerosis.

6. *Consistency*: Consistency of results across epidemiologic studies gets at the heart of inductive reasoning and is highly esteemed by epidemiologists as a guideline to infer causality in observational studies, particularly when ratio-based measures indicate weak associations. Observation of consistent, albeit weak, associations provides the main rationale for the use of meta-analytic techniques for policy decision making (see the next section).

   Consistency among studies, however, should be used as a means to infer causality cautiously, as it may merely reflect consistency of confounding or bias across studies, particularly observational ones.[45] In addition, apparently consistent results across studies may result from publication bias, whereby "positive" results are more likely to be published than null ones (see Section 10.5).

Conversely, lack of consistency does not necessarily constitute evidence against a causal association. The reasons why causal associations may not appear consistent have been described by some authors[46–48] and are summarized as follows.

- *Differences in the specific circumstances of exposure.* Several characteristics of the exposure of interest may cause differences between the results of individual studies, including duration and level. For example, earlier studies of the relationship of estrogen replacement therapy to breast cancer did not take duration into account as accurately as more recent studies[49] and were thus not able to establish firmly the presence of the association.
- *Differences in the timing of the study with regard to the exposure's latency (incubation) period.* When studies are done at different points in time after introduction of a given exposure, they may yield inconsistent results. Plotting the distribution of cases by time after exposure initiation (i.e., constructing an epidemic curve[50,51]) may assist in ascertaining at which point in the curve the study was done. When the minimum latency (incubation) period has not yet gone by in a given study population, investigation of a recently introduced agent cannot detect associations between the agent and the outcome of interest (Figure 10-8).
- *Differences in design and analytic strategies.* Inconsistent results between studies may also result from differences in the confounders included in the statistical models used in data analyses, the sensitivity and specificity of the definitions of exposure and outcome variables, the power of the study, and the length of follow-up (in cohort studies). Use of broad categories of relevant variables is another problem, as it may hide differences in exposure levels between studies; for example, by using merely the categories "yes" and "no" for smoking, differences may occur in the level of tobacco use from study to study, thus resulting in inconsistent values of the measure of association.
- *Differences in the distribution of a component cause.* Differences in results across studies may also reflect differences in the presence of component cause of a sufficient cause constellation. This notion is best understood in the context of effect modification. For example, if a susceptibility gene for salt-induced hypertension varies from population to population, studies conducted in different populations will detect average ("main") effects of high salt intake on hypertension of different magnitudes. Assume the extreme example of a qualitative interaction, in which the relative risk is 3.0 when the susceptibility gene (effect modifier) is present, but is null (1.0) when the gene is absent (Figure 10-9). In this hypothetical example, for the population in which everyone carries the susceptibility gene (a), the relative risk will be 3.0. On the other hand, for populations without the susceptibility gene, the relative risk for hypertension in heavy salt consumers will be 1.0 (b). The lower the prevalence of gene carriers, the nearer the average ("main effect") relative risk will be to 1.0, a phenomenon that has been coined "drowning of susceptibles" (Correa A., personal communication). Consider, for example, the results of the study by Yu et al.[52] on the relationship between smoking and liver cirrhosis in chronic hepatitis B surface antigen carriers (see Section 6.10.2, Table 6-26). In this study, there was marked heterogeneity of the association according to presence of alcohol drinking. Thus, in drinking individuals, the adjusted relative risk for

10.2 Causality: Application to Public Health and Health Policy   405

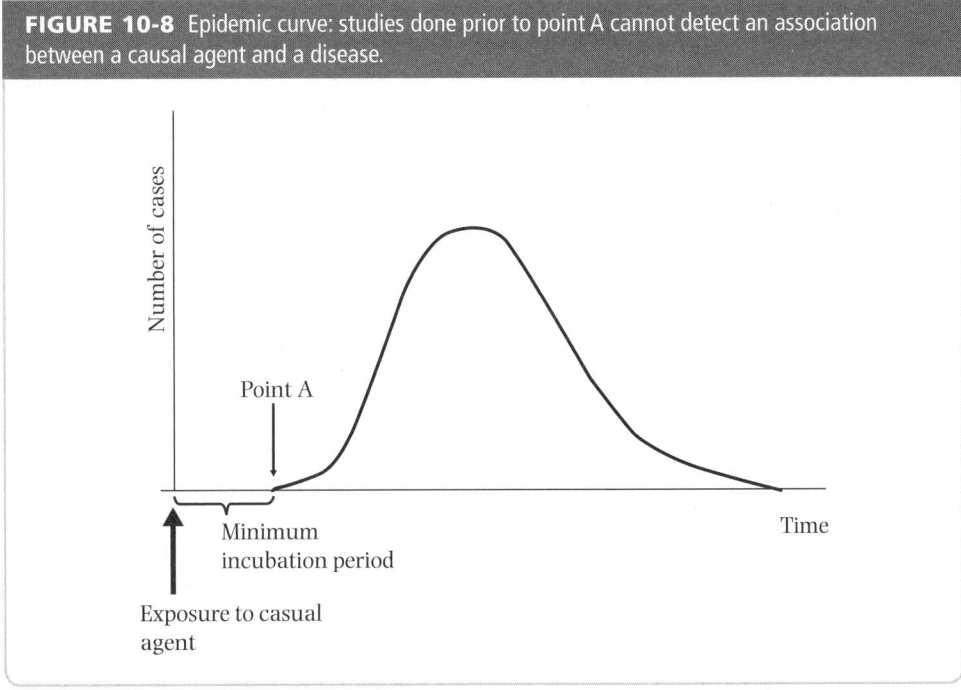

FIGURE 10-8 Epidemic curve: studies done prior to point A cannot detect an association between a causal agent and a disease.

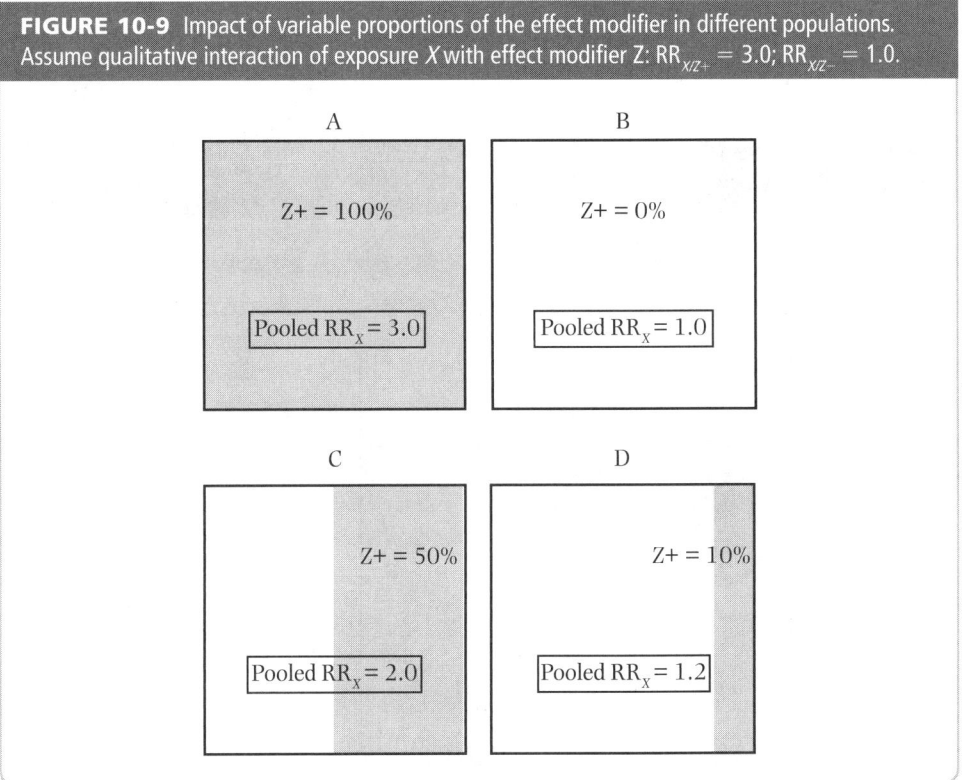

FIGURE 10-9 Impact of variable proportions of the effect modifier in different populations. Assume qualitative interaction of exposure X with effect modifier Z: $RR_{X/Z+} = 3.0$; $RR_{X/Z-} = 1.0$.

heavy smoking was about 9.0, whereas in nondrinkers, it was only 1.9. As a result (and assuming that these adjusted point estimates are the true values), it can be inferred that among hepatitis B surface antigen carriers with a high, compared with those with a low prevalence of drinking, heavy smoking will be a much stronger risk factor for liver cirrhosis.

- *Differences in the stage of the natural history of the underlying process.* The natural history of a given disease is often a lengthy process that starts many years before its clinical manifestations. An example is atherosclerosis, which may begin as early as the first or second decade of life.[53,54] Its clinical expression (e.g., myocardial infarction), however, is not common until the sixth and later decades. Traditional risk factors for clinical atherosclerotic disease include high serum cholesterol levels, hypertension, smoking and diabetes. The role of smoking as a key risk factor had been established early on in the landmark Framingham study.[55] Its association with CHD, however, was not of uniform magnitude in all locations of the Seven Countries Study.[56] In the latter study, the relationship of heavy smoking ($\geq$ 20 cigarettes/day) to CHD was clearly seen in the Northern European but not in the cohort from former Yugoslavia (Figure 10-10). This finding possibly reflects the fact that smoking appears to have a more important role in the development of later (rather than earlier) stages of atherosclerosis (Figure 10-11),[57] which were more prevalent in Northern Europe than in the former Yugoslavia. Thus, when assessing differences in association strengths across populations, it is crucial to consider the natural history of the disease and the fact that the role of each risk factor may be not be equally important in all of its stages.
- *Differences in the effectiveness of interventions.* The applied epidemiologist is often interested in studying the effectiveness of a given preventive intervention, such as a smoking cessation program. A crucial issue usually ignored in evaluating consistency of effectiveness values across studies is that this measure is more

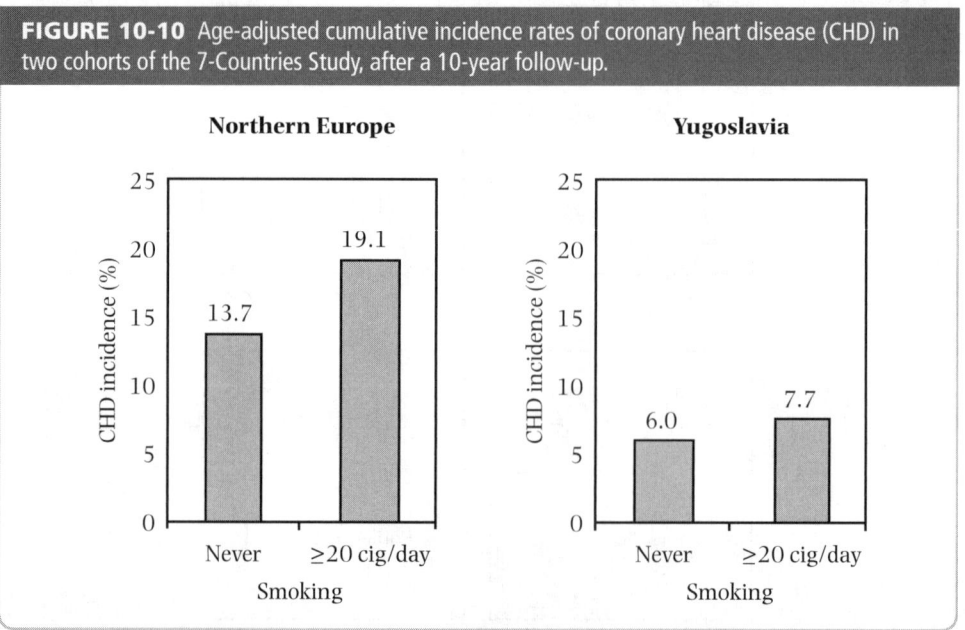

FIGURE 10-10 Age-adjusted cumulative incidence rates of coronary heart disease (CHD) in two cohorts of the 7-Countries Study, after a 10-year follow-up.

Source: Courtesy of the Harvard University Press. A Keys, *Seven Countries Study*, Cambridge, MA, Harvard University Press, 1980.

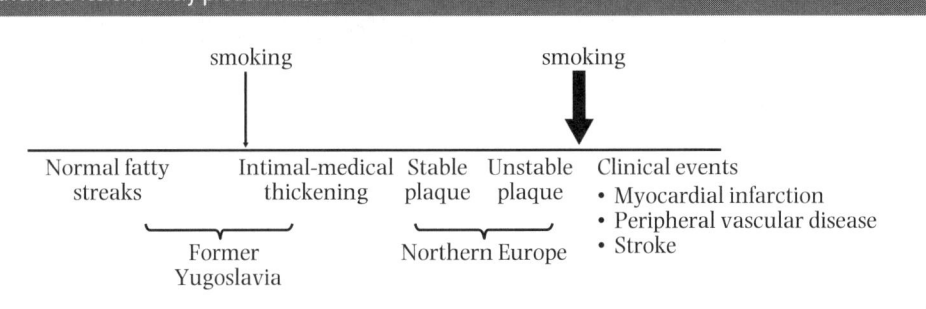

FIGURE 10-11 Smoking seems to be particularly important in later stages of the natural history of atherosclerosis. In the former Yugoslavia, earlier atherosclerotic lesions seemed to predominate, and thus smoking appeared to be a less important risk factor than in Northern Europe, where more advanced lesions likely predominated.

context specific—and thus less generalizable—than efficacy. The use of vaccines in the field underscores the sharp distinction between efficacy and effectiveness. The efficacy of a vaccine may be high, but if the field conditions are not ideal—due, for example, to deterioration of the vaccine because of lack of refrigeration or poor acceptance by the target population—its effectiveness will be compromised.

Another key consideration is that, as persuasively demonstrated by Comstock,[58] observational studies of interventions yield effectiveness, not efficacy estimates. An example is given by an observational study that suggested a negative effectiveness of a needle exchange program (NEP) for prevention of HIV infection in the Montreal area.[59] The explanation for this paradoxical finding, offered by the authors of this study, was that "... because of the availability of clean equipment through pharmacies ... needle exchange programs may have attracted existing core groups of marginalized, high risk individuals ..." and that "in view of the high risk population NEPs, the number of needles may have been less than the actual number needed," which in turn may have led to the use of contaminated needles."[59(p.1001)] An obvious conclusion is that a positive effectiveness may have been achieved under different circumstances than those encountered in this particular study population.

- *Differences in the variability of the risk factor.* As aptly stated by Wynder and Stellman[60(p.459)] with regard to case-control studies, "If cases and controls are drawn from a population in which the range of exposures is narrow, then a study may yield little information about potential health effects." The issue of little variability in the exposure levels is also applicable to cohort studies. For example, as discussed in Chapter 1, Section 1.3, observational studies using individuals as analytic units have been unable to show consistent relationships between salt intake and hypertension (Figure 10-12A); on the other hand, because of the marked interpopulation variability in average salt intake, ecologic studies using country as the unit of analysis have clearly demonstrated a correlation[61] (Figure 10-12B).

Thus, the variability of the risk factor level within a population is a key determinant of whether an association can be found in that population.

Readers might notice the absence of three of the original Hill's guidelines, *coherence*, *analogy*, and *specificity*, of an association from the preceding discussion; we, like others,[13,33] believe that these three guidelines are not too useful for the following reasons: *coherence*

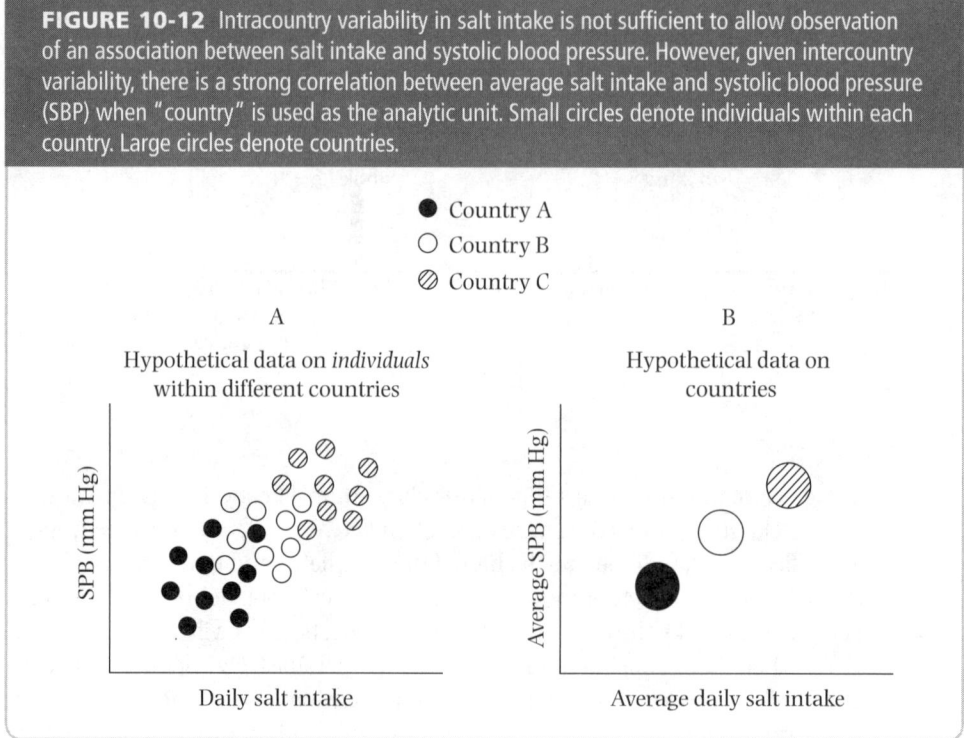

FIGURE 10-12 Intracountry variability in salt intake is not sufficient to allow observation of an association between salt intake and systolic blood pressure. However, given intercountry variability, there is a strong correlation between average salt intake and systolic blood pressure (SBP) when "country" is used as the analytic unit. Small circles denote individuals within each country. Large circles denote countries.

is hard to distinguish from biologic plausibility; *specificity* is inconsistent with state-of-the art knowledge, as it erroneously postulates that a given agent is always associated with only one disease and that the agent can always be found for that disease; and finally, with regard to *analogy*, as aptly pointed out by Rothman and Greenland,[33] "Whatever insight might be derived from analogy is handicapped by the inventive imagination of scientists who can find analogies everywhere."

In the next three sections, four topics closely related to the evaluation of the previous guidelines are briefly discussed: *decision tree*, an approach that is useful when estimating overall effectiveness of a program or intervention; *sensitivity analysis*, a technique to evaluate the impact of errors on study results or of alternative levels of factors influencing effectiveness; *meta-analysis*, an important tool for the evaluation of strength of a given association and consistency across different studies; and *publication bias*, which may strongly affect results of systematic reviews, including meta-analyses.

10.3 DECISION TREE AND SENSITIVITY ANALYSIS

Epidemiologists consistently focus on the quantitative assessment of the impact of random error on the precision (reliability) of effect estimates (e.g., hypothesis testing and calculation of confidence intervals). However, generally little attention is given to the quantitative analysis of the impact of errors—systematic or random—on the estimates' validity. This is the focus of *sensitivity analysis*. Broadly used in fields such as econometrics, environmental sciences, cybernetics, and statistics, sensitivity analysis is a tool to examine the changes in the output (results) of a given model resulting from varying certain model parameters (or assumptions) over a reasonable range. In epidemiology, because of its primary focus on validity, the term *sensitivity analysis* is generally used to refer to the "quantitative assessment of systematic error on an effect estimate."[62(p.451)] It is, however, important to realize that random errors can also affect validity (e.g., regression dilution bias and nondifferential misclassification resulting in bias toward the null hypothesis; see Section 4.3.3); consequently, sensitivity analysis can also be used to assess the impact of such errors on validity (see, e.g., Peppard et al.[63]).

Whether differential or nondifferential, misclassification is one of the primary sources of systematic error that complicates the validity of epidemiologic inference. As discussed in Chapter 4 (Section 4.3.3), when the sensitivity/specificity of exposure/outcome measures are known, estimates of the "corrected" (unbiased) relative risks (or any other measure of association) can be obtained. Misclassification parameters are often unknown, however; in this situation, sensitivity analysis can be used to estimate the association measure under varying (more or less plausible) assumptions regarding these parameters, as illustrated in the following example.

The relative risk expressing the relationship of passive smoking in nonactive smokers (second-hand smoking) to coronary heart disease (CHD) has been found to be around 1.15 to 1.30.[64,65] It could be hypothesized, however, that this excess risk is due to misclassification resulting from the fact that some active smokers self-report as passive smokers. A sensitivity analysis could be based on the assumptions that 5% of active smokers are classified as passive smokers and that all excess risk associated with self-reported passive smoking originate from active smokers misclassified as passive smokers. Under these assumptions, the relative risk for the relationship of active smoking to CHD would have to be 7.0 in order to entirely explain an observed odds ratio of 1.3 for passive smoking.[66] As the relative risk for active smoking and CHD is around 2.0,[67] it can be concluded that, under the stated assumptions, this type of misclassification is unlikely to explain entirely an odds ratio of 1.3 reflecting the association of passive smoking with CHD. (Similar calculations could be done using other reasonable assumptions, e.g., that 10% of active smokers are misclassified as passive smokers.)

In addition to etiologic studies, sensitivity analysis can also be readily applied to studies of effectiveness. Using a hypothetical example, assume that a policy maker wishes to compare the effectiveness of a *new* vaccine with that of a *standard* vaccine. Vaccine *New* is less expensive than vaccine *Standard*, but clinical trials have shown that 30% of those who receive it develop serious adverse effects. The incidence of adverse effects associated with vaccine *Standard*, which has been in use for some time, is 10%. Assuming that it is possible to identify in advance those in whom adverse effects will occur (e.g., pregnant women, individuals with poor nutritional status), only 70% and 90% of the target population are, therefore, eligible to receive vaccines *New* and *Standard*, respectively (Table 10-2, column I). Probabilities of the event (E) that each vaccine is expected to prevent are as follows: for vaccine *New*, 0.08 and 0.40 for those who are and are not eligible to receive it, respectively; for vaccine *Standard*, 0.10 and 0.40 for those who are and are not eligible to receive it, respectively (Table 10-2, column II). The joint probability of E can be estimated by multiplying the proportion of the target population who can or cannot receive the vaccine times the incidence in each stratum (Table 10-2, column III). The sum of these joint probabilities provides the total incidence of E in the target population and is estimated at 17.5% for vaccine *New* and 13% for vaccine *Standard*, thus reflecting a greater effectiveness for *Standard* than for *New* in this example.

Assume that vaccine *New* is less expensive than vaccine *Standard*. Thus, policy makers may wish to know whether further efforts by the laboratory that developed *New*, aiming at achieving the same incidence of adverse effects as that associated with *Standard*,

TABLE 10-2 Probability of event that vaccines *Standard* and *New* are expected to prevent, according to whether or not target population receives the vaccine, assuming a prevalence of eligibility associated with the *Standard* vaccine, *New*, and *Improved* new vaccines of 90%, 70%, and 90% respectively (see text).

			Probability of disease (E) that vaccine is expected to prevent	Joint probability of the event that vaccine is expected to prevent
		(I)	(II)	(III) = (I) × (II)
Eligible to receive *Standard* vaccine	Yes	0.90	0.10	0.90 × 0.10 = 0.09
	No	0.10	0.40	0.10 × 0.40 = 0.04
	Total	1.00		0.09 + 0.04 = 0.13 or 13.0%
Eligible to receive *New* vaccine	Yes	0.70	0.08	0.70 × 0.08 = 0.056
	No	0.30	0.40	0.30 × 0.40 = 0.12
	Total	1.00		0.056 + 0.12 = 0.176 or 17.6%

Effectiveness* of *New* vs *Standard*: [(0.13 − 0.176) ÷ 0.13] × 100 = −35.4%

Imputed values for vaccine *New* (sensitivity analysis)

Eligible to receive *Improved New* vaccine	Yes	0.90	0.08	0.90 × 0.08 = 0.072
	No	0.10	0.40	0.10 × 0.40 = 0.04
Total		1.00		0.072 + 0.04 = 0.112 or 11.2%

Effectiveness* of New (*Improved*) vs Standard: [(0.13 − 0.112) ÷ 0.13] × 100 = 113.8%

*Effectiveness calculated using the formula for *efficacy* (Equation 3.7) applied to the total population that includes both vaccine recipients and nonrecipients.

would make it as, or even more effective than *Standard*. Assuming this new incidence of adverse effects for *New*, a sensitivity analysis (Table 10-2, bottom panel) indicates a slightly lower total incidence of E for vaccine *New* in the target population than that seen for *Standard* (11.2% and 13%, respectively). It can, therefore, be concluded that at the imputed adverse effect levels, although vaccine *New* would be only slightly more effective than vaccine B, its lower cost would likely make it more cost-effective.

In the vaccine example, effectiveness was affected by only one general factor: adverse effects. In most situations, however, there are more than one factor influencing the level of effectiveness. When this happens, a decision tree is a useful tool to estimate the overall effectiveness of an intervention or program. A detailed description of how to construct a decision tree is beyond the scope of this textbook and can be found elsewhere.[69(pp.19–28)] Here, only a simple description and example will be given.

A decision tree, which is part of a decision analysis, has 2 types of nodes: *decision nodes*, which are under the investigator's or policy maker's control, and *chance* (or *probability*) *nodes*, which are not under the investigator's or policy maker's control. In the previous example, assignment of the vaccine to participants is under the epidemiologist's or public health worker's control (control node) whereas the adverse reactions are not (chance node). In the example that follows there is one control node –the decision to implement or not implement intervention A or B—and two chance nodes: tolerance to each intervention and social class. The outcome is mortality. Figure 10-13 displays the decision tree as well as its associated probabilities. Note that,

FIGURE 10-13 Example of decision tree with two chance nodes. Proportions and probabilities shown in parentheses. SC, social class (see text and Exhibit 10-3).

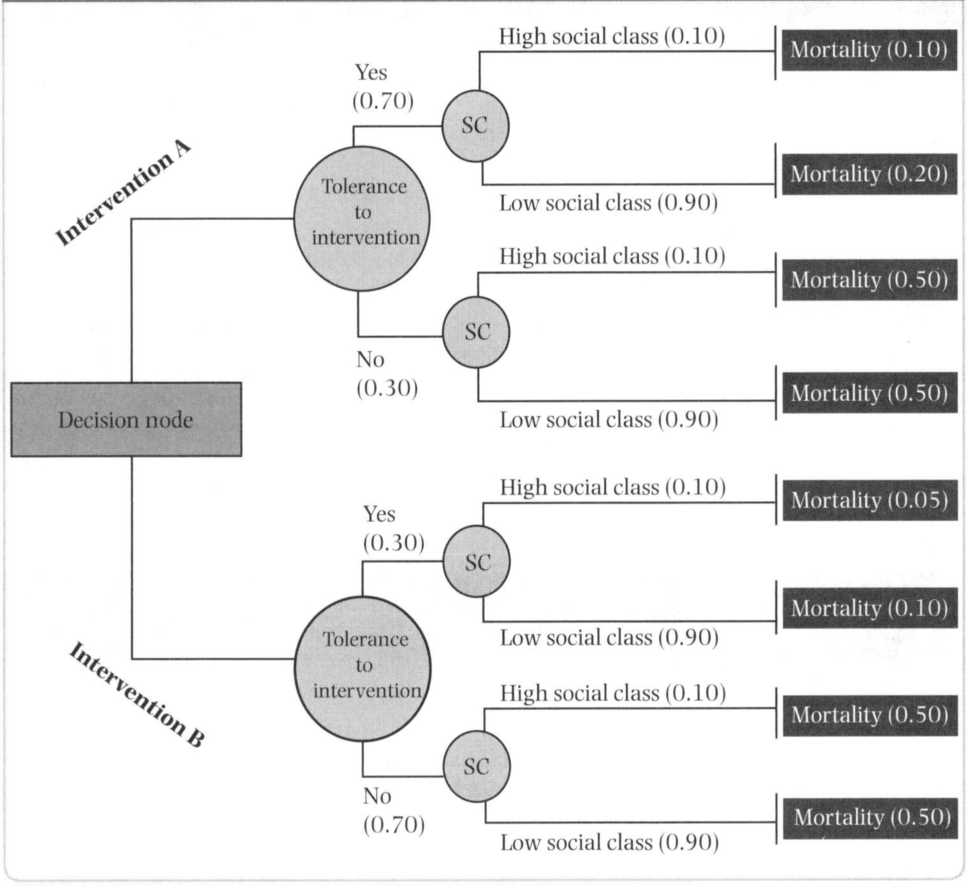

[Decision tree diagram: Decision node branches into Intervention A and Intervention B. Intervention A: Tolerance to intervention — Yes (0.70) → SC → High social class (0.10) → Mortality (0.10); Low social class (0.90) → Mortality (0.20). No (0.30) → SC → High social class (0.10) → Mortality (0.50); Low social class (0.90) → Mortality (0.50). Intervention B: Tolerance to intervention — Yes (0.30) → SC → High social class (0.10) → Mortality (0.05); Low social class (0.90) → Mortality (0.10). No (0.70) → SC → High social class (0.10) → Mortality (0.50); Low social class (0.90) → Mortality (0.50).]

for those who tolerate the intervention, intervention B has a lower mortality than intervention A: for high social class, mortality rates are 0.10 for intervention A and 0.05 for intervention B; for low social class, these rates are, respectively, 0.20 and 0.10. A greater proportion of participants, however, tolerate intervention A (70%) than B (30%). As a result, the overall probability of death—calculated by multiplying the proportions in each pathway shown in Exhibit 10-3—is lower for intervention A than for intervention B: 28.3% vs. 37.85%, respectively. Thus, the effectiveness of A compared with B can be calculated as,

$$\{[(37.85\% - 28.30\%)] \div 37.85\%\} \times 100 = 25.2\%$$

Here, too, a sensitivity analysis can be done, assuming that tolerance to intervention B can be increased to, say, 50% (see Exercise No. 7).

An example of a decision tree based on published results is given in Figure 10-14. In this example, the decision node is to offer drug therapy to hypertensive patients. Chance nodes include whether or not the patients accept the drug therapy, and hypertension control. Incidence of coronary heart disease (CHD) is the outcome of interest. For the patients who do not accept the drug therapy, hypertension control is sometimes achieved by other means (e.g., weight loss or lowering salt intake). CHD incidence rates are identical for those in whom hypertension is controlled, regardless of acceptance of

EXHIBIT 10-3 Effectiveness of Intervention A Compared with Intervention B (Figure 10-13). Intervention B is more efficacious (i.e., those who tolerate the drug have a lower mortality than under Intervention A), but because tolerance to Intervention A is higher, its overall effectiveness is higher. Effectiveness of A (compared with B) = {[37.85% − 28.30%] ÷ 37.85%} × 100 = 25.2%.

Intervention A: less efficacious but better drug tolerance (70%)		Intervention B: more efficacious but less drug tolerance (30%)	
Tolerance	Joint probality of death	Tolerance	Joint probality of death
Yes	0.70 × 0.10 × 0.10 = 0.007	Yes	0.30 × 0.10 × 0.05 = 0.0015
	0.70 × 0.90 × 0.20 = 0.126		0.30 × 0.90 × 0.10 = 0.027
No	0.30 × 0.10 × 0.50 = 0.015	No	0.70 × 0.10 × 0.50 = 0.035
	0.30 × 0.90 × 0.50 = 0.135		0.70 × 0.90 × 0.50 = 0.315
	0.007 + 0.126 + 0.015 + 0.135 = 0.283 (or 28.30%)		0.0015 + 0.027 + 0.035 + 0.315 = 0.3785 (or 37.85%)

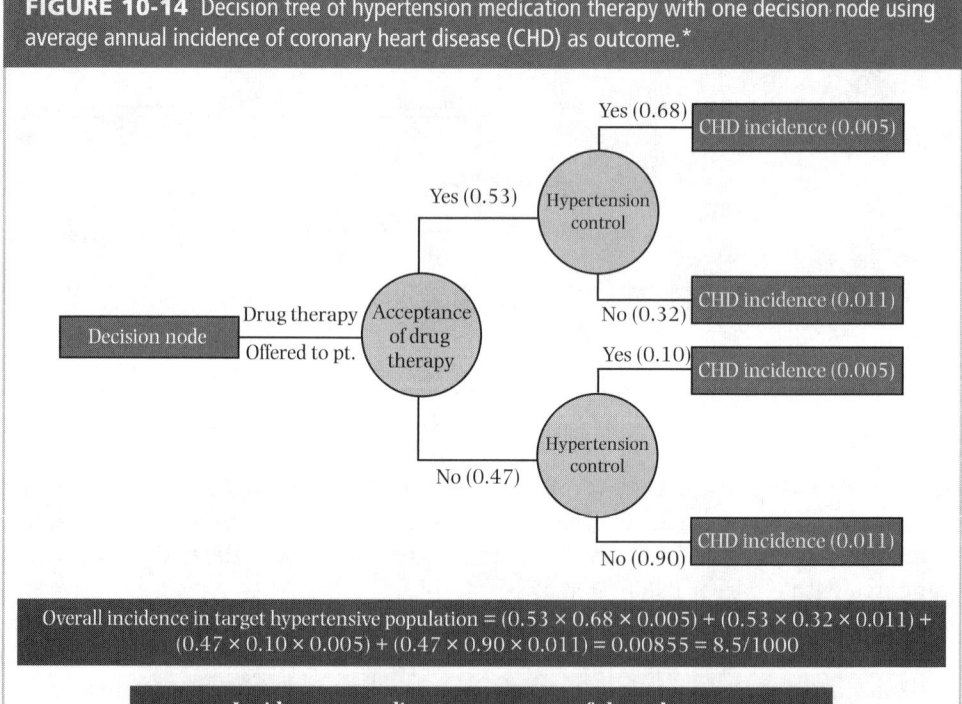

FIGURE 10-14 Decision tree of hypertension medication therapy with one decision node using average annual incidence of coronary heart disease (CHD) as outcome.*

Overall incidence in target hypertensive population = (0.53 × 0.68 × 0.005) + (0.53 × 0.32 × 0.011) + (0.47 × 0.10 × 0.005) + (0.47 × 0.90 × 0.011) = 0.00855 = 8.5/1000

Incidence according to acceptance of drug therapy
Yes: (0.53 × 0.68 × 0.005) + (0.53 × 0.32 × 0.011) = 0.0037 = 3.7/1000
No: (0.47 × 0.10 × 0.005) + (0.47 × 0.90 × 0.011) = 0.0049 = 4.9/1000

*This example is based on real data, but from several studies with different population frames. Thus, it should not be applied to a given target population.
Source: Based on data from FJ Nieto, et al. Population Awareness and Control of Hypertension and Hypercholesterolemia. *Archives of Internal Medicine*, 1995;155:677–684; LE Chambless, et al. Association of Coronary Heart Disease Incidence with Carotid Arterial Wall Thickness and Major Risk Factors. *American Journal of Epidemiology*, 1997;146:483–494; J Moore, Hypertension Catching the Silent Killer. *The Nurse Practitioner*, 2005;30:16–35.

drug therapy (5/1000). However, the proportion of patients achieving hypertension control is much higher in those who accept the drug therapy than in those who do not (68% vs. 10%). As a result, the overall incidence of CHD is 3.7/1000 in the drug therapy acceptance group, and 4.9/1000 in the nonacceptance group. Effectiveness associated with drug acceptance is, thus, (4.9 − 3.7) ÷ 4.9 = 24.5%. Note that, as the figures shown in Figure 10-14 come from different target populations, they must be confirmed. Ideally, the data on the outcome should come from a systematic review and meta-analysis. Thus, for the decision maker, the ideal sequence should be {[meta analysis] → [decision analysis] → [cost-effectiveness analysis]}. The two initial steps are in the realm of epidemiology, whereas the last step (cost-effectiveness) requires the input of health economists.[69]

By using different hypothetical levels of tolerance to interventions, misclassification or other parameters of interest over a reasonable range, an array of plausible values of the effect estimate can be obtained. As an alternative, automated methods to assess the impact of misclassification and other sources of systematic errors and confounding are available.[62,69] These methods are based on multiple iterative reconstructions of the data based on varying selection bias, misclassification, or confounding parameters (or combinations of them), and provide estimates of a distribution of possible "corrected" effect estimates.

10.4 META-ANALYSIS

As aptly defined by Petitti,[69(p.2)] meta-analysis is a "quantitative approach for systematically assessing the results of previous research in order to arrive at conclusions about the body of research" on a given subject. Meta-analysis uses "study" as the unit of analysis, rather than "individual." Its steps include a thorough review of the results of studies dealing with the hypothesis of interest, as well as the statistical analyses of these results. An in-depth discussion of the statistical approaches used by meta-analysts is beyond the scope of this textbook and can be found elsewhere.[68–72] The main features of this technique, however, are briefly described later.

Meta-analysis may be considered as the epidemiologic study of epidemiologic studies (Dr. Bruce Psaty, University of Washington, personal communication). Studies included in a meta-analysis are subjected to predefined inclusion or exclusion criteria, a process that is analogous to that of eligibility for inclusion of individuals in a single study.

Results are typically presented as a summary pooled measure of association that is displayed in a graphic form along with the individual estimates of studies included in the analysis. As an example, Lorant et al.[73] conducted a meta-analysis of the relationship of social class to major depression. When searching the literature addressing the topic, the authors found 743 studies that matched the selected search keywords (e.g., depression, socioeconomic status); however, after the eligibility criteria for inclusion were applied, only a fraction (less than 10%) of these studies were used in the meta-analysis. The results are presented in Figure 10-15 for 51 studies of prevalence done after 1979. The horizontal and vertical axes in this graph correspond, respectively, to the odds ratios (plotted on a logarithmic scale) and the studies included in the meta-analysis. The odds ratio point estimates and their 95% confidence intervals (95% CI) are represented, respectively, by the square black boxes and corresponding horizontal lines. By convention, the area of each black box showing the point estimate is proportional to the precision of the estimate. The solid vertical line is set at the null value (odds ratio = 1.0), denoting the hypothetical lack of association between social class and depression (null hypothesis). When the horizontal lines do not cross this solid vertical line (i.e., when the 95% CIs interval do not include the null value), the odds ratios for those particular studies are statistically significant at an alpha level of 5%.

A diamond (or, in other meta-analyses, an open box or a circle) represents the summary (pooled) measure of association. Meta-analysis can pool both absolute (e.g., attributable risk) and relative (e.g., odds ratio, hazards ratio) measures of association. When a relative measure of association is meta-analyzed, its pooled value can be estimated by using a stratified method akin to that used to estimate adjusted odds ratios or relative risks (see Chapter 7, Section 7.3.3). For example, the Mantel-Haenszel method can also be used to meta-analyze odds ratio data. The weighing scheme used when applying this method of meta-analysis is the same as that used for adjustment of odds ratio in individual case-control studies (i.e., the inverse of the variance of each stratum). Thus, considering each study as a separate stratum and using the notations found in Table 7-9 (Chapter 7), the weight for each stratum is $(b_i \times c_i/N_i)$. The calculation is identical to that shown for individual case-control studies (see Section 7.3.3), providing a weighted pooled estimate of the odds ratio (taking into account the statistical power of each study), as well as allowing estimation of its variance and confidence intervals.

In the example displayed in Figure 10-15, two pooled odds ratios are shown: one uses a random-effects model and another uses a fixed-effects model (akin to the Mantel-Haenszel method just described). There is debate among statisticians as to which of these two meta-analytic strategies is best.[69,74,75] The difference between these models relates to the extent to which results can be generalized: only the specific study populations used in the meta-analysis for the fixed-effects model or a hypothetical "population of studies" for the random-effects model. The latter is more conservative than the former from the statistical precision viewpoint, as it takes into account not only the within-study variance but also the variance between studies.[69] Like the pooling of strata in single studies, the main assumption when pooling measures of association is that results from different studies (the strata)—particularly their directions—are consistent (homogeneous). Homogeneity tests are available to evaluate consistency, and neither method (fixed- or random-effects) is advisable when there is substantial heterogeneity between studies.[76]

In the example shown in Figure 10-15, results are fairly consistent—with all but a handful of the 51 studies showing odds of major depression to be higher in the low than in the high socioeconomic status individuals (denoted as "favor the rich" in the figure).

In another example of meta-analysis, Engel et al.[77] examined the association of Glutathione S-Transferase M1 (GSTM1) null status with bladder cancer (Figure 10-16). GSTM1 is the product of the GSTM1 gene and is involved in the metabolism of polycyclic aromatic hydrocarbons found in tobacco smoke. A null status is related to a reduced clearance of smoking products. This meta-analysis included 17 case-control studies, for a total of about 2150 cases and 3650 controls, and used a random-effects model to estimate the pooled odds ratio at 1.44 (95% confidence interval, 1.23, 1.68). In Figure 10-16 the open circle and its corresponding vertical line represent the pooled odds ratio along with its 95% confidence interval. Note that both in the previous example (Figure 10-15) and in the example shown in Table 10-16, the 95% confidence intervals for the meta-analytic (pooled) odds ratios are very narrow, reflecting the large gain in statistical precision resulting from pooling study results.

Notwithstanding the appeal of a quantitative approach to summarize data from several studies, numerous problems must be considered when conducting a meta-analysis, including the difficulties related to the variable quality of the studies and the

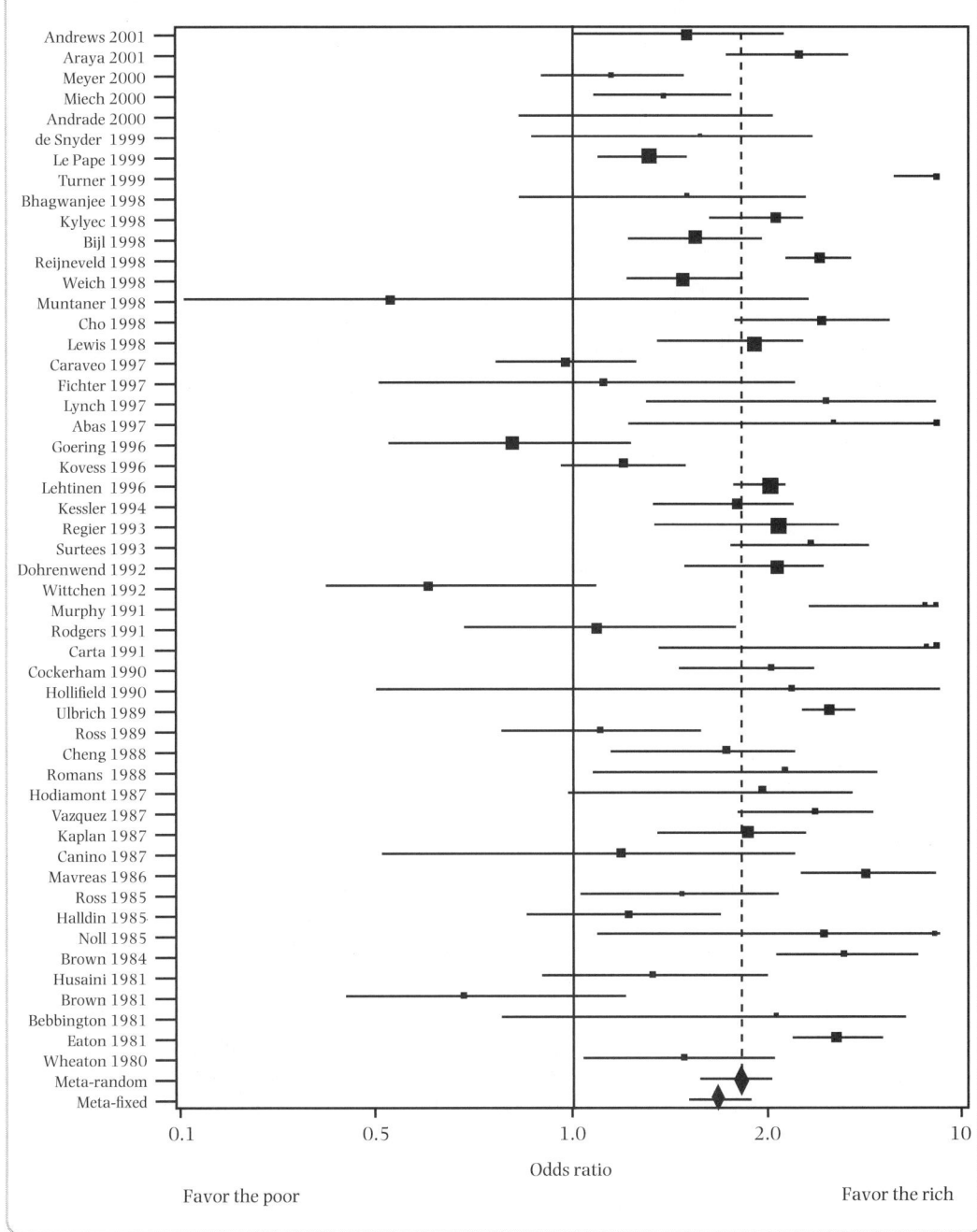

FIGURE 10-15 Odds ratios for major depression by socioeconomic status group in 51 prevalence studies published after 1979. Horizontal lines, 95% confidence intervals. Squares show original estimates; diamonds show meta-analyzed results. The expression "favor the rich" denotes a greater odds of depression in low SES than in high SES individuals.

Source: Data from V Lorant, D Deliege, W Eaton, et al., Socioeconomic Inequalities in Depression: A Meta-Analysis. *American Journal of Epidemiology*, Vol 157, pp. 98–112, © 2003.

fact that different studies use different participant selection and data collection methods, which may result in bias. For these reasons, the use of meta-analytic techniques has been criticized, particularly when applied to observational data. Used judiciously along

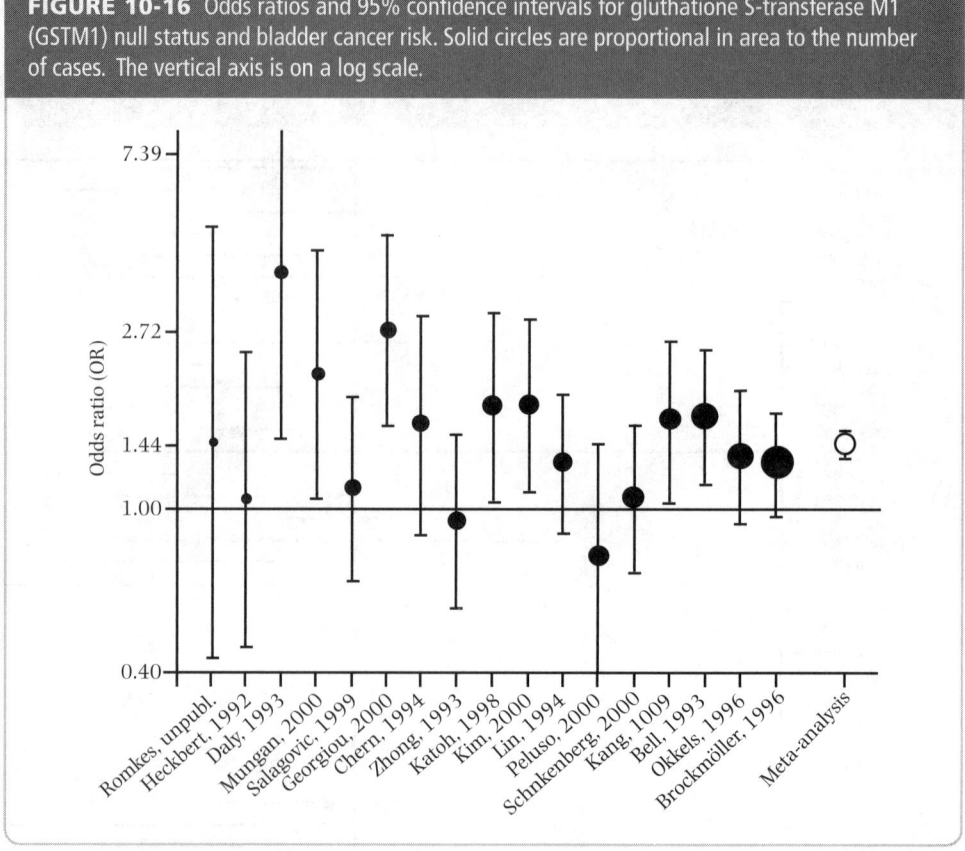

FIGURE 10-16 Odds ratios and 95% confidence intervals for gluthatione S-transferase M1 (GSTM1) null status and bladder cancer risk. Solid circles are proportional in area to the number of cases. The vertical axis is on a log scale.

Source: Data from M Romkes. In LS Engel, E Taioli, R Pfeiffer, et al. Pooled Analysis and Meta-Analysis of Glutathione S-Transferasa M1 and Bladder Cancer: A HuGE Review. *American Journal of Epidemiology.* Vol 156, pp. 95–109, © 2002.

with qualitative reviews of the literature, however, results of meta-analysis may be helpful in decision analysis and analysis of cost-effectiveness of interventions.[69]

10.5 PUBLICATION BIAS

Some common problems that may influence the quality of reporting of epidemiologic studies and that could potentially create reporting biases are discussed in detail in Chapter 9. In this section, we focus on a special type of reporting bias: publication bias.

Assessment of consistency of results of multiple studies and the application of meta-analytic techniques rely heavily on published reports of research results. If papers that favor (or do not favor) a given hypothesis are more likely to be submitted and published, this results in an apparent (biased) consistency and a biased estimation of the pooled measure of association.

Acceptance of the validity of published findings is conditional on two important assumptions: (1) that each published study used unbiased methods (see Chapter 4) and (2) that published studies constitute an unbiased sample of a theoretical population of unbiased studies. When these assumptions are not met, a literature review based on either meta-analytic or conventional narrative approaches will give a distorted view of the exposure–outcome association of interest. Whether these assumptions are met depends on several factors, including the soundness of the study designs and the quality of peer reviews. Publication bias, as conventionally defined, occurs when assumption (2) cannot be met because, besides the quality of the report, other factors dictate acceptability for publication. Direction of findings is one such factor. For example, a study carried out a few decades ago[78] demonstrated that 97% of papers published in four psychology journals showed statistically significant results at the alpha level of 5%, thus strongly suggesting that results were more likely to be published if they had reached this conventional significance level.

Subsequent research[79–83] has confirmed the tendency to publish "positive" results. In a study comparing published randomized clinical trials with completed yet unpublished randomized trials, 55% of the published but only 15% of the unpublished studies favored the new therapy being assessed.[81]

A possible reason for publication bias is the reluctance of journal editors and reviewers to accept negative ("uninteresting"?) results. For example, in a study by Mahoney,[84] a group of 75 reviewers were asked to assess different versions (randomly assigned) of a fictitious manuscript. The "Introduction" and "Methods" sections in all versions were identical, whereas the "Results" and "Discussion" sections were different, with results ranging from "positive" to "ambiguous" to "negative." Reviewers were asked to evaluate the methods, the data presentation, the scientific contribution, and the publication merit. Compared with negative or ambiguous results, the manuscripts with "positive" results systematically received higher average scores for all categories, including the category for evaluation of methods, even though the "Methods" sections were identical in all sets.

Interestingly, however, editors and reviewers may not be the only or even the most important source of publication bias. For example, in Dickersin et al.'s study,[81] publication was intended by the authors for only 12% of unpublished yet completed studies. Reasons given by the authors of why publication was not intended for the remaining 88% included "negative results" (28%), "lack of interest" (12%), and "sample size problems" (11%).

Even source of support seems to interfere with the likelihood of publication. Davidson,[85] for example, found that clinical trials favoring a new over a traditional therapy funded by the pharmaceutical industry had a publication odds 5.2 times greater than that of trials supported by other sources, such as the National Institutes of Health. A similar finding was reported subsequently by Lexchin et al.[86]

Some forms of publication bias are rather subtle, such as "language bias" (e.g., publication in an English language journal versus publication in a journal in another language). For example, Egger et al.[87] compared randomized clinical trials published by German investigators in either German journals or English journals from 1985 through 1994. When articles with the same first author were compared, no evidence of differences in quality between the papers written in German or English was found. In contrast, a strong, statistically significant difference with regard to the significance of findings was present: 63% of the articles published in English reported a statistically significant result compared with only 35% of articles published in German (odds ratio = 3.8; 95% confidence limits 1.3, 11.3). These results strongly suggest that using language as one of the criteria to select studies to be included in a systematic literature review (a criterion that is frequently adopted because of practical reasons or reasons related to access) can seriously undermine the representativeness of published reviews, including those using meta-analytic methods.

Strategies suggested to prevent publication bias include the development of study registers[82,88] and advance publication of study designs.[89] The latter has increasingly found its niche in some peer-reviewed journals (see, e.g., Bild et al.[90]). Prevention of publication bias obviously requires efforts on the part of the scientific community as a whole, including researchers, peer reviewers, and journal editors. The latter should be aware that direction of findings and absence of statistically significant results should not be used as criteria for rejection or acceptance of a paper.

An approach that has been proposed to evaluate the possible presence of publication bias is the "funnel plot."[88,91] To construct the "funnel plot," the values of the measure of association are plotted on one of the graph's axis and the study sample sizes or measures of statistical precision (e.g., standard errors) on the other axis. When there is no publication bias, the graph should have the shape of a funnel, reflecting the sampling variability of studies. The larger, more precise studies will tend to appear close to the center of the "funnel," that is, close to the overall pooled (weighted) estimate; smaller, less precise studies will be expected to appear *symmetrically* distributed on both sides of the average estimate, increasingly distant as their precision decreases (and, thus, the funnel shape). As an example, the funnel plot constructed by Engel et al. for the meta-analysis of GSTM1 null status and bladder cancer is shown in Figure 10-17. Notwithstanding the relatively small number of studies, their odds ratio logarithms (plotted on the vertical axis) fall both in the upper and the lower half of the "funnel" across the precision range of the studies (measured by their standard errors); the plot is, thus, approximately symmetric, thus suggesting that publication bias is not a likely explanation for the findings shown in Figure 10-16.

In contrast, when there is a tendency toward favoring the publication of "positive" results, an asymmetric funnel plot will result. For example, in a systematic review of studies of the genetic epidemiology of stroke, Flossmann et al.[92] presented the funnel

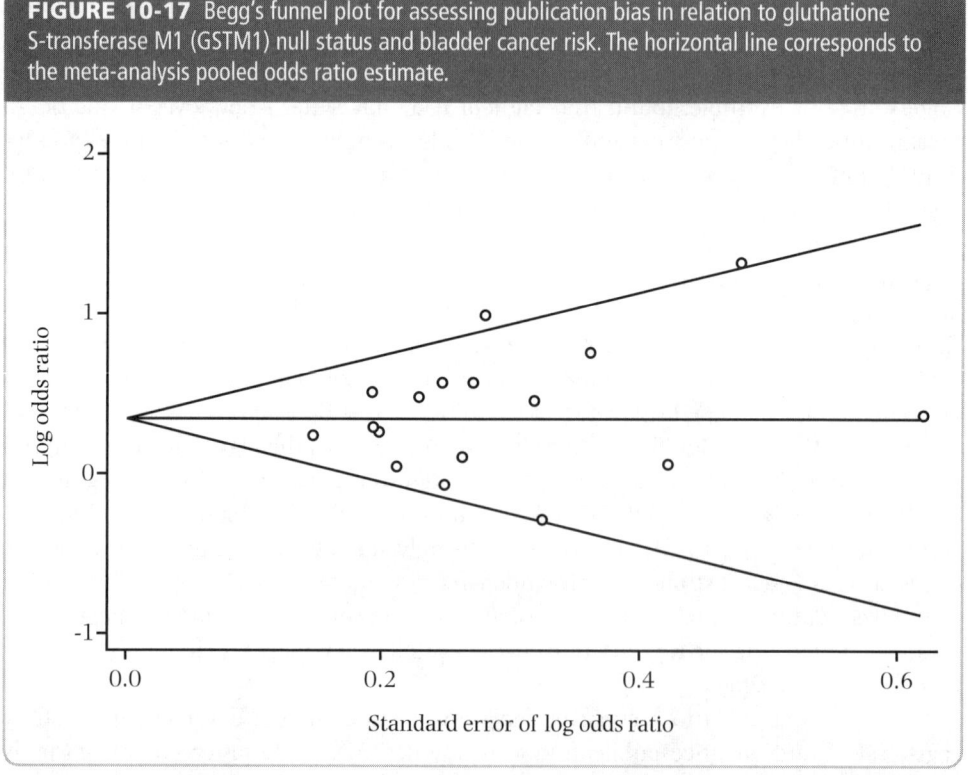

FIGURE 10-17 Begg's funnel plot for assessing publication bias in relation to gluthatione S-transferase M1 (GSTM1) null status and bladder cancer risk. The horizontal line corresponds to the meta-analysis pooled odds ratio estimate.

Source: Data from M Romkes. In LS Engel, E Taioli, R Pfeiffer, et al., Pooled Analysis and Meta-Analysis of Glutathione S-Transferasa M1 and Bladder Cancer: A HuGE Review. *American Journal of Epidemiology*, Vol 156, pp. 95–109, © 2002.

plot shown in Figure 10-18 where the odds ratios are plotted in a logarithmic scale, against a measure of precision (1/standard error). The distribution of odds ratios from the individual studies shows a clearly asymmetric plot, whereby the lower the precision, the more distant is the odds ratio from the null hypothesis. Because, in addition, most studies in this example show odds ratios higher than 1.0, the funnel plot strongly suggests that "negative" studies are not being published. The meta-analytic pooled odds ratio estimate based on this analysis was 1.76, and its 95% CI was 1.7, 1.9, denoting a highly significant result that is nonetheless called into question because of the evidence of publication biased illustrated in Figure 10-18.

Tests of the null hypothesis that the distribution of study results in a funnel plot is homogeneous are available.[93]

A special type of publication bias, which is particularly relevant to clinical trial results, is the selective reporting of outcomes, which occurs when the findings related to the primary endpoints are deemed by the investigators to be "uninteresting"; as a result, the report may address only results pertaining to secondary endpoints that conform to authors' *a priori* expectations. As an example, Chan et al.[94] recorded the number and characteristics of both reported and unreported trial outcomes from protocols, journal articles, and a survey of trialists. An outcome was considered by these authors as incompletely reported if published articles had insufficient information for carrying out a meta-analysis. Overall, about one half of efficacy values and two thirds of harm outcomes per trial were incompletely described. The odds ratios of reporting statistically significant efficacy and harm endpoints (compared with reporting nonstatistically significant results) were, respectively, 2.4 (95% CI, 1.4, 4.0) and 4.7 (1.8, 12.0). More than 60% of the trials had at least one primary endpoint changed, introduced, or omitted. Based

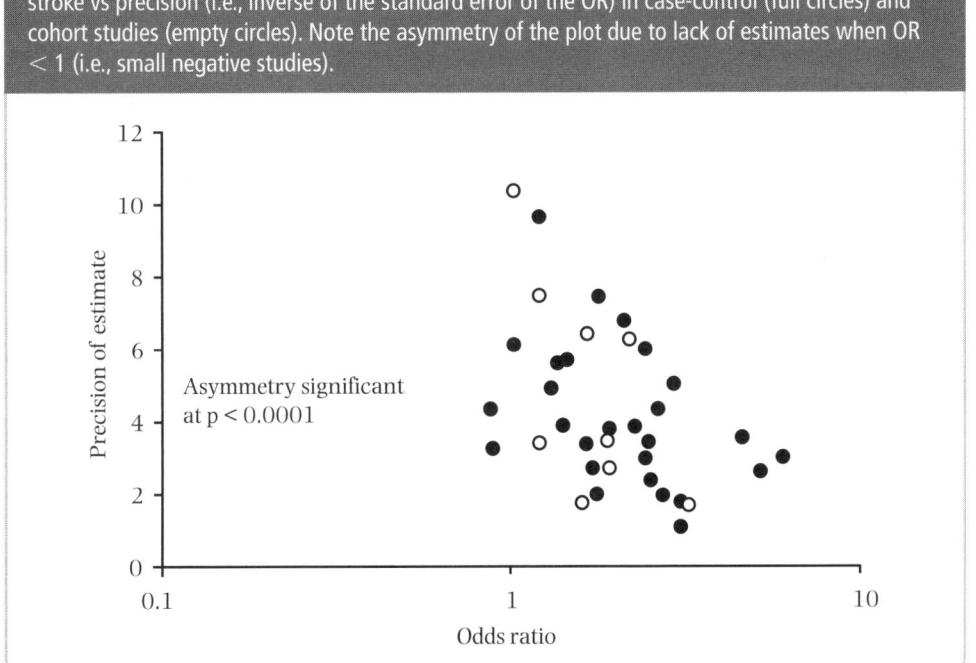

FIGURE 10-18 Funnel plot of odds ratio (OR) of family history of stroke as a risk factor for stroke vs precision (i.e., inverse of the standard error of the OR) in case-control (full circles) and cohort studies (empty circles). Note the asymmetry of the plot due to lack of estimates when OR < 1 (i.e., small negative studies).

Source: Data from E Flossman, UG Schulz, PM Rothwell, Systematic Review of Methods and Results of Studies of the Genetic Epidemiology of Ischemic Stroke. *Stroke*, Vol 35, pp. 212–227, © 2004.

on these findings, the authors concluded that reporting of outcomes in clinical trials is incomplete, biased, and inconsistent with protocols, and recommended that trials be registered and protocols made available before trial completion.

10.6 SUMMARY

The process of translating epidemiologic findings into policy involves careful consideration of issues such as bias and confounding as well as the ability to extrapolate results obtained in one or more study populations to other target populations. Although consideration of issues such as cost-effectiveness, and political and logistical problems in the implementation of programs is a key step in the development of health policy, they were not discussed in this chapter, which focused instead on epidemiologic issues that are routinely dealt with by the applied epidemiologist.

Translation to health policy is best made on the basis of results of experimental studies—in view of their optimal control of bias and confounding—but these studies are often not feasible for logistical and/or ethical reasons. In addition, the experimental design may not lend itself to operationalizing and evaluating certain interventions related to complex component causes—particularly those related to the social milieu. In addition, effectiveness data, commonly obtained from experimental studies, are frequently not generalizable, in view of the influence of between-population differences in sociocultural, economic, and other characteristics.

The observation of ratio-based (e.g., relative risk) weak associations poses another challenge to the policy expert, as even small increases in odds ratios or relative risks may translate into large absolute excesses of incident disease if the exposures are common. Consideration of consistency across studies and the use of meta-analysis to arrive at pooled estimates of the measure of association are useful strategies when weak associations are detected (e.g., those based on incidence ratios below 2.0). Caution must be exercised, however, when relying on consistency of results, as bias and confounding may also be consistent across studies and be the real reasons why associations of similar strengths and direction are observed in different populations. In addition, an apparent consistency among studies may be the result of publication bias.

The type of association—causal versus noncausal—should also be considered. The importance of confounded (as opposed to biased) associations to prevention was emphasized in Chapter 5, Section 5.5.8. For primary prevention, a causal connection between the risk factor or trait and the outcome of interest is a *sine qua non* condition. Given the purpose of making this book as practical as possible, we focused on only one causality model (Rothman's) and one set of guidelines to infer causality (Hill's). Although the latter remain as the main strategy to infer causality from epidemiologic studies, particularly observational ones, the policy expert must be cautious when considering these guidelines, as failure to meet them does not necessarily constitute evidence against causality.

Another issue of great importance to the translation of epidemiologic findings into public health practice and health policy is the choice of the preventive strategy: *high risk* versus *population based*. In this chapter, examples were provided that illustrate why the population-based approach, when feasible, is the strategy of choice to reduce disease incidence in the population as a whole. Whereas the population attributable risk is the ideal measure to assess the potential effectiveness of a population-based prevention strategy, the high-risk strategy is better evaluated through the attributable risk in the exposed, as it usually focuses on the excess risk in individuals exposed to proximal causes (see Chapter 3, Section 3.2.2).

As mentioned at the beginning of this chapter, it focused on a discussion of traditional epidemiologic themes that interface with health policy and public health. The reader with a specific interest on the health policy side of the interface is referred to other textbooks dealing with the cultural, legal, and cost-effectiveness issues specifically relevant to health policy.[95,96]

REFERENCES

1. Paneth N. Assessing the contributions of John Snow to epidemiology: 150 years after removal of the Broad Street pump handle. *Epidemiology*. 2004;15:514–516.
2. Lin JS, O'Connor E, Whitlock EP, et al. Behavioral counseling to promote physical activity and a healthful diet to prevent cardiovascular disease in adults: update of the evidence for the U.S. Preventive Services Task Force. Rockville (MD): Agency for Healthcare Research and Quality (US); 2010 Dec. Report No.: 11-05149-EF-1.
3. The Canadian Task Force on the Periodic Health Examination: Canadian Guide to Clinical Preventive Health Care. *Health Canada*. 1994.
4. *Guide to Clinical Preventive Services*: U.S. Prevention Services Task Force, U.S. Department of Health and Human Services, Office of Disease Prevention and Health Promotion; 2003. Concord, NH.
5. Goodman SN. The mammography dilemma: A crisis for evidence-based medicine? *Ann Intern Med*. 2002;137(5 Pt 1):363–365.
6. van Veen WA, Knottnerus JA. Screening mammography. *Lancet*. 2002;359:1701.
7. Rothman K, Greenland S. *Modern Epidemiology*, 3rd ed. Philadelphia, PA: Wolters Kluwer Health Lippincott; 2008.
8. Hill AB. The environment and disease: Association or causation? *Proc Royal Soc Med*. 1965;58:295–300.
9. Rothman KJ, Lanes S, Robins J. Casual inference. *Epidemiology*. 1993;4:555–556.
10. Koch R. Die aetiologie der tuberkulose. *Mitt Kais Gesundheitsamt*.1884;2:1–88.
11. Porta, M. *A Dictionary of Epidemiology*, 5th ed. New York, NY: Oxford University Press; 2008.
12. MacMahon B, Pugh TF, Ipsen J. *Epidemiology: Principles and Methods*. Boston, MA: Little, Brown and Co.; 1960.
13. Gordis L. *Epidemiology*, 4th ed. Philadelphia, PA: Elsevier Saunders; 2008.
14. Brenner H, Arndt V, Stegmaier C, et al. Is Helicobacter pylori infection a necessary condition for noncardia gastric cancer? *Am J Epidemiol*. 2004;159:252–258.
15. Nomura A. Stomach cancer. In: Schottenfeld D, Fraumeni JF Jr, eds. *Cancer Epidemiology and Prevention*. New York, NY, and Oxford, England: Oxford University Press; 1996:707–724.
16. Menaker RJ, Sharaf AA, Jones NL. Helicobacter pylori infection and gastric cancer: Host, bug, environment, or all three? *Curr Gastroenterol Rep*. 2004;6:429–435.
17. Wynder EL. Invited commentary: Studies in mechanism and prevention: Striking a proper balance. *Am J Epidemiol*. 1994;139:547–549.
18. Goldberger J, Wheeler GA, Sydenstricker E. A study of the relation of family income and other economic factors to pellagra incidence in seven cotton-mill villages of South Carolina in 1916. *Public Health Rep*. 1920;35:2673–2714.
19. Susser M, Susser E. Choosing a future for epidemiology: I: Eras and paradigms. *Am J Public Health*. 1996;86:668–673.
20. Diez-Roux AV. On genes, individuals, society, and epidemiology. *Am J Epidemiol*. 1998;148:1027–1032.
21. Rose G. Sick individuals and sick populations. *Int J Epidemiol*. 1985;14:32–38.
22. Rose G. *The Strategy of Preventive Medicine*. Oxford, England: Oxford University Press, 1992.

23. Chobanian AV, Bakris GL, Black HR, et al. The seventh report of the Joint National Committee on prevention, detection, evaluation and treatment of high blood pressure: the JNC 7 report. *J Am Med Assoc.* 2003;289:2560–2572.

24. Law MR, Frost CD, Wald NJ. By how much does dietary salt reduction lower blood pressure? III: Analysis of data from trials of salt reduction. *Br Med J.* 1991;302:819–824.

25. Szklo M. Selective screening: When should screening be limited to high-risk individuals? *J Gen Intern Med.* 1990;5(5 suppl):S47–S49.

26. Hartmann LC, Sellers TA, Frost MH, et al. Benign breast disease and the risk of breast cancer. *N Engl J Med.* 2005;353:229–237.

27. Mushlin AI, Kouides RW, Shapiro DE. Estimating the accuracy of screening mammography: A meta-analysis. *Am J Prev Med.* 1998;14:143–153.

28. Cassel J, Tyroler HA. Epidemiological studies of culture change: I: Health status and recency of industrialization. *Arch Environ Health.* 1961;3:25–33.

29. Syme SL. Sociological approach to the epidemiology of cerebrovascular disease. *Public Health Monogr.* 1966;76:57–63.

30. Duncan C, Jones K, Moon G. Context, composition and heterogeneity: Using multilevel models in health research. *Soc Sci Med.* 1998;46:97–117.

31. Diez-Roux AV. Bringing context back into epidemiology: Variables and fallacies in multilevel analysis. *Am J Public Health.* 1998;88:216–222.

32. U.S. Department of Health, Education, and Welfare. Smoking and Health: Report of the Advisory Committee to the Surgeon General of the Public Health Service. Washington, DC: U.S. Department of Health, Education, and Welfare, Public Health Service, Centers for Disease Control; 1964. PHS Publication No. 1103.

33. Rothman KJ, Greenland S. Causation and causal inference in epidemiology. *Am J Public Health.* 2005;95(suppl 1):S144–S150.

34. Greenland S, Brumback B. An overview of relations among causal modelling methods. *Int J Epidemiol.* 2002;31:1030–1037.

35. Albanes D, Heinonen OP, Taylor PR, et al. Alpha-Tocopherol and beta-carotene supplements and lung cancer incidence in the alpha-tocopherol, beta-carotene cancer prevention study: Effects of base-line characteristics and study compliance. *J Natl Cancer Inst.* 1996;88:1560–1570.

36. Wells AJ. Passive smoking and coronary heart disease. *N Engl J Med.* 1999;341:697–698; author reply 699–700.

37. Wells AJ. Passive smoking and lung cancer: A publication bias? *Br Med J (Clin Res Ed).* 1988;296:1128.

38. Glantz SA, Parmley WW. Passive smoking and heart disease: Epidemiology, physiology, and biochemistry. *Circulation.* 1991;83:1–12.

39. Thompson WD. Statistical analysis of case-control studies. *Epidemiol Rev.* 1994;16:33–50.

40. Li R, Chambless L. Tests for additive interaction in proportional hazards models. *Ann Epidemiol.* 2007;17:227–236.

41. Hjalgrim LL, Westergaard T, Rostgaard K, et al. Birth weight as a risk factor for childhood leukemia: A meta-analysis of 18 epidemiologic studies. *Am J Epidemiol.* 2003;158:724–735.

42. Hill JA. In vino veritas: Alcohol and heart disease. *Am J Med Sci.* Mar. 2005;329:124–135.

43. Dawber TR. *The Framingham Study: The Epidemiology of Atherosclerotic Disease.* Cambridge, MA: Harvard University Press; 1980.

44. Weed DL, Hursting SD. Biologic plausibility in causal inference: Current method and practice. *Am J Epidemiol.* 1998;147:415–425.

45. Schlesselman JJ. "Proof" of cause and effect in epidemiologic studies: Criteria for judgment. *Prev Med.* 1987;16:195–210.
46. Shapiro S. Meta-analysis/Shmeta-analysis. *Am J Epidemiol.* 1994;140:771–778.
47. Szklo M. Evaluation of Epidemiologic Information. In: Gordis L, ed. *Epidemiology and Health Risk Assessment.* New York, NY: Oxford University Press; 1988:268–272.
48. Szklo M. Population-based cohort studies. *Epidemiol Rev.* 1998;20:81–90.
49. Colditz GA. Estrogen, estrogen plus progestin therapy, and risk of breast cancer. *Clin Cancer Res.* 2005;11(2 Pt 2):909s–917s.
50. Sartwell PE. The incubation period and the dynamics of infectious disease. *Am J Epidemiol.* 1966; 83:204–206.
51. Armenian HK, Lilienfeld AM. Incubation period of disease. *Epidemiol Rev.* 1983;5:1–15.
52. Yu MW, Hsu FC, Sheen IS, et al. Prospective study of hepatocellular carcinoma and liver cirrhosis in asymptomatic chronic hepatitis B virus carriers. *Am J Epidemiol.* 1997;145:1039–1047.
53. Strong JP, Malcom GT, McMahan CA, et al. Prevalence and extent of atherosclerosis in adolescents and young adults: Implications for prevention from the Pathobiological Determinants of Atherosclerosis in Youth Study. *J Am Med Assoc.* 1999;281:727–735.
54. Strong JP, McGill HC Jr. The pediatric aspects of atherosclerosis. *J Atheroscler Res.* 1969;9:251–265.
55. Dawber TR, Kannel WB, Revotskie N, et al. Some factors associated with the development of coronary heart disease: Six years' follow-up experience in the Framingham Study. *Am J Public Health.* 1959;49: 1349–1356.
56. Keys A. *Seven Countries: A Multivariate Analysis of Death and Coronary Heart Disease.* Cambridge, MA: Harvard University Press; 1980.
57. Sharrett AR, Coady SA, Folsom AR, et al. Smoking and diabetes differ in their associations with subclinical atherosclerosis and coronary heart disease: The ARIC Study. *Atherosclerosis.* 2004;172:143–149.
58. Comstock GW. Evaluating vaccination effectiveness and vaccine efficacy by means of case-control studies. *Epidemiol Rev.* 1994;16:77–89.
59. Bruneau J, Lamothe F, Franco E, et al. High rates of HIV infection among injection drug users participating in needle exchange programs in Montreal: Results of a cohort study. *Am J Epidemiol.* 1997;146: 994–1002.
60. Wynder EL, Stellman SD. The "over-exposed" control group. *Am J Epidemiol.* 1992;135:459–461.
61. Elliott P. Design and analysis of multicentre epidemiological studies: The INTERSALT Study. In: Marmot M, Elliott P, eds. *Coronary Heart Disease Epidemiology: From Aetiology to Public Health.* Oxford, England: Oxford University Press; 1992:166–178.
62. Lash TL, Fink AK. Semi-automated sensitivity analysis to assess systematic errors in observational data. *Epidemiology.* 2003;14:451–458.
63. Peppard PE, Young T, Palta M, Skatrud J. Prospective study of the association between sleep-disordered breathing and hypertension. *N Engl J Med.* 2000;342:1378–1384.
64. Chen Z, Boreham J. Smoking and cardiovascular disease. *Semin Vasc Med.* 2002;2:243–252.
65. Kaur S, Cohen A, Dolor R, et al. The impact of environmental tobacco smoke on women's risk of dying from heart disease: A meta-analysis. *J Womens Health (Larchmt).* 2004;13:888–897.
66. Szklo M. The evaluation of epidemiologic evidence for policy-making. *Am J Epidemiol.* 2001;154(12 suppl):S13–S17.
67. Glynn RJ, Rosner B. Comparison of risk factors for the competing risks of coronary heart disease, stroke, and venous thromboembolism. *Am J Epidemiol.* 2005;162:975–982.

68. Fox MP, Lash TL, Greenland S. A method to automate probabilistic sensitivity analyses of misclassified binary variables. *Int J Epidemiol*. Dec 2005;34:1370–1376.

69. Petitti DB. *Meta-Analysis, Decision Analysis, and Cost-Effectiveness Analysis: Methods for Quantitative Synthesis in Medicine*, 2nd ed. New York, NY: Oxford University Press; 2000.

70. Berlin JA, Laird NM, Sacks HS, Chalmers TC. A comparison of statistical methods for combining event rates from clinical trials. *Stat Med*. 1989;8:141–151.

71. Lau J, Ioannidis JP, Schmid CH. Quantitative synthesis in systematic reviews. *Ann Intern Med*. 1997;127:820–826.

72. Greenland S. Quantitative methods in the review of epidemiologic literature. *Epidemiol Rev*. 1987;9:1–30.

73. Lorant V, Deliege D, Eaton W, et al. Socioeconomic inequalities in depression: A meta-analysis. *Am J Epidemiol*. 2003;157:98–112.

74. Demets DL. Methods for combining randomized clinical trials: Strengths and limitations. *Stat Med*. 1987;6:341–350.

75. Fleiss JL, Gross AJ. Meta-analysis in epidemiology, with special reference to studies of the association between exposure to environmental tobacco smoke and lung cancer: A critique. *J Clin Epidemiol*. 1991;44:127–139.

76. Thompson SG. Why sources of heterogeneity in meta-analysis should be investigated. *Br Med J*. 1994;309:1351–1355.

77. Engel LS, Taioli E, Pfeiffer R, et al. Pooled analysis and meta-analysis of glutathione S-transferase M1 and bladder cancer: A HuGE review. *Am J Epidemiol*. 2002;156:95–109.

78. Sterling TD. Publication decisions and their possible effects on inferences drawn from tests of significance or vice versa. *J Am Stat Assoc*. 1959;54:30–34.

79. Dickersin K, Hewitt P, Mutch L, et al. Perusing the literature: Comparison of MEDLINE searching with a perinatal trials database. *Control Clin Trials*. 1985;6:306–317.

80. Dickersin K, Chan S, Chalmers TC, et al. Publication bias and clinical trials. *Control Clin Trials*. 1987;8:343–353.

81. Dickersin K, Min YI, Meinert CL. Factors influencing publication of research results: Follow-up of applications submitted to two institutional review boards. *J Am Med Assoc*. 1992;267:374–378.

82. Dickersin K. Report from the panel on the Case for Registers of Clinical Trials at the Eighth Annual Meeting of the Society for Clinical Trials. *Control Clin Trials*. 1988;9:76–81.

83. Easterbrook PJ, Berlin JA, Gopalan R, Matthews DR. Publication bias in clinical research. *Lancet*. 1991; 337:867–872.

84. Mahoney MJ. Publication prejudices: an experimental study of confirmatory bias in the peer review system. *Cog Ther Res*. 1977;1:161–175.

85. Davidson RA. Source of funding and outcome of clinical trials. *J Gen Intern Med*. 1986;1:155–158.

86. Lexchin J, Bero LA, Djulbegovic B, Clark O. Pharmaceutical industry sponsorship and research outcome and quality: Systematic review. *Br Med J*. 2003;326:1167–1170.

87. Egger M, Zellweger-Zahner T, Schneider M, et al. Language bias in randomised controlled trials published in English and German. *Lancet*. 1997;350:326–329.

88. Dickersin K, Berlin JA. Meta-analysis: State-of-the-science. *Epidemiol Rev*. 1992;14:154–176.

89. Piantadosi S, Byar DP. A proposal for registering clinical trials. *Control Clin Trials*. 1988;9:82–84.

90. Bild DE, Bluemke DA, Burke GL, et al. Multi-ethnic study of atherosclerosis: Objectives and design. *Am J Epidemiol*. 2002;156:871–881.

91. Light RJ, Pillemer DB. *Summing Up: The Science of Reviewing Research*. Beverly Hills, CA: Sage Publications; 1984.
92. Flossmann E, Schulz UG, Rothwell PM. Systematic review of methods and results of studies of the genetic epidemiology of ischemic stroke. *Stroke*. 2004;35:212–227.
93. Egger M, Davey Smith G, Schneider M, Minder C. Bias in meta-analysis detected by a simple, graphical test. *Br Med J*. 1997;315:629–634.
94. Chan AW, Hrobjartsson A, Haahr MT, et al. Empirical evidence for selective reporting of outcomes in randomized trials: Comparison of protocols to published articles. *J Am Med Assoc*. 2004; 291:2457–2465.
95. Armenian HK, Shapiro, S, eds. *Epidemiology and Health Services*. New York, NY: Oxford University Press; 1998.
96. Brownson RC, Petitti, DB, eds. *Applied Epidemiology*. New York, NY: Oxford University Press; 1998.

EXERCISES

1. Women who report nausea sometimes or daily seem to be *less* likely to have a spontaneous abortion than those who do not. On the other hand, caffeine intake appears to be related to an increased risk of spontaneous abortion, which is substantially attenuated when adjusting for occurrence of nausea.* The relationships between caffeine intake, nausea, and spontaneous abortion seem to be complex, but for the purposes of this exercise, assume that many women in whom nausea occurs develop an aversion to coffee (and tea) intake and that nausea, not caffeine intake abstention, is causally related to a decrease in risk of spontaneous abortion.

   How can the relationship between caffeine intake and spontaneous abortion be defined, and what is its practical application?

2. In the study by Haffner et al.,[†] which was the basis for Exercise 2 in Chapter 6, histories of diabetes and of a prior episode of myocardial infarction (MI) were assessed with regard to from CHD risk. Selected results from this study are shown in the table.

   Cumulative fatal or nonfatal myocardial infarction incidence (MI) (%) during a 7-year follow-up, according to a history of prior MI and presence of type 2 diabetes at baseline.

Type 2 diabetes status	Prior MI	Incidence (%)	Relative risk	Attributable risk in those reporting prior MI (%)
Present	Yes	45.0	2.23	24.8
	No	20.2	Reference	Reference
Absent	Yes	18.8	5.37	15.3
	No	3.5	Reference	Reference

   If you had very limited resources, and assuming a homogeneous distribution of the population among the four categories based on diabetes and a prior MI, would you favor the 'diabetes present' or the 'diabetes absent' group to focus your efforts aimed at reducing CHD risk? Justify your answer.

3. The following histogram shows the distribution of a hypothetical population according to levels of a given risk factor (x). This distribution has the typical log-normal shape characteristic of many biological parameters in populations. The number of people in each category of x is shown in the second column of the following table. This table also shows the relative risk of disease y associated with each increasing category of x (in comparison with the lowest category).

---

*Cnattingius S, Signorello LB, Anneren G, et al. Caffeine intake and the risk of first trimester spontaneous abortion. *N Engl J Med.* 2000;343:1839–1845.
[†]Haffner SM, Lehto S, Ronnemaa T, et al. Mortality from coronary heart disease in subjects with type 2 diabetes and in nondiabetic subjects with and without prior myocardial infarction. *N Engl J Med.* 1998;339: 229–234.

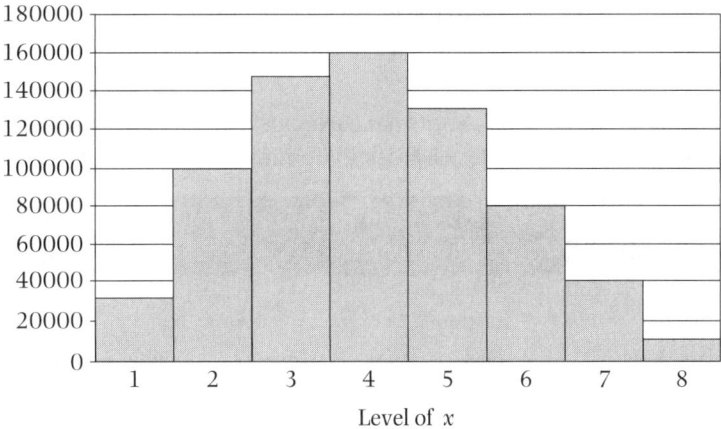

	Population				Cases	
Risk Factor x Level	No. of People	%	Relative risk	Risk	Number	Excess Cases
1 (lowest)	30,000	4.3	Reference	0.05	....	Reference
2	100,000	14.3	1.50	....	....	....
3	150,000	21.4	1.75	....	....	....
4	160,000	22.9	2.00	....	....	....
5	130,000	18.6	2.50	....	....	....
6	80,000	11.4	3.00	....	....	....
7	40,000	5.7	4.00	....	....	....
8	10,000	1.4	5.00	....	....	....
Total	700,000	100.0				

a. Assuming that the risk of y in the lowest category of x is 5%, for each category of x, calculate the total number of cases as well as the excess number of cases (i.e., the excess above the number that would be expected if the risk in each category were equal to that in the lowest category) (complete the last three columns of the table).

Calculations: examples for category $x = 2$

Number of cases: $100{,}000 \times (0.05 \times 1.5) = 7500$

Excess number of cases: $100{,}000 \times (0.05 \times [1.5 - 1.0]) = 2500$

b. What proportion of cases in the population occur in the high risk group ($x = 8$)?

c. Assume that a high-risk strategy for the prevention of those at the highest level of risk factor x (category 8, associated with a RR = 5.0) were to be implemented. A population-wide survey is implemented, and all individuals in that category of exposure are identified and successfully "treated" (moved down to category 7). How many total number of cases would be expected to be prevented with this strategy?

d. Assume that a population-based strategy for prevention is implemented. Measures to reduce exposure in the entire population are implemented and result in a shift to the left of the entire distribution: 15% of individuals in each category are moved to the category immediately below (except for those in the bottom category). How many total number of cases would be expected to be prevented with this strategy?

4. The table shows average annual coronary heart disease incidence rates from the multicenter Atherosclerosis Risk in Communities (ARIC) cohort study.[‡]

Age, field center, and race-adjusted average coronary heart disease incidence rates/1000 person-years (PYs), ARIC.

Smoking	Rate		Rate Ratio		Attributable risk in the exposed/1000 PYs	
	Women	Men	Women	Men	Women	Men
Current	5.3	11.5	4.1	2.5	4.0	6.8
Former	1.6	5.8	1.2	1.2	0.3	1.1
Never	1.3	4.7	Reference	Reference	Reference	Reference

What can be inferred from these results, assuming that they are valid, free of confounding, and precise?

5. Renehan et al. conducted a meta-analysis of cohort studies to examine the relationship of body mass index (measured as weight in kilograms divided by the square of height in meters) to colon cancer. Results for men are shown in the following figure. The abscissa shows the relative risks.[§]

   a. Are the results homogeneous across studies (please justify your answer)?

   b. Are the summary risk ratios similar for North American, European and Australian, and Asia-Pacific cohorts?

   c. To estimate the summary risk ratios shown in the figure, the authors used a random effects model. When they used a fixed effects model, results were virtually the same. Why?

   d. What are the main threats to inferring that the association of body mass index with colon cancer is true?

[‡]Chambless LE, Heiss G, Folson AR, et al. Association of coronary heart disease incidence with *caroid* arterial wall thickness and major risk factors: the Atherosclerosis Risk in Communities (ARIC) Study, 1987–1993. *Am J Epidemiol*. 1997; 146: 483–494.
[§]Renehan AG, Tyson M, Egger M, et al. Body mass index and incidence of cancer: a systematic review and meta-analysis of prospective observational studies. *Lancet* 2008;371:569–578.

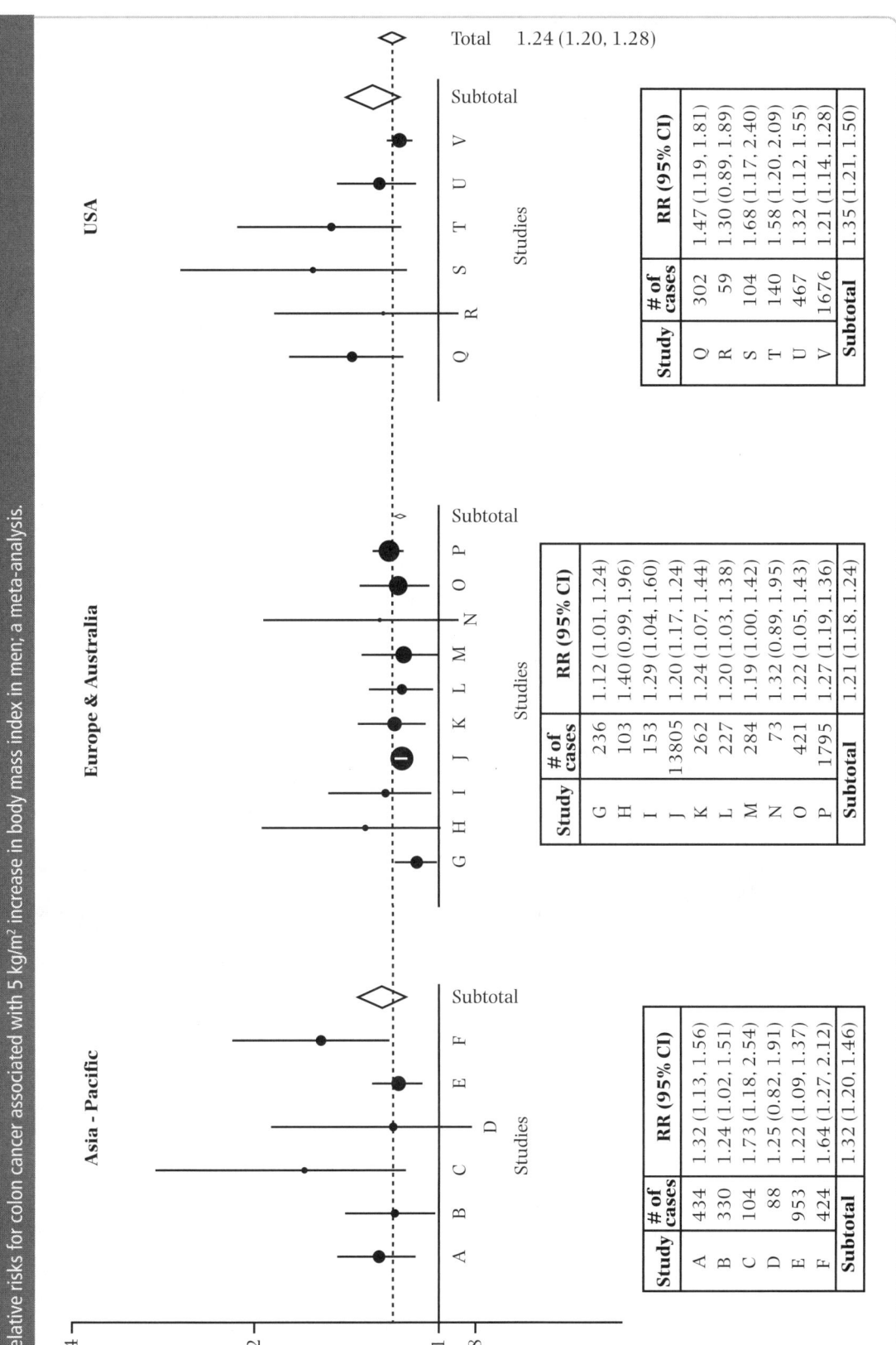

Relative risks for colon cancer associated with 5 kg/m² increase in body mass index in men; a meta-analysis.

430 CHAPTER 10 | Epidemiologic Issues in the Interface with Public Health Policy

The figure below shows a funnel plot for the papers included in Renehan et al.'s meta-analysis on the relation between BMI and colon cancer risk.

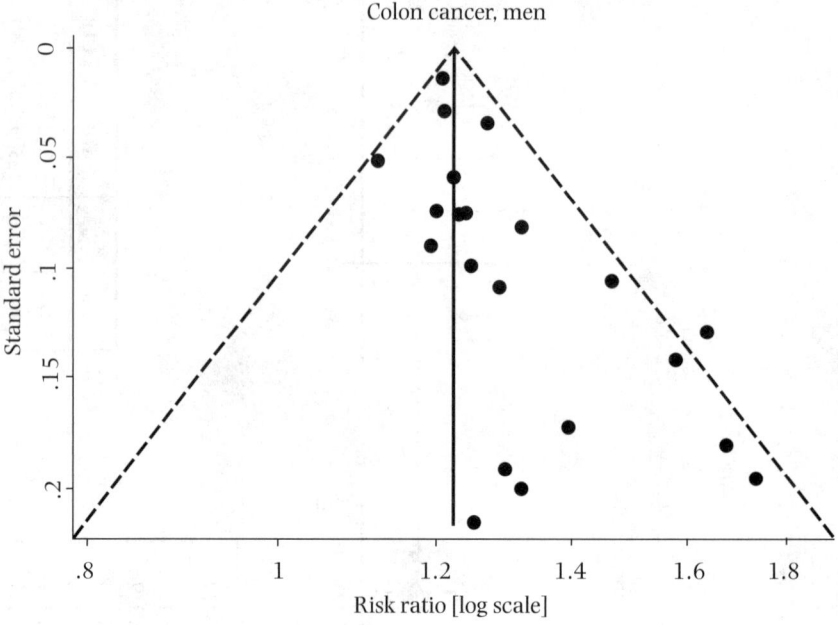

e. What is the usefulness of a funnel plot?

f. Interpret the funnel plot results shown in the figure.

6. A trial was conducted in a specific study population to compare the effectiveness of two interventions (A and B). The table shows the percentage distributions of compliance (yes vs. no) and socioeconomic status (SES, high or low) in the groups assigned to A or B as well as the mortality probabilities associated with the strata formed by these variables.

	Intervention A			Intervention B		
Compliance	SES	Mortality	Compliance	SES	Mortality	
Yes = 0.95	High = 0.20	0.10	Yes = 0.50	High = 0.20	0.05	
	Low = 0.80	0.20		Low = 0.80	0.10	
No = 0.05	High = 0.10	0.40	No = 0.50	High = 0.10	0.40	
	Low = 0.90	0.60		Low = 0.90	0.60	

a. Based on this table, construct a decision tree.

b. How many decision and chance (probability) nodes are there in this setting?

c. Calculate the overall mortality of interventions A and B.

e. Calculate the *effectiveness* of intervention A vis-à-vis B.

7. In the decision tree shown in Figure 10-13 and Exhibit 10-3, assume that the tolerance to intervention B can be increased to 50%, and recalculate the effectiveness of intervention A when compared with intervention B.

Standard Errors, Confidence Intervals, and Hypothesis Testing for Selected Measures of Risk and Measures of Association

APPENDIX A

CONTENTS

Introduction		441
A.1	Cumulative Survival Estimate	443
A.2	Incidence Rate (per Person-Time)	443
A.3	Relative Risk and Rate Ratio	445
A.4	Odds Ratio (Unmatched and Matched)	448
A.5	Attributable Risk	451
A.6	Difference Between Two Adjusted Rates or Probabilities (Direct Method)	453
A.7	Standardized Mortality Ratio	454
A.8	Mantel-Haenszel Odds Ratio (and Rate Ratio)	455
A.9	Regression Coefficient	457
A.10	Sensitivity, Specificity, and Percent Agreement	459
A.11	Youden's J Statistic	460
A.12	Kappa	461

INTRODUCTION

In this appendix, methods for calculating confidence intervals for selected measures of risk and measures of association presented in this textbook are described. For some of the measures, common methods for hypothesis testing are also presented.

This appendix is not intended to represent a comprehensive review of all of the statistical inference methods used in epidemiology. Methods for only some of the epidemiologic parameters are presented, and only one commonly used method for the calculation of standard error is described for each—sometimes among other alternatives. Moreover, it is not our intention to discuss the methodological and conceptual limitations of these methods, which have been thoroughly discussed elsewhere.[1,2] Our intention is pragmatic: to provide a brief description of the methods of statistical inference that we believe are most commonly used in relation to the epidemiologic parameters presented in this textbook.

It is assumed that the reader of this appendix is familiar with basic biostatistical concepts, including standard normal distribution (z-score), t-test, standard deviation, standard error, confidence intervals, hypothesis testing, and the p value. (For a review of these basic concepts, the reader should refer to biostatistics books such as Armitage and Berry[3] or Altman[4]).

The general purpose for the calculation of confidence intervals and hypothesis testing is to estimate the statistical uncertainty around the measure of risk or association obtained in the study (the so-called *point estimate*) in relation to the (unknown) true value of the *parameter* in the reference population. Although shortcuts are provided in specific cases, the general structure of the presentation for most of these measures is as follows:

1. The method for calculating the *variance* and/or its square root, the *standard error*, of the estimate is presented in most instances. However, in cases where the calculation of the standard error is more mathematically cumbersome (e.g., for regression coefficients), it is assumed that the standard error can be obtained from a computer-assisted statistical analysis, and thus this step is skipped.

2. Based on the point estimate of the parameter in question and its standard error (SE), the formula for the 95% confidence interval is provided. The general structure of this formula is as follows:

$$\text{Point estimate} \pm [1.96 \times \text{SE (estimate)}]$$

Notice that 1.96 is the z-score (standard normal score) corresponding to the 95% confidence level (i.e., an alpha error of 5%). Confidence intervals for different levels of alpha error can be obtained by simply replacing this value with the corresponding z-score value (e.g., 1.64 for 90% confidence intervals, 2.58 for 99% confidence intervals, etc.).

3. The test of the null hypothesis is presented for some of the indices (depending on our assessment of its relevance in each particular case and the frequency of its use in the literature). The logic and structure of these tests of hypothesis are also fairly homogeneous across different measures. The standard test of hypothesis is designed to test the *null hypothesis*—that is, the absence of a difference (absolute or relative) or a correlation. Thus, for *absolute* measures of association (e.g., a difference between two means or two rates), the null hypothesis is formulated as follows:

$$H_0: \text{True parameter} = 0$$

For *relative* measures of association (e.g., a relative risk, a rate ratio, an odds ratio), the null hypothesis is formulated as

$$H_0: \text{True parameter} = 1$$

Specific formulations for statistical testing approaches are presented in a few cases. In others, the general approach for a test of hypothesis is to calculate a z-score by dividing the point estimate by its standard error:

$$\frac{\text{Point estimate}}{\text{SE (estimate)}} \approx z\text{-score}$$

Or equivalently, the square of the z-score has a distribution approximate to a chi-square with 1 degree of freedom.

4. An example of each of the above calculations (usually based on one of the examples in the textbook) is presented in most cases.

Finally, a note on "notation": throughout this appendix, the symbol "log x" refers to the natural logarithm of x—that is, the logarithm on base e. The corresponding antilog is the exponential function, which is denoted by either exp[x] or e^x.

A.1 CUMULATIVE SURVIVAL ESTIMATE

As described in Chapter 2, Section 2.2.1, the cumulative survival estimate is the product of the conditional survival probabilities for all preceding intervals (in the case of the classical actuarial life table) or for all preceding events (in the case of the Kaplan-Meier method; see Chapter 2, Table 2-3).

Variance and Standard Error (Greenwood Formula)

In 1926, Greenwood[5] described the following formula, which approximates the variance of a cumulative survival estimate at time i:

$$\text{Var}(S_i) \approx (S_i)^2 \times \sum_{j=1}^{i} \left(\frac{d_j}{n_j(n_j - d_j)} \right)$$

where j indexes all the previous event times (or intervals) up to and including time i, d is the number of deaths at each time (typically 1 in the Kaplan-Meier method, any number in the classical life table), and n is the denominator—that is, the number of individuals at risk at each time (or the "corrected" denominator in the life table—see Equation 2.1 in Chapter 2, Section 2.2.1).

The standard error (SE) can be obtained as the square root of the variance:

$$\text{SE}(S_i) \approx S_i \times \sqrt{\sum_{j=1}^{i} \left(\frac{d_j}{n_j(n_j - d_j)} \right)}$$

95% Confidence Interval

This can be obtained from the point estimate (S_i) and the SE (S_i) as follows:

$$S_i \pm [1.96 \times \text{SE}(S_i)]$$

Example

To calculate the standard error for the cumulative survival estimate at time 9 months in Chapter 2, Table 2-3, we need the estimate of S_9 from the table (0.675) and the number of events and individuals at risk at all previous times up to 9 months (i.e., 1, 3, and 9 months):

$$\text{SE}(S_9) \approx 0.675 \times \sqrt{\left(\frac{1}{10(10-1)} + \frac{1}{8(8-1)} + \frac{1}{7(7-1)} \right)} = 0.155$$

Thus, the 95% confidence interval can be obtained as follows:

$$0.675 \pm (1.96 \times 0.155) = 0.675 \pm 0.304$$

or 0.371 to 0.979.

A.2 INCIDENCE RATE (PER PERSON-TIME)

A person-time incidence rate is obtained by dividing the number of events by the sum of person-time units contributed to by all individuals in the study population over the time interval of interest. Because rates are usually calculated for rare events (i.e., the numerator is usually a small number compared to the denominator), the number of events can be assumed to follow a Poisson distribution.[3] Procedures to calculate variance and standard error of the rate are based on this assumption.

95% Confidence Interval

A simple way to calculate the confidence limits for a rate is based on the table provided by Haenszel et al.[6] (see also Breslow and Day[7(p.70)]):

The process involves two steps:

1. Estimate a confidence interval for the number of events (the numerator of the rate): multiply the number of observed events times the lower and upper limit factors shown in the table. (Note that, for large numbers, an approximate interpolation can be made—e.g., if the number of events is 95, the limit factors would be approximately 0.813 and 1.23.)

Tabulated values of 95% confidence limit factors for a Poisson-distributed variable.

Observed no. of events on which estimate is based	Lower limit factor	Upper limit factor	Observed no. of events on which estimate is based	Lower limit factor	Upper limit factor	Observed no. of events on which estimate is based	Lower limit factor	Upper limit factor
1	.0253	5.57	21	.619	1.53	120	.833	1.200
2	.121	3.61	22	.627	1.51	140	.844	1.184
3	.206	2.92	23	.634	1.50	160	.854	1.171
4	.272	2.56	24	.641	1.49	180	.862	1.160
5	.324	2.33	25	.647	1.48	200	.868	1.151
6	.367	2.18	26	.653	1.47	250	.882	1.134
7	.401	2.06	27	.659	1.46	300	.892	1.121
8	.431	1.97	28	.665	1.45	350	.899	1.112
9	.458	1.90	29	.670	1.44	400	.906	1.104
10	.480	1.84	30	.675	1.43	450	.911	1.098
11	.499	1.79	35	.697	1.39	500	.915	1.093
12	.517	1.75	40	.714	1.36	600	.922	1.084
13	.532	1.71	45	.729	1.34	700	.928	1.078
14	.546	1.68	50	.742	1.32	800	.932	1.072
15	.560	1.65	60	.770	1.30	900	.936	1.068
16	.572	1.62	70	.785	1.27	1000	.939	1.064
17	.583	1.60	80	.798	1.25			
18	.593	1.58	90	.809	1.24			
19	.602	1.56	100	.818	1.22			
20	.611	1.54						

Source: Data are from W Haenszel, DB Loveland, and MG Sirken. Lung Cancer Mortality as Related to Residence and Smoking Histories I. White males. *Journal of the National Cancer Institute.* 1962;28:947–1001.

2. Use these lower and upper limits of the number of events to calculate the confidence limits of the rate, using the number of person-time units as the denominator.

Example

In the hypothetical example cited in Chapter 2, at the beginning of Section 2.2.2, 12 events are observed for a total follow-up time of 500 days. The incidence rate in this example is $12/500 = 0.024$ per person-day, or 2.4 per 100 person-days. The 95% confidence interval for that count, assuming a Poisson distribution, is

$$\text{Lower Limit} = 12 \times 0.517 = 6.2$$

$$\text{Upper Limit} = 12 \times 1.75 = 21.0$$

Thus, the 95% confidence interval for the rate is then calculated as follows:

$$\text{Lower Limit} = 6.2/500 = 0.0124 \text{ per person-day}$$

$$\text{Upper Limit} = 21/500 = 0.042 \text{ per person-day}$$

That is, the 95% confidence interval for the observed rate (2.4 per 100 person-days) is 1.24 to 4.2 per 100 person-days.

A.3 RELATIVE RISK AND RATE RATIO

Relative Risk (Ratio of Probabilities)

The relative risk is the ratio of two incidence cumulative probabilities: the ratio of the proportion of exposed individuals with the event of interest out of the total exposed divided by the proportion of unexposed individuals with the event out of the total number of unexposed subjects (see Chapter 3, Table 3-2, Equation 3.1). Consider the following notation:

	Diseased	Nondiseased	Total
Exposed	a	b	$a+b$
Unexposed	c	d	$c+d$
Total	$a+c$	$b+d$	T

The relative risk (RR) (from Equation 3.1) is

$$\text{RR} = \frac{q_+}{q_-} = \frac{\dfrac{a}{a+b}}{\dfrac{c}{c+d}}$$

Standard Error

Because the relative risk is a multiplicative measure and thus asymmetrically distributed, its standard error (SE) needs to be calculated in a logarithmic scale. Thus, the standard error of the logarithm of the relative risk is[8]

$$\text{SE}(\log \text{RR}) = \sqrt{\frac{b}{a(a+b)} + \frac{d}{c(c+d)}}$$

95% Confidence Interval

The 95% confidence interval should also be calculated in the logarithmic scale:

$$95\% \text{ CI (log RR)} = \log RR \pm 1.96 \times SE(\log RR)$$

$$= \log RR \pm \left(1.96 \times \sqrt{\frac{b}{a(a+b)} + \frac{d}{c(c+d)}}\right)$$

The confidence interval for the relative risk can be obtained taking the antilog (exponentiation) of these numbers:

$$95\% \text{ CI (RR)} = \exp\left[\left(\log RR \pm 1.96 \times \sqrt{\frac{b}{a(a+b)} + \frac{d}{c(c+d)}}\right)\right]$$

Note: A shortcut for this calculation is as follows:

$$\text{Lower Limit } 95\% \text{ CI(RR)} = RR \times e^{-[1.96 \times SE(\log RR)]}$$

$$\text{Upper Limit } 95\% \text{ CI(RR)} = RR \times e^{[1.96 \times SE(\log RR)]}$$

Hypothesis Testing

The null hypothesis is

$$H_0: RR = 1$$

Use usual chi-square or Fisher's exact test for two-by-two contingency tables.

Example

From the data in Chapter 3, Table 3-3, the relative risk of myocardial infarction is estimated as

$$RR = \frac{0.018}{0.003} = 6.0$$

The standard error of the log of this estimate is

$$SE(\log RR) = \sqrt{\frac{9820}{180(10,000)} + \frac{9970}{30(10,000)}} = 0.197$$

Thus, the 95% confidence interval can be obtained as follows:

$$95\% \text{ CI(RR)} = \exp[\log(6.0) \pm (1.96 \times 0.197)] = \exp[1.792 \pm 0.386]$$

$$\text{Lower Limit} = \exp[1.406] = 4.08$$

$$\text{Upper Limit} = \exp[2.178] = 8.83$$

Note: The alternative shortcut is

$$\text{Lower Limit } 95\% \text{ CI(RR)} = 6.0 \times e^{-[1.96 \times 0.197]} = 4.08$$

$$\text{Upper Limit } 95\% \text{ CI(RR)} = 6.0 \times e^{[1.96 \times 0.197]} = 8.83$$

Rate Ratio (Ratio of Incidence Densities)

Approximate procedures to calculate the confidence interval of a rate ratio have been proposed by Ederer and Mantel.[9] Definitions for the notations that will be used are

O_1 = observed events in group 1
O_2 = observed events in group 2
L_1 = person-time observed in group 1
L_2 = person-time observed in group 2
$R_1 = O_1/L_1$ = event rate in group 1
$R_2 = O_2/L_2$ = event rate in group 2
$RR = R_1/R_2$

95% Confidence Interval

Perform the following two steps:

1. Set limits on the ratio of observed events in one group (e.g., group 1) to the total number of observed events:

$$\hat{P} = \frac{O_1}{O_1 + O_2}$$

Using the general formula for the standard error of a binomial proportion, the lower (P_L) and upper (P_U) limits of the 95% confidence interval for this ratio are

$$P_L = \hat{P} - \left[1.96 \times \sqrt{\frac{\hat{p}(1-\hat{p})}{O_1 + O_2}}\right]; \quad P_U = \hat{P} + \left[1.96 \times \sqrt{\frac{\hat{p}(1-\hat{p})}{O_1 + O_2}}\right]$$

2. Convert to limits on rate ratio:

$$RR_L = \left[\frac{P_L}{1 - P_L}\right] \times \frac{L_2}{L_1}; \quad RR_U = \left[\frac{P_U}{1 - P_U}\right] \times \frac{L_2}{L_1}$$

Hypothesis Testing

For testing H_0: RR = 1, an approximate chi-square test with 1 degree of freedom can be used:

$$\chi_1^2 = \frac{(O_1 - E_1)^2}{E_1} + \frac{(O_2 - E_2)^2}{E_2}$$

where

$$E_1 = (O_1 + O_2) \times \frac{L_1}{L_1 + L_2}$$

$$E_2 = (O_1 + O_2) \times \frac{L_2}{L_1 + L_2}$$

Example

$$O_1 = 60, L_1 = 35{,}000, R_1 = 0.00171$$
$$O_2 = 45, L_2 = 30{,}000, R_2 = 0.0015$$
$$RR = 0.00171/0.0015 = 1.14$$
$$\hat{P} = \frac{60}{105}$$

The 95% confidence limits are

$$P_L = \frac{60}{105} - \left(1.96 \times \sqrt{\frac{60}{105} \times \frac{45}{105} \times \frac{1}{105}}\right) = 0.4768$$

$$P_U = \frac{60}{105} + \left(1.96 \times \sqrt{\frac{60}{105} \times \frac{45}{105} \times \frac{1}{105}}\right) = 0.6661$$

$$RR_L = \frac{0.4768}{0.5232} \times \frac{30{,}000}{35{,}000} = 0.78$$

$$RR_U = \frac{0.6661}{0.3339} \times \frac{30{,}000}{35{,}000} = 1.71$$

Hypothesis testing is performed as follows:

$$E_1 = (60 + 45) \times \frac{35{,}000}{65{,}000} = 56.54$$

$$E_2 = (60 + 45) \times \frac{30{,}000}{65{,}000} = 48.46$$

$$\chi_1^2 = \frac{(60 - 56.54)^2}{56.54} + \frac{(45 - 48.46)^2}{48.46} = 0.46; p > 0.5$$

A.4 ODDS RATIO (UNMATCHED AND MATCHED)

Unmatched Case-Control Study

Based on the notation from Chapter 3, Table 3-6 (or from the table in Section A.3, assuming a case-control sampling scheme), in which the controls (cells b and d) are a sample of noncases, the odds ratio can be calculated as the cross-product ratio:

$$OR = \frac{a \times d}{b \times c}$$

Standard Error

As with the relative risk (see Section A.3), because of its multiplicative nature, the standard error for the odds ratio is calculated in a logarithmic scale, as described by Woolf:[10]

$$SE(\log OR) = \sqrt{\frac{1}{a} + \frac{1}{b} + \frac{1}{c} + \frac{1}{d}}$$

95% Confidence Interval

The 95% confidence interval is also calculated in the logarithmic scale:

$$95\% \text{ CI (log OR)} = \log \text{OR} \pm [1.96 \times \text{SE (log OR)}]$$

$$= \log \text{OR} \pm \left(1.96 \times \sqrt{\frac{1}{a} + \frac{1}{b} + \frac{1}{c} + \frac{1}{d}}\right)$$

The limits of the confidence interval for the odds ratio can be obtained taking the antilog of (exponentiating) these numbers:

$$95\% \text{ CI (OR)} = \exp\left[\log \text{OR} \pm \left(1.96 \times \sqrt{\frac{1}{a} + \frac{1}{b} + \frac{1}{c} + \frac{1}{d}}\right)\right]$$

Note: a shortcut for these calculations is as follows:

$$\text{Lower Limit 95\% Confidence interval} = \text{OR} \times e^{-[1.96 \times \text{SE(log OR)}]}$$

$$\text{Upper Limit 95\% Confidence interval} = \text{OR} \times e^{[1.96 \times \text{SE(log OR)}]}$$

Hypothesis Testing

For testing H_0: OR = 1, the usual chi-square or Fisher's exact test for two-by-two contingency tables can be used.

Example

From the data in Chapter 3, Table 3-6:

$$\text{OR} = \frac{180 \times 997}{982 \times 30} = 6.09$$

The standard error of the logarithm of this estimate is

$$\text{SE (log OR)} = \sqrt{\frac{1}{180} + \frac{1}{982} + \frac{1}{30} + \frac{1}{997}} = 0.202$$

The 95% confidence interval can be obtained as follows:

$$95\% \text{ CI(OR)} = \exp[\log 6.09 \pm (1.96 \times 0.202)] = \exp[1.807 \pm 0.396]$$

$$\text{Lower Limit} = \exp[1.411] = 4.10$$

$$\text{Upper Limit} = \exp[2.203] = 9.05$$

Note: The alternative shortcut is

$$\text{Lower Limit 95\% CI(RR)} = 6.09 \times e^{-[1.96 \times 0.202]} = 4.10$$

$$\text{Upper Limit 95\% CI(RR)} = 6.09 \times e^{[1.96 \times 0.202]} = 9.05$$

Matched Case-Control Study

In a case-control study in which cases and controls are individually matched (paired), the odds ratio is estimated as the number of pairs in which the case is exposed and the control is not exposed, divided by the number of pairs in which the case is unexposed and the control is exposed. Thus, based on the notation in Chapter 7, Table 7-12:

$$\text{OR} = \frac{b}{c}$$

Standard Error

The standard error for the logarithm of the paired odds ratio is

$$\text{SE (log OR)} = \sqrt{\frac{1}{b} + \frac{1}{c}}$$

95% Confidence Interval

The 95% confidence interval is also calculated in the logarithmic scale:

$$\text{95\% CI(log OR)} = \log \text{OR} \pm [1.96 \times \text{SE (log OR)}]$$
$$= \log \text{OR} \pm \left(1.96 \times \sqrt{\frac{1}{b} + \frac{1}{c}}\right)$$

The confidence limits for the OR can be obtained, taking the antilog of (exponentiating) these numbers:

$$\text{95\% CI(OR)} = \exp\left[\log \text{OR} \pm \left(1.96 \times \sqrt{\frac{1}{b} + \frac{1}{c}}\right)\right]$$

The same shortcut as for the unmatched OR can be used.

Hypothesis Testing

For testing H_0: OR = 1, use McNemar's chi-square test (corrected for continuity), with 1 degree of freedom:

$$\chi_1^2 = \frac{(|b - c| - 1)^2}{b + c}$$

Example

From the data in Chapter 7, Table 7-12:

$$\text{OR} = \frac{65}{42} = 1.55$$

The standard error of the logarithm of estimate is

$$\text{SE (log OR)} = \sqrt{\frac{1}{65} + \frac{1}{42}} = 0.198$$

The 95% confidence interval is obtained as follows:

$$\text{95\% CI(OR)} = \exp[\log 1.55 \pm (1.96 \times 0.198)] = \exp[0.438 \pm 0.388]$$

$$\text{Lower Limit} = \exp[0.050] = 1.05$$

$$\text{Upper Limit} = \exp[0.826] = 2.28$$

Note: The alternative shortcut is

$$\text{Lower Limit 95\% CI(OR)} = 1.55 \times e^{-[1.96 \times 0.198]} = 1.05$$

$$\text{Upper Limit 95\% CI(OR)} = 1.55 \times e^{[1.96 \times 0.198]} = 2.28$$

Hypothesis testing is performed as follows:

$$\chi_1^2 = \frac{(|65 - 42| - 1)^2}{65 + 42} = 4.52, p < 0.05$$

A.5 ATTRIBUTABLE RISK

Attributable Risk in the Exposed

For the simple excess attributable fraction—that is, the difference in incidence between exposed and unexposed individuals (Chapter 3, Equation 3.4)—the variance can be estimated as the sum of the variances of each of the incidence estimates. For example, if the incidence estimates are based on cumulative survival, the variance of the attributable risk will be the sum of the individual variances obtained using Greenwood's formula (see Section A.1). The standard error is then the square root of the variance, from which 95% confidence limits can be estimated and hypothesis testing can be carried out using the general approach outlined in the introduction to this appendix.

Percent Attributable Risk in the Exposed (% AR_{exp})

Because the %AR_{exp} (Chapter 3, Equation 3.5) reduces to the following equation (Equation 3.6):

$$\%AR_{exp} = \frac{q_+ - q_-}{q_+} \times 100 = \frac{RR - 1}{RR} \times 100$$

this measure is a function of only one parameter (the relative risk, RR). Thus, an estimate of the confidence interval for %AR_{exp} can be based on the confidence interval of the RR (see Section A.3).

Percent Population Attributable Risk (%Pop AR)

Levin's formula for the calculation of the %Pop AR, based on data from a cohort study (Chapter 3, Equation 3.10), is

$$\%\text{Pop AR} = \frac{p_e(RR - 1)}{p_e(RR - 1) + 1} \times 100$$

where RR is the estimated relative risk and p_e is the proportion of individuals exposed in the population [i.e., based on the notation in the table in Section A.3, $p_e = (a + b)/T$]. In a case-control study, assuming that the disease is rare and that the controls are reasonably representative of the total reference population, the relative risk in Levin's formula can be replaced by the odds ratio (see Chapter 3, Section 3.2.2), and p_e can be estimated from the prevalence of exposure in controls.

Standard Error

The following formulas, proposed by Walter,[11] are based on the notation in the table in Section A.3. For %Pop AR calculated from cohort data:

$$SE(\%\text{Pop AR}) = \sqrt{\frac{cT[ad(T-c) + bc^2]}{(a+c)^3(c+d)^3}} \times 100$$

For %Pop AR calculated from case-control data:

$$SE(\%\text{Pop AR}) = \sqrt{\left(\frac{c(b+d)}{d(a+c)}\right)^2 \left(\frac{a}{c(a+c)} + \frac{b}{d(b+d)}\right)} \times 100$$

95% Confidence Interval

The 95% confidence interval can be calculated using the point estimate and the above standard errors:

$$95\% \text{ CI}(\%\text{Pop AR}) = \%\text{Pop AR} \pm 1.96 \times SE(\%\text{Pop AR})$$

Hypothesis Testing

For testing H_0: %Pop AR = 0, the z-score is obtained:

$$\frac{\%\text{Pop AR}}{SE(\%\text{Pop AR})} \approx z\text{-score}$$

Example

According to the hypothetical cohort study data in Chapter 3, Table 3-3, the relative risk of myocardial infarction is 6.0, comparing severe hypertensives to nonhypertensives; the prevalence of exposure (severe systolic hypertension) is 50%. Thus, the population attributable risk is

$$\%\text{Pop AR} = \frac{0.5(6.0 - 1)}{0.5(6.0 - 1) + 1} \times 100 = 71.4\%$$

The standard error of this estimate is

$$SE(\%\text{Pop AR}) = \sqrt{\frac{30 \times 20{,}000 \times [180 \times 9970 \times 19{,}970 + 9820 \times 30^2]}{210^3 \times 10{,}000^3}} \times 100$$

$$= 4.82\%$$

The 95% confidence interval is obtained as follows:

$$95\% \text{ CI}(\%\text{Pop AR}) = 71.4 \pm (1.96 \times 4.82) = 71.4 \pm 9.4$$

$$\text{Lower Limit} = 62.0\%$$

$$\text{Upper Limit} = 80.8\%$$

Hypothesis testing is performed as follows:

$$\frac{71.4}{4.82} = 14.8, \ p < 0.001$$

A.6 DIFFERENCE BETWEEN TWO ADJUSTED RATES OR PROBABILITIES (DIRECT METHOD)

Define $d = I_A^* - I_B^*$—that is, the difference between two adjusted probabilities (see Chapter 7, Section 7.3.1, Table 7-3).

Standard Error

An approximate standard error for d [d being an estimated adjusted difference (e.g., excess incidence) based on $i = 1 \ldots k$ strata] is obtained using the formula:[12]

$$\mathrm{SE}(d) = \frac{\sqrt{\sum_{i=1}^{k} w_i^2 \, p_i (1 - p_i) \left(\frac{1}{n_{Ai}} + \frac{1}{n_{Bi}} \right)}}{\sum_{i=1}^{k} w_i}$$

where p_i are the overall stratum-specific rates (both study groups combined):

$$p_i = \frac{x_{Ai} + x_{Bi}}{n_{Ai} + n_{Bi}}$$

and w_i are the standard population weights used to adjust the study group rates. If the minimum variance method is used (i.e., if these weights are calculated as follows; see Chapter 7, Section 7.3.1),

$$w_i = \frac{n_{Ai} \times n_{Bi}}{n_{Ai} + n_{Bi}}$$

the above formula is substantially simpler:

$$\mathrm{SE}(d_{\text{min variance}}) = \frac{\sqrt{\sum_{i=1}^{k} w_i \, p_i (1 - p_i)}}{\sum_{i=1}^{k} w_i}$$

95% Confidence Interval

The 95% confidence interval can be obtained using the general approach outlined in the introduction to this appendix:

$$d \pm [1.96 \times \mathrm{SE}(d)]$$

Hypothesis Testing

Hypothesis testing also uses the general approach (see above):

$$\frac{d}{\mathrm{SE}(d)} \approx z\text{-score}$$

Example

The data for this example come from the study by Pandey et al.[13] on the comparison of mortality according to dietary vitamin intake in the Western Electric Company Study cohort. These data were used as an example for the techniques to evaluate confounding in Chapter 5 (Tables 5-2 through 5-6). For the purpose of the current example, the category "moderate" is ignored, and the purpose is to calculate the smoke-adjusted difference in mortality rates between the *high* and *low* vitamin intake categories, as well as the corresponding confidence interval for such adjusted difference. Based on the numbers presented in the tables mentioned above, the following working table for the calculation of the adjusted difference (using direct adjustment with the minimum variance method) and its standard error was constructed:

	Low vitamin intake*		High vitamin intake*		Total		Minimum variance standard			
Smoking	N	Rate	N	Rate	N	Rate (p_i)	$N(w_i)^\dagger$	Expected no. of deaths (low)†	Expected no. of deaths (high)†	$w_i p_i (1-p_i)^\dagger$
No	4260	.0134	5143	.0103	9403	.0117	2330.020	31.1763	24.0115	26.9386
Yes	6447	.0214	6233	.0178	12,680	.0196	3169.097	67.8355	56.4367	61.0102
Sum							5499.117	99.0118	80.4482	87.9488

*See Table 5-5, Chapter 5.
†The expected numbers shown in the table are exact and may differ slightly from those obtained using the rates shown for low and high because the latter have been rounded.

Thus, the adjusted rates are:

- For the low vitamin intake group: 99.0118/5499.117 = 0.0180
- For the high vitamin intake group: 80.4482/5499.117 = 0.0146

The adjusted difference between the high and the low vitamin intake groups is therefore: $d = 0.0146 - 0.018 = -0.0034$, or -3.4 per 1000.

The standard error of this estimate can be calculated as:

$$\text{SE}(d_{\text{min variance}}) = \frac{\sqrt{87.9488}}{5499.117} = 0.0017$$

The 95% confidence interval is as follows:

$$-0.0034 \pm 1.96 \times 0.0017$$

$$\text{Lower Limit} = -0.0034 - 0.0033 = -0.0067$$

$$\text{Upper Limit} = -0.0034 + 0.0033 = -0.0001$$

A.7 STANDARDIZED MORTALITY RATIO

The standardized mortality ratio (SMR) and related measures such as the standardized incidence ratio (SIR) are defined as the number of observed events (e.g., deaths, incident cases) in a given population (O) divided by the expected number of events (E) if the study population had the same rates as those in a reference population (see Chapter 7, Section 7.3.2):

$$\text{SMR} = \frac{O}{E}$$

95% Confidence Interval

Assuming that the number of expected events is not subject to random variability, an easy way to obtain the 95% confidence interval for an SMR is to calculate the lower and upper limits for the observed number of events, O (see Section A.2), and then to substitute in the SMR formula. (For alternative methods, see Breslow and Day.[7])

Example

Based on the hypothetical data in Chapter 7, Table 7-8, 70 deaths were observed in study group B. The number of expected events obtained by applying the rates of an external reference population is 110. Thus, the estimated SMR for study group B is $70/110 = 0.64$. According to the table in Section A.2, the lower and upper limit factors for a rate based on 70 observed events (O) are, respectively, 0.785 and 1.27. Thus, the 95% confidence interval limits for O are $O_L = 70 \times 0.785 = 54.95$, and $O_U = 70 \times 1.27 = 88.9$. The resulting limits for the 95% confidence interval for the SMR are thus

$$\text{SMR}_L = \frac{54.95}{110} = 0.50$$

$$\text{SMR}_U = \frac{88.9}{110} = 0.81$$

A.8 MANTEL-HAENSZEL ODDS RATIO (AND RATE RATIO)

Standard Error

For two-by-two contingency tables stratified in k strata ($i = 1, \ldots k$), an approximate formula for the standard error (SE) of the Mantel-Haenszel estimate of the adjusted log odds ratio (OR), based on the notation in Chapter 7, Table 7-9, has been given by Robins et al.:[14]

$$\text{SE}(\log \text{OR}_{MH}) = \sqrt{\frac{\sum_{i=1}^{k}(P_i R_i)}{2\left(\sum_{i=1}^{k} R_i\right)^2} + \frac{\sum_{i=1}^{k}(P_i w_i + Q_i R_i)}{2\left(\sum_{i=1}^{k} R_i\right)\left(\sum_{i=1}^{k} w_i\right)} + \frac{\sum_{i=1}^{k}(Q_i w_i)}{2\left(\sum_{i=1}^{k} w_i\right)^2}}$$

where

$$P_i = \frac{a_i + d_i}{N_i}$$

$$Q_i = \frac{b_i + c_i}{N_i}$$

$$R_i = \frac{a_i \times d_i}{N_i}$$

$$w_i = \frac{b_i \times c_i}{N_i}$$

(Note: Greenland and Robins[15] have derived an analogous equation for the calculation of the SE of the Mantel-Haenszel estimate of the adjusted rate ratio for stratified cohort data—see Chapter 7, Section 7.3.3.)

95% Confidence Interval

The same approach described for the unadjusted OR in Section A.4 should be used: that is, the calculation of the confidence limits in a log scale and the exponentiation of the results to obtain the confidence interval for the OR_{MH}.

Hypothesis Testing

Again, following the notation in Chapter 7, Table 7-9, an approximate chi-square test with 1 degree of freedom (regardless of the number of strata involved) can be calculated as follows:[16]

$$\chi_1^2 = \frac{\left(\left|\sum_{i=1}^{k} a_i - \sum_{i=1}^{k} E_i\right| - 0.5\right)^2}{\sum_{i=1}^{k}\left(\frac{n_{1i} n_{2i} m_{1i} m_{2i}}{N_i^2 (N_i - 1)}\right)}$$

where E_i is the expected value in the "a" cell in each stratum, calculated from the values in the margins as in any chi-square test (e.g., $n_{i1} \times m_{i1}/N_i$).

Example

From the stratified results in Chapter 7, Table 7-1, the estimate of the OR_{MH} was 1.01. The following working table was set to apply the SE formula:

Sex	Case	Cont	N	OR	P	Q	R	w	PR	Pw+QR	Qw
Stratum 1											
M	53	15	81	1.06	0.691	0.309	1.963	1.852	1.357	1.886	0.572
F	10	3									
Stratum 2											
M	35	53	219	1.00	0.521	0.479	12.626	12.584	6.572	12.604	6.034
F	52	79									
			Sum =				14.589	14.436	7.929	14.490	6.606

Thus:

$$SE(\log OR_{MH}) = \sqrt{\frac{7.929}{2 \times 14.589^2} + \frac{14.490}{2 \times 14.589 \times 14.436} + \frac{6.605}{2 \times 14.436^2}}$$

$$= 0.262$$

The 95% confidence interval can be obtained as follows:

$$95\% \ CI(OR) = \exp[\log 1.01 \pm (1.96 \times 0.262)]$$

$$\text{Lower Limit} = \exp[-0.504] = 0.60$$

$$\text{Upper Limit} = \exp[0.525] = 1.69$$

(Note: The same shortcut for the direct calculation of the confidence limits of the OR as that shown for the crude OR—Section A.4—can be used.)

Hypothesis testing is performed as follows:

$$\chi_1^2 = \frac{\left(\left|(53 + 35) - \left(\frac{63 \times 68}{81} + \frac{87 \times 88}{219}\right)\right| - 0.5\right)^2}{\frac{63 \times 18 \times 68 \times 13}{81^2(81 - 1)} + \frac{87 \times 132 \times 88 \times 131}{219^2(219 - 1)}} = 0.008$$

Thus, in this example, the OR_{MH} is not statistically significant.

A.9 REGRESSION COEFFICIENT

In Chapter 7, Section 7.4, several regression models for multivariate analysis of epidemiologic data (linear, logistic, Cox, Poisson) are described. These regression analyses are typically conducted with the help of computers and statistical packages, which provide the estimates of the regression coefficients (b) and of their standard errors (SE(b)). On the basis of these estimates, and following the general approach described in the introduction to this appendix, it is possible to obtain confidence intervals and carry out hypothesis testing.

95% Confidence Interval

The 95% confidence interval for a regression coefficient estimate can be obtained with the following formula:

$$b \pm [1.96 \times SE(b)]$$

The standard errors are scaled to the same units as to those used to calculate the regression coefficient. Thus, in order to calculate the confidence interval for a different unit size, both terms need to be recalibrated. E.g., to calculate the 95% confidence limits corresponding to a 10-unit increment in the independent variable:

$$(b \times 10) \pm [1.96 \times SE(b) \times 10]$$

Likewise, to calculate the 95% confidence limits of an increase in one tenth of the b-value:

$$(b \times 0.1) \pm [1.96 \times SE(b) \times 0.1]$$

(See examples below.)

Hypothesis Testing

The null hypothesis is formulated as follows:

$$H_0: \beta = 0$$

where β denotes the true value of the parameter in the reference population.

The test statistic in this context is known as the Wald statistic:

$$\frac{b}{SE(b)} \approx z\text{-score}$$

Examples
Linear Regression

From the value of the regression coefficient and standard error for systolic blood pressure (10 mm Hg increase) in Chapter 7, Table 7-17, the 95% confidence intervals can be calculated as

$$0.040 \pm (1.96 \times 0.011)$$

That is, the estimated 95% confidence interval for the increase in leucocyte count per 10 mm Hg increase in systolic blood pressure is 0.018 to 0.062 thousand per mm^3. As described above, the 95% confidence interval for an increase in 5 mm Hg (instead of 10) would be estimated as:

$$(0.040 \times 0.5) \pm (1.96 \times 0.011 \times 0.5)$$

Or $0.020 \pm 0.01078 = 0.009$ to 0.031.

The Wald statistic, which approximates the z-score, is calculated as

$$z \approx \frac{0.040}{0.011} = 3.64$$

This value is associated with $p < 0.001$, which allows rejecting the null hypothesis with a probability of type-I error lower than $1/1000$.

Logistic Regression

As with the above linear regression example, in order to calculate the OR corresponding to a different unit of the independent variable, the rescaling of units for both the logistic regression coefficient *and* its standard error need to be done *before* the exponentiation step. For example, according to the results of the logistic regression analysis shown in Chapter 7, Table 7-18 and assuming a standard error for the coefficient of 0.0045 (not shown in Table 7-18), the 95% confidence interval for the OR corresponding to an increase in one mm Hg of systolic blood pressure (OR = $e^{0.0167}$ = 1.017) will be:

Lower Limit = exp $[0.0167 - (1.96 \times 0.0045)] = 1.008$

Upper Limit = exp $[0.0167 + (1.96 \times 0.0045)] = 1.026$

And the 95% confidence limits for the OR associated with an increase in 10 mm Hg:

Lower Limit = exp $[0.0167 \times 10 - (1.96 \times 0.0045 \times 10)] = 1.082$

Upper Limit = exp $[0.0167 \times 10 + (1.96 \times 0.0045 \times 10)] = 1.291$

As an additional example for the case of a categorical variable, in the example in Table 7-19, the estimated logistic regression coefficient associated with hypertension is 0.5103, which translates into an estimated odds ratio of coronary disease of $e^{0.5103} = 1.67$, comparing hypertensives with nonhypertensives (adjusted for all the other variables displayed in Table 7-19). The standard error corresponding to the estimated regression coefficient is 0.1844 (not shown in Table 7-19). Thus, the 95% confidence interval for the regression coefficient is calculated as follows:

$$0.5103 \pm (1.96 \times 0.1844)$$

or 0.1489 (lower limit) and 0.8717 (upper limit). The corresponding confidence interval (CI) of the odds ratio (OR) estimate can be obtained by exponentiating these confidence limits. This can also be done in just one step, as follows:

$$\text{Lower Limit} = \exp[0.5103 - (1.96 \times 0.1844)] = 1.16$$

$$\text{Upper Limit} = \exp[0.5103 + (1.96 \times 0.1844)] = 2.39$$

The corresponding Wald statistic for the regression coefficient estimate is

$$z \approx \frac{0.5103}{0.1844} = 2.767$$

The associated p value for this z-score is 0.006. Note that this statistic tests the null hypothesis (H_0: $\beta = 0$, or the equivalent H_0: OR = 1).

The same approach can be used to obtain confidence limits and conduct hypothesis testing for regression coefficients and derived measures of association from Cox and Poisson regression models.

Wald Statistic for Interaction

If the model contains an interaction term (e.g., the product of two x variables; see Chapter 7, Section 7.4.2, Equation 7.4), the statistical significance of the corresponding regression coefficient estimate (Wald statistic) is a formal test for the interaction between the two variables. In the example in Equation 7.4, which is a variation of model 2 in Table 7-16, allowing for an interaction between age and systolic blood pressure, the estimated b_3 is 0.0000503, with a standard error of 0.0000570, which corresponds to a Wald statistic of 0.882 (not statistically significant). Thus, these data do not support the hypothesis that there is an interaction between age and systolic blood pressure in relation to carotid intimal-medial thickness.

A.10 SENSITIVITY, SPECIFICITY, AND PERCENT AGREEMENT

Statistical inference procedures for these three measures are the same as those for any other simple proportion.

Standard Error, 95% Confidence Interval

The standard formulation to calculate the standard error of a proportion (p) calculated in a sample of N individuals can be used:

$$\text{SE}(p) = \sqrt{\frac{p(1-p)}{N}}$$

Once the standard error is calculated, the general approach for obtaining confidence limits outlined in the introduction to this appendix can be used.

Examples

The following examples are all based on the data from a validation study of self-reported "difficulty in standing up from a chair"[17] (Chapter 8, Table 8-13).

Sensitivity

The estimated sensitivity is $71/(71 + 42) = 0.628$. To calculate the standard error, use as N the total number of true positives ($N = 113$, the denominator for sensitivity):

$$\text{SE (sensitivity)} = \sqrt{\frac{0.628(1 - 0.628)}{113}} = 0.0455$$

Thus, the 95% confidence interval is

$$\text{Lower Limit} = 0.628 - (1.96 \times 0.0455) = 0.539$$

$$\text{Upper Limit} = 0.628 + (1.96 \times 0.0455) = 0.717$$

Specificity

The estimated specificity is $455/(455 + 41) = 0.917$. To calculate the standard error, use as N the total number of true negatives ($N = 496$, the denominator for specificity):

$$\text{SE (specificity)} = \sqrt{\frac{0.917(1 - 0.917)}{496}} = 0.0124$$

Thus, the 95% confidence interval is

$$\text{Lower Limit} = 0.917 - (1.96 \times 0.0124) = 0.893$$

$$\text{Upper Limit} = 0.917 + (1.96 \times 0.0124) = 0.941$$

Percent Agreement

The estimated percent agreement is $(71 + 455)/609 = 0.864$. To calculate the standard error, use as N the total number in the table ($N = 609$):

$$\text{SE (\% Agreement)} = \sqrt{\frac{0.864(1 - 0.864)}{609}} = 0.0139$$

Thus, the 95% confidence interval (using percentage values) is

$$\text{Lower Limit} = 86.4 - (1.96 \times 1.39) = 83.7\%$$

$$\text{Upper Limit} = 86.4 + (1.96 \times 1.39) = 89.1\%$$

A.11 YOUDEN'S J STATISTIC

Standard Error, Confidence Interval

Youden's J statistic is based on the sum of two proportions (sensitivity and specificity) (see Chapter 8, Section 8.4.1). Assuming that these are independent, the standard error (SE) can be calculated as

$$\text{SE}(J) = \sqrt{\frac{\text{Sens}(1 - \text{Sens})}{N_{\text{true}+}} + \frac{\text{Spec}(1 - \text{Spec})}{N_{\text{true}-}}}$$

Once the standard error is calculated, the general approach for obtaining confidence limits outlined in the introduction to this appendix can be used.

Examples

The following example is based on the data from Chapter 8, Table 8-5. The estimated Youden's J statistic is $(18/19) + (11/30) - 1 = 0.314$. Using the above formula, the standard error is as follows:

$$\text{SE}(J) = \sqrt{\frac{\frac{18}{19} \times \frac{1}{19}}{19} + \frac{\frac{11}{30} \times \frac{19}{30}}{30}} = 0.102$$

Thus, the 95% confidence interval is

$$\text{Lower Limit} = 0.314 - (1.96 \times 0.102) = 0.114$$
$$\text{Upper Limit} = 0.314 + (1.96 \times 0.102) = 0.514$$

A.12 KAPPA

The kappa statistic is a useful measure of reliability of categorical variables (see Chapter 8, Section 8.4.1). Formulas for the calculation of the standard error and 95% confidence interval for the *unweighted* kappa are provided as follows.

Standard Error and 95% Confidence Interval

Formulas for the calculation of the standard error of kappa have been published.[18] Consider a situation in which two replicate readings (e.g., readings by two raters, A and B) of a given set of test values have been done. The outcome of the test has k possible values, the number of agreement cells. The following table defines the notation for the observed proportions (p) in each cell and marginal totals of the resulting contingency table of both sets of readings.

		Rater B				
		1	2	...	k	Total
Rater A	1	p_{11}	p_{12}	...	p_{1k}	$p_{1\cdot}$
	2	p_{21}	p_{22}	...	p_{2k}	$p_{2\cdot}$
	...	...	...	...	...	...
	k	p_{k1}	p_{k2}	...	p_{kk}	$p_{k\cdot}$
	Total	$p_{\cdot 1}$	$p_{\cdot 2}$	...	$p_{\cdot k}$	1

Based on the preceding notation, the SE of the estimated kappa (k) can be obtained as follows:

$$\text{SE}(\hat{\kappa}) = \frac{1}{(1 - p_e) \times \sqrt{n}} \times \sqrt{p_e + p_e^2 - \left[\sum_{i=1}^{k} p_{i\cdot} \times p_{\cdot i} \times (p_{i\cdot} + p_{\cdot i})\right]}$$

where p_e is the total expected chance agreement, which is calculated from the product of the symmetrical marginal proportions (see Chapter 8, Section 8.4.1):

$$p_e = \sum_{i=1}^{k} p_{i\cdot} \times p_{\cdot i}$$

Note: Formulas for the standard error of *weighted* kappa have also been derived; see, e.g., Fleiss.[18]

Example

The following example is based on the data from a study of self-reported "difficulty in standing up from a chair"[17] (Chapter 8, Table 8-13) (see also Section A.10):

	Observed difficulty		
Reported difficulty	Yes	No	Total
Yes	71	41	112
No	42	455	497
Total	113	496	609

Source: Data from M Ferrer et al., Comparison of Performance-Based and Self-Rated Functional Capacity in Spanish Elderly. *American Journal of Epidemiology*, Vol 149, pp. 228–235.

Dividing numbers in the table by the total ($N = 609$), the following table shows the proportions as in the notation table shown previously.

	Observed difficulty		
Reported difficulty	Yes	No	Total
Yes	0.1166		0.1839
No		0.7471	0.8161
Total	0.1856	0.8144	1

Note: The proportions in the discordant cells are not shown because they are not used in the calculations that follow.
Source: Data from M Ferrer et al., Comparison of Performance-Based and Self-Rated Functional Capacity in Spanish Elderly,. *American Journal of Epidemiology*, Vol 149, pp. 228–235. © 1999.

The observed agreement is

$$p_o = \sum_{i=1}^{k} p_{ii} = 0.1166 + 0.7471 = 0.8637$$

The expected (chance) agreement is

$$p_e = \sum_{i=1}^{k} p_{i\cdot} \times p_{\cdot i} = (0.1865 \times 0.1839) + (0.8144 \times 0.8161) = 0.6989$$

Thus, the estimated kappa for these data is

$$\kappa = \frac{p_0 - p_e}{1 - p_e} = \frac{0.8637 - 0.6989}{1 - 0.6989} = 0.547$$

Using the above formula, the standard error is as follows:

$$\frac{1}{(1 - 0.6989)\sqrt{609}} \times \sqrt{0.6989 + 0.6989^2 - \left(\begin{array}{c} 0.1839 \times 0.1856 \times (0.1839 + 0.1856) \\ + 0.8161 \times 0.8144 \times (0.8161 + 0.8144) \end{array}\right)} = 0.041$$

Thus, the 95% confidence interval is

$$\text{Lower Limit} = 0.547 - (1.96 \times 0.041) = 0.467$$

$$\text{Upper Limit} = 0.547 + (1.96 \times 0.041) = 0.627$$

REFERENCES

1. Goodman SN. *p* values, hypothesis tests, and likelihood: Implications for epidemiology of a neglected historical debate. *Am J Epidemiol.* 1993;137:485–496.
2. Royal R. *Statistical Evidence: A Likelihood Primer*. London, England: Chapman and Hall; 1997.
3. Armitage P, Berry G, Matthews JNS. *Statistical Methods in Medical Research*, 4th ed. Oxford, UK: Blackwell Publishing; 2002.
4. Altman DG. *Practical Statistics for Medical Students*. London, England: Chapman and Hall; 1991.
5. Greenwood M. A report on the natural duration of cancer. *Rep Public Health Med Subjects.* 1926;33:1–26.
6. Haenszel W, Loveland DB, Sirken MG. Lung cancer mortality as related to residence and smoking histories: I: White males. *J Natl Cancer Inst.* 1962;28:947–1001.
7. Breslow NE, Day NE. *Statistical Methods in Cancer Research*, Vol. 2. The Design and Analysis of Cohort Studies. Lyon, France: IARC Scientific Publications; 1987.
8. Katz D, Baptista J, Azen SP, et al. Obtaining confidence intervals for the risk ratio in cohort studies. *Biometrics.* 1978;34:469–474.
9. Ederer F, Mantel N. Confidence limits on the ratio of two Poisson variables. *Am J Epidemiol.* 1974;100:165–167.
10. Woolf B. On estimating the relation between blood group and disease. *Ann Hum Genet.* 1955;19:251–253.
11. Walter SD. Calculation of attributable risks from epidemiological data. *Int J Epidemiol.* 1978;7:175–182.
12. Kahn HA, Sempos CT. *Statistical Methods in Epidemiology*. 2nd ed. New York, NY: Oxford University Press; 1989.
13. Pandey DK, Shekelle R, Selwyn BJ, et al. Dietary vitamin C and β-carotene and risk of death in middle-aged men: The Western Electric Study. *Am J Epidemiol.* 1995;142:1269–1278.
14. Robins J, Greenland S, Breslow NE. A general estimator for the variance of the Mantel-Haenszel odds ratio. *Am J Epidemiol.* 1986;124:719–723.
15. Greenland S, Robins JM. Estimation of a common effect parameter from sparse follow-up death. *Biometrics.* 1985;41:55–68.
16. Mantel N, Haenszel W. Statistical aspects of the analysis of data from retrospective studies of disease. *J Natl Cancer Inst.* 1959;22:719–748.
17. Ferrer M, Lamarca R, Orfila F, Alfonso J. Comparison of performance-based and self-rated functional capacity in Spanish elderly. *Am J Epidemiol.* 1999;149:228–235.
18. Fleiss JL. *Statistical Methods for Rates and Proportions*, 2nd ed. New York, NY: John Wiley and Sons; 1981.

Test for Trend (Dose Response)

APPENDIX B

When exposure is categorized into multiple *ordinal* categories, it may be of interest to assess whether the observed relation between increasing (or decreasing) levels of exposure and the risk (or odds) of disease follows a *linear* dose-response pattern. One example was provided in Chapter 3 at the end of Section 3.4.1, Table 3-12, in which the odds ratios of craniosynostosis seemed to increase in relation to increasing maternal age in a dose-response fashion.[1] A statistical test to assess whether the observed trend is statistically significant (i.e., whether the null hypothesis that there is no linear trend can be rejected) was developed by Mantel.[2] The formulation below is based on the following notation:

Stratum (i)	Score (x_i)	No. of cases (a_i)	No. of controls (b_i)	Total (n_i)
1	x_1	a_1	b_1	n_1
2	x_2	a_2	b_2	n_2
.	.	.	.	.
.	.	.	.	.
k	x_k	a_k	b_k	n_k
Total		A	B	N

The following statistic has a chi-square distribution with 1 degree of freedom:

$$\chi_1^2 = \frac{\left[\sum_{i=1}^{k}\left(a_i x_i - \frac{n_i x_i A}{N}\right)\right]^2}{\left(\frac{A \times B \times \left[\left(N \times \sum_{i=1}^{k} n_i x_i^2\right) - \left(\sum_{i=1}^{k} n_i x_i\right)^2\right]}{N^2(N-1)}\right)}$$

where the scores (x_i) are values that represent the level of exposure in each subsequent ordinal category (see below).

APPENDIX B | Test for Trend (Dose Response)

EXAMPLE

To illustrate the application of Mantel's trend test, the data from the example in Chapter 3, Table 3-11, are used. For the purpose of making the calculations easier, these data are rearranged in the following work table:

Age (yr)	i	x_i	a_i	b_i	n_i	$\left[a_i x_i - \dfrac{n_i x_i A}{N} \right]$	$n_i x_i$	$n_i x_i^2$
< 20	1	1	12	89	101	−6.748	101	101
20–24	2	2	47	242	289	−13.290	578	1156
25–29	3	3	56	255	311	−5.186	933	2799
> 29	4	4	58	173	231	60.485	924	3696
Total			173	759	932	35.262	2536	7752

Source: Data from BW Alderman et al., An Epidemiologic Study of Craniosynostosis: Risk Indicators for the Occurrence of Craniosynostosis in Colorado. *American Journal of Epidemiology*, Vol 128, pp. 431–438, © 1988.

Thus, applying the above formula:

$$\chi_i^2 = \frac{[35.262]^2}{\left(\dfrac{173 \times 759 \times [(932 \times 7752) - 2536^2]}{932^2 (932 - 1)} \right)} = 9.65$$

corresponding to a *p* value of 0.0019.

NOTES

The null hypothesis corresponding to this trend test is that there is no linear association, or, in other words, that the *slope* of the association with increasing levels of exposure is zero (flat). Thus, a significant *p* value from this test means that the data do not support the hypothesis of a zero slope. Such a result should not replace the examination of the actual odds ratio estimates in order to judge whether a linear trend is indeed present. As for any other statistical test, the *p* value depends strongly on the sample size; thus, if the sample size is large, a *J*-type or a threshold-type association may result in a significant trend test, even though the association is not linear. For example, suppose that the estimated odds ratios for five increasing ordinal categories of a given exposure (e.g., quintiles of a continuous variable) are 1.0 (reference), 0.9, 1.1, 1.0, and 3.0. If the sample size is sufficiently large, the trend test may yield a highly significant result, which simply indicates that the null hypothesis ("slope" = 0) can be rejected with a certain level of confidence, notwithstanding the fact that, in this example, the pattern of the association is practically flat, except for the high odds ratio in the top quintile that is an increase in odds limited to the individuals in the top fifth of the distribution. This phenomenon is analogous to the issues discussed in Chapter 7 on the use of linear models to analyze nonlinear patterns (Section 7.4.7).

The above trend test is analogous to the Wald test for a linear regression coefficient (see Section 7.4.8), except that it is based on a small number of data points (four in the above example), which are *weighted* according to the number of subjects in the corresponding category. Thus, as when using any linear regression model, caution should be exercised when interpreting the results of a trend test.

Alternative formulations of the trend test described have been proposed, based on assessing the linear trends in proportions (see, for example, Cochran[3]). Given the arithmetical equivalence between proportions and odds, all these alternative tests lead to similar results; for additional references and discussion, see Fleiss[4] or Schlesselman.[5]

In the example below, the scores were arbitrarily set as 1, 2, 3, and 4. Note that the exact same chi-square value will be obtained using the scores −1, 0, 1, and 2, while the calculations (if done by hand) will be considerably easier. In the case of ordinal categorizations based on a continuous variable (such as age in the example above), instead of these completely arbitrary scores, it may be more appropriate to choose as scores the midpoints for the variables that define each category. For example, assuming that the ranges for the top and bottom open-ended categories above were 10 to 19 years and 30 to 39 years, respectively, the scores would be 15, 22.5, 27.5, and 35, with the following result:

Age (yr)	i	x_i	a_i	b_i	n_i	$\left[a_i x_i - \dfrac{n_i x_i A}{N} \right]$	$n_i x_i$	$n_i x_i^2$
< 20	1	15	12	89	101	−101.22	1515	22,725
20–24	2	22.5	47	242	289	−149.51	6502.5	146,306.3
25–29	3	27.5	56	255	311	−47.535	8552.5	235,193.8
> 29	4	35	58	173	231	529.244	8085	282,975
Total			173	759	932	230.982	24,655	687,200

Source: Data from BW Alderman et al., An Epidemiologic Study of Craniosynostosis: Risk Indicators for the Occurrence of Craniosynostosis in Colorado. *American Journal of Epidemiology*, Vol 128, pp. 431–438, © 1988.

In this example, the resulting chi-square is 10.08, $p = 0.0015$. (Alternatively, the score for each category could be the mean or median value for the variable in question for all the individuals included in each respective category.)

MULTIVARIATE TREND TEST

As stated previously, the statistical test for trend is the analogue to the Wald test assessing the statistical significance of a linear regression coefficient (see Chapter 7, Section 7.4.8 and Appendix A.9). In fact, a regression approach can be used to test the statistical significance of a linear dose-response trend (using odds ratios or another measure of association, depending on the statistical model at hand; see Chapter 7, Table 7-14) corresponding to an ordinal variable *while adjusting for additional covariates* included in the model. For example, it may be of interest to assess whether the risk of craniosynostosis increases linearly with age (categorized as above) while adjusting for additional covariates (e.g., socioeconomic status, family history). In that situation, to carry out the multivariate analogue of the above trend test in the example, a logistic regression model can be used entering the variable AGEGROUP as a single ordinal term (with values 1, 2, 3, and 4, or any other meaningful alternative, as discussed above), along with any other variables in the model that need to be controlled for. The Wald statistic for the regression coefficient corresponding to this variable can be interpreted as a statistical test for linear dose response for adjusted data. As for the trend test for unadjusted data, it is important to examine whether there is an actual dose response trend by inspection of stratum-specific estimates (e.g., by examining the estimates based on a model using dummy variables) before interpreting this statistical trend test on the basis of regression (see Chapter 7, Section 7.4.7).

REFERENCES

1. Alderman BW, Lammer EJ, Joshua SC, et al. An epidemiologic study of craniosynostosis: Risk indicators for the occurrence of craniosynostosis in Colorado. *Am J Epidemiol.* 1998;128:431–438.
2. Mantel N. Chi-square tests with one degree of freedom: extensions of the Mantel-Haenszel procedure. *J Am Stat Assoc.* 1963;58:690–700.
3. Cochran WG. Some methods for strengthening the common chi-square tests. *Biometrics.*1954; 10:417–451.
4. Fleiss JL. *Statistical Methods for Rates and Proportions*, 2nd ed. New York, NY: John Wiley and Sons; 1981.
5. Schlesselman JJ. *Case Control Studies*. New York, NY: Oxford University Press; 1982.

APPENDIX C

Test of Homogeneity of Stratified Estimates (Test for Interaction)

As discussed in Chapter 6, interaction or effect modification is present when the association between a given exposure and an outcome is modified by the presence or level of a third variable (the *effect modifier*). The different aspects that need to be considered when judging whether an observed heterogeneity of the association is truly interaction or is due to random variability of the stratum-specific estimates were discussed in Chapter 6 (Sections 6.9 and 6.10.1). In this appendix, a general procedure to assess the hypothesis of homogeneity (i.e., lack of interaction) is described. As with any hypothesis test, the *p* value resulting from this homogeneity testing is strongly dependent on sample size. This problem is especially important when stratified data are evaluated. Epidemiologic studies are typically designed to optimize the statistical power to detect associations based on pooled data from the total study sample. However, the power to detect interaction is often limited by insufficient stratum-specific sample sizes.[1]

Consider a situation in which a given measure of association r between exposure and outcome is estimated across k strata of a suspected effect modifier. The general form of a statistical test of the homogeneity hypothesis (i.e., H_0: the strength of association is homogeneous across all strata) is analogous to a familiar type of statistical test to compare stratified survival data (log rank test) and adopts the following general form:[1]

$$\chi^2_{k-1} = \sum_{i=1}^{k} \frac{(R_i - \hat{R})^2}{V_i}$$

where R_i is the stratum-specific measure of association (for $i = 1$ to k strata), V_i is the corresponding variance, and $\hat{R}$ is the estimated "common" underlying value of the measure of association under the null hypothesis. The latter is usually estimated using one of the approaches to obtain weighted averages of stratum-specific estimates of association described in Section 7.3 of Chapter 7 (e.g., direct adjustment, indirect adjustment, Mantel-Haenszel). This test statistic has a chi-square distribution with as many degrees of freedom as the number of strata minus 1.

One important consideration is that for multiplicative (relative) measures of association (e.g., relative risk, odds ratio, rate ratio), the logarithm of the ratio (not the ratio itself) is used in the preceding equation for R_i and $\hat{R}$; consequently, the corresponding variance, V_i, is the variance of the log (ratio).

EXAMPLE: TEST OF HOMOGENEITY OF STRATIFIED ODDS RATIOS

This test uses the following formula:

$$\chi^2_{k-1} = \sum_{i=1}^{k} \frac{(\log \text{OR}_i - \log \hat{\text{OR}})^2}{\text{var}(\log \text{OR}_i)}$$

APPENDIX C | Test of Homogeneity of Stratified Estimates (Test for Interaction)

The following example of the application of this test uses data from Table 7-2, which displayed the association between oral contraceptive use and myocardial infarction stratified by age.[2] The Mantel-Haenszel estimate of the overall odds ratio for these data is $OR_{MH} = 3.97$ (Section 7.3.3). The following table is organized to facilitate the calculations of the homogeneity test statistic:

Stratum no. (age, yr)	OC	No. of cases (a) (c)	No. of controls (b) (d)	OR $(a \times d)$ $(b \times c)$	Log OR	Var (Log OR) $\left(\frac{1}{a} + \frac{1}{b} + \frac{1}{c} + \frac{1}{d} \right)^*$
1 (25–29)	Yes	4	62	7.226	1.978	0.771
	No	2	224			
2 (30–34)	Yes	9	33	8.864	2.182	0.227
	No	12	390			
3 (35–39)	Yes	4	26	1.538	0.431	0.322
	No	33	330			
4 (40–44)	Yes	6	9	3.713	1.312	0.296
	No	65	362			
5 (45–49)	Yes	6	5	3.884	1.357	0.381
	No	93	301			

Note: OC, oral contraceptive use.
*See Appendix A, Section A.4.
Source: Data from S Shapiro et al., Oral-Contraceptive Use in Relation to Myocardial Infarction. *Lancet*, Vol 1, pp. 743–747, © 1979.

Thus, applying the above formula:

$$\chi_4^2 = \frac{[1.978 - \log(3.97)]^2}{0.771} + \frac{[2.182 - \log(3.97)]^2}{0.227} + \ldots + \frac{[1.357 - \log(3.97)]^2}{0.381}$$

$$= 0.4655 + 2.8382 + 2.7925 + 0.0151 + 0.0013$$

$$= 6.113$$

This chi-square value with 4 degrees of freedom is associated with a $P > 0.10$ and thus is nonsignificant at conventional levels.

REFERENCES

1. Rothman KJ, Greenland S. *Modern Epidemiology*, 3rd ed. Philadelphia, PA: Wolters Kluwer Health Lippincott; 2008.
2. Shapiro S, Slone D, Rosenberg L, et al. Oral-contraceptive use in relation to myocardial infarction. *Lancet*. 1979;1:743–747.

Quality Assurance and Quality Control Procedures Manual for Blood Pressure Measurement and Blood/Urine Collection in the ARIC Study

Appendix D

The following is a verbatim transcription of two sections of the Atherosclerosis Risk in Communities (ARIC) Study Quality Assurance/Quality Control Manual of operations. These are included as examples for some of the procedures discussed in Chapter 8. For more detail on the ARIC Study design and protocol (including the entire Quality Control Manual and other manuals cited in the following text), see the ARIC Study Web page (http://www.cscc.unc.edu/aric).

SITTING BLOOD PRESSURE

1. Brief Description of Sitting Blood Pressure Procedures and Related Quality Assurance and Quality Control Measures

The following equipment is used for measuring sitting blood pressure: a standard Littman stethoscope with bell; standardized Hawksley random-zero instrument; standard Baum manometer for determining peak inflation level; four standardized cuffs (from Baum). After the technician explains the procedure to the participant, measures the arm circumference and wraps the arm with the correct cuff, the participant sits quietly for 5 minutes, and then the technician makes two readings, with at least 30 seconds between reading one measure and beginning the next. The average of the two readings is reported to the participant.

From the detailed protocol for sitting blood pressure in ARIC Manual 11, the various data transfer points and other possible sources of error have been considered, and needed quality assurance and control measures have been derived. Important elements in quality assurance are training and certification programs, observation of data collection by supervisors, biannually simultaneous blood pressure measurements using Y-tubes by two technicians, and standard equipment maintenance procedures performed and entered into logs.

2. Maintenance of Equipment

a. *Availability of all sizes cuffs*: The field center blood pressure supervisor makes certain that the field center always has the full range of blood pressure cuffs available at each blood pressure station. Field center staff report immediately to the blood pressure supervisor if they cannot find all cuff sizes at the station.

b. *Sphygmomanometers*: Regular inspections of random-zero and standard sphygmomanometers are described in ARIC Manual 11, Section 1.13.1 and Appendices I, II, and V. A log sheet is kept by the field center blood pressure supervisor, who records the performance of these checks and comments on any problems found (see copy of log sheet in Manual 11, Appendix IV). By the end of each January and July, the summary form for the checklists should be filled and mailed to the Coordinating Center.

c. *Measuring tape*: Each week the blood pressure supervisor checks the condition of the measuring tape used to measure arm circumference at the blood pressure station(s), and replaces any that have become worn. The results of this check are recorded on the anthropometry weekly log. (See the anthropometry section for details.)

3. Field Center Monitoring of Technician Performance

a. *Double stethoscoping*: To help assess the accuracy and precision of blood pressure measurements, once each January and July each blood pressure technician takes part in measuring blood pressure simultaneously with another technician, using a Y-tube. *This procedure should be carried out using volunteers or other field center staff members, not ARIC study participants.* The two technicians also perform independent measurements of arm circumference, which they record on the forms. If the two technician measurements lead to a disagreement on which blood pressure cuff to use, then both remeasure the arm together and use the cuff size determined by that measurement. Each records this disagreement on the Sitting Blood Pressure form. Each technician separately records all blood pressure measurements on paper on a standard Sitting Blood Pressure form. The two paper forms are given to the field center blood pressure supervisor, who compares the results.

The field center blood pressure supervisor reviews the results of these duplicate examinations, calculating the disagreement between technicians on the blood pressure measurements and recording it on the form. The two technicians should agree on each of the two measurements of diastolic and systolic blood pressure within 4 mm Hg, and their average should agree within 3 mm Hg, as is required by the standards for certification. If they do not, further duplicate readings are taken to determine if either or both technicians require recertification. These further measurements should again be recorded as described in the previous paragraph.

The IDs of each set of technicians paired for simultaneous measurement of blood pressure are recorded in the Report on Use of Observation and Equipment Checklist, which is mailed to the Coordinating Center at the end of each January and July.

b. *Biannual observation*: Once every January and July, the field center's blood pressure supervisor observes each blood pressure technician performing the entire measurement procedure with a study participant. The field center supervisor notes any problems with technique and discusses them with the technician after the examination has been completed. Also, another technician observes the field center blood pressure supervisor perform the entire measurement process. After the examination, the two of them discuss any questions that come up in the course of this observation. In performing these observations, the supervisor and technicians use the checklist given in Appendix III of ARIC Manual 11. For each technician, the date that the technician was observed and the observer's ID number are recorded in the Report on Use of Observation and Equipment Checklist.

4. Recording of Participant ID Data

In filling out the Sitting Blood Pressure screen, the technician verifies that the name and ID number on the DES screen which accompanies the participant match the participant's to avoid ID errors. If the PC is down and a paper form is used, the technician verifies the name on the folder accompanying the participant before using the ID labels in the folder on the forms.

5. Measurement of Arm Circumference and Choice of Blood Pressure Cuff

As described above, once every 6 months duplicate measurements of blood pressure are performed on a volunteer or field center staff member (not an ARIC participant). During the course of this procedure, both technicians measure arm circumference and record their results. The field center blood pressure supervisor compares these results, and if they differ by more than 1 cm, the measurement technique is reviewed with both technicians.

Both the arm measurement and the cuff size chosen are recorded on the SBP form. The data entry system checks for the consistency of cuff size and arm circumference.

6. Participant Posture and Rest Before Blood Pressure Measurement

The field center blood pressure supervisor monitors that the station(s) used for blood pressure measurement continue to meet the conditions specified in the protocol, for example, that blood pressure measurements are done in a quiet room away from other field center activities. Coordinating Center staff on monitoring visits also take note whether this condition is being maintained.

The field center blood pressure supervisor is responsible for seeing that the protocol is followed by timing blood pressure measurements early in the visit, before blood drawing or other stressful activities. Each month the field center supervisor reviews a sample of participant itinerary forms for the previous month to confirm that this is done.

To assist in judging that a full 5-minute rest is allowed before taking the first blood pressure measurement, the blood pressure technician uses a handheld timer or other means of accurately timing the rest period. Biannually, the field center blood pressure supervisor observes each technician performing the full blood pressure procedure and notes whether the correct rest period is being allowed.

7. Coordinating Center Quality Control Analyses

The Coordinating Center analyzes data from each technician for digit preference in reading systolic or diastolic blood pressure. This check is performed annually, unless problems detected call for more or less intensive monitoring. The Coordinating Center reports these results to the field center, and the field center blood pressure supervisor reviews these results with each technician.

The Coordinating Center checks that correct data entry procedures are used for recording missing data. The Coordinating Center communicates with the field centers when problems are identified.

BLOOD AND URINE COLLECTION AND PROCESSING

1. Brief Description of Blood Collection and Processing and Related Quality Assurance and Quality Control Measures

At the time of the telephone contact participants are requested to fast for 12 hours before field center visit, unless they are diabetics taking insulin or have other medical reasons that make fasting inadvisable. A detailed protocol, set out in ARIC Manual 7 (*Blood Collection and Processing*) has been developed, which describes the preparation of blood tubes, the anticoagulants to be used for samples for each laboratory, and the specific steps to be taken in blood drawing and processing. After the blood is drawn, the sample tubes go through further processing at the field center. Blood samples used for lipid and hemostasis analyses are frozen at $-70°C$ for weekly shipment to the ARIC central laboratories. Samples for hematology analyses are sent to local laboratories. All shipments to Central Laboratories are by overnight delivery services. All of these steps are performed by technicians trained in the ARIC protocol and certified to have adequately mastered its details.

The first step in quality assurance for blood drawing consists in this training and certification process. Other steps include maintaining logs of equipment checks; observation of technicians (by other technicians and by monitors on visits) as they go through the sequence of steps in blood drawing and processing; review of the condition of samples received at central laboratories for problems in shipment; and periodic analysis of the study data for participant compliance with fasting and for signs of problems in drawing or processing, such as hemolysis or delays in completing processing.

2. Maintenance of Equipment

Each field center performs daily temperature checks on refrigerators, freezers, the refrigerated centrifuge, and the heating block (see ARIC Manual 7). The actual speed of the centrifuge is checked and recorded monthly with a tachometer. The results of these checks are recorded on a log sheet kept at the blood processing station and are summarized onto the Report on the Use of Observation and Equipment Checklist at the end of each January and July. A copy of the report is sent to the Coordinating Center at that time.

3. Participant Compliance with Protocol

In contrast to previous visits, venipuncture is performed on all cohort members, regardless of their fasting status (Manual 2, Section 3.9.2), and includes three plasma samples for the Lipid and Hemostasis labs; two serum samples for the Hemostasis and Dental labs; and an optional sample for a local Hematology lab. In addition, a second venipuncture is performed on OGTT eligible participants. The post glucola blood draw must occur within 2 hours (plus or minus 10 minutes) of administration of the glucola drink. Failure to meet criteria can affect the values of various measurements (e.g., lipids, glucose) and compromise their value to the study. ARIC participants should also abstain from smoking and vigorous physical effort before the visit to the field center, since smoking may affect electrocardiograms or blood pressure and vigorous activity may activate fibrinolysis and alter blood levels of tPA and FPB8. Interviewers are trained to explain the importance of compliance with these restrictions. When field centers contact participants before their appointment to remind them about the scheduled visit, they repeat these instructions.

The Coordinating Center analyzes study data for information on length of time fasting and time since smoking and hard exercise, broken down by field center, to obtain the number and percent of participants at each field center each month who do not comply with these restrictions.

4. Maintaining Proficiency

To maintain their proficiency, technicians are urged to perform blood drawing and processing at least once each week (or eight times each 2 months). The Coordinating Center analyzes the study data to report on the number of times that technicians collect and process blood in the field centers.

5. Periodic Observation

Periodically (each month in the beginning) each field center technician performing blood drawing and processing is observed performing the entire procedure by either another trained technician or a supervisor, using a detailed checklist to verify that the technician is continuing to follow all parts of the ARIC protocol. Carrying out this observation also provides a review of the protocol for the person doing the observation (see ARIC Manual 7 for further details and for a copy of the ARIC Venipuncture and Processing Procedure Certification Checklist). This checklist is also used for observations by monitors from the Coordinating Center performing monitoring. The IDs of observer and observed are recorded in the ARIC Venipuncture and Processing Procedure Certification Checklist. They are also recorded on the Report on the Use of Observation and Equipment Checklist, which is mailed to the Coordinating Center by the end of each January and July.

6. The Laboratory Form

To avoid ID errors in which information regarding a given participant's samples is written down on the wrong form, the technician should begin filling out each Laboratory Form (LABB) as the blood is drawn, verifying the ID from the folder that accompanies the participant.

7. Quality Control Replicate Data

The system of drawing extra tubes of blood for QC replicate analysis is fully explained in ARIC Manual 7. In this system specified extra tubes of blood are drawn from a number of participants and matched to one "phantom participant" per week. The post-glucola blood sample is designated as Tube 6 on the Phantom Participant and Non-Participant ID form. See also Chapter 2 of Manual 12 for an explanation of the QC phantom system.

Persons who are nonfasting and indicate that they would like to be rescheduled for another blood draw should never be used as a QC blood phantom.

The field center blood drawing station maintains a schedule of which tubes should be drawn for phantoms each day (see ARIC Manual 7) to help fit the QC phantom sets into the work flow and make it easy to keep track of what is required. The Coordinating Center reviews each month, broken down by field center, the number of QC phantom forms for which blood drawing is indicated. If field centers fail to provide sufficient sets of QC phantom blood, the Coordinating Center contacts the field centers to discuss the problem. To reduce the risk of labeling a QC phantom blood tube with the wrong ID or of recording the wrong match between phantom and participant IDs on the QC Phantom Participant Forms, QC blood is drawn from no more than one member of each pair of participants whose blood is processed together. To help make certain that the correct match is recorded between real participant ID and QC phantom ID, as soon as blood-drawing has been completed an ID label for the real participant ID is added to the appropriate space on the QC Phantom Participant and Non-Participant ID Form in the QC phantom folder.

8. Analysis of Venipuncture and Processing Data for Quality Control

The Coordinating Center analyzes the study data annually to determine the frequencies of filling time, number of stick attempts and reported presence of hemolysis, and selected markers of lack of adherence to protocol during phlebotomy and/or processing of specimens at the field center laboratory. These analyses include field center tabulations by the ID of the technician performing the blood drawing or processing. (Standards for time needed for various processing steps are given in ARIC Manual 7.) Adherence to the 2-hour post-glucola blood draw window is assessed quarterly and reported to field centers.

9. Packing Samples for Shipment to Laboratories

All vials of blood samples as well as the plastic bags in which the samples for a given participant are packed for shipment to the several laboratories are labeled with the participant's ID. A shipping list is enclosed with each shipment to the Central Laboratories giving the IDs for all sets of samples that are enclosed. The person unpacking these samples at the Central Laboratories verifies that the IDs on the vials match the IDs on the plastic bag and checks both against the shipping list. If any discrepancies are detected, the Central Laboratory contacts the field center to resolve the problem.

Blood vials shipped to the Central Laboratories must be packed securely to avoid both breakage and warming. Full instructions for packing samples are specified in ARIC Manual 7, Sections 5.1–5.3. The laboratories monitor the arrival condition of the samples sent from each field center. If problems are encountered, the laboratories notify the field centers involved. If a pattern of sample damage becomes apparent that suggests a need to modify the materials used to ship samples (e.g., excessive leakage of a certain type of vial) or how samples are packed, the Laboratory Subcommittee takes appropriate action.

ARIC blood samples are mailed promptly to the Central Laboratories at the start of the week after they are drawn. The laboratories monitor the dates of blood drawing on samples which they receive and notify the field center and the Coordinating Center if they receive samples that were shipped at a later date than that called for under this schedule. (Note: quality control phantom blood tubes are held over one week before shipping, but the date of drawing on these samples that is reported to the laboratory is altered to conceal their identity as QC.) The field centers should phone the central laboratories to notify them if they are shipping on a day other than Monday.

To avoid delays in transit to the laboratories that might cause samples to be warmed or thawed in shipping, all samples are shipped by an overnight delivery service. To avoid delays over weekends or holidays in delivering samples or in moving them to the Central Laboratory freezer once they are delivered to the receiving area, all samples are shipped out at the beginning of the working week, on Monday or Tuesday. The laboratories notify the Coordinating Center and the field center if a shipment is received that was shipped out on a later day in the week, and the field center reports to the Coordinating Center on the reasons for this deviation from protocol. The laboratories notify the Field Centers if sets of samples are received late. If a pattern of delays is encountered with the delivery service a field center is using, the field center will change to an alternate delivery service.

10. Description of Urine Collection and Processing and Related Measures for Quality Assurance and Quality Control

After a participant is greeted at the clinic, he or she is asked to provide a urine specimen at the participant's convenience (e.g., when the participant expresses the need to void). When the participant is ready to void, a specimen cup (labeled with the participant's ID and TIME VOIDED) is provided, and the participant is instructed to fill the cup if possible. If the sample is insufficient for processing, the participant is requested to void again in a clean container prior to leaving the field center. Prior to processing, the technician records on the participant's Laboratory Form whether a urine sample was obtained, the collection time of the initial (if more than one) urine sample, and adequacy of volume.

11. QC Sample Preparation

The following instructions describe specific additions to urine collection and processing protocols in order to meet QC requirements. These instructions assume that the normal procedures for collecting, processing, and shipping creatinine and albumin samples (see Manual 7, Section 6.0–6.3) are being followed.

12. Urine QC Schedule

The Visit 4 schedule for urine QC sampling parallels the blood QC sampling protocol: a minimum of one sample is required each week. QC specimens should be taken from the first participant either Tuesday or Thursday who provides sufficient urine. If no participant on Tuesday (or Thursday) provides a sufficient amount, the first participant to do so on Wednesday (or Friday) should be selected.

Urine QC sample collection should be added to the weekly checklist maintained by the field center venipuncture technicians. As with blood QC samples, each urine sample should be checked off as it is prepared. On Wednesday or Friday mornings, the checklist is consulted to see if an additional urine sample is still needed.

13. QC Sample Requirements

Each participant's urine specimen is divided into three separate sample tubes and frozen at the field centers until shipping. Aliquots for creatinine and albumin on each participant (3.5 ml each) are shipped to the Minneapolis ARIC Field Center. The 50–ml conical tube (one per participant) for the hemostatic metabolites is shipped to the ARIC Hemostasis Laboratory; this tube must contain a minimum of 40 ml. When the schedule calls for collection of a QC sample (phantom) for creatinine and albumin, the participant's specimen cup must contain at least 54 ml (14 ml for a total of four 3.5-ml vials and one 40-ml hemostasis sample). For a hemostasis laboratory phantom, 87 ml (7 ml for two 3.5-ml vials and two 40-ml hemostasis samples) are needed.

14. Laboratory and Phantom Forms

To ensure that the correct match is recorded between the real participant ID and the QC phantom ID, as soon as it can be ascertained that sufficient urine for a QC sample has been provided, an ID label for the real participant ID is added to the appropriate space on the QC Phantom Participant and Nonparticipant ID Form.

To avoid ID errors in which information regarding a given participant's urine sample is entered on the wrong form, the technician should begin filling out a URINE SAMPLE section of the Laboratory Form for the phantom ID at the same time the participant's URINE SAMPLE section of this form is completed.

15. Sample Preparation

When creatinine and albumin phantom urine specimens are to be prepared, a total of four 3.5-ml aliquoting vials are required. Two vials are labeled with the participant ID and the remaining two with the phantom ID.

The two CREATININE and two ALBUMIN specimen vials are distinguished by cap inserts: YELLOW for CREATININE, and BLUE for ALBUMIN. The creatinine participant and phantom cryovials are filled first by the lab technician. Then the procedure for pH balancing of the albumin sample is executed (Manual 7, Section 6.1.2), and the pH balanced specimen is pipetted into the participant and phantom cryovials.

The phantom hemostasis urine specimen is prepared at the same time and manner as the participant hemostasis urine sample.

16. Procedure for Small Samples

For QC purposes, the pairs of participant and phantom creatinine, albumin, and hemostasis urine samples must come from the same batch. If a single batch is inadequate for both the participant and phantom samples, then the specimens should be combined prior to drawing the samples.

17. Storage Instructions

Storage instructions (Manual 7, Section 6.2) stipulate that samples be packed in the order of the date drawn, putting a single participant's two specimens (CREATINE and ALBUMIN) side by side in the row. Since the phantom and participant specimens are drawn on the same date, they will likely be on the same row, possibly next to each other.

Record the box and position numbers on the participant's Laboratory Form, and be sure to do the same for the phantom.

Finally, record the IDs of all participants and phantoms in each box on a Box Log Form.

18. Quality Assurance and Quality Control

In addition to annual recertification authorized by the Hemostasis Laboratory, protocol adherence in the performance of each procedure is reviewed at least biannually by the lead technician, and annually by Coordinating Center field center monitors. Deviation from protocol and possible remedial actions are discussed with study coordinators and staff at that time. Major deviations are brought to the attention of the Cohort Operation Committee.

The CC will produce reports based on replicate data from the labs. Results of these reports will be examined by the QC Committee, and recommended corrective actions will be implemented. The Coordinating Center will provide to the QC Committee and field centers a report based on the procedural data recorded on the Laboratory Form. This report will evaluate data for consistency, and for missing or out of range values.

Calculation of the Intraclass Correlation Coefficient

APPENDIX E

The intraclass correlation coefficient (ICC) is the proportion of the total variability in the measured factor that is due to the variability between individuals (see Chapter 8, Section 8.4.2). In this appendix, two approaches for the calculation of the ICC are described: one is based on analysis of variance (ANOVA) results[1] and the other on a shortcut formula described by Deyo et al.[2] Both techniques are illustrated using as an example the between-scorer reliability data from the Sleep Heart Health Study quality control study (see Chapter 8, Table 8-20).

ANALYSIS OF VARIANCE

To carry out an ANOVA on a set of replicate observations (e.g., the between-scorer apnea-hypopnea index (AHI) reliability data from Table 8-20), the data need to be arranged so that *all* AHI values (from both sets of replicate observations) are contained in a single variable. Additional indicator variables denote the identifier for both the study number (1 through 30) and the scorer (A or B). Thus, in this example, the data can be arranged for a total of 60 observations, as follows:

Study no.	Scorer	AHI
1	A	1.25
1	B	1.38
2	A	1.61
2	B	2.05
3	A	5.64
3	B	5.50
.	.	.
.	.	.
.	.	.
29	A	2.09
29	B	2.35
30	A	11.09
30	B	9.25

A similar approach is used to arrange the arousal index (AI) data, also shown in Table 8-20.

An ANOVA of these data can be conducted using any standard statistical package. From the output of the analysis conducted using SAS (SAS Institute, Cary, NC), the following tables are obtained:

For AHI:

Source of variation	Sum of squares (SS)	Degrees of freedom (DF)*	Mean square SS/DF	Label
Observer	2.023	1	2.023	MSO
Study	2477.991	29	85.448	MSS
Error	7.169	29	0.247	MSE

*Degrees of freedom: for *observer*, $k - 1$, where k is the number of times each observation is made; for *study*, $n - 1$, where n is the number of observations; for *error*, $(k - 1) \times (n - 1)$.

For AI:

Source of variation	Sum of squares (SS)	Degrees of freedom (DF)*	Mean square SS/DF	Label
Observer	166.010	1	166.010	MSO
Study	4436.759	29	152.992	MSS
Error	1087.749	29	37.509	MSE

*Degrees of freedom: for *observer*, $k - 1$, where k is the number of times each observation is made; for *study*, $n - 1$, where n is the number of observations; for *error*, $(k - 1) \times (n - 1)$.

In these tables, "observer" relates to the variability due to the scorer in this example (or to the specific set of repeat readings in a within-observer reliability study), and "study" refers to the variability related to the participant, study, or specimen that is being repeatedly studied, read, or determined.

The formula for the calculation of the ICC is[1]

$$ICC = \frac{MSS - MSE}{MSS + MSE(k - 1) + k(MSO - MSE)/n}$$

where k is the number of repeat readings (e.g., 2 in the above example) and n is the number of individual studies or specimens being studied (e.g., 30 in the above example).

Applying this formula to the above data, the following results are obtained:

For AHI:

$$ICC_{AHI} = \frac{85.448 - 0.247}{85.448 + 0.247(2 - 1) + 2(2.023 - 0.247)/30} = 0.993$$

For AI:

$$ICC_{AI} = \frac{152.992 - 37.509}{152.992 + 37.509(2 - 1) + 2(166.01 - 37.509)/30} = 0.580$$

DEYO'S METHOD

An equivalent formula described by Deyo et al.[2] can easily be applied using a pocket calculator or a standard computer spreadsheet. The layout for this calculation requires obtaining the difference between the values (e.g., scores) for each pair of repeated observations, as shown in the following table for both the AHI and AI data from Table 8-20.

Study no.	AHI			AI		
	Scorer A	Scorer B	Difference	Scorer A	Scorer B	Difference
1	1.25	1.38	−0.13	7.08	8.56	−1.48
2	1.61	2.05	−0.44	18.60	19.91	−1.31
3	5.64	5.50	0.14	20.39	25.17	−4.78
.	.	.	.	.	.	.
.	.	.	.	.	.	.
.	.	.	.	.	.	.
29	2.09	2.35	−0.26	18.66	18.02	0.64
30	11.09	9.25	1.84	12.50	23.25	−10.74
Mean	5.748	5.381	**0.367**	17.306	20.632	**−3.327**
s	6.702	6.386	0.703	7.682	11.467	8.661
s^2	**44.918**	**40.777**	**0.494**	**59.017**	**131.483**	**75.017**

s: standard deviation.

Deyo's formula uses the numbers shown in bold in the table, namely the mean difference ($\bar{x}_{diff}$), the variances (standard deviations squared) for the measurements by each scorer (s_A^2 and s_B^2), and the variance of the differences (s_{diff}^2):

$$ICC = \frac{s_A^2 + s_B^2 - s_{diff}^2}{s_A^2 + s_B^2 + \bar{x}_{diff}^2 - s_{diff}^2/n}$$

where n is the total number of studies (paired observations).
For the above data:

$$ICC_{AHI} = \frac{44.918 + 40.777 - 0.494}{44.918 + 40.777 + 0.367^2 - 0.494/30} = 0.993$$

$$ICC_{AI} = \frac{59.017 + 131.483 - 75.017}{59.017 + 131.483 + 3.327^2 - 75.017/30} = 0.580$$

These results are identical to the values obtained from the ANOVA, shown above.

REFERENCES

1. Armitage P, Berry G. *Statistical Methods in Medical Research*, 3rd ed. London, England: Blackwell; 1994.
2. Deyo RA, Diehr P, Patrick DL. Reproducibility and responsiveness of health statistics measures: Statistics and strategies for evaluation. *Controlled Clin Trials.* 1991;12:142S–158S.

Answers to Exercises

APPENDIX F

CHAPTER 1

1a. No. In order to examine incidence trends as a given birth cohort ages, one needs to look along the diagonals. It is clear that the incidence rates increase with age within each birth cohort. See the example below, shown in shaded cells for the cohort born around 1933—that is, those who were, on average, 22 years in 1955.

As rates within each age group have consistently increased from birth cohort to birth cohort, in each cross-sectional set of incidence rates the older ages seem to have unusually low rates, as they originate from the older cohorts, which had lower rates.

Age	Calendar Year							
	1950	1955	1960	1965	1970	1975	1980	1985
20–24	10	15	22	30	33	37	41	44
25–29	8	17	20	24	29	38	40	43
30–34	5	12	22	25	28	35	42	45
35–44	3	12	15	26	30	32	39	42
45–49	2	10	17	19	28	32	39	42
50–54	2	12	15	18	21	33	40	42
55–59	2	10	16	20	25	32	42	44
60–64	2	15	17	19	22	27	43	44

1b. Birth cohort: allows the examination of how rates in the population change over time in individuals born at approximately the same time, and thus how these rates change with age in a longitudinal fashion, regardless of calendar time.

Cross-sectional: allows assessment of the patterns of disease (or condition) burden according to age or any other characteristic at a given point in time. Cross-sectional rates provide a 'snapshot' of a given point in time, which may be useful for various reasons (e.g., policy, budget, outreach), but can be misleading if extrapolated beyond that snapshot (e.g., trying to establish a pattern with aging, or causality).

2a. Not for age, because the age ranges are very broad. For calendar time, the 5-year intervals are fairly narrow and, thus, use of the midpoint is reasonable. When intervals are broad, information on trends is lost, as it is assumed that the changes within each interval are uniform.

2b. Using the midpoint for age, individuals dying at age 10 years in 1973 belong to the 1963 birth cohort. However, as 0–19 years is a fairly broad category, it would be more accurate to say that individuals aged 0–19 who died in 1973 belong to cohorts born from 1954 through 1973 (that is, from [1973 − 19] years old through [1973 − less than 1 year old]).

2c. Birth cohorts are examined by looking at the same age grouping over calendar years. For ages 20–69 years, mortality does not seem to have changed much across birth cohorts (as the curve is pretty flat). However, for ages 0–19 years, it looks like the birth cohort mortality rates decreased a bit across cohorts, starting in 1986–1990 (a slight increase is seen in more recent cohorts). The broad age groupings, however, render this analysis fairly crude.

2d. Yes. The rates are higher for those aged 20–69 years than for those aged 0–19 years in all cohorts. The age differences seem to have become more pronounced with time.

3a. Yes. Within each birth cohort and across the birth cohorts, the incidence increases with age.

3b. No. The separate lines for each birth cohort seem to overlap. For example, in the dementia plot, for age ~78 years, there are two data points (for two different birth cohorts, 1900 and 1905), indicating that the rate at age 78 years is similar in the two cohorts. The same phenomenon is largely seen for many other ages and birth cohorts.

3c. Yes. When there is no cohort effect, the age pattern within each cohort and that observed in a cross-sectional analysis tend to be the same.

4a. A case-cohort design would be ideal, as the same control group, represented by a sample of the total cohort at baseline, could be used as a comparison group to multiple case groups. If a nested case-control study design were chosen, a different control group would have to be selected for each case group, which would not be cost-effective.

4b. In a cohort study, cross-sectional associations can be sought at baseline between exposures and prevalent outcomes. Its advantages are that they allow identification of associations that can later be confirmed in longitudinal analyses (that is, they allow generation of hypotheses). The disadvantage is that point prevalence ratios may not be good estimates of the relative risks, as prevalence is a reflection of both incidence and duration of the disease after diagnosis (see also Chapter 4). Although cross-sectional results may also inform decisions about what measures to add or drop from follow-up exams, epidemiologists should be mindful of the prevalence-incidence bias.

5a. By matching on ethnic background, the investigators will also match on variables related to ethnic background, which may include residence area. As a result, cases and controls may be "overmatched," that is, they may be matched on the exposure of interest.

5b. Probably not. Little additional efficiency (statistical power) is achieved when the ratio of controls to cases is greater than 4:1 or 5:1.

CHAPTER 2

1a. Survival analysis of 20 participants of a hypothetical prospective study:

Follow-up time (months)	Event	Probability of death at exact time when death occurred	Probability of survival beyond point when death occurred	Cumulative probability of survival beyond time when death occurred
2	Death	1/20 = 0.050	0.950	0.950
4	Censored	–	–	–
7	Censored	–	–	–
8	Death	1/17 = 0.059	0.941	0.894
12	Censored	–	–	–
15	Death	1/15 = 0.067	0.933	0.834
17	Death	1/14 = 0.071	0.929	0.775
19	Death	1/13 = 0.077	0.923	0.715
20	Censored	–	–	–
23	Death	1/11 = 0.091	0.909	0.650

1b. Cumulative survival probability = 0.65
1c. See graph:

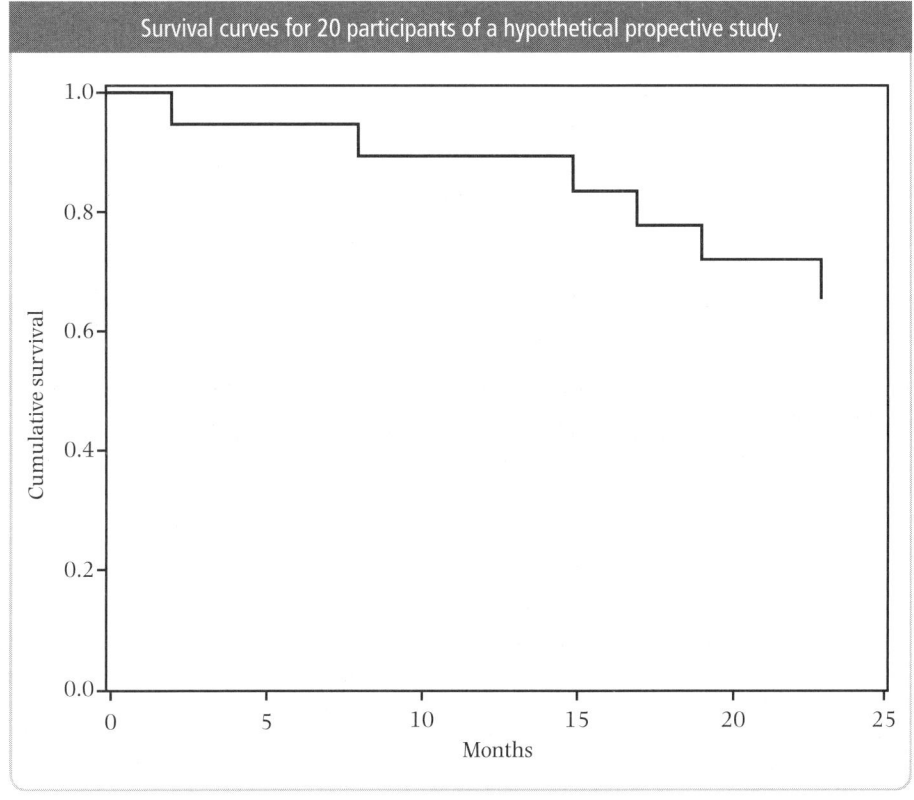

Survival curves for 20 participants of a hypothetical propective study.

1d. Of the 20 alive at the beginning of the study, 14 are alive at the end of the follow-up period; thus, the proportion surviving is 14 ÷ 20 = 0.70 = 70%.

1e. The survival analysis adjusts for varying lengths of follow-up, i.e., it takes into account that not all individuals are observed for the entire follow-up period. In other words, the simple proportion does not take into consideration the censored observations, whereas the survival analysis does.

1f. 10 individuals who were neither censored nor died contributed with 24 person-months of follow-up. Thus, the total number of person-months for these individuals was 24 × 10 = 240, or 240 ÷ 12 = 20 person-years of follow-up. Those who either died or were censored contributed to the following person-months of follow-up:

Person	Event	Total follow-up (months)
1	Death	2
2	Censored	4
3	Censored	7
4	Death	8
5	Censored	12
6	Death	15
7	Death	17
8	Death	19
9	Censored	20
10	Death	23
Total		127

Person-time: 2 + 4 + 7 + 8 + 12 + 15 + 17 + 19 + 20 + 23 = 127 person-months, or 127 ÷ 12 = 10.6 person-years

Thus, the total number of person-years of observation (including those who were followed up for the 2-year total period) = 20 + 10.6 = 30.6

Death rate per 100 person-years = 6 ÷ 30.6 = 19.6

1g. No. of person-years in the *first year* = (15 × 12) + 2 + 4 + 7 + 8 + 12 = 213 person-months = 17.75 person-years

Rate in *first year* = 2 ÷ 17.75 = 0.113 = 11.3/100 person-years

No. of person-years in the *second year* = (10 × 12) + 3 + 5 + 7 + 8 + 11 = 154 person-months = 12.83 person-years

Rate in *second year* = 4 ÷ 12.83 = 0.312 = 31.2/100 person-years

1h. No. The rates do not appear to be homogenous within the 2-year period (the rate in the second year is almost 3 times that in the first year). Thus, it is not appropriate to calculate the rate per person-year for the total two-year period; rates should be reported separately for the first and for the second year of follow-up.

1i. Participants lost to follow-up (censored observations) have the same probability of survival as those who are not lost to follow-up. In other words, there is independence between censoring and survival.

1j.   Proportion dying = 6 ÷ 20 = 0.30 = 30%

              Odds of dying = 6:14 = 0.43:1 = 43:100 (43%)

Note that the odds are usually reported as a percent (in the example, 43%). However, as the absolute odds is a ratio of events to nonevents, in this example it may make more sense to report it as 43:100, that is, for every 43 deaths, there are 100 people who survived.

1k. As death is fairly frequent in this group of people, the odds of death is much higher than the proportion dying.

2a.

	Number of individuals	Number with probable AD	Person-years	Incidence density of AD per 100 person-years	Average duration of follow-up (years)
All subjects	3,099	263	18933	1.389	6.11
< 80 years	2,343	157	15529	1.011	6.63
≥ 80 years	756	106	3404	3.114	4.50
APOE ε4(+)	702	94	4200	2.238	5.98
APOE ε4(−)	2,053	137	12894	1.063	6.28

2b. Age and perhaps APOE e4 status are also risk factors for death from other causes, thus, decreasing duration of follow-up for those older than 80 years, and individuals with APOE ε4(+). If the older persons and those with APOE ε4(+) ("exposed") are more likely to be lost to follow-up (compared to their counterparts), incidence of AD will be underestimated, more so in the exposed group than in the unexposed group. Duration of follow-up is particularly important for the age-AD association, as older individuals have a shorter mean survival time (shorter duration of follow-up).

2c. No. Because the incidence of AD increases with age, the risk of AD will increase over the follow-up period. The incidence should be reported over relatively short time intervals, within which the risk tends to be homogenous.

3a. Using absolute numbers, odds of hypertension history: cases = 70/248 = 0.28; controls = 30/363 = 0.08

3b. Using percentages, odds of hypertension history: cases = 22:78 = 0.28; controls = 7.6/92.4 = 0.08

3c. Odds can be calculated using either the absolute numbers of exposed and unexposed, or their relative frequencies.

3d. Because the proportion (prevalence) of a history of hypertension is much lower in controls (7.6%) than in cases (22.0%). The odds tends to approximate the proportion when the proportion is low.

4. The relationship of prevalence to duration and incidence is expressed by the formula,

$$\frac{\text{Point Prevalence}}{1 - \text{Point Prevalence}} = \text{Incidence} \times \text{Duration}$$

Thus, average duration can be estimated as,

$$\text{Duration} = \frac{\text{Point Prevalence}}{1 - \text{Point Prevalence}} \times \frac{1}{\text{Incidence}}$$

Thus,

$$\text{Duration} = \frac{0.56}{1 - 0.56} \times \frac{1}{0.05} = 25.45 \text{ years}$$

CHAPTER 3

1a.

Radiation dose (REM)	Total population	Cancer cases	Cumulative* incidence	Relative risk	Odds ratio (comparing cases to noncases)	Odds ratio (comparing cases to total population)
0–0.99	3642	390	0.107	1.0	1.0	1.0
1–4.99	1504	181	0.120	1.12	1.14	1.12
≥5	1320	222	0.168	1.57	1.69	1.57

*Assumes no losses to follow-up.

For the "case vs noncase" analysis, the number of noncases needs to be calculated:

Radiation dose (REM)	Cases	Noncases*
0–0.99	390	3252
1–4.99	181	1323
≥5	222	1098

*Example: For 0–099 = 3642 − 390 = 3252

Using noncases as controls:

$$\text{OR}_{1-4.99} = \frac{181/1323}{390/3252} = 1.14$$

$$\text{OR}_{\geq 5} = \frac{222/1098}{390/3252} = 1.69$$

Using total population as controls:

$$\text{OR}_{1-4.99} = \frac{181/1504}{390/3642} = 1.12$$

$$\text{OR}_{\geq 5} = \frac{222/1320}{390/3642} = 1.57$$

1b. The odds ratio based on noncases as controls is slightly farther away from 1.0 than the RR. When using the total population as the control group, the odds ratio of exposure yields the relative risk. For example, for the category ≥5, the relative risk calculated in a "prospective" mode is identical to the exposure odds ratio when the odds of exposure in cases is divided by the odds of exposure in the total population, as follows:

$$\text{Relative Risk} = \frac{222/1320}{390/3642} = \frac{222/390}{1320/3642} = 1.57$$

1c. #4 (the OR is always farther away from 1 than the RR), as the "built-in" bias is always > 1 when RR > 1 and < 1 when RR < 1. (When the OR is 1.0, the RR is also 1.0)

1d. Dose-response (See also Chapter 10, Section 10.2.4)

2a. A case-cohort study, that is, a case-control study within a defined cohort in which the control group is a random sample of the total cohort at baseline.

2b. Yes, the same control group (cohort sample) could be used; for every type of case, the exposure odds ratio would yield the relative risk.

2c. Prevalence of exposure (IL-6 values in the highest quintile) = 0.20

$$\text{Relative risk} = 1.9$$

Percent population attributable risk using Levin's formula:

$$\text{Percent Population AR} = \frac{0.20(1.9 - 1.0)}{0.20(1.9 - 1.0) + 1.0} \times 100 = \frac{0.18}{1.18} \times 100 = 15.2\%$$

3a. Case-based case-control study using hospital patients as cases and their matched controls.

3b. For age group ≤55, OR = [18÷(163−18)] / [6÷(231−6)] = 4.66
For age group >55, OR = [52÷(237−52)] / [16÷(165−16)] = 2.62

3c. The odds of developing B-NHL is 2.62 times greater for individuals who are positive for HCV than for those without HCV. (Even in a case-control study, the interpretation of the odds ratio is always "prospective").

3d. HCV was tested after B-NHL in cases and the diseases in controls had started. Thus, temporality cannot be determined in this study (see also Chapter 10).

4a. Incidence

$BMI_{<18.5}$: 285/(285 + 1,451) + 0.164

$BMI_{18.5-24.9}$: 304/(304 + 1,684) = 0.153

$BMI_{≥25}$: 21/(21 + 231) = 0.083

Odds

$BMI_{<18.5}$: 285/1451 = 0.196

$BMI_{18.5-24.9}$: 304/1684 = 0.180

$BMI_{≥25}$: 21/231 = 0.091

Odds ratios

$$BMI_{<18.5}: \quad 2.2$$
$$BMI_{18.5-24.9}: \quad 2.0$$

Relative Risks

$$BMI_{<18.5}: \quad 2.0$$
$$BMI_{18.5-24.9}: \quad 1.8$$

4b. The assumption is fairly robust. Even with incidence values as high as near 20% in the BMI categories, < 18.5 and 18.5 − 24.9, the odds ratios are fairly similar to the relative risks.

CHAPTER 4

1a. Observed OR = (162 ÷ 268) / (133 ÷ 418) = 1.9

1b. Total number of cases = 162 + 268 = 430:
Sensitivity of self-report in cases = 0.90. Thus, truly obese = 162/0.90 = 180 and truly nonobese = 430−180 = 250

$$\text{Total number of controls} = 133 + 418 = 551$$

Sensitivity of self-report in controls = 0.95. Thus, truly obese = 133/0.95 = 140 and truly nonobese = 551−140 = 411

$$\text{"Corrected" OR} = (180 \div 250) / (140 \div 411) = 2.1$$

1c. There is differential misclassification of obesity status, resulting from the fact that the sensitivity of self-reported obesity is different between cases and controls. (When there is differential misclassification, the OR can be biased in any direction depending on what the patterns of misclassification in cases and controls are; e.g., closer to 1.0, as in this example).

1d. Individuals in the validation study are not representative of the entire study population (e.g., validation study participants included more females, higher educated, and perhaps they are also different with regard to other variables related to the self-report validity). Thus, it may be inappropriate to generalize the validation results to the entire study population.

Another limitation is that validation results are based on a small sample, and are thus subject to large sample variability.

2. Individuals who undergo vasectomy may have better access to health care, and thus had their subclinical disease more often diagnosed.

In case-control studies, recall bias may occur, whereby cases are more likely to recall past vasectomy than controls (although, given the fact that this exposure is "objective," this is not likely).

Publication bias, whereby only "positive" results are reported in peer-reviewed journals.

(Not discussed in this chapter, there may be differences between vasectomized and nonvasectomized men that are relevant to the observed findings, such as level of sexual activity. This would be an example of confounding, and is discussed in detail in Chapter 5.)

3. Mortality is not subjected to lead time bias. When survival is estimated, lead time bias needs to be known and taken into account.

4a. No. Women with certain characteristics known to be related to breast cancer are more likely to participate in the program—for example those with a family history of breast cancer, those with benign breast disease, and those with a higher socioeconomic status (and thus better educational level and health awareness). Incidence in those taking advantage of the program is therefore expected to be higher than in the total population of women aged 50–59 years.

4b. Cases detected at the first exam are point prevalent cases. Given the low point prevalence, the simplified formula expressing the relation between point prevalence and incidence can be used: Prevalence ≈ Incidence × Duration; thus,

$$\text{Duration} \approx \text{Point Prevalence} \div \text{Incidence}.$$

Using the incidence and point prevalence values above,

$$\text{Duration} \approx 200/100{,}000 \div 100/100{,}000 = 2 \text{ years}$$

Using the more precise, correct formula, Point prevalence = Incidence × Duration × (1 − Point prevalence) and thus,

$$\text{Duration} = (\text{Point prevalence}) \div [\text{Incidence} \times (1 - \text{Point prevalence})]$$

In this example, Duration = 0.002 ÷ [0.001 × (1 − 0.0020)] = 2.004 years (Note the use of three decimal places for the duration of the detectable clinical phase of breast cancer when using the correct formula aimed at highlighting the fact that, when the prevalence is very low, the duration values using either the correct or the simplified formula are virtually identical.)

4c. Lead time is the time between early diagnosis using a screening test (followed by a confirmatory diagnostic test) and the time when the disease would have been diagnosed by usual clinical practice (that is, if screening had not been done).

4d. Survival time appears to be longer in those who undergo the screening procedure (above and beyond any possible true benefits brought about by the screening.) This longer survival reflects the fact that diagnosis was advanced by the application of the screening test (vis-à-vis when it would have occurred without screening).

4e. The average lead time for point prevalent cases is about one-half of the duration of the detectable preclinical phase, i.e., 2 years ÷ 2 = 1 year. This estimation is based on the assumption that the sensitivity of the test is homogeneous throughout the duration of the detectable preclinical phase.

4f. The average lead time for incident cases will increasingly approximate the duration of the detectable preclinical phase when screenings are done more and more frequently. This is because cases are more likely to be detected earlier in the detectable preclinical phase.

CHAPTER 5

1a. The variable needs to be associated with the exposure.
The variable needs to be associated with the outcome.
The variable must not be in the causal pathway between exposure and outcome.

1b. The easiest way to assess confounding is to stratify cases and controls by the potential confounding factor, and then examine the association between case-control status and the potential risk factor in each stratum, as follows:

Smokers		
	Lung cancer	
	cases	Controls
Alcohol drinkers		
Nondrinkers		
	OR =	

Nonsmokers		
	Lung cancer	
	cases	Controls
Alcohol drinkers		
Nondrinkers		
	OR =	

When this table is used, absence of confounding is suggested by the fact that the odds ratios for alcohol stratified by smoking are similar to the pooled (crude) odds ratio (an exception is noncollapsibility–see Chapter 5, section 5.4.2).

Alternatively, the dual relationship between smoking and both exposure (alcohol) and outcome can be assessed:

	Alcohol	
	drinkers	Nondrinkers
Smokers		
Nonsmokers		
	OR =	

	Lung cancer	
	cases	Controls
Smokers		
Nonsmokers		
	OR =	

Note that, if there is no interaction between smoking and drinking, the odds ratios reflecting the relationship of smoking to drinking should be similar in cases and controls. It is, however, customary to assess the relationship between the potential confounder and the potential risk factor of interest in controls, which (theoretically at least) represent a sample of the cases study base, that is, the population from which cases developed.

(Note, in addition, that the suspected confounding variable cannot be in the causal pathway between the potential risk factor of interest and the outcome, that is, it cannot be a mediator. In this example, it does not make sense to consider smoking as a mediator for the relation of alcohol to lung cancer.)

2a. Triglyceride level is a positive confounder of the association between serum dioxin and diabetes but, as the odds ratio remains > 1.0 upon adjustment, the association cannot be entirely explained by the confounding effect of triglycerides.

2b. Serum triglycerides explain part of the association between serum dioxin and diabetes, but other variables may be in the causal pathway of the dioxin $\rightarrow$ diabetes association, explaining the fact that the association did not disappear after adjustment for triglycerides. There could also be a direct effect of dioxin on diabetes by means of, for example, pancreatic damage (that is, without any effects of mediating factors).

3. By Situation No.:
   #1 – Positive confounding
   #2 – Negative confounding
   #3 – Negative confounding
   #4 – Positive confounding

4a. The sentence lengths were longer at the later period. The fact that the suicide rate was attenuated after adjusting for sentence length represents positive confounding, which occurs when the exposure-confounder and the outcome-confounder associations are in the same direction. We know from the footnote to the table that increased sentence length is associated with increased suicide rate, so the confounder-calendar time (exposure) association must be in the same direction, i.e., later time period associated with longer sentences.

4b. Temporal changes in other variables, i.e., characteristics of the population of prisoners that could also be related to suicide risk should also be considered (e.g., whether there are other confounders or selection biases that changed over time). In other words, as with all attempts to infer causal associations, one must consider residual confounding, other potential biases, and other potential causes for the temporal change in suicide rates.

5. Statistical significance is not a good criterion to establish the presence of a confounding effect. Because smoking is very strongly related to the disease, even a small difference between cases and controls may explain an association between X and Y. In this example, it would be important to adjust for smoking in order to see whether the adjusted odds ratio differs from the unadjusted odds ratio.

CHAPTER 6

1a.

Alcohol drinking	Anti-HCV	# of persons	Incidence rates (per 100,000)	Relative risk	Attributable risk (per 100,000)
absent	negative	8968	78.7	Reference	Reference
absent	positive	2352	127.1	1.61	48.4
present	negative	461	309.7	3.94	231.0
present	positive	90	384.9	4.89	306.2

1b. Expected joint relative risk = $1.61 \times 3.94 = 6.34$
Expected joint attributable risk = $48.4 + 231.0 = 279.4$ per 100,000

1c. The expected joint relative risk (6.34) is greater than the *observed* joint relative risk (4.89), thus, denoting negative multiplicative interaction. On the other hand, the expected joint attributable risk in the exposed (279.4/100,000) is lower than the observed joint attributable risk (306.2/100,000), denoting a positive additive interaction.

1d. Using alcohol as the effect modifier, the relative risks and attributable risks for those exposed to HCV are:

Relative Risks for anti-HCV

Alcohol drinking absent: $127.1 \div 78.7 = 1.61$

Alcohol drinking present: $384.9 \div 309.7 = 1.24$

Attributable Risks in Individuals Exposed to HCV

Alcohol drinking absent: 127.1 − 78.7 = 48.4/100,000

Alcohol drinking present: 384.9 − 309.7 = 75.2/100,000

Thus, the homogeneity strategy confirmed the findings obtained from the comparison between expected and observed joint effects: the relative risk for anti-HCV exposure is lower for the alcohol present than for the alcohol absent stratum (negative multiplicative interaction), but the anti-HCV attributable risk is higher for the alcohol present than for the alcohol absent stratum (positive additive interaction).

Note that the same inference pertaining to heterogeneity is made when using anti-HCV as the effect modifier. The relative risks and attributable risks in those exposed to alcohol drinking are:

Relative Risks

Anti-HCV negative: 309.7 ÷ 78.7 = 3.93

Anti-HCV positive: 384.9 ÷ 127.1 = 3.02

Attributable Risks

Anti-HCV negative: 309.7 − 78.7 = 231/100,000

Anti-HCV positive: 384.9 − 127.1 = 257.8/100,000

The relative risk for alcohol drinking is greater in those negative than in those positive for anti-HCV (negative multiplicative interaction), but the attributable risk in those exposed to alcohol drinking shows the inverse pattern (positive additive interaction). These findings confirm the fact that interaction is a reciprocal phenomenon, that is, if alcohol modifies the association of HCV with hepatocellular carcinoma, then, by definition, HCV will modify the association of alcohol with hepatocellular carcinoma.

2a. There is a negative multiplicative interaction and a positive additive interaction between diabetes and a previous MI. The relative risk is smaller in the stratum of diabetes present (negative multiplicative interaction) and the attributable risk in those exposed to a previous MI is greater in the stratum of diabetes present (positive additive interaction).

2b. No. The adjusted relative risk and attributable risk would be averages, which ignore the heterogeneity by presence of diabetes.

2c. When incidence proportions/rates/risks are high in the reference category (individuals without a prior MI), there is a *tendency* for the relative risk to approach 1.0. Note that the incidence is much higher in those without a previous MI in the stratum with diabetes (20.2%) than in the stratum without diabetes (3.5%). As (theoretically) the maximum incidence in any strata is 100%, the maximum relative risk associated with a prior MI for those with diabetes would be 100% ÷ 20.2% = 4.9, whereas in those without diabetes, it could reach 100% ÷ 3.5% = 28.6.

3a. It is the odds ratio of heavy smokers in those unexposed to asbestos, i.e., 45.4.

3b. It is the odds ratio of asbestos exposure ≥ 2.5 fiber-years in never smokers, i.e., 10.2.

3c. Joint expected odds ratio:

$$\text{Additive model: } 10.2 + 45.4 - 1.0 = 54.6$$

$$\text{Multiplicative model: } 10.2 \times 45.4 = 463.1$$

3d. For the additive model, the joint expected odds ratio is lower than the joint observed odds ratio; thus, there is positive additive interaction.
   For the multiplicative model, the joint expected odds ratio is larger than the joint observed odds ratio; thus, there is negative multiplicative interaction.

4a. Because the interaction is qualitative, it is present in both scales.

4b. For smokers only, there was negative confounding by the set of variables adjusted for.

Chapter 7

1a. 1st criteria: Yes, this criterion is met: the odds of engaging in gardening are lower for older than for younger persons.

	Gardening	No gardening
Age < 65 years	70 + 299 = 369	20 + 198 = 218
Age ≥ 65 years	55 + 15 = 70	40 + 25 = 65

$$\text{OR}_{\text{older vs younger}} = 70/65 \div 369/218 = 0.64$$

Note: comparison of proportions (instead of odds) will work as well.
2nd criteria: Yes, the criterion is met.

	Low back pain	No low back pain
Age < 65 years	70 + 20 = 90	299 + 198 = 497
Age ≥ 65 years	55 + 40 = 95	15 + 25 = 40

$$\text{OR}_{\text{older vs younger}} = 95/40 \div 90/497 = 13.1$$

Note: Comparison of proportions will work as well.

3rd criterion: Age is not in the causal pathway and, thus, this criterion is also met here (for age to be in the causal pathway, gardening would have to "cause" age; i.e., gardening → increased age → back pain).

1b.

	Low back pain	No low back pain
Gardening	70 + 55 = 125	299 + 15 = 134
No gardening	20 + 40 = 60	198 + 25 = 233

$$\text{OR} = 125/314 \div 60/223 = 1.48$$

1c. $\text{OR}_{\text{MH}} = (70 \times 198/587 + 55 \times 25/135) / (20 \times 299/587 + 40 \times 15/135) = 2.31$

1d. Yes. Conducting this adjustment is appropriate because the stratified OR's above are 2.32 (for the younger) and 2.29 (for the older), thus approximately equal.

1e. Age is a negative confounder of the association between gardening and low back pain. Thus, the adjusted OR is further away from the null than the crude OR.
Alternative answer: Older age is inversely associated with exposure and positively associated with the outcome.

Note that, because of the homogeneity of stratum specific ORs (about 2.3 in both strata), there is no evidence of age being an effect modifier.

2a. For the highest level of alcohol drinking, there seems to be positive confounding (as the OR becomes closer to 1.0 after multiple adjustment.)

For the category <6 days/week, the adjusted OR is the same as the crude OR, indicating that the set of variables included in the adjusted model did not confound the association.

2b. No, as the shape of the function seems to be an inverted U, rather than linear.

3a.

		Expected number of cases	
Smoking	Standard population	Women	Men
Current	5000	0.0053 × 5000 = 26.5	0.0115 × 5000 = 57.5
Never	2000	0.0013 × 2000 = 2.6	0.0047 × 2000 = 9.4
Total	7000	29.1	66.9
Smoking adjusted rate		29.1/7000 = 4.2/1000	66.9/7000 = 9.5/1000
Rate ratio		Reference	2.3
Absolute difference in rates		Reference	5.3/1000

3b. *Rate ratios*

$$\text{Current smokers: } 0.0115/0.0053 = 2.2$$

$$\text{Never smokers: } 0.0047/0.0013 = 3.6$$

Absolute differences in rates

$$\text{Current smokers: } 11.5 - 5.3 = 6.2/1000 \text{ person-years}$$

$$\text{Never smokers: } 4.7 - 1.3 = 3.4/1000 \text{ person-years}$$

3c. There is a negative multiplicative interaction (rate ratio for gender is lower in current than in never smokers) and a positive additive interaction (absolute difference in rates is higher for current than for never smokers).

3d.

Smoking	Standard population	Expected number of cases	
		Women	Men
Current	500	0.0053 × 500 = 2.7	0.0115 × 500 = 5.8
Never	10,000	0.0013 × 10,000 = 13.0	47.0
Total	10,500	15.7	52.8
Smoking adjusted rate		15.7/10,400 = 1.5/1000	5.1/1000
Rate ratio		Reference	3.4
Absolute difference in rates		Reference	3.6/1000

3e. Because the standard population sample size for never smokers is much larger than that for smokers, both the relative risk and the attributable risk approximate those of never smokers.

3f. When the confounder is also an effect modifier, association measures may not be similar across populations with different distributions of the confounder, and will tend to approximate the value of the measure obtained in the category of the standard population with the larger sample size. In other words, if the rate ratios are not homogeneous across strata of the confounder, the adjusted rate ratio will vary according to the composition of the standard population.

4a.

Age	Pop A	Pop B	Incidence rates	Observed numbers of incident cases		"Standard" rates	Expected numbers of incident cases	
				Pop A	Pop B		Pop A	Pop B
45–54	2000	400	0.01	20	4	0.005	10	2
55–64	800	600	0.015	12	9	0.007	5.6	4.2
65–74	400	2500	0.025	10	62.5	0.02	8	50
Total population	3200	3500	–	–	–	12/1000	–	–
Total number of cases	–	–	–	42	75.5	–	23.6	56.2
Standardized incidence ratio	–	–	–	–	–	–	1.78	1.34

4b. A standardized incidence ratio (SIR) estimates whether the rate (or risk) is the same (SIR = 1.0), greater (SIR > 1.0) or lower (SIR < 1.0) in each study population than in the population that was used as a source of the "standard" rates.

4c. The standardized incidence (or mortality) ratio expresses only the comparison between each population and the population that served as the source of standard rates. Note that the age distributions of populations A and B in this exercise are very different, which renders the comparison between the two standardized incidence ratios inappropriate. In other words, these values are not standardized to the same (standard) population.

5a. Yes. Sunburn score has very different distributions in the groups, and it is also associated with mean number of new nevi on follow-up. Thus, it can be concluded that it is a confounding variable.

5b.

	Sunscreen		Control		"Standard"		
Sunburn score	N	(a) Mean new nevi	N	(b) Mean new nevi	(c)* Total N	$(d) = (a) \times (c)$	$(e) = (b) \times (c)$
Low	50	20	180	50	230	4600.00	11,500.00
High	172	60	56	90	228	13,680.00	20,520.00
Total	–	–	–	–	458	18,280.00	32,020.00

*Standard population

Sunburn score-adjusted mean number of new nevi in sunscreen group = 18,280/458 = 39.91

Sunburn score-adjusted mean number of new nevi in control group = 32,020/458 = 69.91

Sunburn score-adjusted mean [control − sunscreen] difference = 69.91 − 39.91 = 30

5c. Yes. The differences are homogeneous across strata (in this example, mean [control−sunscreen] difference = 30 for both strata of sunscreen score. Thus, any standard set of weights (standard population) would yield the same estimates. When using mean differences of continuous variables, additive interaction is evaluated. In this example, homogeneity of the differences between the control and intervention groups indicates that there is no additive interaction. When there is no additive interaction, any standard population would yield the same adjusted mean differences (or rates/risks).

5d. If only the facial freckle-adjusted mean difference in development of new nevi had been reported, the heterogeneity seen in the table would have been missed. This information is useful for determining which children would be likely to benefit from sunscreen. In this example, and assuming that the results are valid and precise, children with 10% of the face covered by freckles would not benefit from sunscreen use with regard to development of new nevi.

6.

Type of matched set	Exposed?	Case	Cont	Total	No. of matched sets	Num	Den
A	Yes	1	0	4	40	3/4	0
	No	0	3	–	–	–	–
B	Yes	1	1	4	60	2/4	0
	No	0	2	–	–	–	–
C	Yes	1	2	4	12	1/4	0
	No	0	1	–	–	–	–
D	Yes	1	3	4	10	0	0
	No	0	0	–	–	–	–
E	Yes	0	0	4	30	0	0
	No	1	3	–	–	–	–
F	Yes	0	1	4	5	0	1/4
	No	1	2	–	–	–	–
G	Yes	0	2	4	7	0	2/4
	No	1	1	–	–	–	–
H	Yes	0	3	4	20	0	3/4
	No	1	0	–	–	–	–

There are 8 types of matched sets, according to the combination of presence or absence of exposure in cases and controls. Each matched set (one case and three matched controls) should be considered as a separate stratum. For example, for type set A, there is one exposed case and three unexposed controls. Thus, using the Mantel-Haenszel approach, the numerator pertaining to each of this type of matched set is $(1 \times 3) \div 4 = 0.75$. As there are 40 sets of this type, this number should be multiplied by 40. The same approach is used for each type of set in the numerator and in the denominator. Using set F as another example, the denominator is $(1 \times 1) \div 4 = 0.25$. As there are 5 matched sets of this type, this number should be multiplied by 5. And so on.

Numerator = $(40 \times .75) + (60 \times .5) + (12 \times .25) + 0 + 0 + 0 + 0 + 0 = 63$
Denominator = $0 + 0 + 0 + 0 + 0 + (5 \times .25) + (7 \times .5) + (20 \times .75) = 19.75$
OR (M-H) = $63/19.75 = 3.19$

7a. The log odds of impaired glucose tolerance increases by 3.625 per unit increase in waist/hip ratio, after simultaneous control for body mass index, diabetogenic drugs, and regular exercise.

The log odds ratio of impaired glucose tolerance is 1.664 higher in those who don't exercise regularly compared with those who exercise regularly, after simultaneous control for BMI, waist/hip ratio, and use of diabetogenic drugs.

7b. OR = exp (regression coefficient)

95% CI lower limit = exp (regression coefficient − (1.96 × se))

95% CI upper limit = exp (regression coefficient + (1.96 × se))

	Regression coefficient	SE	OR	95% CI lower limit	95% CI upper limit
BMI (per 1)	0.077	0.032	1.08	1.01	1.15
WHR (per 1)	3.625	1.67	37.52	1.42	990.49
Drugs (yes = 1)	0.599	0.302	1.82	1.01	3.29
Exercise (no = 1)	1.664	0.74	5.28	1.24	22.52

7c. Waist/hip ratio: $e^{3.625} = 37.52 \rightarrow$ The odds of impaired glucose tolerance is 37.5 greater per unit difference in waist/hip ratio, after simultaneous control for BMI, regular exercise, and use of diabetogenic drugs. Note that the extraordinarily high magnitude of this OR is a consequence of the extraordinarily large unit that defines it: a difference in one unit in the W/H ratio would correspond to the comparison of two persons with extreme (almost biologically implausible) W/H ratios (e.g., W/H ratio = 1.5—or waist circumference 50% larger than hip circumference—vs a W/H ratio = 0.5—or waist circumference half of the hip circumference). In this particular case, a more reasonable (more realistic and more informative) unit for reporting this association might be, for example, a 0.1 unit difference; i.e:

$$OR_{0.1 \text{ W/H ratio}} = e^{3.625 \times 0.1} = 1.43$$

Regular exercise: $e^{1.664} = 5.28 \rightarrow$ The odds of impaired glucose tolerance is 5.28 greater in those who do not exercise regularly than in those who exercise regularly, after simultaneous control for BMI, waist/hip ratio, and use of diabetogenic drugs.

7d. No. In general, it is not a good idea to compare association strengths based on the values of the coefficients or odds ratios. Not only variables differ in their biological mechanisms, but in addition the magnitude of the coefficients (or derived odds ratios) depend on the units, which are arbitrarily defined.

7e. $$e^{0.01 \times 3.625} = 1.037 \simeq 1.04$$

$$95\% \text{ CI} = e^{\{0.01 \times 3.625 \pm 1.96 \times 0.1 \times 1.670\}} = (1.004, 1.071) \simeq (1.00, 1.07)$$

8a. b_1 = An increase in age of one year corresponds to an average increase in plasma fibrinogen concentration of 0.018 mg/dL, after simultaneously controlling for sex, race, cigarette smoking, and body mass index (BMI).

b_4 = Those who smoke 1–19 cigarettes per day have an average concentration of plasma fibrinogen that is 12.2 mg/dL higher than that of nonsmokers, after simultaneously controlling for age, sex, race, and BMI.

8b. [√] Body mass index but not cigarette smoking is a positive confounder of the association between race and plasma fibrinogen levels.

Chapter 8

1a. Sensitivity = 18/19 = 0.95
Specificity = 11/30 = 0.37
Positive predictive value = 18/37 = 0.49
Negative predictive value = 11/12 = 0.92

1b. The test should not be recommended because the test's validity, particularly its specificity, is poor. The poor validity would result in substantial misclassification. Because of the poor specificity, many people classified as having a cholesterol ≥ 200 mg/dL would in reality have a lower cholesterol concentration (i.e., the test has a low positive predictive value).

1c. Yes. As stated above, there is a graded ("dose-response") relationship of cholesterol with coronary heart disease. Thus, the investigators should have examined cholesterol as a continuous variable, and calculated the intraclass correlation between the results obtained by the finger-stick test and those obtained in the standard laboratory.

2a. Quality assurance: procedures that aim at preventing bias and imprecision, which are conducted prior to data collection activities.

Quality control: procedures that aim at correcting bias and imprecision, which are conducted after the onset of data collection.

Activity	Quality assurance	Quality control
Preparation of manuals of operation	√	
Over-the-shoulder observation of interviews during the study's data collection phase		√
Determination of interobserver reliability during the study's data collection phase		√
Certification of interviewers	√	
Recertification of interviewers		√
Examination of intralaboratory reliability using phantoms based on collection of blood samples from the study participants		√
Assessment of the validity of two data collection instruments to decide which instrument should be used in the study	√	
Duplicate readings (with adjudication by a third reader) of X-rays for confirmation of an outcome in an ongoing cohort study		√
Training of interviewers	√	
Pretest of a questionnaire	√	

3a. *Unweighted kappa*

Observed agreement: $(10 + 12 + 5) \div 30 = 0.90$

Expected agreement: $[(10 \times 10) + (13 \times 14) + (7 \times 6)] \div 30^2 = 0.36$

$$\text{Unweighted Kappa} = \frac{(\text{Observed agreement}) - (\text{Expected agreement})}{1.0 - (\text{Expected agreement})}$$

$$= \frac{0.90 - 0.36}{1.0 - 0.36} = 0.84$$

Weighted kappa

Observed agreement: $[1.0 (10 + 12 + 5) + 0.7(1 + 2)] \div 30 = 0.97$

Expected agreement: $\{1.0 [(10 \times 10) + (13 \times 14) + (7 \times 6)\} + 0.7 [(13 \times 6) + (7 \times 14)]\} \div 30^2 = [1.0 (100 + 182 + 42) + 0.7 (78 + 98)] \div 900 = (324 + 123.2) \div 900 = 0.50$

$$\text{Weighted Kappa} = \frac{(\text{Observed agreement}) - (\text{Expected agreement})}{1.0 - (\text{Expected agreement})}$$

$$= \frac{0.97 - 0.50}{1.0 - 0.50} = 0.94$$

3b. The excellent agreement (as expressed by a high kappa value) is encouraging. However, it would be important to know more about specific reasons why there was some disagreement. Were the procedures used by the observers exactly the same? Did the measurements of height and weight pose difficulties?

3c. When there is a clearly discernible ranking with regard to the different levels of disagreement in a multi-categorical variable, and tolerance for certain levels of disagreement vis-à-vis the purposes of the study.

The use of a weight of 0.7 for a one category disagreement in this example was somewhat arbitrary, although based on the investigators' perception of the need to give some "credit" to this level of disagreement; it seemed reasonable to tolerate the fact that, for 3 participants, classification was discrepant by one category.

4a. For each pair of measurements, the variance is,

$$V_i = \sum_{j=1}^{2} (X_{ij} - X_i)^2$$

and, thus, the standard deviation is

$$SD = \sqrt{V_i}$$

The coefficient of variability is, for each pair of measurements (where $\overline{X}$ is the mean of the two estimates),

$$CV_i = \frac{SD_i}{\overline{X}} \times 100$$

The coefficient of variability is calculated for each pair or measurements and averaged (i.e., divided by 10) to estimate the overall coefficient of variability. The table shows the detailed calculation for the first pair of observations.

Participant no.	Technician A	Technician B	Coefficient of variability (%)
1	122	125	$V_1 = (122 - 123.5)^2 + (125 - 123.5)^2 = 4.5$; SD = 2.12; $V_{\bar{x}} = 123.5$ CV = 2.12/123.5 × 100 = 1.72%
2	130	129	0.55
3	118	116	1.21
4	136	135	0.52
5	114	108	3.82
6	116	118	1.21
7	124	120	2.32
8	110	111	0.64
9	140	130	5.24
10	146	141	2.46
Total			1.97

4b. (1) There does not seem to be a systematic difference between technicians, particularly in view of the small number of observations: In four pairs of observations, technician B records higher levels than technician A, who records higher levels for the six remaining pairs.
   (2) Technician A has a strong digit preference: he/she only records final even digits. The values recorded by technician B are evenly distributed with regard to the final digit (odd or even).
   (3) The overall coefficient of variability is fairly small, but for a few pairs of observations, the differences vis-à-vis means are reasonably large (participants No. 5 and 9, and perhaps 7 and 10 as well). These differences should be investigated and highlight the importance of examining "real" values, rather than just a summary measure (coefficient of variability).

Chapter 9

1. (1) Title is sketchy: information on calendar time, characteristics of the cohort (gender, age, place or source, study period; etc.) is missing.
   (2) It is not clear whether the category "yes" includes drinking irrespective of amount, current or past, ever, etc.
   (3) The relative risk is based on dividing the incidence proportions during the follow-up without adjustment for follow-up time; i.e., there is no indication of whether authors considered time to event. (Alcohol is associated with smoking, which increases the likelihood of death, and thus of a difference in the duration of follow-up between drinkers and non-drinkers.)
   (4) It is not stated whether the relative risks are adjusted for confounding factors.
   (5) The 95% confidence interval, or "p" value should have been provided.

2. Alcohol use was associated with respiratory cancer in unadjusted analyses, but not when controlling for the number of cigarettes smoked (20 words)

3a.

Freckles %	Average number of new nevi on follow-up		Difference in average number of new nevi (sunscreen minus control)	Difference in average number of new nevi (sunscreen minus control) as a percentage of the number of new nevi in controls
	Sunscreen	Control		
10	24	24	0	0
20	20	28	−8	−28.6
30	20	30	−10	−33.3
40	16	30	−14	−46.7

3b.

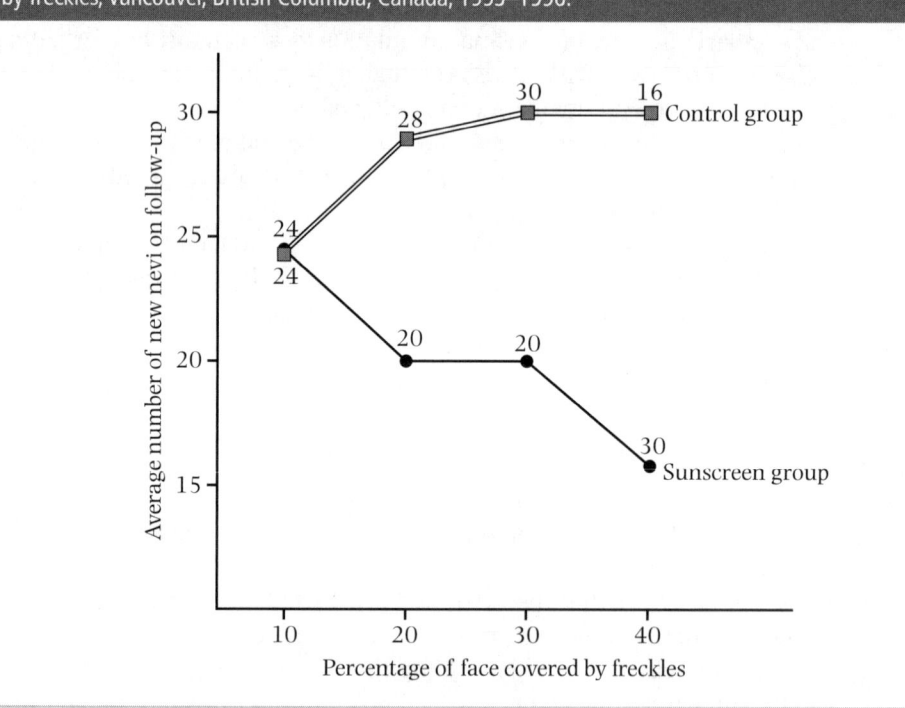

Number of new nevi over a 3-year follow-up in white children in grades 1 and 4, randomly assigned to high-sun protection factor sunscreen or control group, by percentage of face covered by freckles, Vancouver, British Columbia, Canada, 1993–1996.

3c. "The *effectiveness** of the high-sun protection factor sunscreen increased as the percentage of the face covered with freckles increased. It was zero for 10% of the

---

*Effectiveness, rather than efficacy, was likely estimated, as controls were not given a placebo and were not advised about use of a sunscreen. It is, in addition, possible that some children assigned to the control group may have used sunscreen.

face covered by freckles, and almost 50% when the children had 40% of their face covered by freckles. Thus, there seemed to be an additive interaction between freckling and sunscreen use, in terms of reduction of average number of new nevi."

Alternative statement: "The effectiveness of the high-sun protection factor sunscreen in preventing the development of new nevi was modified by the percentage of the face covered by freckling. Because the outcome—development of new nevi—is a continous variable, it can be stated that there was an additive interaction between sunscreen and percent of the face covered by freckles."

4a. See graph. There are two ways to plot these data: (1) using a log scale in the ordinate, or (2) taking the log of the odds ratio values and plotting these in an arithmetic scale.

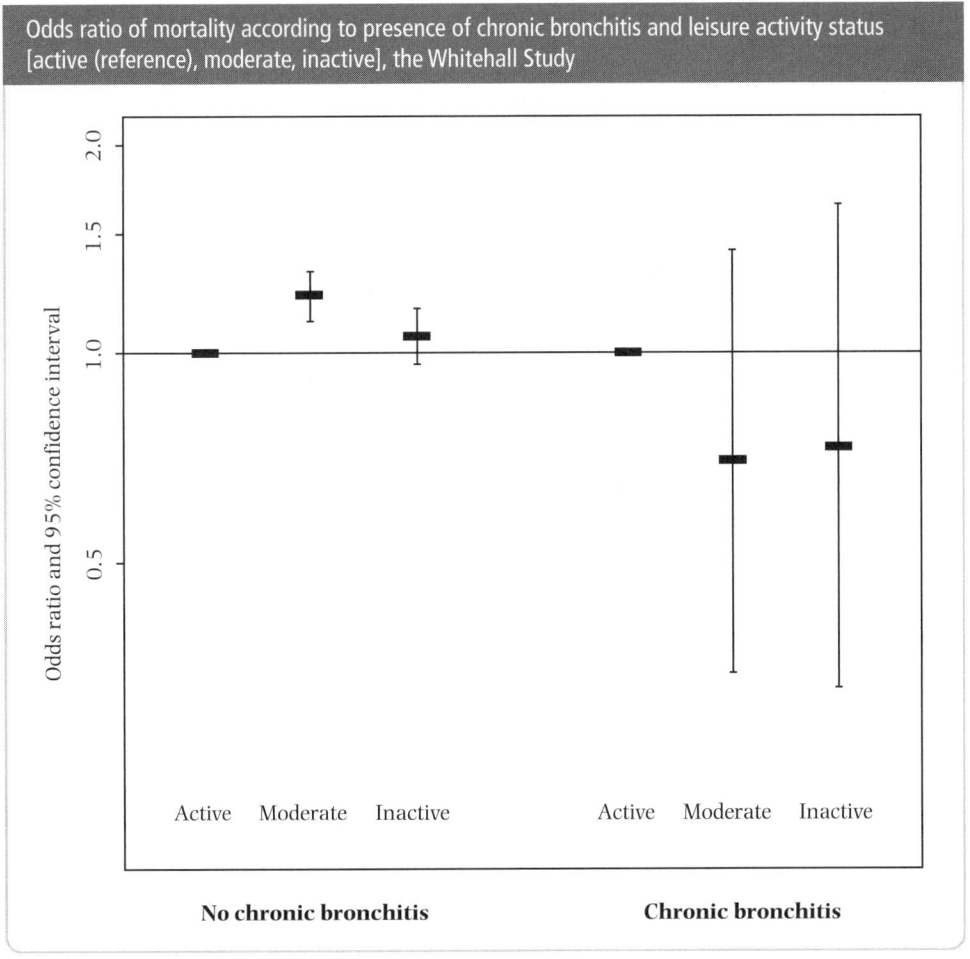

4b. Although confidence intervals largely overlap the null odds ratio (1.0), it is interesting that the point estimates suggest that leisure activity may be beneficial in those with chronic bronchitis—which warrants the "cliché" statement that further studies are necessary.

5a. (1) The order in which variables are described does not follow the order of variables shown in the table.

(2) The authors confuse "no association" with "no statistically significant association." In this table, the strength of the point estimate for current smoking (with a "positive association equivalent" of $1/0.69 = 1.45$, which is described as "no association") is virtually identical to that for family history (1.46, which is described as "significant"); thus, current smoking may be related to colorectal cancer. Judging from the 95% CI for this association, the p value for current smoking may well be of borderline significance.

(3) There is no need to repeat in the text all results shown in the table; otherwise, why bother with presenting the table?

Chapter 10

1. Nausea is a confounder for the relation between caffeine intake and spontaneous abortion. However, even if it is confounded by nausea, caffeine intake defines a high risk group for spontaneous abortion.

2. This study's results emphasize the relevance of additive interaction for prevention. Although the relative risk for a prior history of MI is higher in nondiabetics than in diabetics, the excess absolute risk attributable to a prior MI shows the opposite pattern. Assuming the distributions of diabetes and prior MI to be homogeneous in the population, and (as stated in the question) further assuming limited resources, the presence of a positive (synergistic) additive interaction strongly suggests favoring diabetic patients with history of a prior MI as the group in which prevention of CHD should be especially emphasized—notwithstanding the observation of a negative (antagonistic) multiplicative interaction.

3a.

Risk factor X level	Population				Cases			
	N	Proportion	Relative risk	Risk	Number	Number expected at 5% risk	Excess	
1	30,000	0.043	Reference	0.05	1500	1500	Reference
2	100,000	0.143	1.5	0.075	7500	5000	2500
3	150,000	0.214	1.75	0.0875	13,125	7500	5625
4	160,000	0.229	2	0.1	16,000	8000	8000
5	130,000	0.186	2.5	0.125	16,250	6500	9750
6	80,000	0.114	3	0.15	12,000	4000	8000
7	40,000	0.057	4	0.2	8000	2000	6000
8	10,000	0.014	5	0.25	2500	500	2000
Total	700,000	1			76,875		41,875

3b. $2500/76,875 = 3.25\%$

3c. Calculation: All 10,000 individuals in category 8 are moved to category 7, which now has 50,000 individuals. The number of cases in category 7 is now

10,000 (50,000 × 0.05 × 4.0) (cases no longer occur in category 8). Thus the total number of cases in the population is 76,375 (compared with the total 76,875 before the high risk strategy was implemented). The total number of cases prevented is, thus, 500.

As seen in the revised table below, the new number of cases would be 76,375, or only 500 cases prevented.

Risk factor X level	Population				Cases			
	N	Proportion	Relative risk	Risk	Number	Number expected at 5% risk	Excess
1	30,000	0.043	Reference	0.05	1500	1500	Reference
2	100,000	0.143	1.5	0.075	7500	5000	2500
3	150,000	0.214	1.75	0.0875	13,125	7500	5625
4	160,000	0.229	2	0.1	16,000	8000	8000
5	130,000	0.186	2.5	0.125	16,250	6500	9750
6	80,000	0.114	3	0.15	12,000	4000	8000
7	50,000	0.057	4	0.2	10,000	2500	7500
8	0	0.014	5	0.25	0	0	0
Total	700,000	1			76,375		41,375

3d. Prevented cases = 2118 (rounded down)
Calculation:

Risk factor level	Original population	Population after 15% down shift	New number of cases	Difference between cases before and after shift
1	30,000	45,000	2250	−750
2	100,000	107,500	8062.5	−562.5
3	150,000	151,500	13,256.25	−131.25
4	160,000	155,500	15,550	450
5	130,000	122,500	15,312.5	937.5
6	80,000	74,000	11,100	900
7	40,000	35,500	7100	900
8	10,000	8500	2125	375
Total	700,000	700,000	74,756.25	2118.75

Example of calculation: 1500 persons are shifted from level 8 to level 7, and 6000 persons are shifted from level 7 to level 6; thus, there remain 35,500 in risk factor level 7 (i.e., 40,000 + 1500 − 6000). The new number of cases in level 7, thus, becomes 35,500 × 0.05 × 4.0 = 7100. As previously the number of cases was 8000, the shift resulted in 900 fewer cases.

4. There is a multiplicative interaction between smoking and sex, with rate ratios for current smoking higher in women than in men. There is also heterogeneity in the attributable risks in those exposed to smoking, but in the opposite direction. Also, for both women and men, as the rate in former smokers approximates the rate in those who never smoked, it can be inferred that smoking cessation is effective. (It is never late to stop smoking!)

5a. Yes. Relative risk point estimates do not differ substantially (all are below 1.75 and above 1.0).

5b. Yes, all summary relative risks have approximately the same value.

5c. When results from different studies are relatively homogeneous, fixed and random effects models should yield the same or very similar summary association measures.

5d. (1) The same biases or residual (positive) confounding can be present in all studies, moving the relative risk away from the null value of 1.0.
(2) Publication bias.

5e. Funnel plots are used to evaluate whether publication bias is present.

5f. This funnel plot shows asymmetry around the pooled risk ratio, indicating that publication bias is present. As expected, as precision decreases—as expressed by the increase in standard errors of the risk ratios—the risk ratios get further away from the average risk ratio. (Note that the SE increases as its values move down in the abscissa scale.) The bottom left of the plot is conspicuously bare, although we would expect to see some smaller, less precise studies having reported estimates less than the average risk ratio; this finding suggests that smaller studies are only published if a positive association is found. In other words, there seems to be publication bias.

6a.
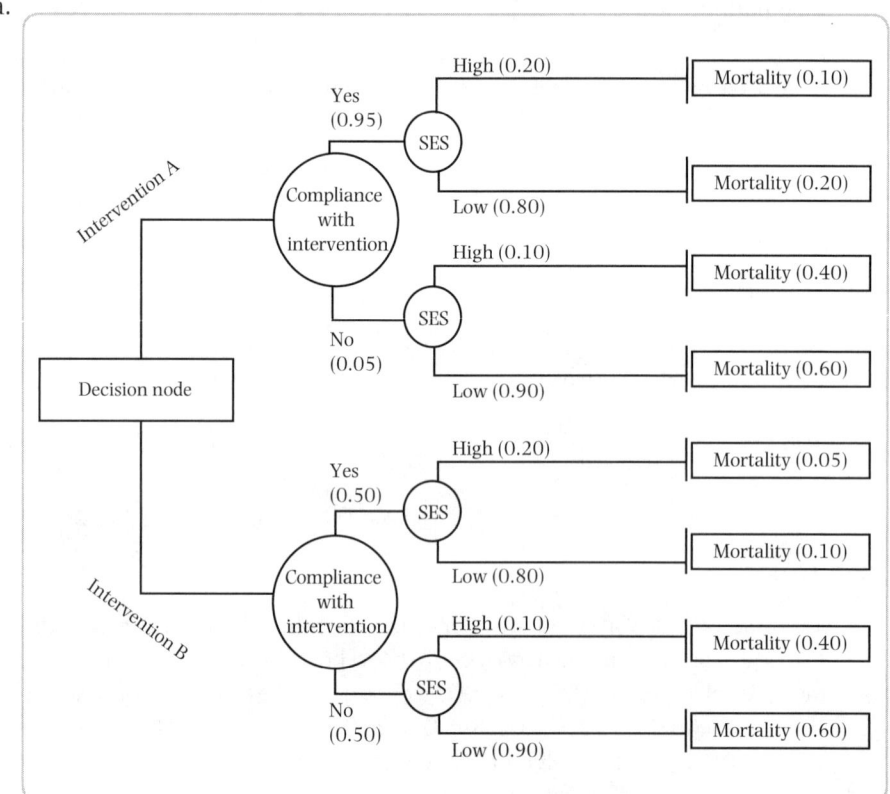

6b. One decision node: assignment to intervention A or B; and two chance nodes: compliance and social class.

6c.

	Intervention A			Intervention B		
Compliance	Socio-economic status	Joint probability of death	Compliance	Socio-economic status	Joint probability of death
Yes	High	$0.95 \times 0.20 \times 0.10 = 0.019$	Yes	High	$0.50 \times 0.20 \times 0.05 = 0.005$
	Low	$0.95 \times 0.80 \times 0.20 = 0.152$		Low	$0.50 \times 0.80 \times 0.10 = 0.040$
No	High	$0.05 \times 0.10 \times 0.40 = 0.002$	No	High	$0.50 \times 0.10 \times 0.40 = 0.02$
	Low	$0.05 \times 0.90 \times 0.60 = 0.027$		Low	$0.50 \times 0.90 \times 0.60 = 0.027$
Total mortality		0.200 or 20%	Total mortality		0.335 or 33.5%

6d. Mortality:
Intervention A: 0.200
Intervention B: 0.335
Effectiveness of A = $[(0.335 - 0.200)/0.335] \times 100 = 40.3\%$

7. Sensitivity analysis: assume that tolerance to the intervention in Intervention A is increased to 50%

Intervention A: Less efficacious but better drug tolerance (70%)		Intervention B: More efficacious but less drug tolerance (50%)	
Tolerance	Joint probability of death	Tolerance	Joint probability of death
Yes	$0.70 \times 0.10 \times 0.10 = 0.007$	Yes	$0.50 \times 0.10 \times 0.05 = 0.0025$
	$0.70 \times 0.90 \times 0.20 = 0.126$		$0.50 \times 0.90 \times 0.10 = 0.045$
No	$0.30 \times 0.10 \times 0.50 = 0.015$	No	$0.50 \times 0.10 \times 0.50 = 0.025$
	$0.30 \times 0.90 \times 0.50 = 0.135$		$0.50 \times 0.90 \times 0.50 = 0.225$
	$0.007 + 0.126 + 0.015 + 0.135$		$0.0025 + 0.045 + 0.025 + 0.225$
	$= 0.283$ (or 28.30%)		$= 0.2975$ (or 29.75%)
			(Before: 37.85%)

Effectiveness of A (vis-à-vis B) = $\{[29.75\% - 28.30\%] + 29.75\%\} \times 100 = 4.9\%$
Intervention A is still a bit more effective than Intervention B, but if the cost of B is lower, it might be cost-effective to implement the latter.

Index

Exhibits, figures, notes, and tables are indicated by exh., f, n, and t following page numbers.

A

Abbreviations, 374
Absolute differences
   of additive interactions, 188–189, 191
   homogeneous stratum-specific, 236–237, 237t
   measures of association and, 79
Absolute measures of disease frequency, 47–48, 47t
Absolute odds of exposure ($Odds_{exp}$), 91
Accuracy, 313. *See also* Validity
Actuarial life table, 49, 52, 55
Additive interactions
   attributable risk and, 186, 188–189, 188t, 189f, 191–193, 193t
   in case-control studies, 199–201, 202t
   detection of, 191
   expected joint effects and, 191–193, 199–201, 202t
   matching and, 36
   model of, 186, 191, 193t
   multiplicative vs., 205–207, 206–207t, 206f
   observed joint effects and, 191–193, 199–201, 202t
   positive, 207, 207t
Adjusted incidence rates, 236
Adjusted odds ratio, 167, 242–243, 272, 272–273t
Adjustment methods, 229–311. *See also* Regression techniques
   assumptions regarding, 233–234
   confounding and, 167, 170, 170t, 211–212, 213t
   covariate, 292
   direct. *See* Direct adjustment
   incomplete, 293–295
   indirect, 239–242, 241t, 242f
   limitations of, 246–248
   Mantel-Haenszel approach, 167, 242–246, 243–247t
   odds ratio, 167, 242–243
   over-adjustment, 173, 295–296
   rate ratio, 244
   selection of, 299–300, 299t
   statistical models for, 229, 233–234
   stratification-based, 234–248
Administrative losses, 56–57
Age effects
   cohorts and, 5–9, 6–7f, 8t, 9f
   cross-sectional studies and, 4f, 4–5t, 4–6, 6f
   defined, 8 *exh.*
   incidence rates and, 10–11, 12f
   mortality data and, 9–10, 10f
   prevalence and, 4–5t, 4–6, 4f, 6f
Agent–host–environment paradigm, 3
Aggregate data, 58–59
Aggregate measures, 14
Aggregation bias, 16, 16f
AHI. *See* Apnea-Hypopnea Index
AI. *See* Arousal index
Alternative modeling techniques for nonlinear relationships, 279–281, 280–281f
Ambidirectional studies, 27
American Cancer Society cohort studies, 20
American Thoracic Society questionnaire to assess respiratory symptoms, 316
Americans' Changing Lives survey, 161
Analogies, 408
Analytical epidemiology
   defined, 3
   differences in strategy, 404
   measures of association used in, 79, 79t
ANOVA (analysis of variance) tables, 355, 469–470
Antagonistic (negative) interactions, 185
Apnea-Hypopnea Index (AHI), 349t, 350, 469, 470, 471
AR. *See* Attributable risk
ARIC Study. *See* Atherosclerosis Risk in Communities Study
Arithmetic scale, 383, 384, 384–385f
Arousal index (AI), 349t, 350, 469, 470, 471
Arrogance, scientific, 373
Associations, 79–106
   across variables, 376–378
   assessing strength of, 101–103
   in case-control studies, 90–101
   causality and, 375
   in cohort studies, 79–90
   in cross-sectional studies, 90

dose-response, 401, 401–403f, 403, 455–458
exposure categories and, 99–100, 100t
lack of, 376
noncausal. *See* Confounding
odds ratio. *See* Odds ratio (OR)
overview, 79
point prevalence rate ratio, 72, 90, 134–135
population controls and, 96–97t, 96–98
random, 159
rarity assumption, 94–96, 95t
representativeness of, 37, 221
risk. *See* Attributable risk (AR);
    Relative risk (RR)
strength of, 101–103, 102 *exh.*, 375–376, 400
types of, 79, 79t
Atherosclerosis Risk in Communities (ARIC) Study
adjusted odds ratio in, 272, 272–273t
case-cohort approach in, 28–29, 30, 273–274, 273t
coefficient of variability (CV) and, 355, 355t, 357
conditional logistic regression analyses of, 271–272, 272t
Cox proportional regression analyses of, 267–268, 268t
cross-sectional approach in, 31, 102 *exh.*
intraclass correlation coefficients (ICCs) and, 355, 355t
kappa statistic in, 347–348, 348t
linear regression analyses of, 249, 249f
matched odds ratio in, 272, 273t
medical surveillance bias and, 133
monitoring of trends in, 318–319
multiple linear regression analyses of, 255, 255t, 258, 258t
multiple logistic regression analyses of, 261–263, 261t, 263t
paired odds ratio in, 244, 245t
percent agreement in, 334–335, 335–336t
Poisson regression analyses of, 270, 271t
Quality Assurance/Quality Control Manual, 461–468
recall bias in, 118
residual confounding in, 293, 293t
Attributable risk (AR)
additive interactions and, 186, 188–189, 188t, 189f, 191–193, 193t
adjusted, 236, 237–238, 237t
in case-control studies, 101
in cohort studies, 84–90, 85f, 88–89f
confidence interval calculation for, 441, 442
expected joint, 191, 193
in exposed individuals, 84–85, 85f
homogeneous, 236–237, 237t
observed joint, 191, 193

percent in exposed individuals, 85–87, 441
population, 87–90, 88–89f, 441–442
standard error calculation for, 441, 442
"Average" susceptibility, 221

B

"Backdoor path," 162
Berksonian bias, 111
Between-observer variability, 325
Bias, 109–151. *See also* Selection bias
aggregation bias, 16, 16f
Berksonian bias, 111
built-in bias, 83
combined selection/information bias, 133–139
compensating bias, 114–115
confounding and, 177–179, 178f
control of, 110
cross-sectional bias, 134–139
defined, 109
detection bias, 133–134
differential bias over time, 321, 321f
duration ratio bias, 135
exposure identification bias, 117–120
heterogeneity due to, 215–217, 216–217t, 218f
incidence-prevalence bias, 134–137, 137f, 139–141
information bias, 111, 111f, 116–133, 116 *exh.*
interviewer bias, 119–120
language bias, 417
lead time bias, 141–145, 142–144f
length bias, 139–141
medical surveillance bias, 110, 133–134
observer bias, 119, 120–121
outcome identification bias, 120–121
over-diagnosis bias, 145–146, 146t
overview, 109–111, 109f
point prevalence complement ratio bias, 135–136
prevention of, 110
publication, 369, 416–420
recall bias, 26, 111, 117–119, 118t
regression dilution, 325
respondent bias, 121
in screening interventions, 139–146
surveillance bias, 110, 133–134
survival bias, 26, 26f, 135, 139
temporal bias, 137–139, 321, 321f, 400
Binary linear regression model, 259
Biologic plausibility, 403
Biostatistics, 234n
Birth cohorts, defined, 5, 5n. *See also* Cohort effects; Cohort studies
Bland-Altman plots, 357–358, 357f

Blood collection, quality assurance for, 463–468
Blood pressure measurement, quality assurance for, 315–316, 325, 326f, 461–463
Built-in bias, 83

C

Calendar time, 9, 64–65, 65f, 65t
Case-based case-control studies, 24–27, 25–26f
Case-based control selection, 114
Case-cohort studies
  examples of, 29–30
  multivariate analyses in, 273–274, 273t
  overview, 27–29, 28f
  population control selection in, 96–97t, 96–99, 100t
  relative risk in, 97
Case-control studies, 23–30
  additive interactions in, 199–201, 202t
  ambidirectional, 27
  analytical approach to, 23, 24f, 299t
  association measures in, 90–101
  attributable risk in, 101
  case-based, 24–27, 25–26f
  cohorts within. *See* Case-cohort studies
  differential misclassification, 125–133, 126t, 127–128 *exh.*, 129–131t
  exposure categories in, 99–100, 100t
  homogeneity of effects in, 196–198, 198–199t
  hybrid, 27
  incidence-prevalence bias in, 136–137
  interaction assessment in, 196–203
  internal validity in, 25
  interviewer bias in, 119–120
  matched, 33, 94, 270–272, 439–441
  medical surveillance bias and, 133–134
  multiplicative interactions in, 196–198, 198–199t, 201–203, 202–204t
  multivariate analyses of, 265–266, 265t, 270–274
  nested, 27–28, 27f, 29, 98–99, 100t, 272–273
  nondifferential misclassification, 121–125, 122–125 *exh.*
  observed and expected joint effects in, 198–203, 200f, 200t, 202t
  odds ratio in, 90–100, 91–93t, 93f, 95–97t, 100t
  paired data in, 244–246, 245–247t
  population control selection in, 96–97t, 96–99, 100t
  rarity assumption in, 94–96, 95t
  recall bias in, 26, 117–119
  relative risk in, 94–96
  selection bias in, 25, 111–115, 112–113t, 115t
  stratification in, 230–231, 230t, 232–233, 232t
  survival bias in, 26, 26f
  temporal bias in, 137
Case-crossover studies, 32, 32t
Categorical variables
  kappa statistic and, 338, 348
  multiple linear regression and, 254
  percent agreement and, 335, 336
  Poisson regression and, 269, 270
  sensitivity and specificity and, 328
Causal diagrams, 162
Causality, 392–408
  associations and, 375
  component causes, 393–394, 393f
  distal causes, 394–395, 395f, 397
  Hill's guidelines for, 399–401, 403–404, 406–408
  intermediate causes, 394–395, 395f, 397
  Koch's postulates and, 392
  patterns of cause-effect relationship, 401, 401f
  proximate causes, 394–395, 395f, 397
  public health policy applications and, 392–408
  relationship to type of prevention, 178–179, 179 *exh.*
  reverse, 138, 400
  Rothman's model, 393–394, 393f
  social determinants of health and, 398–399
  sufficient causes, 393–394, 393f
  web of, 17, 19, 392–393
Censored observations, 21, 49, 55–57, 70, 71 *exh.*
Centers for Disease Control and Prevention (CDC), 319, 320
Chamberlain's percent positive agreement, 338
Chance agreement, 338–339, 340, 343
Classic life table, 49, 51, 52, 55
Classification. *See also* Misclassification
  of individuals, 116
  for interpretation of kappa statistic, 339, 340f
Clinic-based control selection, 114
Coefficient of variability (CV), 356–357
Coherence, 407–408
Cohort data, 19
Cohort effects, 4–14
  aggregates and, 59
  calendar time and, 9
  cross-sectional studies and, 5–8, 6–7f
  defined, 8 *exh.*
  incidence rates and, 10–11, 12f
  interactions and, 9
  in measures of incidence, 57
  mortality data and, 9–10, 10f
  prevalence and, 5–9, 6–7f, 8t, 9f
Cohorts, defined, 19, 19n
Cohort studies
  analytical approach to, 21, 21f, 299t

association measures in, 79–90
attributable risk in, 84–90, 85f, 88–89f
in case-control studies. *See* Case-cohort studies
components of, 19, 20f
concurrent, 22, 23, 23f
cross-tabulation of exposure and disease in, 80, 80t
historical, 22–23, 23f
hypothetical, 20–21, 20f, 22f
incidence-prevalence bias in, 137
interaction assessment in, 194–195, 195–197t
matching in, 33
medical surveillance bias and, 133, 134
mixed design, 23, 23f
multiple logistic regression in, 260–265, 261t, 263t
nonconcurrent, 22–23, 23f
objectives, 19
observer bias in, 120
occupational, 19–20
odds ratio in, 80–84, 81–82t
recall bias in, 119
relative risk in, 80–84, 81–82t, 203, 205t
selection bias in, 116
time scales relevant in, 64–66, 66t
types of, 19–20, 22–23, 23f
Colliders, 164
Collinearity, 172
Communicating results. *See* Reporting results
Comparability, 37
Compensating bias, 114–115
Component causes, 393–394, 393f
Concurrent cohort studies, 22, 23, 23f
Conditional confounding, 177
Conditional logistic regression, 270–273
Conditional probabilities, 51
95% Confidence intervals, 431–453
attributable risk and, 441, 442
cumulative survival estimate and, 433
defined, 375n
direct adjustment and, 443, 444
J statistic and, 450–451
kappa statistic and, 451, 453
Mantel-Haenszel method and, 446
odds ratio and, 439, 440–441
overview, 431–434
percent agreement and, 449, 450
person-time incidence rates and, 434–435
rate ratio and, 437, 438
regression coefficients and, 447–449
of regression estimates, 281–282
relative risk and, 436
results reporting and, 375–376, 376t, 377f
sensitivity and, 449–450
specificity and, 449, 450

standardized mortality ratio (SMR) and, 444–445
Confounding, 153–183. *See also* Residual confounding
adjustment methods and, 167, 170, 170t, 211–212, 213t
as "all-or-none" phenomenon, 165–167 *exh*., 171–172
assessment of, 164–171, 165 *exh*.
bias and, 177–179, 178f
conditional, 177
crude analyses of, 165–167, 166–167 *exh*., 166f, 168t
defined, 33, 153, 185
directed acyclic graphs (DAGs), 162–164, 163f, 371
examples, 153–155
experimental epidemiologic studies, 154 *exh*.
framing of, 162–164
general rule of, 156–157f, 156–162
heterogeneity due to, 214–215, 215–216t
by indication, 155
indirect relationships and, 179
interactions and, 211–212, 213t
matching and, 33, 35–36, 37–38, 38f
negative, 174–175, 175t, 176, 176f, 177t
nonexperimental epidemiologic studies, 154 *exh*.
odds ratio and, 167, 167 *exh*.
overview, 153–155
population attributable risk and, 89–90
positive, 174–175, 175t, 176, 176f, 177t
qualitative, 175–176, 176f, 177t
from random associations, 159
relative risk and, 174–175, 175t, 176f
by severity, 155
statistical significance and, 176–177
stratification and, 166–167, 171, 230–234
types of, 174–176
Confounding variables
association with outcome and exposure, 157–158f, 157–162, 160f, 165–171, 169–170t
correlation with exposure of interest, 172–173, 172–173f
defined, 33, 153
improper definitions of, 293
inclusion of, 294
misclassification of, 131, 294–295, 295t
reporting on selection of, 371
as surrogate markers, 159
time and, 64
Consistency of results, 403–404
Construct validity, 15, 15n, 174
Continuous variables
categorizing, 371

comparing, 377
defined, 47
indices of validity and reliability for, 348
multiple linear regression and, 254
multiple regression methods and, 262
regression to the mean and, 358
Control groups, 118
Control selection
  sampling frame for, 98–99, 100t
  types of, 114
Correlation coefficients
  intraclass, 354–355, 469–472
  Pearson's linear, 250, 350–353, 352–353f
  Spearman's (ordinal, rank), 353
  statistical significance testing of, 353–354
Correlation graphs, 350, 351f
Counterfactual model, 155
Covariates, 66–68, 292
Cox proportional hazards model, 266–269, 267f, 272, 273
Cronbach alpha, 355
Cross-level inferences, 17
Cross-product ratios, 80
Cross-sectional bias, 134–139
Cross-sectional studies
  age effects and, 4–5t, 4–6, 4f, 6f
  analytical approach to, 30–31, 31f, 299t
  association measures in, 90, 102, 102 exh.
  bias in, 134–139
  cohort effects and, 5–8, 6–7f
  period effects and, 8–9, 9f, 30n
Crude analyses, 165–167, 166–167 exh., 166f, 168t, 234n
Cumulative incidence rates, 49–57
  assumptions in estimation of, 55–57, 56t
  comparing with incidence rates, 69–70, 69–70 exh.
  density sampling vs., 98–99
  Kaplan-Meier approach, 52–55, 53–54f, 54t, 71
  life table approach, 49–52
  overview, 49, 50f, 51f
  survival analyses and, 49, 55–57, 56t, 70, 71 exh.
Cumulative incidence ratio, 98
Cumulative (lifetime) prevalence, 48, 72
Cumulative survival estimate, 49, 433
Cutoff points, 371–372
CV (coefficient of variability), 356–357

D

DAGs. *See* Directed acyclic graphs
Data
  aggregate, 58–59
  cohort, 19

collection instruments, 316–317
experimental evidence, 399–400
gold standard data, 319–320, 321, 323, 399
grouped, 62–63, 63t
incidence density, 58, 60, 62–63, 63t
modeled, 372–373
paired case-control data, 244–246, 245–247t
"phantom" measurements, 325–326, 327f
results. *See* Reporting results
unmodeled, 372–373
Decision trees, 410–411, 411–412f, 412 exh.
Denominators, 380
Density. *See* Incidence density
Dependent variables, 250
Descriptive epidemiology, 3
Design strategies. *See* Study designs
Detectable preclinical phase (DPCP), 140–141, 140–141f, 142t, 143–145, 144–145f
Detection bias, 133–134
Deyo's method, 471–472
Diagrams
  causal, 162
  scatter, 350, 351f
Dichotomous variables, 259
Differences
  absolute, 79, 188–189, 191
  mean, 356
  relative, 79, 189–190, 193–194
Differential bias over time, 321, 321f
Differential losses to follow-up, 116
Differential misclassification, 117, 120, 125–133, 126t, 127–128 exh., 129–131t
Direct adjustment
  attributable risk and, 236, 237–238, 237t
  confidence interval calculation for, 443, 444
  hypothesis testing for, 443, 444
  for incidence rate comparison, 234, 235t, 236
  overview, 234
  practical considerations for, 238–239
  relative risk and, 236, 237, 238, 238t
  standard error calculation for, 443, 444
  standardized mortality ratio and, 240t, 241–242, 242f
Directed acyclic graphs (DAGs), 162–164, 163f, 371
Directionality, 162
Disease
  cross-tabulation with exposure, 80, 80t, 96, 96t
  detectable preclinical phase (DPCP) of, 140–141, 140–141f, 142t, 143–145, 144–145f
  frequency, 47–48, 47t
  natural history of, 140, 140f, 142t, 406
  occurrence measures of. *See* Incidence rates; Prevalence rates

odds ratio of, 99
status, 117
susceptibility to, 118, 186, 214, 221
Distal causes, 394–395, 395*f*, 397
Dose-response associations, 401, 401–403*f*, 403, 455–458
Double stethoscoping, 318
DPCP. *See* Detectable preclinical phase
"Drift," 321, 321*f*
Dummy variables. *See* Indicator variables
Duration ratio bias, 135
Dynamic cohorts, 59

E

Ecologic fallacy, 16, 16*f*
Ecologic studies, 14–19, 15–16*f*
Effect modification, 185, 186, 187
Effect modifiers, 185, 186, 187, 209–210
Effects. *See* Age effects; Cohort effects; Heterogeneity of effects; Homogeneity of effects; Period effects
Efficacy, 86
Emergent risk factors, 220
Environmental measures, 14
Epidemic curve, 404, 405*f*
Epidemiology
analytical, 3, 79, 79*t*, 404
defined, 3
descriptive, 3
experimental, 153
genetic, 289
observational, 3, 19, 33, 153
occupational, 23, 66, 239
Errors. *See* Standard errors (SE)
Etiologic fractions, 84
Events, defined, 48, 48*t*
Event times. *See* Kaplan-Meier approach
Evidence
experimental, 399–400
levels of, 391 *exh.*
for prevention purposes, 178–179
Excess fractions, 84
Expected joint effects
additive interactions and, 191–193, 199–201, 202*t*
attributable risk and, 191, 193
in case-control studies, 198–203, 200*f*, 200*t*, 202*t*
multiplicative interactions and, 193–194, 201–203
overview, 190–191
relative risk and, 194, 201, 204
Experimental epidemiology, 153, 154 *exh.*
Experimental evidence, 399–400

Exposure
association with confounding and outcome, 157–158*f*, 157–162, 160*f*, 165–171, 169–170*t*
correlation with confounding variables, 172–173, 172–173*f*
cross-tabulation with disease, 80, 80*t*, 96, 96*t*
differences in, 404
heterogeneity due to intensity of, 217, 219
latency period of, 404, 405*f*
measuring. *See* Associations
objective markers of, 118
statistical models for, 298–299
subjective markers of, 118
verification of information, 117
Exposure categories
misclassification and, 122, 125, 126*t*
odds ratio and, 99–100, 100*t*
Exposure identification bias, 117–120
interviewer bias, 119–120
overview, 117
recall bias, 26, 111, 117–119, 118*t*
Exposure intensity, 101, 217, 219
Exposure prevalence, 124–125, 125*t*
Exposure status, 117
External validity, 37

F

Fallacy
ecologic, 16, 16*f*
interaction, 198
False negatives, 122
False positives, 121, 122
Feldstein's binary linear regression model, 259
Field center monitoring, 462
Figures, 378, 380, 382–385, 382–385*f*
Follow-up
differential losses to, 116
person-time incidence rates and, 63–68, 64–67*t*, 65*f*, 67–68*f*
Food frequency questionnaire, 321, 324, 327
Force of morbidity/mortality, 70
Framingham Study, 19, 133, 264, 300, 401, 406
Frequency matching, 34
Frequency of disease measures, 47–48, 47*t*
Frost, Wade Hampton, 9, 10*f*
Funnel plots, 418–419, 418–419*f*

G

Generalized linear models, 249
Genetic epidemiology, 289
Global measures, 15
Gold standard data
experimental evidence and, 399

in validity studies, 319–320, 321, 323
Graded patterns, 401, 403
Graphs
  correlation, 350, 351*f*
  directed acyclic graphs (DAGs), 162–164, 163*f*, 371
  interaction assessment with, 188–189, 188*t*
Greenwood formula, 433
Grouped data, 62–63, 63*t*

H

Hazard rates, 70–71, 266–269, 267*f*, 272, 273
Headings on tables, 379
Health and Retirement Study, 283–285, 284*f*
Health Insurance Plan Study, 140, 208
Health policy. *See* Public health policy applications
Health Professionals Study cohort, 20
Healthy worker effects, 116
Heterogeneity of effects
  bias and, 215–217, 216–217*t*, 218*f*
  confounding and, 214–215, 215–216*t*
  defined, 185
  exposure intensity and, 217, 219
  random variability and, 214
High-risk groups, 179
High-risk prevention strategies, 394, 395, 396*f*, 397, 398*t*
Hill's guidelines for causality, 399–401, 403–404, 406–408
Hispanic Health and Nutrition Examination Survey, 277, 278*t*, 279
Historical cohort studies, 22–23, 23*f*
Homogeneity of effects
  absolute differences and, 236–237, 237*t*
  assessment of, 186–190, 187*f*, 196–198
  attributable risk and, 236–237, 237*t*
  in case-control studies, 196–198, 198–199*t*
  defined, 185
  relative risk and, 237, 238*t*
  statistical tests of, 212, 459–460
Hospital-based control selection, 114
Host factors, 217, 219
Hybrid studies, 27
Hypertension Detection and Follow-up Program, 358
Hypotheses, 369–370
Hypotheses testing, 431–453
  direct adjustment and, 443, 444
  Mantel-Haenszel method and, 446, 447
  for null hypothesis, 447, 456
  odds ratio and, 439, 440–441
  overview, 431–434
  rate ratio and, 437, 438
  regression coefficients and, 447
  relative risk and, 436

I

ICCs (intraclass correlation coefficients), 354–355, 469–472
Incidence density
  based on individual data, 58, 60, 62–63, 63*t*
  ratio, 99
  sampling, 27–28, 27*f*, 99
Incidence odds, 73
Incidence-prevalence bias
  in case-control studies, 136–137
  in cohort studies, 137
  in cross-sectional studies, 134–137, 137*f*
  length bias, 139–141
  in screening interventions, 139–141
  survival bias, 26, 26*f*, 135, 139
Incidence proportion, 49
Incidence rates, 47–71
  adjusted, 236
  cohort-age-period analyses and, 10–11, 12*f*
  comparing, 69–70, 69–70 *exh.*
  cumulative, 49–57, 98–99
  defined, 47–48, 47*t*
  density sampling, 28
  direct adjustment for comparing, 234, 235*t*, 236
  hazard rates and, 70–71, 266–269, 267*f*, 272, 273
  odds and, 73
  person-time, 57–68, 433–435
  standardized, 236
  stratification and, 63–68
  yearly, 62
Incomplete adjustment, 293–295
Independent variables, 250
Indicator variables, 275–277, 276*t*, 279
Indirect adjustment, 239–242, 241*t*, 242*f*
Indirect relationships, 179
Individual data, 58, 60, 62–63, 63*t*
Individual matching, 34
Inferences, 17, 375–378
Information bias, 116–133
  combined selection/information bias, 133–139
  defined, 111, 111*f*
  differential misclassification and, 117, 120, 125–131
  exposure identification bias, 117–120
  interviewer bias, 119–120
  medical surveillance bias, 133
  nondifferential misclassification and, 117, 121–125, 125–126*t*, 131
  outcome identification bias, 120–121
  overview, 116–117
  recall bias, 26, 111, 117–119, 118*t*

temporal bias, 137–139, 321, 321f, 400
Initial population, 99
Instantaneous conditional incidence, 70
Instrumental variable method, 282–289
    applications of, 283–285, 284f
    conditions for using, 283, 283f
    limitations of, 285–287, 287f, 289
    Mendelian randomization, 287–289, 288f
    overview, 282–283
    randomization approach, 285, 286f, 287–289, 288f
Intention-to-treat approach, 285
Interaction fallacy, 198
Interactions, 185–226. *See also* Additive interactions; Multiplicative interactions
    antagonistic (negative), 185
    in case-control studies, 196–203
    cohort effects and, 9
    in cohort studies, 194–195, 195–197t
    confounding and, 211–212
    definitions of, 185, 186, 203–205
    evaluation strategies, 186–195, 187f
    fallacy, 198
    host factors and, 217, 219
    interpreting, 214–219
    negative, 185, 220, 220t
    observed and expected joint effects, 190–194
    overview, 185–186
    positive, 185
    quantitative vs. qualitative, 207–209, 208f, 209t, 210f
    reciprocity of, 209, 211, 211t
    reporting of, 373
    representativeness of associations and, 37, 221
    risk factors and, 219–221, 220t
    statistical modeling and tests for, 212–213
    synergistic (positive), 185
    terms used regarding, 256–257
    testing for, 459–460
Intercept, 250, 252
Intermediate causes, 394–395, 395f, 397
Intermethod reliability estimates, 328
Internal comparisons, 22
Internal validity, 25, 37
Inter-observer variability, 325
Interval-based life table, 49
Interval cases, 140
Interventions. *See* Screening interventions
Interviewer bias, 119–120
Intraclass correlation coefficients (ICCs), 354–355, 469–472
Intra-observer variability, 324

J

J statistic, 333–334, 450–451
Jargon, 374
Joint effects. *See* Expected joint effects; Observed joint effects
J-shape relationships, 274, 275f, 279, 401, 401f

K

Kaplan-Meier approach, 52–55, 53–54f, 54t, 71
Kappa statistic
    agreement measures for, 338–340, 341t
    applications for, 339–340, 342
    calculation of, 338
    classifications for interpretation of, 339, 340f
    confidence interval calculation for, 451, 453
    prevalence and, 345–348, 346–347t
    standard error calculation for, 451–452
    weighted, 342–345, 344t, 345n
Koch's postulates, 392

L

Labels
    on figures, 382, 383f
    on tables, 379
Laboratory forms, 465, 467, 468
Laboratory measurements, 319–321, 320f
Language bias, 417
Latency period of exposure, 404, 405f
Lead time bias, 141–145, 142–144f
Least-squares method, 250–251, 251f, 281, 282
Length bias, 139–141
Levin, M. L., 87, 88, 89–90
Lexis diagrams, 65, 67f
Life table approach, 49–52
Lifetime (cumulative) prevalence, 48, 72
Likelihood ratio test, 282
Linear correlation, 350
Linear correlation coefficient, 250, 350–353, 352–353f
Linear function, 248
Linear regression
    binary, 259
    confidence interval calculation and, 448
    general concepts, 249–254
    graphical representations of, 249–252, 249f, 251–252f, 253
    interpretation of, 253–254
    least-squares method, 250–251, 251f, 281, 282
    in log odds scale, 266
    modeling nonlinear relationships with, 274–277, 275f, 279–281, 280–281f

multiple, 254–259
  reliability indices and, 354
  trends tests and, 455–457
Linkage disequilibrium, 289
Lipid Research Clinics (LRC) Family Study, 322, 328–329, 337, 337t
Logarithmic scale, 383, 384, 384–385f
Log-binomial regression model, 266
Logistic function, 259, 261
Logistic regression
  conditional, 270–273
  confidence interval calculation and, 448–449
  multiple, 259–266
Log-linear models, 269
Log odds (*logit*), 260, 266
Losses, 56–57, 116
Low data-ink ratio, 382
Low-risk groups, 219–221
LRC Family Study. *See* Lipid Research Clinics Family Study

M

Mantel-Haenszel method, 167, 242–246, 243–247t, 414, 445–447
Mantel's trend test, 455–458
Manuals of operation, 315–316
Markers, 153
Masking of interviewers, 120
Masking of observers, 120
Matched case-control studies, 33, 94, 270–272, 439–441
Matched odds ratio, 94, 272, 273t, 439–441
Matching, 33–38, 35f, 38f
  additive interactions and, 36, 186, 188–189, 188t, 189f
  advantages of, 36
  in case-control studies, 33, 94, 270–272, 439–441
  in cohort studies, 33
  confounding and, 33, 35–36, 37–38, 38f
  disadvantages of, 36–37
  frequency, 34
  minimum Euclidean distance measure method, 34–35, 35f
  odds ratio and, 94
  overmatching, 37, 173, 296
  overview, 33
  propensity scores and, 290–292, 291t
  types of, 34–35
  validity and, 37
Maximum likelihood method (MLE), 282
Mean difference, 356
Mean values, 14, 14*n*
Medical surveillance bias, 110, 133–134

Mendelian randomization, 287–289, 288f
Meta-analyses, 413–416, 415f
Minimum Euclidean distance measure method, 34–35, 35f
Minimum-variance standard population, 239
Minnesota Heart Survey (MHS), 320, 321
Misclassification, 111, 121–133
  of confounding variables, 131, 294–295, 295t
  differential, 117, 120, 125–131
  exposure categories and, 122, 125, 126t
  nondifferential, 117, 121–125, 125–126t, 131
  odds ratio and, 123–125, 126–128, 130
  overview, 121
  prevention of, 131–133
Mixed design cohort studies, 23, 23f
MLE (maximum likelihood method), 282
Modeled data, 372–373
Monitoring
  field center, 462
  of observations, 318–319
  of trends, 318–319
Morbidity data, 70, 240
Mortality data
  cohort–age–period analyses and, 9–10, 10f
  force of, 70
  standardized mortality ratio (SMR), 240–242, 241t, 242f, 444–445
Multicenter AIDS Cohort Study, 20, 160
Multi-Ethnic Study of Atherosclerosis, 103, 103f, 118, 378
Multilevel analyses, 15–16
Multiple linear regression, 254–259
  examples of, 254–255, 255t, 258–259, 258t
  graphical representations of, 255–258, 257f
  overview, 254
Multiple logistic regression, 259–266
  in case-control studies, 265–266, 265t
  in cohort studies, 260–265, 261t, 263t
  Framingham risk equation, 264
  graphical representations of, 260, 260f
  overview, 259
Multiple Risk Factor Intervention Trial, 214
Multiplicative interactions
  additive vs., 205–207, 206–207t, 206f
  in case-control studies, 196–198, 198–199t, 201–203, 202–204t
  expected joint effects and, 193–194, 194 *exh.*, 201–203
  observed joint effects and, 193–194, 194 *exh.*, 201–203
  ratio model of, 189–190, 193–194
  relative risk and, 186, 189–190, 189f, 190t, 193–194

Multivariate analyses, 229–311. *See also* Adjustment methods; Regression techniques; Stratification
   of case-cohort studies, 273–274, 273*t*
   of case-control studies, 265–266, 265*t*, 270–274
   defined, 229, 234*n*
   instrumental variable method, 282–289
   limitations of, 246–248
   propensity scores, 290–292, 291*t*
   techniques, 299–300, 299*t*
   trend tests and, 457–458

N

National Death Index, 57
National Health and Nutrition Examination Survey (NHANES), 71, 316, 322, 332
Natural history of disease, 140, 140*f*, 142*t*, 406
Negative confounding, 174–175, 175*t*, 176, 176*f*, 177*t*
Negative interactions, 185, 220, 220*t*
Negative multiplicative interactions, 207, 207*t*
Negative predictive value (NPV), 330*n*
Nested case-control studies, 27–28, 27*f*, 29, 98–99, 100*t*, 272–273, 299*t*
Netherlands OC Study, 336, 336*t*
NHANES. *See* National Health and Nutrition Examination Survey
95% Confidence intervals. *See* Confidence intervals
Noncausal association measures. *See* Confounding
Noncollapsibility, 167, 171
Nonconcurrent cohort studies, 22–23, 23*f*
Nondifferential misclassification, 117, 121–125, 122–125 *exh.*, 125–126*t*, 131
Nonexchangeability, 155
Nonexperimental epidemiology. *See* Observational epidemiology
Nonexposure. *See also* Exposure
   case-control study, 23, 24*f*, 29
   cohort study, 21–22, 21–22*f*
   cross-sectional study, 31
   hazard rates, 267*f*
   Levin's population attributable risk, 87
   types of matching, 34, 35*f*
Nonlinear relationships, 274–277, 275*f*, 279–281, 280–281*f*
NPV (negative predictive value), 330*n*
Null hypothesis, 447, 456
Nurses Health Study
   as cohort, 20
   differential misclassification and, 128–130, 129–130*t*, 132
   recall bias and, 117
   reliability and, 327
   validity and, 321

O

Objective markers of exposure, 118
Objectives of studies, 369–370
Observational epidemiology, 3, 19, 33, 153, 154 *exh.*
Observations
   censored, 21, 49, 55–57, 70, 71 *exh.*
   monitoring of, 318–319
Observed agreement, 338, 339, 340, 343, 344*t*
Observed joint effects, 190–193
   additive interactions and, 191–193, 199–201, 202*t*
   attributable risk and, 191, 193
   in case-control studies, 198–203, 200*f*, 200*t*, 202*t*
   compared with expected effects, 190–191, 192–193 *exh.*
   multiplicative interactions and, 193–194, 194 *exh.*, 201–203
   overview, 190–191
   relative risk and, 194, 201, 204–205
Observer bias, 119, 120–121
Occupational cohort studies, 19–20
Occupational epidemiology, 23, 66, 70, 239
Occurrence of disease measures. *See* Incidence rates; Prevalence rates
Odds
   based on initial population, 99
   defined, 73
   of exposure, 91
   point prevalence, 73, 134–135
Odds ratio (OR)
   adjusted, 167, 242–243, 272, 272–273*t*
   as antilogarithm of regression coefficient, 261
   case-cohort studies and, 98–99, 100*t*
   in case-control studies, 90–100, 91–93*t*, 93*f*, 95–97*t*, 100*t*
   in cohort studies, 80–84, 81–82*t*
   confidence interval calculation for, 439, 440–441
   confounding variable and, 167, 167 *exh.*
   defined, 80
   density, 99
   differential misclassification and, 126–128, 130
   of disease, 99
   exposure categories and, 99–100, 100*t*
   hypothesis testing for, 439, 440–441
   Mantel-Haenszel method, 167, 242–246, 243*t*, 245–247*t*, 414, 445–447
   matched, 94, 272, 273*t*, 439–441
   meta-analysis of, 413–414, 415–416*f*
   nested case-control studies and, 98–99, 100*t*

nondifferential misclassification and, 123–125
for paired data, 244–246, 245–247t
population controls and, 96–97t, 96–98
probability odds ratio, 80–81
rarity assumption and, 94–96, 95t
relative risk and, 80–84, 81–82t, 94–96, 95t
standard error calculation for, 438–439, 440
stratum-specific, 242
Open cohorts, 59
Operational definitions of events, 48, 48t
OR. *See* Odds ratio
Ordinal correlation coefficient, 353
Ordinal variables, 371
Ordinary least-squares method, 281, 282
Ordinate scale, 382–385, 384–385f
Outcome identification bias, 120–121
Outcomes
   association with confounding and exposure, 157–158f, 157–162, 160f, 165–171, 169–170t
   measuring. *See* Associations
   risk factors association with, 82, 101–102
   selective reporting of, 419
   statistical models for, 298–299
   stratified analyses, 166–167
   systematic assessment of, 133
Over-adjustment, 173, 295–296
Over-diagnosis bias, 145–146, 146t
Over-estimation, 174
Over-matching, 37, 173, 296

P

P values, 354
Paired case-control data, 244–246, 245–247t
Paired *t* test, 356
Pair-wise comparison, 350
Participants. *See* Study participants
Pearson's linear correlation coefficient, 250, 350–353, 352–353f
Percent agreement, 334–337, 335–336t, 335f, 449, 450
Percent attributable risk, 85–87, 441
Percent positive agreement (PPA), 337–338
Period effects
   cross-sectional studies and, 8–9, 9f
   defined, 8 *exh.*
   incidence rates and, 10–11, 12f
   in measures of incidence, 57
   mortality data and, 9–10, 10f
   prevalence and, 8–9, 9f
Period prevalence, 48, 71–72
Person-time incidence rates, 57–68, 433–435
   aggregate data and, 58–59
   assumptions in estimation of, 60, 61f, 62

confidence interval calculation for, 434–435
covariates and, 66–68
density and, 58, 60, 62–63, 63t
follow-up time and, 63–68, 64–67t, 65f, 67–68f
individual data and, 60, 61t
overview, 57–58, 58t
standard error calculation for, 433–434
stratification of, 64, 65, 65–67t
Person-years, 58, 58t
"Phantom" measurements, 320f, 325–326, 327f
Pilot testing, 317–318
Point estimates, 432
Point prevalence, 71–73, 72n
Point prevalence complement ratio bias, 135–136
Point prevalence odds, 73, 134–135
Point prevalence rate ratio, 72, 90, 134–135
Poisson regression model, 269–270
Population, standard, 236–239, 240
Population attributable risk, 87–90, 88–89f, 441–442
Population controls, 96–97t, 96–98
Population-level implications, 17
Population stratification, 289
Population-wide prevention strategies, 395, 397f
Positive additive interactions, 207, 207t
Positive confounding, 174–175, 175t, 176, 176f, 177t
Positive interactions, 185
Positive predictive value (PPV), 330n
PPA (percent positive agreement), 337–338
Predictive values, 329–330, 330n
Predictor variables, 250
Pretesting, 317
Prevalence rates
   age effects and, 4–5t, 4–6, 4f, 6f
   cohort effects and, 5–9, 6–7f, 8t, 9f
   cumulative (lifetime), 48, 72
   defined, 47t, 48, 71
   incidence-prevalence bias, 134–137, 137f, 139–141
   kappa statistic and, 345–348, 346–347t
   measuring, 71–73
   odds and, 73
   period effects and, 8–9, 9f
   period prevalence, 48, 71–72
   point prevalence, 71–73, 72n
   point prevalence rate ratio, 72, 90, 134–135
   standardized, 240
Prevention
   high-risk strategies, 394, 395, 396f, 397, 398t
   population-wide strategies, 395, 397f
   primary, 178–179, 179 *exh.*
   secondary, 179, 179 *exh.*
Primary prevention, 178–179, 179 *exh.*

Probability
  conditional, 51
  estimating, 263–264
  odds ratio, 80–81
Product terms, 256
Propensity scores, 290–292, 291t
Proportional hazards model (Cox), 266–269, 267f, 272, 273
Proportions, 14n
Prospective studies. *See* Cohort studies
Protocol, 315
Proximate causes, 394–395, 395f, 397
Publication bias, 369, 416–420
Public health policy applications, 391–430
  causality and, 392–408
  decision trees and, 410–411, 411–412f, 412 *exh.*
  meta-analyses and, 413–416, 415f
  overview, 391–392
  publication bias and, 369, 416–420
  sensitivity analyses and, 300, 322, 408–411, 410t

Q

Qualitative confounding, 175–176, 176f, 177t
Qualitative interactions, 207–209, 208f, 209t, 210f
Quality assurance, 313, 315–318
  for blood pressure measurement, 315–316, 325, 326f, 461–463
  data collection instruments and, 316–317
  manuals of operation and, 315–316
  overview, 313, 315
  pretesting and pilot studies, 317–318
  steps involved in, 318 *exh.*
  study protocol and, 315
  training of staff and, 317
  for urine and blood collection, 463–468
Quality Assurance/Quality Control Manual (ARIC Study), 461–468
Quality control, 313, 318–328
  for blood pressure measurement, 461–463
  monitoring of observations and trends, 318–319
  overview, 313, 318
  reliability studies and, 324–328
  for urine and blood collection, 463–468
  validity studies and, 319–324
Quantitative interactions, 207

R

Random associations, 159
Randomization
  instrumental variable approach and, 285, 286f
  Mendelian, 287–289, 288f
  simulated, 290
Random variability, 214
Rank correlation coefficient, 353
Rarity assumption, 94–96, 95t
Rate ratio
  adjusted, 244
  confidence interval calculation for, 437, 438
  hypothesis testing for, 437, 438
  Mantel-Haenszel method, 244, 244–245t, 445–447
  in Poisson regression model, 270
Ratio model of multiplicative interactions, 189–190, 193–194
Readability of results, 374–375
Recall bias, 26, 111, 117–119, 118t
Reciprocity of interactions, 209, 211, 211t
Reductionism, 18, 18n
Redundancy in tables, 379
Regression coefficients, 250, 252–253, 259, 270, 377–378, 447–449
Regression dilution bias, 325
Regression techniques, 248–282. *See also* Linear regression
  confidence intervals of, 281–282
  Cox proportional hazards model, 266–269, 267f, 272, 273
  log-binomial model, 266
  logistic, 259–266, 270–273, 448–449
  overview, 234, 248, 248t
  Poisson model, 269–270
  statistical testing of estimates, 281–282
Regression to the mean, 358, 359f
Relative differences, 79, 189–190, 193–194
Relative odds. *See* Odds ratio (OR)
Relative risk (RR)
  adjusted, 236, 237, 238, 238t
  in case-control studies, 94–96
  in cohort studies, 80–84, 81–82t, 203, 205t
  confidence interval calculation for, 436
  confounding effects and, 174–175, 175t, 176f
  expected joint effects and, 194, 201, 204
  formula, 36–37
  homogeneous, 237, 238t
  hypotheses testing and, 436
  multiplicative interactions and, 186, 189–190, 189f, 190t, 193–194
  observed joint effects and, 194, 201, 204–205
  odds ratio and, 80–84, 81–82t, 94–96, 95t
  population controls and, 96–97t, 96–98
  prevalence rate ratio as estimate of, 135
  preventative strategy geared to, 393 *exh.*, 395
  rarity assumption and, 94–96, 95t
  standard error calculation for, 435, 436
Reliability
  defined, 116 *exh.*
  inter-method estimates, 328

Index

overview, 313
reporting, 371
Reliability coefficient, 354
Reliability indices, 328–358
   coefficient of variability (CV), 356–357
   correlation coefficients, 350–355
   kappa statistic and, 338–340, 342, 342*f*, 345–348
   linear regression and, 354
   mean difference and paired *t* test, 356
   overview, 328, 329*t*, 348, 350
   percent agreement, 334–336, 335–336*t*, 335*f*
   percent positive agreement (PPA), 337–338
   scatter diagrams, 350, 351*f*
Reliability studies
   data from previous studies, 327–328
   paired, 356
   "phantom" measurements and, 325–326, 327*f*
   quality control and, 324–328
   sub-studies, 119
   variability in, 324–326
Repeatability. *See* Reliability
Repeat measurements, 325, 327
Reporting results, 369–390
   confidence intervals and, 375–376, 376*t*, 377*f*
   confounding variable selection, 371
   consistency of, 403–404
   cutoff points, 371–372
   data collection procedures, 371
   figures, 378, 380, 382–385, 382–385*f*
   how to report, 373–385
   inferential mistakes in, 375–378
   interaction assessment, 373
   modeled and unmodeled data, 372–373
   overview, 369
   readability and, 374–375
   scientific arrogance and, 373
   statistical significance and, 375–376
   study objectives and hypotheses, 369–370, 447, 456
   tables, 378–380, 380–381*t*
   validity and reliability, 371
   verbosity and, 373–374
   what to report, 369–373, 370 *exh.*
Representativeness of associations, 37, 221
Reproducibility. *See* Validity
Research. *See* Study designs
Residual confounding
   defined, 173
   examples of, 173–174
   lack of, 233
   matching and, 37–38, 38*f*
   sources of, 293–295, 293*t*, 295*t*
Respondent bias, 121
Restriction techniques, 36
Results. *See* Reporting results

Retrospective cohort studies, 22–23, 23*f*
Reverse causality, 138, 400
Risk. *See also* Attributable risk; Relative risk (RR)
   high-risk groups, 179
   high-risk strategies, 394, 395, 396*f*, 397, 398*t*
   low-risk groups, 219–221
   percentage excess risk explained, 161, 161*n*
Risk factors
   emergent, 220
   in low-risk groups, 219–221
   negative interactions between, 220, 220*t*
   outcome association with, 82, 101–102
   variability of, 407, 408*f*
Risk-set sampling, 28, 99
Rose questionnaire, 316
Rothman's causality model, 393–394, 393*f*
RR. *See* Relative risk

S

Sampling
   controls, 30
   density, 27–28, 27*f*, 99
   errors, 109
   frame for control selection, 98–99, 100*t*
   reliability and validity sub-studies in, 119
   risk-set, 28, 99
Scatter diagrams, 350, 351*f*
Scientific arrogance, 373
Screening interventions
   bias in, 139–146
   detectable preclinical phase (DPCP) and, 140–141, 140–141*f*, 142*t*, 143–145, 144–145*f*
   high-risk strategies and, 397, 398*t*
SE. *See* Standard errors
Secondary prevention, 179, 179 *exh.*
Secular trends, 56, 57
Selection bias
   in case-control studies, 25, 111–115, 112–113*t*, 115*t*
   in cohort studies, 116
   combined selection/information bias, 133–139
   confounding and, 177–178, 178*f*
   defined, 110–111, 110*f*
   incidence-prevalence bias, 134–137, 137*f*, 139–141
   medical surveillance bias, 110, 133
   prevention of, 139
   in screening interventions, 139
Selective reporting of outcomes, 419
Self-reporting, 132, 332, 334*t*
Sensitivity
   analyses of, 300, 322, 408–411, 410*t*
   for binary variables, 328, 330*t*
   calculation of, 328–331, 330–331*t*, 333*f*

confidence interval calculation for, 449–450
defined, 116 *exh.*, 117
differential misclassification and, 125–131, 129–131*t*
J statistic, 333–334
kappa statistic and, 345–346
limitations of, 331–333, 334*t*
nondifferential misclassification and, 122–125, 123*f*, 125*t*, 131
percent agreement and, 337
of self-reporting, 332, 334*t*
standard error calculation for, 449–450
of tests used in studies, 322, 322*t*
Seven Countries Study, 406, 406–407*f*
Simulated randomization, 290
SIR (standardized incidence ratio), 240
Sleep Heart Health Study (SHHS) project, 348, 349*t*, 350, 355
SMOG grading formula, 374
SMR. *See* Standardized mortality ratio
Social determinants of health, 398–399
Spearman's correlation coefficient, 353
Specificity
for binary variables, 328, 330*t*
calculation of, 328–331, 330–331*t*, 333*f*
confidence interval calculation for, 449, 450
defined, 116 *exh.*, 117
differential misclassification and, 125–131, 129–131*t*
in Hill's guidelines, 408
J statistic, 333–334
kappa statistic and, 345–346
limitations of, 331–333
nondifferential misclassification and, 122–125, 123*f*, 125*t*, 131
percent agreement and, 337
standard error calculation for, 449, 450
of tests used in studies, 322, 322*t*
SPR (standardized prevalence ratio), 240
Staff training, 317
Standard errors (SE), 431–453
attributable risk and, 441, 442
cumulative survival estimate and, 433
direct adjustment and, 443, 444
J statistic and, 450–451
kappa statistic and, 451–452
linear regression and, 253
Mantel-Haenszel method and, 445–446
odds ratio and, 438–439, 440
overview, 431–434
percent agreement and, 449, 450
person-time incidence rates and, 433–434
relative risk and, 435, 436
sensitivity and, 449–450
specificity and, 449, 450

Standardization of procedures, 316
Standardized incidence rates, 236
Standardized incidence ratio (SIR), 240
Standardized mortality ratio (SMR), 240–242, 241*t*, 242*f*, 444–445
Standardized pools for laboratory measurements, 319–321, 320*f*
Standardized prevalence ratio (SPR), 240
Standardized regression coefficients, 377–378
Standard population, 236–239, 240
Statistical adjustment, 229
Statistical compatibility, 250
Statistical models
adjustment methods for, 229, 233–234
for exposures and outcomes, 298–299
for interactions, 212–213
linear regression and, 250
selection of, 299–300, 299*t*
as sketches or caricatures, 296–297, 297*f*
Statistical significance testing
in confounding assessment, 176–177
of correlation coefficients, 353–354
for interactions, 212–213
of regression estimates, 281–282
results reporting and, 375–376
Storage instructions, 468
Stratification, 229–311
adjustment methods based on, 234–248. *See also* Direct adjustment; Indirect adjustment
assumptions regarding, 233
in case-control studies, 230–231, 230*t*, 232–233, 232*t*
confounding and, 166–167, 171, 230–234
defined, 229
incidence rates and, 63–68
limitations of, 246–248
Mantel-Haenszel method, 167, 242–246, 243–247*t*
medical surveillance bias and, 134
of person-time incidence rates, 64, 65, 65–67*t*
population, 289
on propensity scores, 292
test of homogeneity of, 459–460
Stratum-specific odds ratio, 242
Study designs, 3–44. *See also* Case-control studies; Cohort studies; Cross-sectional studies
age effects and, 4–5*t*, 4–14, 4*f*, 6–7*f*, 8*t*, 9–13*f*
ambidirectional, 27
case-crossover, 32, 32*t*
cohort effects and, 5–14, 6–7*f*, 8*t*, 9–13*f*
differences in strategy, 404
ecologic, 14–19, 15–16*f*
features of, 313, 314–315*t*
hybrid, 27
matching in. *See* Matching

Index

overview, 3
period effects and, 8–14, 9–13f
Study objectives, 369–370
Study participants
   compliance with protocols, 464
   recording data of, 462–463
   selection of, 79
   variability within, 325, 326f
Study protocol, 315
Subcohorts, 273
Subjective markers of exposure, 118
Sufficient causes, 393–394, 393f
Surveillance bias, 110, 133–134
Survival analyses, 49, 55–57, 56t
   assumptions necessary for, 70, 71 exh.
Survival bias
   in case-control studies, 26, 26f
   defined, 135
   in screening interventions, 139
Survival function, 49, 54
Susceptibility to disease, 118, 186, 214, 221
Synergistic interactions, 185
Systematic errors, 109

T

Tables, 378–380, 380–381t
Temporal bias, 137–139, 321, 321f
Temporal "drift," 321, 321f
Temporality, 399, 400
Threshold phenomenon, 274
Time scales, 64–66, 66t. See also Person-time incidence rates
Titles on figures, 382
Training of staff, 317
Trends
   linear regression and, 455–457
   monitoring of, 318–319
   secular, 56, 57
   testing for, 455–458

U

Underestimation, 174
Unmodeled data, 372–373
Urine collection, quality control for, 463–468
U.S. National Health Surveys, 30n
U-type relationships, 274

V

Validity. See also Bias; Confounding; Interactions
   approaches to, 321
   construct, 15, 15n, 174
   defined, 116 exh., 117, 313
   external, 37
   internal, 25, 37

matching and, 37
overview, 313
of published findings, 416
reporting, 371
sub-studies in samples, 119
Validity indices, 328–358. See also Sensitivity; Specificity
   correlation coefficients, 350–355
   J statistic, 333–334
   kappa statistic and, 338–340, 342, 348
   mean difference and paired t test, 356
   overview, 328, 329t, 348, 350
   percent agreement, 336
Validity studies
   data from previous studies, 322
   importance and limitations of, 322–324
   quality control and, 319–324
   standardized pools for laboratory measurements, 319–321, 320f
   sub-studies, 119
Variability
   between-observer (inter-observer), 325
   coefficient of, 356–357
   in reliability studies, 324–326
   of risk factors, 407, 408f
   sources of, 324–325
   within study participants, 325, 326f
   within-observer (intra-observer), 324
Variables. See also Categorical variables; Confounding variables; Continuous variables
   across association measures, 376–378
   dependent, 250
   dichotomous, 259
   independent, 250
   indicator (dummy), 275–277, 276t, 279
   ordinal, 371
   predictor, 250
Verbosity, 373–374

W

Wald statistic, 282, 447, 449, 456, 457
Walter, S. D., 89–90
Web of causality, 17, 19, 392–393
Weighted kappa, 342–345, 344t, 345n
Western Electric Company study, 168, 169t, 170, 170t
Willett's food frequency questionnaire, 321, 324, 327
Withdrawals, 21
Within-observer variability, 324
Women's Health Initiative, 292

Y

Yearly average rates, 69
Youden's J statistic, 333–334, 450–451